Lecture Notes in Electrical Engineering

Volume 269

For further volumes:
http://www.springer.com/series/7818

Shaozi Li · Qun Jin · Xiaohong Jiang
James J. (Jong Hyuk) Park
Editors

Frontier and Future Development of Information Technology in Medicine and Education

ITME 2013

Volume 2

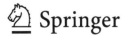

Editors
Shaozi Li
Cognitive Science
Xiamen University
Xiamen
People's Republic of China

Qun Jin
Networked Information Systems Lab,
  Human Informatics and Cognitive
  Sciences
Waseda University
Waseda
Japan

Xiaohong Jiang
School of Systems Information Science
Future University Hakodate
Hakodate, Hokkaido
Japan

James J. (Jong Hyuk) Park
Department of Computer Science and
  Engineering
Seoul National Universityof Science and
  Technology (SeoulTech)
Seoul
Korea, Republic of South Korea

ISSN 1876-1100 ISSN 1876-1119 (electronic)
ISBN 978-94-007-7617-3 ISBN 978-94-007-7618-0 (eBook)
DOI 10.1007/978-94-007-7618-0
Springer Dordrecht Heidelberg New York London

Library of Congress Control Number: 2013948373

© Springer Science+Business Media Dordrecht 2014
This work is subject to copyright. All rights are reserved by the Publisher, whether the whole or part of the material is concerned, specifically the rights of translation, reprinting, reuse of illustrations, recitation, broadcasting, reproduction on microfilms or in any other physical way, and transmission or information storage and retrieval, electronic adaptation, computer software, or by similar or dissimilar methodology now known or hereafter developed. Exempted from this legal reservation are brief excerpts in connection with reviews or scholarly analysis or material supplied specifically for the purpose of being entered and executed on a computer system, for exclusive use by the purchaser of the work. Duplication of this publication or parts thereof is permitted only under the provisions of the Copyright Law of the Publisher's location, in its current version, and permission for use must always be obtained from Springer. Permissions for use may be obtained through RightsLink at the Copyright Clearance Center. Violations are liable to prosecution under the respective Copyright Law.
The use of general descriptive names, registered names, trademarks, service marks, etc. in this publication does not imply, even in the absence of a specific statement, that such names are exempt from the relevant protective laws and regulations and therefore free for general use.
While the advice and information in this book are believed to be true and accurate at the date of publication, neither the authors nor the editors nor the publisher can accept any legal responsibility for any errors or omissions that may be made. The publisher makes no warranty, express or implied, with respect to the material contained herein.

Printed on acid-free paper

Springer is part of Springer Science+Business Media (www.springer.com)

Message from the ITME 2013 General Chairs

ITME 2013 is the 5th International Symposium on IT in Medicine and Education. This conference took place in July 19–21, 2013, in Xining, China. The aim of the ITME 2013 was to provide an international symposium for scientific research on IT in Medicine and Education. It was organized by Qinghai University, Future University Hakodate, Xiamen University, Shandong Normal University. ITME 2013 is the next event in a series of highly successful international symposia on IT in Medicine and Education, ITME-12 (Hokkaido, Japan, August 2012), ITME-11 (Guangzhou, China, December 2011), ITME-09 (Jinan, China, August 2009), ITME-08 (Xiamen, China, December 2008).

The papers included in the proceedings cover the following topics: IT Application in Medicine Education, Medical Image Processing and compression, e-Health and e-Hospital, Tele-medicine and Tele-surgery, Standard in Health Informatics and cross-language solution, Computer-Aided Diagnostic (CAD), Health informatics education, Biomechanics, modeling and computing, Digital Virtual Organ and Clinic Application, Three Dimension Reconstruction for Medical Imaging, Hospital Management Informatization, Construction of Medical Database, Medical Knowledge Mining, IT and Biomedicine, IT and Clinical Medicine, IT and Laboratory Medicine, IT and Preclinical Medicine, IT and Medical Informatics, Architecture of Educational Information Systems, Building and Sharing Digital Education Resources on the Internet, Collaborative Learning/ Training, Computer Aided Teaching and Campus Network Construction, Curriculum Design and Development for Open/Distance Education, Digital Library, e-Learning Pedagogical Strategies, Ethical and Social Issues in Using IT in Education, Innovative Software and Hardware Systems for Education and Training, Issues on University Office Automation and Education Administration Management Systems, Learning Management Information Systems, Managed Learning Environments, Multimedia and Hypermedia Applications and Knowledge Management in Education, Pedagogical Issues on Open/Distance Education, Plagiarism Issues on Open/Distance Education, Security and Privacy issues with e-learning, Software Agents and Applications in Education. Accepted and presented papers highlight new trends and challenges of Medicine and Education. The presenters showed how new research could lead to novel and innovative applications. We hope you will find these results useful and inspiring for your future research.

We would like to express our sincere thanks to Steering Chair: Zongkai Lin (Institute of Computing Technology, Chinese Academy of Sciences, China). Our special thanks go to the Program Chairs: Shaozi Li (Xiamen University, China), Ying Dai (Iwate Prefectural University, Japan), Osamu Takahashi (Future University Hakodate, Japan), Dongqing Xie (Guangzhou University, China), Jianming Yong (University of Southern Queensland, Australia), all program committee members, and all the additional reviewers for their valuable efforts in the review process, which helped us to guarantee the highest quality of the selected papers for the conference.

We cordially thank all the authors for their valuable contributions and the other participants of this conference. The conference would not have been possible without their support. Thanks are also due to the many experts who contributed to making the event a success.

June 2013

Yongnian Liu
Xiaohong Jiang
James J. (Jong Hyuk) Park
Qun Jin
Hong Liu

Message from the ITME 2013 Program Chairs

Welcome to the 5th International Symposium on IT in Medicine and Education (ITME 2013), which will be held on July 19–21, 2013, in Xining, China. ITME 2013 will be the most comprehensive conference focused on the IT in Medicine and Education. ITME 2013 will provide an opportunity for academic and industry professionals to discuss the recent progress in the area of Medicine and Education. In addition, the conference will publish high-quality papers which are closely related to the various theories and practical applications on IT in Medicine and Education. Furthermore, we expect that the conference and its publications will be a trigger for further related research and technology improvements in these important subjects.

For ITME 2013, we received many paper submissions, after a rigorous peer review process; only very outstanding papers will be accepted for the ITME 2013 proceedings, published by Springer. All submitted papers have undergone blind reviews by at least two reviewers from the technical program committee, which consists of leading researchers around the globe. Without their hard work, achieving such a high-quality proceeding would not have been possible. We take this opportunity to thank them for their great support and cooperation. We would like to sincerely thank the following keynote speakers who kindly accepted our invitations, and, in this way, helped to meet the objectives of the conference: Prof. Qun Jin, Department of Human Informatics and Cognitive Sciences, Waseda University, Japan, Prof. Yun Yang, Swinburne University of Technology, Melbourne, Australia, Prof. Qinghua Zheng, Department of Computer Science and Technology, Xi'an Jiaotong University, China. We also would like to thank all of you for your participation in our conference, and also thank all the authors, reviewers, and organizing committee members.

Thank you and enjoy the conference!

Shaozi Li, China
Ying Dai, Japan
Osamu Takahashi, Japan
Dongqing Xie, China
Jianming Yong, Australia

Organization

General Conference Chairs

Prof. Yongnian Liu (QHU, China)
Prof. Xiaohong Jiang (FUN, Hakodate, Japan)
Prof. James J. (Jong Hyuk) Park, Seoul National University of Science and Technology, Korea
Prof. Qun Jin (Waseda, Japan)
Prof. Hong Liu (SDNU, China)

General Conference Co-Chairs

Prof. Yu Jianshe (GZHU, China)
Prof. Ramana Reddy (WVU, USA)
Dr. Bin Hu (UCE Birmingham, UK)
Prof. Dingfang Chen (WHUT, China)
Prof. Junzhong Gu (ECNU, China)

Program Committee Chairs

Prof. Shaozi Li (XMU, China)
Prof. Ying Dai (Iwate Prefecture University, Japan)
Prof. Osamu Takahashi (FUN, Hakodate, Japan)
Prof. Dongqing Xie (GZHU, China)
Dr. Jianming Yong (USQ, Australia)

Organizing Committee Chairs

Prof. Mengrong Xie (QHU, China)
Prof. Gaoping Wang (HAUT, China)

Dr. Jiatuo Xu (SHUTCM, Shanghai, China)
Prof. Zhimin Yang (Shandong University)

Local Arrangement Co-Chairs

Prof. Jing Zhao (QHU, China)
Prof. Peng Chen (QHU, China)

Publication Chairs

Prof. Hwa Young Jeong, Kyung Hee University, Korea
Dr. Min Jiang (XMU, Xiamen, China)

Program Committee

Ahmed Meddahi, Institute Mines-Telecom/TELECOM Lille1, France
Ahmed Shawish, Ain Shams University, Egypt
Alexander Pasko, Bournemouth University, UK
Angela Guercio, Kent State University
Bob Apduhan, Kyushu Sangyo University, Japan
Cai Guorong, Jimei University, China
Cao Donglin, Xiamen University, China
Changqin Huang, Southern China Normal University, China
Chaozhen Guo, Fuzhou University, China
Chensheng Wang, Beijing University of Posts and Telecommunications, China
Chuanqun Jiang, Shanghai Second Polytechnic University, China
Cui Lizhen, Shandong University, China
Cuixia Ma, Institute of Software Chinese Academy of Sciences, China
Feng Li, Jiangsu University, China
Fuhua Oscar Lin, Athabasca University, Canada
Hiroyuki Mituhara, Tokushima University, Japan
Hongji Yang, De Montfort University, UK
Hsin-Chang Yang, National University of Kaohsiung, Taiwan
Hsin-Chang Yang, National University of Kaohsiung, Taiwan
I-Hsien Ting, National University of Kaohsiung, Taiwan
Jens Herder, University of Applied Sciences, Germany
Jian Chen, Waseda University, Japan
Jianhua Zhao, Southern China Normal University, China
Jianming Yong, University of Southern Queensland, Australia
Jiehan Zhou, University of Oulu, Finland

Jungang Han, Xi'an University of Posts and Telecommunications, China
Junqing Yu, Huazhong University of Science and Technology, China
Kamen Kanev, Shizuoka University, Japan
Kiss Gabor, Obuda University, Hungary
Lei Yu, The PLA Information Engineering University, China
Li Xueqing, Shandong University, China
Luhong Diao, Beijing University of Technology, China
Masaaki Shirase, Future University Hakodate, Japan
Masashi Toda, Future University, Japan
Mohamed Mostafa Zayed, Taibah University, KSA
Mohammad Tariqul Islam, Multimedia University, Malaysia
Mohd Nazri Ismail, Universiti Kuala Lumpur, Malaysia
Neil Y. Yen, University of Aizu, Japan
Osamu Takahashi, Future University Hakodate, Japan
Paolo Maresca, University Federico II, Italy
Pierpaolo Di Bitonto, University of Bari, Italy
Ping Jiang, University of Hull, UK
Qiang Gao, Beihang University, China
Qianping Wang, China University of Mining and Technology, China
Qingguo Zhou, Lanzhou University, China
Qinghua Zheng, Xi'an Jiao Tong University, China
Rita Francese, University of Salerno, Italy
Roman Y. Shtykh, Waseda University, Japan
Rongrong Ji, Columbia University, USA
Shaohua Teng, Guangdong University of Technology, China
Shufen Liu, Jilin University, China
Su Songzhi, Xiamen University, China
Tianhong Luo, Chongqing Jiaotong University, China
Tim Arndt, Cleveland State University, USA
Tongsheng Chen, Comprehensive Information Corporation, Taiwan
Wei Song, Minzu University of China, Tsinghua University, China
Wenan Tan, Shanghai Second Polytechnic University, China
Wenhua Huang, Southern Medical University, China
Xiaokang Zhou, Waseda University, Japan
Xiaopeng Sun, Liaoning Normal University, China
Xiaosu Zhan, Beijing University of Posts and Telecommunications, China
Xinheng Wang, Swansea University, UK
Xiufen Fu, Guangdong University of Technology, China
Yaowei Bai, Shanghai Second Polytechnic University, China
Yingguang Li, Nanjing University of Aeronautics and Astronautics, China
Yinglong Wang, Shandong Academy of Sciences, China
Yinsheng Li, Fudan University, China
Yiwei Cao, IMC AG, Germany
Yong Tang, South China Normal University, China
Yoshitaka Nakamura, Future University Hakodate, Japan

Yuichi Fujino, Future University, Japan
Yujie Liu, China University of Petroleum, China
Zhang Zili, Southwestern University, China
Zhao Junlan, Inner Mongolia Finance and Economics College, China
Zhaoliang Jiang, Shandong University, China
Zhendong Niu, Beijing Institute of Technology, China
Zhenhua Duan, Xidian University, China
Zhongwei Xu, Shandong University at Weihai, China
Zonghua Zhang, Institute Mines-Telecom/TELECOM Lille1, France
Zongmin Li, China University of Petroleum, China
Zongpu Jia, Henan Polytechnic University, China

Contents

Volume 1

1. The Anti-Apoptotic Effect of Transgenic Akt1 Gene on Cultured New-Born Rats Cardiomyocytes Mediated by Ultrasound/Microbubbles Destruction 1
   Dongye Li, Xueyou Jiang, Tongda Xu, Jiantao Song, Hong Zhu and Yuanyuan Luo

2. Logic Operation in Spiking Neural P System with Chain Structure 11
   Jing Luan and Xi-yu Liu

3. A Mathematical Model of the Knee Joint for Estimation of Forces and Torques During Standing-up 21
   Zhi-qiang Wang, Yu-kun Ren and Hong-yuan Jiang

4. Adaptive Online Learning Environment for Life-Long Learning 29
   Zhao Du, Lantao Hu and Yongqi Liu

5. A Membrane Bin-Packing Technique for Heart Disease Cluster Analysis 39
   Xiyu Liu, Jie Xue and Laisheng Xiang

6. Teaching Chinese as a Foreign Language Based on Tone Labeling in the Corpus and Multi-Model Corpus 51
   Zhu Lin

7. A Systematically Statistical Analysis of Effects of Chinese Traditional Setting-up Exercise on Healthy Undergraduate Students 61
   Tiangang Li, Yongming Li and Xiaohong Gu

8	Sample-Independent Expression Stability Analysis of Human Housekeeping Genes Using the GeNORM Algorithm .... Li Li, Xiaofang Mao, Qiang Gao and Yicheng Cao	73
9	Development of a One-Step Immunochromatographic Strip Test for Rapid Detection of Antibodies Against Classic Swine Fever .... Huiying Ren, Shun Zhou, Jianxin Wen, Xinmei Zhan, Wenhua Liu and Shangin Cui	81
10	Cramer-Von Mises Statistics for Testing the Equality of Two Distributions.............................. Qun Huang and Ping Jing	93
11	Establishment of Craniomaxillofacial Model Including Temporomandibular Joint by Means of Three-Dimensional Finite Element Method .... Zhang Jun, Zhang Wen-juan, Zhao Shu-ya, Li Na, Li Tao and Wang Xu-xia	103
12	The Teaching and Practice for Neutral Network Control Course of Intelligence Science and Technology Specialty ..... Lingli Yu	113
13	A New ACM/ICPC-Based Teaching Reform and Exploration of "Design and Analysis of Algorithms" .... Yunping Zheng and Mudar Sarem	123
14	Application Studies of Bayes Discriminant and Cluster in TCM Acupuncture Clinical Data Analysis.............. Xiangyang Feng, Youqun Shi, Qinfeng Huang, Wenli Cheng, Houqin Su and Jie Liu	133
15	Implanting Two Fiducials into the Liver with Single Needle Insertion Under CT Guidance for CyberKnife® SBRT....... Li Yu, Xu Hui-jun and Zhang Su-jing	145
16	On the Statistics and Risks of Fiducial Migration in the CyberKnife Treatment of Liver Cancer Tumors ...... Li Yu, Hui-jun Xu and Su-jing Zhang	157

17	The Comparative Analysis with Finite Element for Cemented Long- and Short-Stem Prosthetic Replacement in Elderly Patients with a Partial Marrow Type I Intertrochanteric Fracture Wang Shao-lin, Tan Zu-jian and Zhou Ming-quan	165
18	The Exploration of Higher Undergraduate Education Mode Based on University-Enterprise Cooperation Yunna Wu, Jianping Yuan and Qing Wang	185
19	Higher Education Quality Supervision System Research Yunna Wu, Jinying Zhang, Zhen Wang, Jianping Yuan and Yili Han	195
20	Micro-blog Marketing of University Library Based on 4C Marketing Mix Feng Qing, Shang Wei and Chen Huilan	205
21	On Ethics and Values with Online Education Jiayun Wang and Jianian Zhang	213
22	What? How? Where? A Survey of Crowdsourcing Xu Yin, Wenjie Liu, Yafang Wang, Chenglei Yang and Lin Lu	221
23	Hierarchical Clustering by a P System with Chained Rules Jie Sun and Xiyu Liu	233
24	Design and Implementation of Key Techniques in TCM Clinical Decision Support System Mingfeng Zhu, Bin Nie, Jianqiang Du, Chenghua Ding and Qinglin Zha	243
25	The Effect of a Simulation-Based Training on the Performance of ACLS and Trauma Team of 5-Year Medical Students Jie Zhao, Shuming Pan, Yan Dong, Qinmin Ge, Jie Chen and Lihua Dai	253
26	A Novel Enhancement Algorithm for Non-Uniform Illumination Particle Image Liu Weihua	265
27	Research on Predicting the Number of Outpatient Visits Hang Lu, Yi Feng, Zhaoxia Zhu, Liu Yang, Yuezhong Xu and Yingjia Jiang	273

28	Acute Inflammations Analysis by P System with Floor Membrane Structure Jie Xue and Xiyu Liu	281
29	Different Expression of P_{53} and Rb Gene in the Experimental Neuronal Aging with the Interference of Cholecystokinin Feng Wang, Xing-Wang Chen, Kang-Yong Liu, Jia-Jun Yang and Xiao-Jiang Sun	293
30	Attitudes Toward and Involvement in Medical Research: A Survey of 8-year-Program Undergraduates in China Jie-Hua Li, Bin Yang, Jing-Xia Li, Yan-Bo Liu, Hui-Yong Chen, Kun-Lu Wu, Min Zhu, Jing Liu, Xiao-Juan Xiao and Qing-Nan He	307
31	Study the Effect of Different Traditional Chinese Medicine Treatment which to the Elasticity Modulus of Asthma Rats' Lung Zhao-xia Xu, Xue-liang Li, Na Li, Peng Qian, Jin Xu, Yi-qin Wang and Jun-qi Wang	321
32	Cloning and Characterization of Two cDNA Sequences Coding Squalene Synthase Involved in Glycyrrhizic Acid Biosynthesis in *Glycyrrhiza uralensis* Ying Liu, Ning Zhang, Honghao Chen, Ya Gao, Hao Wen, Yong Liu and Chunsheng Liu	329
33	Ontology-Based Multi-Agent Cooperation EHR Semantic Interoperability Pattern Research Jian Yang and Jiancheng Dong	343
34	Visual Analysis on Management of Postgraduate Degrees Chen Ling and Xue-qing Li	353
35	An Energy-Saving Load Balancing Method in Cloud Data Centers Xiao Li and Mingchun Zheng	365
36	Application of a New Association Rules Mining Algorithm in the Chinese Medical Coronary Disease Feng Yuan, Hong Liu and ShouQiang Chen	375
37	Design and Development of a Clinical Data Exchange System Based on Ensemble Integration Platform Wang Yu, Guo Long, Tian Yu and Jing-Song Li	385

38	The Management and Application of a Radio Frequency Identification System in Operating Rooms Jun-Der Leu, Yu-Hui Chiu and Hsueh-Ling Ku	393
39	Exploiting Innovative Computer Education Through Student Associations Wei Hu, Daikun Zou, Wenfei Li, Hong Guo and Ning Li	403
40	Traditional Chinese Medicine Literature Metadata: A Draft Technical Specification Developed by the International Organization for Standardization Tong Yu, Meng Cui, Haiyan Li, Shuo Yang, Yang Zhao and Zhang Zhulu	413
41	A Visualization Method in Virtual Educational System Guijuan Zhang, Dianjie Lu and Hong Liu	421
42	Moral Education with the Background of Information Globalization Liying Xiang	431
43	A Bayes Network Model to Determine MiRNA Gene Silence Mechanism Hao-yue Fu, Xiao-jun Lu and Xiang-de Zhang	441
44	The Novle Strategy for the Recognition and Classification of the Red Blood Cell in Low Quality Form Images Qiyou Cao, Xueqing Li and Qi Zhang	449
45	Scalable and Explainable Friend Recommendation in Campus Social Network System Zhao Du, Lantao Hu, Xiaolong Fu and Yongqi Liu	457
46	Application of Virtual Reality Technology in Medical Education Yan-Li Shi	467
47	An Improved Outlier Detection Algorithm Based on Reverse K-Nearest Neighbors of Adaptive Parameters Xie Fangfang, Xu Liancheng, Chi Xuezhi and Zhu Zhenfang	477
48	A Practical Study on the Construction of Diversified Network Monitoring System for Teaching Quality Jia Bing, Jiang Fengyan and Li Di	489

49	Reformation and Application of "Project-Tutor System" in Experimental Course Teaching of Fundamental Medicine .... Li-fa Xu and Jian Wang	501
50	A Knowledge-Based Teaching Resources Recommend Model for Primary and Secondary School Oriented Distance-Education Teaching Platform .... Meijing Zhao, Wancheng Ni, Haidong Zhang, Ziqi Lin and Yiping Yang	511
51	A Fast and Simple HPLC–UV Method for Simultaneous Determination of Emodin and Quinalizarin from Fermentation Broth of *Aspergillus. ochraceus* lp_0429 .... ShaoMei Yu and Ping Lv	523
52	Alteration of Liver MMP-9/TIMP-1 and Plasma Type IV Collagen in the Development of Rat Insulin Resistance .... Jun-feng Hou, Xiao-di Zhang, Xiao-guang Wang, Jing Wei and Kai Jiao	531
53	Evaluation Method for Software System Reliability .... Han Lu, Shufen Liu, Zhao Jin and Xue Fan	545
54	P System Based Particle Swarm Optimization Algorithm ..... Qiang Du, Laisheng Xiang and Xiyu Liu	553
55	Specifying Usage of Social Media as a Formative Construct: Theory and Implications for Higher Education .... Tao Hu, Ping Zhang, Gongbu Gao, Shengli Jiao, Jun Ke and Yuanqiang Lian	565
56	Unsupervised Brain Tissue Segmentation by Using Bias Correction Fuzzy C-Means and Class-Adaptive Hidden Markov Random Field Modelling .... Ziming Zeng, Chunlei Han, Liping Wang and Reyer Zwiggelaar	579
57	An Adaptive Cultural Algorithm Based on Dynamic Particle Swarm Optimization. .... Liu Peiyu, Ren Yuanyuan, Xue Suzhi and Zhu Zhenfang	589
58	A Modified Approach of Hot Topics Found on Micro-blog. ... Lu Ran, Xue Suzhi, Ren Yuanyuan and Zhu Zhenfang	603

59	Computational Fluid Dynamics Simulation of Air Flow in the Human Symmetrical Six-Generation Bifurcation Bronchial Tree Model................................ Shouliang Qi, Zhenghua Li and Yong Yue	615
60	Discrimination of Solitary Pulmonary Nodules on CT Images Based on a Novel Automatic Weighted FCM.............. Zhang Xin, Jiaxing Li, Wang Bing, Ming Jun, Yang Ying and Zhang Jinxing	625
61	Investigation of Demands on On-Campus Health Information Education Services........................ Zhao-feng Li, Xuan Li, Xi-peng Han, Xing Tu, Tong Li and Wen-bin Fu	635
62	Suicidality in Medication-Native Patients with Single-Episode Depression: MRSI of Deep White Matter in Frontal Lobe and Parietal Lobe.................................. Xizhen Wang, Hongwei Sun, Shuai Wang, Guohua Xie, Shanshan Gao, Xihe Sun, Yanyu Wang and Nengzhi Jiang	647
63	Relating Research on ADC Value and Serum GGT, TBil of Lesions in Neonatal Hypoxic Ischemic Encephalopathy .... Yue Guan, Anhui Yan, Yanming Ge, Yanqi Xu, Xihe Sun and Peng Dong	659
64	Design and Implementation of the Regional Health Information Collaborative Platform .... Kong Hua-Ming, Qin Yao, Peng-Fei Li and Jing-Song Li	669
65	A Multi-objective Biogeography-Based Optimization with Mean Value Migration Operator................... Xiang-wei Zheng, Kai-ge Gao, Xiao-guang Wang and Chi-zhu Ma	679
66	Observation of Curative Effect on 200 Cases of Myasthenia Gravis Treated with Traditional Chinese Medicine .... Wang Di and Wang Zhenqiu	687
67	Integrating Social Question–Answer Sites in Learning Management System................................ Yongqi Liu, Zhao Du, Lantao Hu and Qiuli Tong	695
68	The Study of Dynamic Threshold Strategy Based-On Error Correction .... Zhimin Yang, Jie Li, Gaofeng Han, Yue Wang and Songnan Zhao	705

69	**Identification of Evaluation Collocation Based on Maximum Entropy Model** LingYun Zhao, FangAi Liu and Zhenfang Zhu	713
70	**Comparison of Beta Variable Gene Usage of T Cell Receptor in Peripheral Blood and Synovial Fluid of Rheumatoid Arthritis Patients** Jianwei Zhou, Cui Kong, Xiukui Wang, Zhaocai Zhang, Chengqiang Jin and Qin Song	723
71	**New Impossible Differential Cryptanalysis on Improved LBlock** Xuan Liu, Feng Liu and Shuai Meng	737
72	**Speckle Noise Reduction in Breast Ultrasound Images for Segmentation of Region Of Interest (ROI) Using Discrete Wavelets** S. Amutha, D. R. Ramesh Babu, M. Ravi Shankar, R. Mamatha and S. Vidhya Suman	747
73	**Sonic Hedgehog Signaling Molecules Expression in TGF-β1-Induced Chondrogenic Differentiation of Rat Mesenchymal Stem Cells In Vitro** Yingchao Shi, Ying Jia, Shanshan Zu, Yanfei Jia, Xueping Zhang, Haiji Sun and Xiaoli Ma	755
74	**A FCA-Based Approach to Data Integration in the University Information System** Yong Liu and Xueqing Li	763
75	**Research and Design on Agent-Based Collaborative Learning Model for Sports Students** Zhaoxia Lu, Lei Zhang and Dongming Liu	773
76	**Toxicology Evaluation and Properties of a New Biodegradable Computer Made Medical Biomaterial** Jinshu Ma, Chao Zhang, Jingying Sai, Guangyu Xu, Xiaotian Zhang, Chao Feng, Fan Li and Fang Wang	783
77	**Investigation and Analysis on Ear Diameter and Ear Axis Diameter in Maize RIL Population** Daowen He, Hongmei Zhang, Changmin Liao, Qi Luo, Guoqiang Hui, Zhirun Nan, Yi Sun and Yongsi Zhang	795

Contents

78	**Descriptive Statistics and Correlation Analysis of Three Kernel Morphology Traits in a Maize Recombinant Inbred Line Population**............................. Changmin Liao, Daowen He and Xiaohong Liu	803
79	**Study on Two Agronomic Traits Associated with Kernel Weight in a Maize RIL Segregation Population**............. Changmin Liao	811
80	**Improved Single-Key Attack on Reduced-Round LED**........ Feng Liu, Pei-li Wen, Xuan Liu and Shuai Meng	819
81	**Automatic Screening of Sleep Apnea-Hypopnea Syndrome by ECG Derived Respiration**......................... Qing Qiao, Guangming Tong and Rui Chen	829
82	**Research on the Informatization Top-level Design Methods**... Zhang Huilin, Tong Qiuli and Xie Suping	837
83	**Research on Optimization of Resources Allocation in Cloud Computing Based on Structure Supportiveness**...... Wei-hua Yuan, Hong Wang and Zhong-yong Fan	849
84	**Ambidextrous Development Model of University Continuing Education in Yunnan Province Based on CRM**............ Hong-wu Zuo, Ze-jian Li and Ming Pan	859
85	**Bibliometric Analysis on the Study of Education Informatization**...................................... Qiaoyun Chen	869
86	**A Method for Integrating Interfaces Based on Cluster Ensemble in Digital Library Federation**................. Peng Pan, Qingzhong Li and XiaoNan Fang	879
87	**Long Term Web Service Oriented Transaction Handling Improvement of BTP Protocol**....................... Zhi-Lin Yao, Lu Han, Jin-Ting Zhang and Shu-Fen Liu	889
88	**The Verification of a Newly Discovered Hepatitis B Virus Subtype Based on Sequence Analysis**............... Qingqing Yi, Lei Ma, Qinan Jia and Jianfeng He	899
89	**A Primary Study for Cancer Prognosis based on Classification and Regression Using Support Vector Machine**............ Jia Qinan, Ma Lei, He Jianfeng, Yi QingQing and Zhang Jun	909

Volume 2

90 Feature Extraction and Support Vector Machine Based Classification for False Positive Reduction in Mammographic Images............................ 921
Q. D. Truong, M. P. Nguyen, V. T. Hoang, H. T. Nguyen, D. T. Nguyen, T. D. Nguyen and V. D. Nguyen

91 Research on Distributed Synchronous CAD Collaborative Design System 931
Chen Li

92 Enterprise Evolution with Molecular Computation 941
Xiuting Li, Laisheng Xiang and Xiyu Liu

93 Research and Implementation of Auxiliary System for Waken-up Craniotomy 951
Liu Yu, Feng Wu, Hongmin Bai and Weimin Wang

94 Investigation Performance on Electrocardiogram Signal Processing based on an Advanced Algorithm Combining Wavelet Packet Transform (WPT) and Hilbert-Huang Transform (HHT)*.................................. 959
Jin Bo, Xuewen Cao, Yuqing Wan, Yuanyu Yu, Pun Sio Hang, Peng Un Mak and Mang I Vai

95 Study on Self-Adaptive Clinical Pathway Decision Support System Based on Case-Based Reasoning........... 969
Gang Qu, Zhe Liu, Shengnan Cui and Jiafu Tang

96 Wireless Body Sensor Networks with Cloud Computing Capability for Pervasive Healthcare: Research Directions and Possible Solutions................................ 979
Xiaoya Xu and Miao Zhong

97 Robust Predictive Control of Singular Systems with Structured Feedback Uncertainty 989
Xiaohua Liu and Rong Gao

98 Image Enhancement Methods for a Customized Videokeratography System Designed for Animals with Small Eyes 1001
Bin Chen, Shan Ling, Hongfei Cen, Wenfu Xu, Kee Chea-su, Yongjin Zhou and Lei Wang

99	Cloning and Expression of Catechol 2,3-dioxygenase from *Achromobacter Xylosoxidans* LHB21 .... Shuang Yu, Naiyu Chi and QingFang Zhang	1011
100	Design of Trust Model Based on Behavior in Cloud Computing Environment........................ Yong Sheng Zhang, Ming Tian, Shen Juan Lv and Yan Dong Zhang	1021
101	The Study of Community–Family Remote Health Supervisory System Based on IOT .... Dongxin Lu and Wei Li	1029
102	Consistent Metric Learning for Outcomes of Different Measurement Tools of Cervical Spondylosis: Towards Better Therapeutic Effectiveness Evaluation .... Gang Zhang, Ying Huang, Yingchun Zhong and Wuwei Wang	1039
103	Design and Creation of a Universal Model of Educational Process with the Support of Petri Nets .... Zoltán Balogh, Milan Turčáni and Martin Magdin	1049
104	The Application of MPC-GEP in Classification Rule Mining....................................... Min Yao, Zhepeng Xu and Zenhong Wu	1061
105	Effects of Informationization on Strategic Plan of Regional Universities .... Guilin Chen, Shenghui Zhao and Chunyan Yu	1073
106	A Survey on Wireless Camera Sensor Networks .... Xiaolan Liu	1085
107	A Modified Hexagon-Based Search Algorithm for Fast Block Matching Motion Estimation.................... Yun Cheng, Tiebin Wu and Minlei Xiao	1095
108	Protection of Xi Lei Powder to Intestinal Mucosa in Enema-Microstructure Observation by TEM and Light Microscope............................. Feng Zhang, DuanYing Cai and Juan Xu	1105
109	Study on the Theory Building of Relationship Between National Culture Benefit and Language Education Policy..... Jingying Ma	1113

110	Study on the Defect and Research About Discipline Speech Act Theory of Educator. Li Ying	1119
111	Study on the Nature of Education Information: The Education of Digital Virtual World Zhang Junmei	1125
112	Study on the Construction of General Framework of Educational Cost Management Mode in Colleges and Universities Xiu Hongbo	1131
113	Study on the Risk Identification and Warning of Tax Administration. Liu Weidong	1137
114	Study on the System Design of Sports Public Service Performance Evaluation Weidong Liu	1143
115	Research on the Construction of Teaching Resources Platform in Universities Qian Meng	1149
116	Applications of Virtualization Technology to Digital Library. Yu Xiaoyi, Wang Zhengjun, Yu Zhenguo, Jin Yuling, Wang Hong, Liang Yufang, Wang Quanhong, Gao Jian and Wang Haiyin	1155
117	The Health Status Among College Teachers: Taking Jiangxi Local Colleges as Example. Kaiqiang Guo, Weisong Bu and Fangping Li	1163
118	Research on Students' Perception and Expectations of Printed Materials in Online Education Jin Yiqiang	1175
119	Task Driven is an Effective Teaching Model of Discrete Mathematics in High Education Liu Shuai, Fu Weina, Li Qiang, Zhao Yulan and Duan Chanlun	1183

120	Evaluation on Application of Scene-Simulation Teaching Method in Oral Medicine Teaching.................. Xiaoli An, Qianqian Lin, Wu Fanbieke, YuLin Zhang, Bin Liu and Wang Jizeng	1189
121	Research on Three Convolutions Related Issues in Signal Processing .... Wei Song	1195
122	Evaluation of College Students' Self-Regulated Learning Based on the IT Technology .... X. Wang, B. Qu and Ch. Y. Jia	1201
123	The Association Analysis of P16 in Transitional Cell .... Yu Hui	1207
124	Problem-Based Learning (PBL) in Eight-Year Program of Clinical Medicine in Xiangya School of Medicine: New Mode Needs Exploration .... Jieyu He, Qingnan He, Xiaoqun Qin, Yongquan Tian, Donna Ambrozy and Aihua Pan	1213
125	Design of Virtual Reality Guide Training Room Based on the Modern Education Technology .... Zhang Pengshun	1221
126	Exploration and Practice of Teaching Mode of Mechanical Engineering Control Foundation Based on Project Driving ... Tao Wu and Xiao-Bin Duan	1229
127	Wireless Sensor Network Distributed Data Collection Strategy Based on the Regional Correlated Variability of Perceptive Area........................ Yongjun Zhang and Enxiu Chen	1235
128	The System Design of the Network Teaching Platform of Learning Based on the Concept of Development Evaluation .... Liu Yong	1241
129	3-Dimensional Finite Element Analysis on Periodontal Stress Distribution of Impacted Teeth During Orthodontic Treatment .... Xu-xia Wang, Na Li, Jian-guang Xu, Xu-sheng Ren, Shi-liang Ma and Jun Zhang	1247

130	A Score-Analysis Method Based on ID3 of NCRE . . . . Zeng Xu	1253
131	Education Cloud: New Development of Informationization Education in China. . . . . Liangtao Yang	1259
132	CRH5 EMU Fault Diagnosis Simulation Training System Development. . . . . Jian Wang, Zhiming Liu, Fengchuan Jiao and Xinhua Zhang	1267
133	A Study on Recruitment Requirements of Small and Medium-Sized Enterprises and the Talent Training of Local Colleges . . . . Zhang Weiwei	1277
134	Simultaneous Determination of Atractylenolide II and III in *Rhizoma Atractylodes Macrocephalae* and Chinese Medicinal Preparation by Reverse-Phase High-Performance Liquid Chromatography. . . . . Xiao-hong Sun and Jian Ge	1283
135	Research on the Pharmacokinetics and Elimination of Epigallocatechin Gallate (EGCG) in Mice . . . . Yang Liu, Jian Ge, Meng-xin Wang, Lin Cui and Bao-yu Han	1291
136	Simultaneous Determination of Five Phthalic Acid Esters (PAEs) in Soil and Air . . . . Tian-yu Hu, Yang Liu, Hua-jun Hu, Meng-xin Wang, Bao-yu Han and Jian Ge	1299
137	The Relationship Between Employability Self-Efficacy and Growth: The Mediator Role of e-Recruiting Perceived . . . Chun-Mei Chou, Chien-Hua Shen, Hsi-Chi Hsiao, Hui-Tzu Chang, Su-Chang Chen, Chin-Pin Chen, Jen-Chia Chang, Jing-Yi Chen, Kuan-Fu Shen and Hsiang-Li Shen	1307
138	A Study to Analyze the Effectiveness of Video-Feedback for Teaching Nursing Etiquette. . . . . Xiaoling Zhu, Mulan Wei, Ruoyan Chen, Daolin Jian and Xiaofei Chen	1315

139	A Biomedical Microdevice for Quantal Exocytosis Measurement with Microelectrodes Arrays .... Liguo Sun, Zhimeng Zou, Haifei Li, Peizheng Liu, Keping Tan and Jun Li	1321
140	The Construction of Comprehensive Financial Evaluation System in Higher Vocational Colleges Based on Connotation Construction......................... Zhongsheng Zhu and Fei Gao	1325
141	Spatial Covariance Modeling Analysis of Hypertension on Cognitive Aging................................ Lan Lin, Wei-wei Wu, Shui-cai Wu and Guang-yu Bin	1331
142	A New Practice Mode and Platform Based on Network Cooperation for Software Engineering Specialty .... Ling He	1337
143	Post-newborn: A New Concept of Period in Early Life ...... Long Chen, Jie Li, Nan Wang and Yuan Shi	1343
144	Analysis of the Characteristics of Papillary Thyroid Carcinoma and Discussion on the Surgery (Experience of 392 Cases)........................... Jia Liu, Guimin Wang, Guang Chen, Shuai Xue and Su Dong	1351
145	Skills of Minimally Invasive Endoscopic Thyroidectomy via Small Incision of Neck (Experience of 1,226 Cases) ...... Jia Liu, Su Dong, Xianying Meng, Shuai Xue and Guang Chen	1359
146	Research on the Contemporary College Students' Information Literacy .... Zhong Wenjuan, Wang Jing, Wang Mei and Guan Yanwen	1365
147	The CEMS Research Based on Web Service .... Wenke Zang and Xiyu Liu	1373
148	Enterprise Development with P Systems .... Xiuting Li, Laisheng Xiang and Xiyu Liu	1383
149	Application of Microblog in Educational Technology Practice Teaching................................. Jiugen Yuan and Ruonan Xing	1389

150	Ultrasound Image Segmentation Using Graph Cuts with Deformable Prior Lin Li, Yue Wu and Mao Ye	1395
151	Classifying and Diagnosing 199 Impacted Permanent Using Cone Beam Computed Tomography Xu-xia Wang, Jian-guang Xu, Yun Chen, Chao Liu, Jun Zheng, Wan-xin Liu, Rui Dong and Jun Zhang	1401
152	Research Status and Development Tendency of Multi-campus and Two Level Teaching Quality Monitoring and Security System Mu Lei, Liu Xilin, Wang Keqin and Sun Ye	1407
153	Analysis of the Research and Trend for Electronic Whiteboard Guiying Guo and Baishuang Qiu	1413
154	Study on Multi-faceted Teaching Model of Common Courses in Stomatology: Taking Curriculums of "The Oral Prevention and Health Care" as an Example Yanyang Xu, Qian Zheng, Yuting Du, XueLi Gou, Guilong Gu, Jianhua Huang and Bin Liu	1419
155	Teaching Discussion on Pattern Matching Algorithm in the Course of Data Structure Yang An and Bo Zhao	1425
156	The Optimal Medical Device Order Strategy: An Improved EOQ Model in Hospital Wei Yan, Yong Jiang and Huimin Duan	1431
157	Improve Effectiveness and Quality of Course Practices by Opening, Reusing and Sharing Rao Lan and Xinjun Mao	1437
158	Application of PBL Teaching Method in the Experimental Teaching of Hematologic Examination Min Sun, Ya Li Zhang, LiJun Gao and XinYu Cui	1443
159	Study on Bilingual Teaching of Heat Transfer Curriculum Assisted by Distance Education Shunyu Su, Chuanhui Zhou and Xiongbing Ruan	1449

160	Nonlinear Analysis of Bioprosthetic Heart Valve on Suture Densities.................................... Quan Yuan, Xia Zhang, Xu Huang and Hua Cong	1455
161	Reflections on Primary PostCapacity-Oriented Integrated Practice Teaching of Oral Courses in Higher Vocational Colleges.. Chun-feng Wang, Jin Ling, Jian-guo Yi, Min-jiang Huang and Guang-ye Zhao	1463
162	Excellent Man Marathon Runners and Plateau, Plateau Training Period Portion of the Blood in the Index Comparison Analysis .... Zhang Sheng-lin	1473
163	The Implication of Collaborative Learning in College English..................................... Yan Sufeng and Song Runjuan	1481
164	Bilingual Teaching Efficiency of Prosthodontics in Different Teaching Methods .... Liangjiao Chen, Ting Sun, Hua Fan, Yaokun Zhang, Ruoyu Liu and Longquan Shao	1487
165	Practice of Paradigm Teaching on Circuit Theory........... Yumin Ge and Baoshu Li	1493
166	The Study of Relationship Between the Nature and Other Properties of Traditional Chinese Medicines Based on Association Rules..................................... Wang Zhe and Yu Hong-Yan	1501
167	Usage of Turbine Airflow Sensor in Ventilator.............. Yaoyu Wu, Feng Chang and Dongmin Liu	1507
168	Study on the Model of Double Tutors System in Postgraduate Education .... Jian Wang and Zhongyan Han	1515
169	Research on the Mobile Learning Resources Based on Cellphone .... Huang Lehui and Xing Ruonan	1521

170	Data Structure Teaching Practice: Discussion on Non-recursive Algorithms for the Depth-First Traversal of a Binary Tree.................................... Zhong-wei Xu	1527
171	Contrast Analysis of Standardized Patients and Real Patients in Clinical Medical Teaching .... Zhang Yali, Xi Bo, Zhou Rui, Chunli Wu, Feng Jie, Jiping Sun, Jing Lv, Qingzhi Long and Bingyin Shi	1533
172	Effect of Jiangtang Fonglong Capsule on Expressions of Insulin of Deaf Animal Models of Diabetes .... Ruiyu Li, Kaoshan Guo, Lizhen Tang, Yanzhuo Zhang, Meng Li and Bin Li	1539
173	The Discussion for the Existence of Nontrivial Solutions About a Kind of Quasi-Linear Elliptic Equations........... Bingyu Kou, Lei Mao, Xinghu Teng, Huaren Zhou and Chun Zhang	1547
174	A Team-Learning of Strategies to Increase Students' Physical Activity and Motivation in Sports Community............. Hongyv Wu, Xiabing Fan and Dinghong Mou	1555
175	Research on Feet Health of College Students.............. Pan Meili	1561
176	Uncertain Life .... Shao-lin Wang and Dian-ming Jiang	1569
177	Large-Scale Clinical Data Management and Analysis System Based on Cloud Computing..................... Ye Wang, Lin Wang, Hong Liu and Changhai Lei	1575
178	Satisfaction Changes Over Time Among Dentists with Outpatient Electronic Medical Record............... Hong-wei Cai, Yu Cao, Hong-bo Peng, Bo Zhao and Wan-hui Ye	1585
179	Discussion on English Collaborative Learning Mode in Vocational Schools Under the IT-Based Network Environment............................... X. Yang and H. H. Tan	1591

180	The Design of Learner-Centered College Teaching Resource Libraries .... Cui Wei, Liang Lijing and Hua Wei	1597
181	Research on Practice Teaching of Software Engineering ..... Lianying Sun, Chang Liu, Baosen Zhang, Tao Peng and Yuting Chen	1603
182	Construction of Transportation Professional Virtual Internship Platform .... Zhao Jianguang and Lui Ruijun	1609
183	Chronic Suppurative Otitis Media Bacteriology Culturing and Drug Sensitive Experiment of Er Yannig .... Wu Liping, Hu Xiaoqian, Li Meng, Hou Jinjie and Li Ruiyu	1615
184	Research Hotspots Analysis of Hypertension Receptor by PubMed....................................... Chaopeng Li, Qinting Zhang, Yang Liu, Shuangping Wei, Jungai Li, Jinjie Hou, Ruijuan Zhang, Weiya Guo, Lijun Wang, Yuhong Liu and Ruiyu Li	1619
185	Creative Approaches Combined with Computer Simulation Technology in Teaching Pharmacology .... Chuang Wang and Jiejie Guo	1625
186	Problems and Counterplans of College English Independent Study Under Network Environment .... Zhai Fengjie	1633
187	Integrity Verification of Cloud Data .... Fan-xin Kong and Li Liu	1639
188	Establishing Automotive Engineering School-Enterprise Practice Training Model Based on Excellent Engineer Plan ... Geng Guo-qing, Zhu Mao-tao and Xu Xing	1645
189	Mechanical Finite Element Analysis to Two Years Old Children's Orbital-Bone Based on CT .... Jing liu, He Jin, Tingting Ning, Beilei Yang, Juying Huang and Weiyuan Lu	1651
190	Study on Digitalized 3D Specimen Making of Pathologic Gross Specimen Basing on Object Panorama.............. Ran Hua-quan, Jiang Jun and Zeng Zhao-fang	1659

191	Ontology-Based Medical Data Integration for Regional Healthcare Application Yu-Xin Wen, Hua-Qiong Wang, Yi-Fan Zhang and Jing-Song Li	1667
192	The Application of Positive Psychology in Effective Teaching Yu Lin, Yu Jing, He Zhifang and Li Wuiguo	1673
193	The Exploration of Paramilitary Students Management in Vocational Colleges Wang Haohui	1683
194	Research on a New DNA-GA Algorithm Based on P System Shuguo Zhao and Xiyu Liu	1691
195	Study on the Assistance of Microblogging in English Literature Teaching Haixia Fang	1699
196	Problem-Based Learning of Food Hygiene in Higher University of Traditional Chinese Medicine Daozong Xia	1707
197	Education Security of Bridgehead Strategic in Southwest China: Concept, Problems and Solutions Jing Tian and Ling Wang	1713
198	Applications of Network-Based Education in Lifelong Medical Education Liyuan Sun, Mingcheng Li and Yundong Zhao	1719
199	The Application of Informatics Technology in Foreign Medical Undergraduates Teaching Limei Liu, Taiguang Piao and Wei Li	1725
200	Discussion on the Reform of Teaching Software Development Training Curriculum Based on Application Store Yan-jun Zhu, Wen-liang Cao and Jian-xin Li	1731
201	Research on Construction of Bilingual-Teaching Model Course for Bioinformatics Dong Hu, Jiansheng Wu, Han Wei, Meng Cui and Qiuming Zhang	1737

202	Research on Endpoint Information Extraction for Chemical Molecular Structure Images Zhao-man Zhong and Yan Guan	1747
203	Using Video Recording System to Improve Student Performance in High-Fidelity Simulation Wangqin Shen	1753
204	Exploration of Vocational Talents Culture Model of "Promote Learning with Competition, Combine Competition with Teaching" Wen-liang Cao and Xuan-zi Hu	1759
205	Research of Training Professionals in Computer Application Major from the Perspective of the Connection Between Middle and Higher Vocational Education Xuan-zi Hu and Wen-liang Cao	1765
206	Meta Analysis of Teachers' Job Burnout in China Jian-ping Liu, Zhi-fang He and Lin Yu	1771
207	Similar Theory in Material Mechanics Problem Luo Mao and Song Shaoyun	1779
208	Some Reflections on the Course Teaching of Physical Oceanography Hao Liu and Song Hu	1785
209	A Neural Tree Network Ensemble Mode for Disease Classification Feng Qi, Xiyu Liu and Yinghong Ma	1791
210	Application of PBL Model in the Teaching of Foreign Graduate Student Songzhu Xia, Xiaoyong Cao, Guisheng Yin, Haibo Liu and Jianguo Sun	1797
211	The Influence in Bone Mineral Density of Diabetes with Deafness in Different Syndrome Types by Prescriptions of Hypoglycemic Preventing Deafness Ruiyu Li, Kaoshan Guo, Meng Li, Jianqiao Li, Junli Yan, Liping Wu, Weihua Han, Qing Gu, Shuangping Wei and Yanfu Sun	1803

Volume 3

212 Application of Data Mining in the Assessment
of Teaching Quality 1813
Huabin Qu and Xueqing Li

213 A Data Mining System for Herbal Formula
Compatibility Analysis 1821
Li Jinghua, Feng Yi, Yu Tong, Liu Jing, Zhu Ling, Dong Yan,
Shuo Yang, Lirong Jia, Bo Gao and Gao Hongjie

214 The Analysis of the Chronic Patients' Demand of the Hospital
Health Information Service 1829
Guiling Li, Liqun Yang, Lin Ding, Runbin Wu,
Chundi Zhang, Limei Guo and Xiumei Ma

215 Learning from Errors and Learning from Failures:
A Study on the Model of Organizational Learning
from Errors 1833
Yangqun Xie, Jianian Zhang and Xiangzhi Zhuo

216 Employment-Oriented Web Application Development
Course Design Reform 1841
Chong-jie Dong

217 A Process Model of User Reactions to IT System Features 1847
Yan Yu and Zou Jin

218 Application of Modified PBL Mode on Pathophysiology
Courses 1855
Tang Hua, Chen Rong, Zhang Chun-Mei,
Li Zhu-Hua and Zou Ping

219 Meditations on the Semantic Net: Oriented Library
Information Service in Cloud Computing Era 1863
Yumei Liu

220 Synthesis and Antibacterial Activity
of Resveratrol Derivatives 1871
Yuanmou Chen, Fei Hu, Yinghao Gao, Na Ji and Shaolong Jia

221	Comparison of Intravenous Propofol Using Target-Controlled Infusion and Inhalational Sevoflurane Anesthesia in Pediatric Patients .... Dong Su, Haichun Ma, Wei Han, Limin Jin and Jia Liu	1883
222	Effect of Different Fluids on Blood Volume Expansion in Epidural Anesthesia of Elderly Patients................ Dong Su, Lei Pang, Haichun Ma, Wei Han and Jia Liu	1891
223	The Application of Association Rule Mining in the Diagnosis of Pancreatic Cancer .... Song Shaoyun	1899
224	Meta-Analysis of Chinese Herbs in the Treatment of Nephropathy: Huangqi and Danggui Type Formulations ... Ming-gang wei and Xiao-feng Cai	1905
225	Establishment and Significance of Digital Embryo Library for Enhancing Embryology Teaching Effect............... Bai Sheng-Bin, Chen Hong-Xiang, Tang Li, Liao Li-Bin, Li Tian, Feng Shu-Mei, Qin Wen, Zhong Jin-Jie and Luo Xue-Gang	1913
226	3D Reverse Modeling and Rapid Prototyping of Complete Denture................................ Dantong Li, Xiaobao Feng, Ping Liao, Hongjun Ni, Yidan Zhou, Mingyu Huang, Zhiyang Li and Yu Zhu	1919
227	Simulation Training on Improving Basic Laparoscopic Skills of Medical Students .... Ni Hong, Song Ge and Junfang Qin	1929
228	Research on Reforming of Vocational Colleges for Music Majors in Education................................ Liu Li	1935
229	Research on Badminton Sports in National Fitness Activities................................... Yanling Dong and Qiang Ji	1941
230	University Students' Humanity Quality Education of Tai Ji Quan to Cultivate Influence .... Ji Qiang and Dong YanLing	1947

231	**Study Progress of Traditional Chinese Massage Treatment of Lumbar Disc Herniation** Qing Lan and Weihong Deng	1953
232	**Chinese Anti-Inflammatory Herb May Postpone the Forming and Exacerbating of Diabetic Nephropathy (DN)*** Hongjie Gao, Huamin Zhang, Haiyan Li, Jinghua Li, Junwen Wang, Meng Cui and Renfang Yin	1961
233	**Analysis of Electromagnetic Radiation Effect on Layered Human Head Model** Lanlan Ping, Dongsheng Wu, Hong Lv and Jinhua Peng	1971
234	**A Study on Potential Legal Risks of Electronic Medical Records and Preventing Measures** Hu Shengli, Feng Jun and Chi Jinqing	1979
235	**Fostering the Autonomous Learning Ability of the Students Under the Multimedia Teaching Environment** Zhao-ying Chen and Xiu-qing Wang	1987
236	**Pattern Matching with Flexible Wildcard Gaps** Zhang Junyan and Yang Chenhui	1993
237	**Establishment and Practice of the New Teaching Model of Maxillofacial Gunshot Injuries** Zhen Tang, Xiaogang Xu, Zhizhong Cao and Dalin Wang	1999
238	**Research of Database Full-Text Retrieval Based on Related Words Recognition** Gao Pei-zhi and Li Xue-qing	2007
239	**Construction and Application of High Quality Medical Video Teaching Resources** Chu Wanjiang, Zhuang Engui, Wang Honghai, Xu Zhuping, Bai Canming, Wang Jian and Li Lianhong	2013
240	**Research and Construction of Mobile Development Engineer Course System** Xiufeng Shao and Xuemei Liu	2023
241	**Backward Direction Link Prediction in Multi-relation Systems** Wang Hong, Yuan Wei Hua and Zhou Qian	2031

242	The Innovation of Information Service in University Library Based on Educational Informationization .... Liu Fang	2037
243	Speculate the Teaching of Medical Microbiology Network Resource .... Wang Hongying, Zhang Tao, Zhang Chuntao, Ma Haimei, Ding Jianbing and Ma Xiumin	2043
244	Clinical Significance of the Detection of Serum Procalcitonin in Patients with Lung Infection After Liver Transplantation .... Juan Guo, Wei Cao, Xiao Yang and Hui Xie	2049
245	Exploration of Teaching Strategies in Medical Network Teaching .... Bing Li, Jian Tan, Zhi Dong, Chen Xu, Zhaohui Zhong and Xiaoli He	2055
246	The Application of Information Technology Means During Clinical Medical Education in China .... Ying Xing, Shu-lai Zhu and Chun-di Chang	2061
247	Research Hotspots Analysis of Hypertension Treatment by PubMed .... Hou Jinjie, Chen Lianqun and Li Ruiyu	2067
248	Research Hotspots Analysis of Hepatitis Receptor by PubMed .... Hou Jinjie and Li Ruiyu	2073
249	The Application of Information Technology in Modern Sports Teaching .... Xiao Hong Li and Tuan Ting Zhang	2079
250	How to Use Multimedia Technology for Improvement of the Teaching Effect of Medical Immunology .... Ding Jianbing, Wang Song, Zhou Xiao Tao, Fulati Rexiti, Dilinar Bolati, Wei Xiaoli and Xu Qian	2085
251	Application of Mind Map in Teaching and Learning of Medical Immunology .... Song Wang, Jianbing Ding, Qi Xu, Xiaoli Wei, Qi Xu and Bolati Dilinar	2091

252	**Electron Microscopy Technology and It's Application in the Morphology** Caili Sun, Xiaohong Li, Zhou Li and Tuanting Zhang	2095
253	**Empirical Study on the Relationship Between Financial Structure and Economic Growth: An Example of Zhejiang Province** Songyan Zhang	2103
254	**The Teaching Design of Digital Signal Processing Based on MATLAB and FPGA** Xiaoyan Tian, Lei Chen and Jiao Pang	2109
255	**The Design of an Management Software for High Value Medical Consumables** Zhou Longfu, Hu Yonghe, Fan Quanshui, Zhao Ming, Zhang Chaoqun and Li Zheng	2115
256	**Libraries Follow-Up Services in the Era of Fragmentation Reading** Lu Yanxiang	2123
257	**Research on Construction of Green Agriculture Products Supply Chain Based on the Model Differentiation** Bo Zhao	2129
258	**Visualization Analysis and Research of Scientific Papers and Thesis in University** Jiangning Xie, Xueqing Li, Lei Wang and Ye Tao	2135
259	**Multimedia Assisted Case-Based Teaching Application in Intercultural Communication** Huang Fang and Zhao Chen	2143
260	**The Informatization Reform and Practice of the Humanities Courses in Nursing Profession** Ying Wang	2149
261	**A Modified Minimum Risk Bayes and It's Application in Spam Filtering** Zhenfang Zhu, Peipei Wang, Zhiping Jia, Hairong Xiao, Guangyuan Zhang and Hao Liang	2155

262	Research of CRYPTO1 Algorithm Based on FPGA .... Zhang Haifeng, Yang Zhu and Zhang Pei	2161
263	Change of Plasma Adrenomedullin and Expression of Adrenomedullin and its Receptor in Villus of Normal Early Pregnancy .... Lihong Ruan, Zhenghui Fang, Jingxia Tian, Yan Dou, Wenyu Zhong, Xiue Song, Wei Shi, Aiying Lu, Lizhi Sun, Guihua Jia, Haifeng Yu, Shuyi Han and Hongqiao Wu	2169
264	A Summary of Role of Alveolar Epithelial Type II Cells in Respiratory Diseases........................... Xueliang Li, Yiqin Wang and Zhaoxia Xu	2177
265	Application of Inquiry Teaching in Econometrics Course..... Songyan Zhang	2183
266	Extract Examining Data Using Medical Field Association Knowledge Base .... Li Wang, Yuanpeng Zhang, Danmin Qian, Min Yao, Jiancheng Dong and Dengfu Yao	2189
267	The Analysis and Research on Digital Campus Construct Model.................................. Liu Xiaoming and Jiang Changyun	2195
268	Emotional Deficiency in Web-Based Learning Environment and Suggested Solutions.................... Cai Li-hua	2201
269	Mapping Knowledge Domain Analysis of Medical Informatics Education............................... Danmin Qian, Yuanpeng Zhang, Jiancheng Dong and Li Wang	2209
270	Negation Detection in Chinese Electronic Medical Record Based on Rules and Word Co-occurrence .... Yuanpeng Zhang, Kui Jiang, Jiancheng Dong, Danmin Qian, Huiqun Wu, Xinyun Geng and Li Wang	2215
271	Design and Implementation of Information Management System for Multimedia Classroom Based on B/S Structure.... Xian Zhu, Yansong Ling and Yongle Yang	2221

272	The Application of E-Learning in English Teaching of Non-English Major Postgraduate Education .... Qu Daqing	2233
273	The Construction of Semantic Network for Traditional Acupuncture Knowledge............................. Ling Zhu, Feng Yang, Shuo Yang, Jinghua Li, Lirong Jia, Tong Yu, Bo Gao and Yan Dong	2239
274	The New Training System for Laboratory Physician .... Rong Wang, Xue Li, Yunde Liu, Yan Wu, Xin Qi, Weizhen Gao and Lihong Yang	2247
275	The Investigation on Effect of Tele-Care Combined Dietary Reminds in Overweight Cases.......................... Y.-P. Chen, C.-K. Liu, C.-H. Chen, T.-F. Huang, S.-T. Tu and M.-C. Hsieh	2253
276	A Training System for Operating Medical Equipment .... Ren Kanehira, Hirohisa Narita, Kazinori Kawaguchi, Hideo Hori and Hideo Fujimoto	2259
277	The Essential of Hierarchy of E-Continuing Medical Education in China................................ Tienan Feng, Xiwen Sun, Hengjing Wu and Chenghua Jiang	2267
278	The Reverse Effects of Saikoside on Multidrug Resistance .... Huiying Bai, Jing Li, Kun Jiang, Xuexin Liu, Chun Li and Xiaodong Gai	2273
279	Research and Practice on "Three Steps of Bilingual Teaching" for Acupuncture and Moxibustion Science in Universities of TCM .... Xiang Wen Meng, Dan Dan Li, Hua Peng Liu, Sheng Ai Piao, Cheng Hui Zhu and Karna Lokesh Kumar	2281
280	Current Status of Traditional Chinese Medicine Language System .... Meng Cui, Lirong Jia, Tong Yu, Shuo Yang, Lihong liu. Ling Zhu, Jinghua Li, Bo Gao and Yan Dong	2287
281	The Selection Research of Security Elliptic Curve Cryptography in Packet Network Communication .... Yuzhong Zhang	2293

282	Improvement of Medical Imaging Course by Modeling of Positron Emission Tomography.................... Huiting Qiao, Libin Wang, Wenyong Liu, Yu Wang, Shuyu Li, Fang Pu and Deyu Li	2301
283	The Research of Management System in Sports Anatomy Based on the Network Technology.................... Hong Liu, Dao-lin Zhang, Xiao-mei Zhan, Xiao-mei Zeng and Fei Yu	2307
284	Innovation of Compiler Theory Course for CDIO.......... Wang Na and Wu YuePing	2315
285	The Design and Implementation of Web-Based E-Learning System................................. Chunjie Hou and Chuanmu Li	2321
286	Complex System Ensuring Outstanding Student Research Training in Private Universities....................... YueYu Xu	2325
287	The Influence of Short Chain Fatty Acids on Biosynthesis of Emodin by *Aspergillus ochraceus* **LP-316**............... Xia Li and Lv Ping	2331
288	Relationship Between Reactive Oxygen Species and Emodin Production in *Aspergillus ochraceus*..................... Ping Lv	2337
289	A Studies of the Early Intervention to the Diabetic Patients with Hearing Loss by Hypoglycemic Anti-deaf Party........ Kaoshan Guo, Ruiyu Li, Meng Li, Jianqiao Li, Liping Wu, Junli Yan, Jianmei Jing, Weiya Guo, Yang Liu, Weihua Han, Yanfu Sun and Qing Gu	2345
290	Effect of T Lymphocytes PD-1/B7-H1 Path Expression in Patients with Severe Hepatitis Depression from Promoting Liver Cell Growth Hormone Combinations from Gongying Yinchen Soup.................................... Zhang Junhui, Gao Junfeng, Zhao Xinguo, Li Meng, Ma Limin, Hou Jinjie, Sun Yanfu, Gu Qing and Li Ruiyu	2353

291	**The Influence of Hepatocyte Growth-Promoting Factors Combined with Gongying Yinchen Soup for Depression in Patients with Fulminant Hepatitis Peripheral Blood T Lymphocyte Subsets and Liver Function** .... Liping Wu, Junfeng Gao, Xinguo Zhao, Huilong Li, Jianqiao Li, Limin Ma, Meng Li, Weihua Han, Qing Gu and Ruiyu Li	2361
292	**The Impact of Hepatocyte Growth-Promoting Factors Combined with Gongying Yinchen Soup on Peripheral Blood SIL-2R of Depression in Fulminant Hepatitis Patients** .... Guo Kaoshan, Gao Junfeng, Li Jianqiao, Zhao Xinguo, Li Huilong, Ma Limin, Li Meng, Sun Yanfu, Gu Qing, Han Weihua and Li Ruiyu	2367
293	**Design and Development of Learning-Based Game for Acupuncture Education** .... Youliang Huang, Renquan Liu, Mingquan Zhou and Xingguang Ma	2375
294	**Clinical Research on Using Hepatocyte Growth-Promoting Factors Combined with Gongying Yinchen Soup to Cure Depression in Patients with Fulminant Hepatitis** .... Guo Kaoshan, Hou Shuying, Gao Junfeng, Zhao Xinguo, Li Jianqiao, Li Huilong, Hou Jinjie, Ma Limin, Li Meng, Sun Yanfu, Gu Qing and Li Ruiyu	2381
295	**The Development of Information System in General Hospitals: A Case Study of Peking University Third Hospital** .... Jiang Xue and Jin Changxiao	2389
296	**Several Reflections on the Design of Educational Computer Games in China** .... Nie Yun and L. V. Ping	2397
297	**A Rural Medical and Health Collaborative Working Platform** .... Jiang Yanfeng, Yin Ling, Wang Siyang, Lei Mingtao, Zheng Shuo and Wang Cong	2403
298	**Application of Internet in Pharmacological Teaching** .... Chen Jianguang, Li He, Wang Chunmei, Sun Jinghui, Sun Hongxia, Zhang Chengyi and Fan Xintian	2413

299	Assessing Information Literacy Development of Undergraduates .... Fei Li, Bao Xi and Hua Jiang	2419
300	Improved Access Control Model Under Cloud Computing Environment............................... Yongsheng Zhang, Jiashun Zou, Yan Gao and Bo Li	2425
301	Research on Regional Health Information Platform Construction Based on Cloud Computing .... Zhimei Zhang, Xinping Hu, Jiancheng Dong, Jian Yang and Tianmin Jiang	2431
302	Detection of Fasciculation Potentials in Amyotrophic Lateral Sclerosis Using Surface EMG .... Boling Chen and Ping Zhou	2437
303	Biological Performance Evaluation of the PRP/nHA/CoI Composite Material .... Ning Ma, Li Zhang, Di Ying, Pan He, Ming-guang Jin, He Liu and Chun-yu Chen	2443
304	An Integrated Service Model: Linking Digital Libraries with VLEs .... Deng Xiaozhao and Ruan Jianhai	2453
305	The Research and Application of Process Evaluation Method on Prosthodontics Web-Based Course Learning ..... Min Tian, Zhao-hua Ji, Guo-feng WU, Ming Fang and Shao-feng Zhang	2461
306	Application of Multimedia in the Teaching of Pharmacological Experiment Course................... Wang Chunmei, Li He, Sun Jinghui, Sun Hongxia, Zhang Chengyi, Fan Xintian and Chen Jianguang	2469
307	THz Imaging Technology and its Medical Usage .... Yao Yao, Guanghong Pei, Houzhao Sun, Rennan Yao, Xiaoqin Zeng, Ling Chen, Genlin Zhu, Weian Fu, Bin Cong, Aijun Li, Fang Wang, Xiangshan Meng, Qiang Wu, Lingbo Pei, Yiwu Geng, Jun Meng, Juan Zhang, Yang Gao, Qun Wang, Min Yang, Xiaoli Chong, Yongxia Duan, Bei Liu, Shujing Wang, Bo Chen and Yubin Wang	2475

308	Effects of Project-Based Learning in Improving Scientific Research and Practice Capacity of Nursing Undergraduates .... Ruiling Li, Dongmei Dou and Yuanyuan Wang	2481
309	Research on an Individualized Pathology Instructional System .... Kai Hu and Zhiqian Ye	2487
310	Security Problems and Strategies of Digital Education Resource Management in Cloud Computing Environment .... Li Bo	2495
311	Vocabulary Learning Strategies in Computer-Assisted Language Learning Environment .... Liming Sun and Ni Wang	2501
312	Bioinformatics Prediction of the Tertiary Structure for the Emy162 Antigen of *Echinococcus multilocularis* ...... Yanhua Li, Xianfei Liu, Yuejie Zhu, Xiaoan Hu, Song Wang, Xiumin Ma and Jianbing Ding	2507
313	IT in Education Application of Computer in Teaching Flavor and Fragrance Technology...................... Guangyong Zhu, Zuobing Xiao, Rujun Zhou, Yalun Zhu and Yunwei Niu	2513
314	Building an Effective Blog-Based Teaching Platform in Higher Medical Education .... Bailiu Ya, Qun Ma and Chuanping Si	2519
315	Design and Implementation of Educational Administration Information Access System Based on Android Platform...... Yifeng Yan, Shuming Xiong, Xiujun Lou, Hui Xiong and Qishi Miao	2525
316	The Application of Information Technology and CBS Teaching Method in Medical Genetics................... Yang Sun, Fang Xu, Yanjie Wang, Mingzhu Li, Ying Liang and Boyan Wu	2535
317	Research on Practice Teaching of Law in the Provincial Institutions of Higher Learning....................... Haiying Zheng	2541

318	Path Selection for Practice Teaching of Law in Institutions of Higher Learning............................ Rongxia Zhang	2547
319	Inhibition Effects of Celery Seed Extract on Human Stomach Cancer Cell Lines Hs746T.................. Lin-Lin Gao, Chang-Xiang Zhou, Xiu-Feng Song, Ke-Wei Fan and Fu-Rong Li	2553
320	Research on the Practice of Teaching Auto Selective Course While China Stepping into Automobile Society....... Zhang Tiejun and Guan Ying	2561
321	An Integrated Research Study of Information Technology (IT) Education and Experimental Design and Execution (EDE) Courses........................ Guoying Wang and Yunsheng Zhang	2567
322	Empirical Study of Job Burnout Among Higher Vocational College Teachers......................... Cheng Wang	2575
323	Appeals on College Moral Education: Based on Open Environment of Laboratories Under Campus Network....... Jun-Yan Zhang	2581
324	Intercultural Pragmatics Research on Written Emails in an Academic Environment .... Su Zhang	2589
325	Construction of a Differentiated Embryo Chondrocyte 1 Lentiviral Expression Vector and Establishment of its Stably Transfected HGC27 Cell Line .... Rui Hu, Yun-Shan Wang, Yi Kong, Pin Li, Yan Zheng, Xiao-Li Ma and Yan-Fei Jia	2599
326	Construction of Expression Vector of miRNA Specific for FUT3 and Identification of Its Efficiency in KATO-III Gastric Cancer Cell Line .... Yong-Hong Xin, Yan-Fei Jia, Qiang Liu, Hong Zhang, Hai-ning Zhu, Xiao-li Ma, Yong-Jun Cai and Yun-Shan Wang	2607

327 Molecular Cloning, Sequence Analysis of Thioesterases from Wintersweet (*Chimonanthus Praecox*) 2615
Li-Hong Zhang, Qiong Wu, Xian-Feng Zou, Li-Na Chen, Shu-Yan Yu, Chang-Cheng Gao and Xing Chen

328 Effects of Bodymass on the SDA of the Taimen 2623
Guiqiang Yang, Liying Zhang and Shaogang Xu

329 Effects of Temperature on the SDA of the Taimen 2631
Guiqiang Yang, Ding Yuan and Shaogang Xu

330 Wireless Heart Rate Monitoring System of RSS-Based Positioning in GSM 2637
Hongfang Shao, Jingling Han, Jianhua Mao and Zhigang Xuan

331 Research of Separable Polygraph Based on Bluetooth Transmission 2643
Zhan-ao Wu, Tingting Cheng, Jianhun Mao and Feifei Wang

332 The Design of Intelligent Medicine Box 2649
Jianhua Mao, Xiubin Yuan and Hongfang Shao

333 The Questionnaire Survey about the Video Feedback Teaching Method for the Training of Abdominal Examination in the Medical Students 2655
Liu Juju, Ma Huihao, Xie Yuanlong, Qin Lu and Jian Daolin

334 Correlation Analysis on the Nature of Traditional Chinese Medicine 2663
Zhang Pei-Jiang

335 The Classification of Meningioma Subtypes Based on the Color Segmentation and Shape Features 2669
Ziming Zeng, Zeng Tong, Zhonghua Han, Yinlong Zhang and Reyer Zwiggelaar

336 An Extraction Method of Cerebral Vessels Based on Multi-Threshold Otsu Classification and Hessian Matrix Enhancement Filtering 2675
Xiangang Jiang and Yunli Qiu

337 Architecture of a Knowledge-Based Education System for Logistics 2683
Dianjun Fang and Xiaodu Hu

Volume 4

338 Research and Practice of University Statistics Sharing Scheme 2693
Suping Xie, Huaichu Chen, Shixue Yin and Zou Xiangrong

339 A Formal Framework for Domain Software Analysis Based on Raise Specification Language 2699
Yuanzheng Zhao, Tie Bao, Lu Han, Shufen Liu and Qu Chen

340 Video Feedback Teaching Method in Teaching of Abdominal Physical Examination 2707
Huihao Ma, Wang Bo, Juju Liu, Daoling Jian and Yuanlong Xie

341 Evaluation of EHR in Health Care in China: Utilizing Fuzzy AHP in SWOT Analysis 2715
Ying Xiang and Jinchang Li

342 A Method of Computing the Hot Topics' Popularity on the Internet Combined with the Features of the Microblogs 2721
Yongqing Wei, Zhen Zhang, Shaodong Fei and Wentao Du

343 The Value of CBL Autonomous Learning Style for the Postgraduate of Medical Imageology: Promoting Professional Knowledge Learning Based on the PACS 2729
Peng Dong, Ding Wei-yi, Wang Bin, Wang Xi-zhen, Long Jin-feng, Zhu Hong and Sun Ye-quan

344 Web-Based Information System Construction of Medical Tourism in South Korea 2735
Yinghua Chen and Jaekwang Lee

345 Quantitative Modeling and Verification of VANET 2743
Jing Liu, Xiaoyan Wang, Shufen Liu, Han Lu and Jing Tong

346 Study on the Financial Change of the Primary Health Care Institutions After the Implementation of Essential Drug System 2749
Changchun Zhan and Yasai Ge

347	Construction of a Recombinant Plasmid for Petal-Specific Expression of HQT, a Key Enzyme in Chlorogenic Acid Biosynthesis .... Yuting Bi, Wei Tian, Wen Zeng, Yushan Kong, Yanhong Xue and Shiping Liu	2755
348	Explorations on Strengthening of Students' Programming Capabilities in Data Structure Teaching .... Song Yucheng, Jin Shaoli and Xu Fasheng	2765
349	A Study of the Effect of Long-Term Aerobic Exercise and Environmental Tobacco Smoke (ETS) on Both Growth Performance and Serum T-AOC, Ca^{2+}, BUN in Rat .... Xiao Xiao-ling, Huang Wen-ying, Wu Tao, Yu Chun-lian and Xu Chun-ling	2771
350	Research on Multimedia Teaching and Cultivation of Capacity for Computational Thinking .... Yongsheng Zhang, Yan Gao, Jiashun Zou and Aiqin Bao	2779
351	The Algorithm of DBSCAN Based on Probability Distribution .... Ma Yu, Gao Yuling and Song Shaoyun	2785
352	Exploration and Practice on Signal Curriculum Group Construction of Instrument Science .... Wang Rui, Liang Yu, Li Hui and Zhou Hao-min	2793
353	On Improving the E-Learning Adaptability of the Postgraduate Freshmen .... Ruan Jianhai and Deng Xiaozhao	2799
354	Construction of a Network-Based Open Experimental Teaching Management System .... Yan-Rong Tong and Peng-Bo Song	2807
355	Prediction of Three-Dimensional Structure of PPARγ Transcript Variant 1 Protein .... Cong Sun, Qiang Wu, Ye-chao Han, Ting-ting Tang and Li-li Wang	2813

356	Interactive Visualization of Scholar Text .... Ming Jing and Xueqing Li	2821
357	Date-driven Based Image Enhancement for Segmenting of MS Lesions in T2-w and Flair MRI .... Ziming Zeng, Zhonghua Han, Yitian Zhao and Reyer Zwiggelaar	2827
358	On Aims and Contents of Intercultural Communicative English Teaching .... Diao Lijing and Wang Huanyun	2833
359	Research on the Cultivation of Applied Innovative Mechanical Talents in Cangzhou...................... Wang Huanyun	2839
360	On Feasibility of Experiential English Teaching in Higher Vocational Institutes .... Diao Lijing	2845
361	Vi-RTM: Visualization of Wireless Sensor Networks for Remote Telemedicine Monitoring System............. Dianjie Lu, Guijuan Zhang, Yanwei Guo and Jue Hong	2851
362	The Effect of T-2 Toxin on the Apoptosis of Ameloblasts in Rat's Incisor................................... Sha-fei Zhai, Zhu Yong, Ma Zheng and Yaochao Zhang	2857
363	A Preliminary Study of the Influence of T-2 Toxin on the Expressions of Bcl-2 and Bax of Ameloblasts in Rat's Incisor................................... Sha-fei Zhai, Zhu Yong, Ma Zheng and Yaochao Zhang	2865
364	PET Image Processing in the Early Diagnosis of PD .... Kai Ma, Zhi-an Liu, Ya-ping Nie and Dian-shuai Gao	2871
365	"4 Steps" in Problem Based Teaching in the Medical Internship: Experiences from China .... Huasheng Liu, Mei Zhang, Richard Bae, Muxing Li, Xiaoping Xi, Qin Gao, Yan Li, Di Wu and Bingyin Shi	2879

366	Applications of Pitch Pattern in Chinese Tone Learning System.................................... Song Liu and Peng Liu	2887
367	Detection of Onset and Offset of QRS Complex Based a Modified Triangle Morphology........................ Xiao Hu, Jingjing Liu, Jiaqing Wang and Zhong Xiao	2893
368	Ecological Characters of Truffles........................ Hai-feng Wang, Yan-ling Zhao and Yong-jun Fan	2903
369	A Study on Mobile Phone-Based Practice Teaching System... Tiejun Zhang	2909
370	Study on Application of Online Education Based on Interactive Platform............................... Li Fengyun	2919
371	Analysis on Curative Effect of Exercise Therapy Combined with Joint Mobilization in the Treatment of Knee Osteoarthritis .... Wang Hongliang	2927
372	Predictions with Intuitionistic Fuzzy Soft Sets .... Sylvia Encheva	2935
373	Eliciting the Most Desirable Information with Residuated Lattices............................... Sylvia Encheva	2941
374	Research on Data Exchange Platform Based on IPSec and XML.................................. Li Bo	2947
375	Integration and Utilization of Digital Learning Resources in Community Education .... Liangtao Yang	2953
376	Correlation of Aberrant Methylation of APC Gene to MTHFR C677T Genetic Polymorphisms in Hepatic Carcinoma................................. Lian-Hua Cui, Meng Liu, Hong-Zong Si, Min-Ho Shin, Hee Nam Kim and Jin-Su Choi	2961

377	The Application of Humane Care in Clinical Medical Treatment .... Chunhua Su	2969
378	Chinese EFL Learners' Metacognitive Knowledge in Listening: A Survey Study .... Zeng Yajun and Zeng Yi	2975
379	Research on Mobile Learning Games in Engineering Graphics Education .... Huang Chen, Liang Chen, Jinchang Chen and Jin Xu	2981
380	Design and Implementation of a New Generation of Service-Oriented Graduate Enrollment System .... Shao Zhenglong, Li Yanxia and Zhong Wenfeng	2987
381	Research on the Quality of Life of Cancer Patients Based on Music Therapy............................ He Wei	2995
382	Design, Synthesis and Biological Evaluation of the Novel Antitumor Agent 2H-benzo[b][1, 4]oxazin-3(4H)-one and Its Derivatives .... Huanhuan Li, Kailin Han, Qiannan Guo, Fengxi Liu, Peng Yu and Yuou Teng	3003
383	On Structural Model of Knowledge Points in View of Intelligent Teaching .... Jun Li	3013
384	Evaluation Model of Medical English Teaching Effect Based on Item Response Theory .... Lanfen Ji, Dianjun Lu and Dianxiang Lu	3019
385	Discussion on Intervention of Chinese Culture in Chinese College Students' English Writing and Dealing Strategies .... Ruxiang Ye	3025
386	Investigation and Analysis of Undergraduate Students' Critical Thinking Ability in College of Stomatology Lanzhou University.................................. Li ZhiGe, Wang Xuefeng, Zhang Yulin, Weng Wulian, WuFan Bieke, Na Li and Liu Bin	3033

387	Surgeons' Experience in Reviewing Computer Tomography Influence the Diagnosis Accuracy of Blunt Abdominal Trauma .... Sun Libo, Xu Meng, Chen Lin, Su Yanzhuo, Li Chang and Shu Zhenbo	3039
388	Analysis of Face Recognition Methods in Linear Subspace.... Hongmei Li, Dongming Zhou and Rencan Nie	3045
389	Energy Dispersive X-Ray Spectroscopy of HMG-CoA Synthetase During Essential Oil Biosynthesis Pathway in *Citrus grandis* .... She-Jian Liang, Ping Zheng, Han Gao and Ke-Ke Li	3053
390	The Method Research on *Tuber* spp. DNA in Soil .... Yong-jun Fan, Fa-Hu Li, Yan-Lin Zhao and Wei Yan	3059
391	The Impact of Modern Information Technology on Medical Education.............................. Zifen Guo, Yong Feng and Honglin Huang	3065
392	In the Platform of the Practice Teaching Link, Study on Environmental Elite Education..................... Yu Caihong, Huang Ying, Xu Dongyao, He Xuwen, Wang Jianbing and Yu Yan	3071
393	The Application of a Highly Available and Scalable Operational Architecture in Course Selection System........ Yanxia Li, Zhang Yu, Peng Yu, Chun Yu and Zhenglong Shao	3077
394	Network Assisted Teaching Model on Animal Histology and Embryology.................................... Xin Ma, Yunjiao Zhao, Limin Wang, Aidong Qian and Winmin Luan	3083
395	Research on Application of Artificial Immune System in 3G Mobile Network Security....................... Dongming Zhao	3089
396	Neuromorphology: A Case Study Based on Data Mining and Statistical Techniques in an Educational Setting .... F. Maiorana	3095

397	Construction and Practice of P.E. Network Course Based on Module Theory in University Xin-Ping Zhang and Dong-Hai Wu	3103
398	Application and Practice of LAMS-Based Intercultural Communication Teaching Bin Long and Jinxi Li	3111
399	A Study on Using Authentic Video in Listening Course Yan Dou	3117
400	Comparison of Two Radio Systems for Health Remote Monitoring Systems in Rural Areas Manuel García Sánchez, Rubén Nocelo López and José Antonio Gay-Fernández	3125
401	3D Ear Shape Feature Optimal Matching Using Bipartite Graph Xiaopeng Sun, Wang Xingyue, Guan Wang, Feng Han and Lu Wang	3133
402	Research on Anti-Metastasis Effect of Emodin on Pancreatic Cancer Haishuai Yu	3139
403	Research on Chronic Alcoholic Patients with Nerve Electrophysiology He Wei	3145
404	Genetic Dissection of *Pax6* Through GeneNetwork Hong Lu and Lu Lu	3151
405	Impact of Scan Duration on PET/CT Maximum Standardized Uptake Value Measurement Qiuping Fan, Minggang Su and Luyi Zhou	3157
406	16-Slice Spiral Computer Tomography and Digital Radiography: Diagnosis of Ankle and Foot Fractures Hanqing Zhang, Liangzhou Xu, Peng Wang, Huang Bo, Jian Liu, Xiaojun Dong, Nianzu Ye, Wang Fei and Peng Gu	3163

407	Structural SIMilarity and Spatial Frequency Motivated Atlas Database Reduction for Multi-atlas Segmentation Yaqian Zhao and Aimin Hao	3169
408	Some Reflections on Undergraduate Computer Graphics Teaching Shanshan Gao and Caiming Zhang	3175
409	The Application of the Morris Water Maze System to the Effect of Ginsenoside Re on the Learning and Memory Disorders and Alzheimer's Disease Tie Hong, Shunan Liu, Liangjiao Di, Ning Zhang and Xiangfeng Wang	3181
410	The Application of HYGEYA in Hospital's Antimicrobial Drugs Management Xiangfeng Wang, Xiujuan Fu, Dasheng Zhu, Yadan Chen, Tie Hong, Shunan Liu, Liangjiao Di and Ning Zhang	3191
411	The Analysis of Wavelet De-Noising on ECG Dongxin Lu, Qi Teng and Da Chen	3197
412	Research of Education Training Model by Stages for College Students' Information Literacy Jinyuan Zhou and Tianling Zhou	3205
413	Effect of Bufei Granules on the Levels of Serum Inflammatory Markers in Rats with Chronic Obstructive Pulmonary Disease Stable Phase Sijia Guo, Zengtao Sun, Enshun Liu, Jihong Feng, Wei Liu, Peng Guan and Jingshen Su	3213
414	Design of Remote Medical Monitoring System Dongxin Lu and Yuanbo Qin	3221
415	Development of University Information Service Chun Yu, Fang Yuan and JunYang Feng	3227
416	Adaptive Tracking Servo Control for Optical Data Storage Systems Zhizheng Wu, Yang Li, Fei Peng and Mei Liu	3235

Contents

417	Optimal Focus Servo Control for Optical Data Storage Systems .... Zhizheng Wu, Qingxi Jia, Lu Wang and Mei Liu	3241
418	Curriculum Design of Algorithms and Data Structures Based on Creative Thinking .... Chen Weiwei, Li Zhigang, Chen Weidong, Li Qing, Tang Yanqin, Wu Yongfen and Shi Lei	3247
419	Questionnaire Design and Analysis of Online Teaching and Learning: A Case Study of the Questionnaire of "Education Online" Platform of Beijing University of Technology............................ Shidong Xu, Shuyi Zhou, Qian Cao, Jin Lei, Xiaoyong Li and Yuhu He	3253
420	The Application of Telemedicine Technology.............. Ming-gang Wang, Ying-jun Mao and Wei Li	3261
421	A Method of Data Flow Diagram Drawing Based on Word Segmentation Technique..................... Shuli Yuwen and Kaifei Wang	3269
422	Chemical Reaction Optimization for Nurse Rostering Problem .... Ziran Zheng and Xiaoju Gong	3275
423	Survey of Network Security Situation Awareness and Key Technologies............................. Zhang Xuan	3281
424	Mining ESP Teaching Research Data Using Statistical Analysis Method: Using One-Sample t Test as an Example ... Yicheng Wang and Mingli Chen	3287
425	Research on the Impact of Experiential Teaching Mode on the Cultivation of Marketing Talents .... Jia Cai and Hui Guan	3293
426	Lung Segmentation for CT Images Based on Mean Shift and Region Growing................................ Huang Zhanpeng, Yi Faling and Zhao Jie	3301

427	The Application of Psychological Teaching Combined with Daily Life: The Role of the Internet. Chuanhua Gu	3307
428	Developing a Pilot Online Learning and Mentorship Website for Nurses. Sue Coffey and Charles Anyinam	3313
429	Estrogenic and Antiestrogenic Activities of Protocatechic Acid. Fang Hu, Junzhi Wang, Huajun Luo, Ling Zhang, Youcheng Luo, Wenjun Sun, Fan Cheng, Weiqiao Deng, Zhangshuang Deng and Kun Zou	3319
430	A Study on Learning Style Preferences of Chinese Medical Students. Yuemin Ding, Jianxiang Liu and Xiong Zhang	3329
431	Design and Implementation of the Virtual Experiment System. Liyan Chen, Qingqi Hong, Beizhan Wang and Qingqiang Wu	3335
432	Application of Simulation Software in Mobile Communication Course. Fangni Chen and Zhongpeng Wang	3341
433	Study on the Effect of Astragalus Polysaccharide on Function of Erythrocyte in Tumor Model Mice. Chen-Feng Ji, Yu-bin Ji and Zheng Xiang	3347
434	Anti-Diabetes Components in Leaves of Yacon. Zheng Xiang, Chen-Feng Ji, De-Qiang Dou and Kuo Gai	3353
435	Nitric Oxide Donor Regulated mRNA Expressions of LTC4 Synthesis Enzymes in Hepatic Ischemia Reperfusion Injury Rats. FF Hong, CS He, GL Tu, FX Guo, XB Chen and SL Yang	3359
436	An Optimal In Vitro Model for Evaluating Anaphylactoid Mediator Release Induced by Herbal Medicine Injection. Zheng Xiang, Chen-Feng Ji, De-Qiang Dou and Hang Xiao	3367

437	Change Towards Creative Society: A Developed Knowledge Model for IT in Learning M. Yu, C. Zhou and W. Xing	3373
438	TCM Standard Composition and Component Library: Sample Management System Erwei Liu, Yan Huo, Zhongxin Liu, Lifeng Han, Tao Wang and Xiumei Gao	3379
439	The Teaching Method of Interrogation in Traditional Chinese Diagnostics Jingjing Fu, Haixia Yan and He Jiancheng Ding Jie	3389
440	Designing on system of Quality Monitoring on Instruction Actualizing Zhang Yan	3395
441	Comparisons of Diagnosis for Occult Fractures with Nuclear Magnetic Resonance Imaging and Computerized Tomography Ying Li, Huo-Yan Wu, Zhi-Qiang Jiang and Zhang-Song Ou	3401
442	Identifying Questions Written in Thai from Social Media Group Communication Chadchadaporn Pukkaew and Kanchana Kanchanasut	3409
443	A Programming Related Courses' E-learning Platform Based on Online Judge Xiaonan Fang, Huaxiang Zhang and Yunchen Sun	3419
444	Leading and Guiding Role of Supervisors in Graduate Education Administration Huaqiang Zhang, Xinsheng Wang and Hannan Fang	3425
445	Development of Dental Materials Network Course Based on Student-Centered Learning Shibao Li, Xinyi Zhao, Lihui Tang and Xu Gong	3429
446	Research and Practice of Practical Teaching Model Based on the Learning Interest Tao Gao, Bo Long, Pingan Du and Yefei Li	3435

447	Developing and Applying Video Clip and Computer Simulation to Improve Student Performance in Medical Imaging Technologist Education. . . . . Lisha Jiang, Houfu Deng and Luyi Zhou	3441
448	Research on the Quality of Life of Patients with Depression Based on Psychotherapy . . . . Zhou Xiaoqiu	3447
449	On Systematic Tracking of Common Problems Experienced by Students . . . . Sylvia Encheva	3453
450	Research on Nerve Electrophysiology of Chronic Pharyngitis Based on Automobile Exhaust Pollution . . . . Chunxin Dong	3457
451	The Status and Challenge of Information Technology in Medical Education . . . . Jun Li, Ming Zhao and Guang Zhao	3463
452	The Comparison of Fetal ECG Extraction Methods. . . . . Zhongliang Luo, Jingguo Dai and Zhuohua Duan	3469
453	Study on Evaluation Index System of Hotel Practice Base Based on Bias Analysis and Reliability and Validity Test . . . . . Changfeng Yin	3475
454	Improvement on Emergency Medical Service System Based on Class Analysis on Global Four Cases . . . . Zhe Li and Feng Hai	3483
455	Educational Data Mining for Problem Identification . . . . Sylvia Encheva	3491
456	Statistics Experiment Base on Excel in Statistics Education: Taking Zhejiang Shuren University as Example. . . . . Wenjie Li, Yitao Wang and Guowei Wan	3495
457	Simulating the Space Deep Brain Stimulations Using a Biophysical Model . . . . Yingyuan Chen, Fei Su, Jiang Wang, Xile Wei and Bin Deng	3501

458	Strategy and Analysis of Emotional Education into the Cooperative Learning in Microcomputers Teaching Dongxing Wang	3507
459	Construction and Practice of Network Platform for Training of GPs Gang Liu, Guochun Xiang, Heqing Huang, Junsheng Ji, Hong Chen, Haitao Guo, Biyuan Li, You Li, Guangqiong Liu, Zegui Li and Kehou Wang	3513
460	Research on the Construction of Regional Medical Information Service Platform Qun Wang, Chuang Ma, Yong Yu and Gen Zhu	3519
461	Study on the Application of Simulation Technology in the Medical Teaching Yong Yu, Xiaolin Chen, Qun Wang and Gen Zhu	3525
462	Desynchronization of Morris: Lecar Network via Robust Adaptive Artificial Neural Network Yingyuan Chen, Jiang Wang, Xile Wei, Bin Deng, Haitao Yu, Fei Su and Ge Li	3531
463	Building and Sharing of Information Resources in Radio and TV Universities Libraries Under Network Environment Liu Juan and Wang Jing-na	3537
464	Research on Network Information Resources Integration Services in Medicine Library Zhang Li-min	3543
465	Applied Research of Ultrasound Microbubble in Tumor-Transferred Lymph Node Imaging and Treatment Xin Zhao and Guijie Li	3549
466	The Examination of Landau-Lifshitz Pseudo-Tensor Under Physical Decomposition of Gravitational Field Peng-Cheng Zhang, Jia Guo, Jun Zhao and Ben-Chao Zhu	3555

467 Exploring of the Integration Design Method of Rectal Prolapse TCM Clinical Pathway System 3561
Zhihui Huang

Author Index 3567

Chapter 90
Feature Extraction and Support Vector Machine Based Classification for False Positive Reduction in Mammographic Images

Q. D. Truong, M. P. Nguyen, V. T. Hoang, H. T. Nguyen,
D. T. Nguyen, T. D. Nguyen and V. D. Nguyen

Abstract In this paper, we propose a new method for massive false positive reduction in. Our goal is to distinguish between the true recognized masses and the ones which actually normal parenchyma. Our proposal is based on Block Difference Inverse Probability (BDIP) and Support Vector Machine (SVM) for classifying the detected masses. The proposed approach is evaluated in about 2700 ROIs detected from Mini-MIAS database. An accuracy of $A_z = 0.91$ (area under the curve) is obtained.

Keywords Mammography · Computer aided detection · Mass detection · Feature extraction · Support vector machine

90.1 Introduction

One of the most common types of cancer among women all over the world is breast cancer. According to a survey conducted by the American Cancer Society, one out of 8–12 American women will suffer from breast cancer during her lifetime. It is exceeded only by lung cancer [1]. In European Community, breast cancer represents 19 % of cancer deaths and 24 % of all cancer cases [2]. The World Health Organization's International Agency for Research on Cancer

---

The authors would like to thank Vietnam National Foundation for Science and Technology Development (NAFOSTED) for their financial support to publish this work.

Q. D. Truong (✉) · M. P. Nguyen · V. T. Hoang · H. T. Nguyen · D. T. Nguyen · T. D. Nguyen · V. D. Nguyen
School of Electronics and Telecommunications, Hanoi University of Science and Technology, Hanoi, Vietnam
e-mail: dong.kstn@gmail.com

(IARC) estimated more than one million cases of breast cancer occur annually and reported that more than 400, 000 women die each year from this fatal disease [3].

A crucial issue for a high survival rate in breast cancer treatment is the detection of the cancer at early stage. However, it is not an easy task. Commonly used imaging modality for breast cancer is mammogram, which has significantly enhanced the radiologists' ability to detect and diagnose cancer at an early stage and take immediate precautions for its earliest prevention [4].

The introduction of digital mammography gave the opportunity of increasing the number of Computer-Aided Detection (CAD) systems for detecting and diagnosing the breast cancer at an early stage [5–7]. However, CAD system in its present form does not have significant impact on the detection of breast cancer [8]. The main reason for the mistrust of radiologists on the role of CAD system in breast cancer detection is due to a large number of false positives (FP) usually arises when high sensitivity is desired [9]. A FP is a Region of Interest (RoI)—a sub-image containing the suspicious region—being normal tissue but interpreted by the CAD as an abnormal one. Therefore, almost all works trying to detect masses in mammography need a final step in order to reduce the number of false positives [10] (as shown on Fig. 90.1).

In this paper, we propose an FPR procedure based on statistical and textural features of detected ROIs. Our aim is to reduce the number of False Positive per Image (FPpI) while preserving the sensitivity value the highest possible. Here, we propose the use of FOS (First Order Statistical), GLCM-based (Gray Level Co-occurrence Matrix) and BDIP (Block Difference Inverse Probability) features to characterize the ROIs. Once the characterization is done, Support Vector Machine (SVM) is utilized to classify the ROIs into real mass or normal parenchyma. To our knowledge, this is the first attempt to use BDIP in the field of mammographic mass detection.

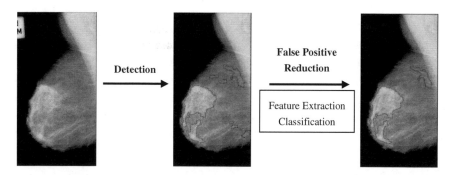

Fig. 90.1 CAD block scheme

90.2 Materials and Methods

In this section, we present the detail of the proposed method for massive false positive reduction. First, we give brief introduction to mass identification. Next, feature extraction method is given. Finally, we overview the classification technique used in our method.

90.2.1 Mass Detection

In this first step, CAD system extracts, from the original mammogram, suspicious regions on which the radiologists have to focus their attention. The steps of this procedure are fully described in our previous paper [11]. Here below, we only recall the basic ideas.

- Unwanted parts removal
- Morphological top-hat and bottom-hat enhancement
- Contour-based ROI detection
- Marking detected ROIs as true positive ROIs (TP-ROIs) or false positive ROIs (FP-ROIs).

90.2.2 Feature Extraction

Six FOS features, twelve GLCM-based features and BDIP feature are extracted. Hence, there are total nineteen features are used to characterize the ROIs

90.2.2.1 FOS Features

Six used FOS features [12] include average value of gray level (μ_f), standard deviation (σ_f), coefficient of variance (cv), entropy (ent), skewness (sk), kurtosis (kur). They are calculated as follow

$$\mu_f = \sum_{l=0}^{L-1} l.p(l) \qquad \sigma_f = \sqrt{m_2} = \sqrt{\sum_{l=0}^{L-1} (l - \mu_f)^2 . p(l)}$$

$$cv = \frac{\sigma_f}{\mu_f} \qquad ent = -\sum_{l=0}^{L-1} p(l).\log[p(l)]$$

$$sk = \frac{m_3}{(m_2)^{3/2}} \qquad kur = \frac{m_4}{(m_2)^2}$$

where $p(l)$ is the probability of each gray level l appeared in the ROI and m_k is m-order momentum of the ROI

$$p(l) = \frac{N(l)}{\sum N(l)} \qquad m_k = \sum_{l=0}^{L-1}(l-\mu_f)^k \cdot p(l)$$

and $N(l)$ is frequency of gray level l in the ROI.

90.2.2.2 GLCM-Based Features

The GLCM $p_{d,\theta}(l_1,l_2)$ represents the probability of occurrence of a pair of gray levels (l_1,l_2) separated by a given distance d at angle θ. We consider specific distance d = 1 at quantized angles $\theta = k\pi/4$ with k = 0,1,2,3. So there are 4 GLCMs for each ROI.

For each GLCM, 4 features that are invariant under monotonic gray tone transformation are calculated [13]. They are

- Energy: $f_1 = \sum_{ij} p_{ij}^2$
- Entropy: $f_2 = -\sum_{ij} p_{ij} \cdot \ln(p_{ij})$
- Information measures of correlation

$$f_3 = \frac{f_2 - H_1}{\max\{H_x, H_y\}} \qquad f_4 = [1 - \exp\{-2(H_2 - f_2)\}]^{1/2}$$

where

$$P_x(i)$$

$$H_1$$

From three types of properties, average value, range and variance are computed for each $\theta = k\pi/4$, therefore there are total 12 textural features.

90.2.2.3 BDIP Feature

In the spatial domain, BDIP [14] for a block B of an image I is defined as

$$BDIP = M^2 - \frac{\sum_{i,j \in B} I(i,j)}{\max_{i,j \in B} I(i,j)}$$

where M^2 is area of the block.

90.2.3 Classification

The number of features in each region are quite large bring about the number of dimension of vector space which we should consider to classify the data are sketching out. In addition, there is always the overlapping of the data class corresponding to the features in the sample region. Applying Support Vector Machine, a state-of-the-art classification method introduced in 1992 [15] to solve this problem takes many advantages in this case. In machine learning, support vector machines (SVMs, also support vector networks) are supervised learning models with associated learning algorithms that analyze data and recognize patterns, used for classification and regression analysis. The basic SVM takes a set of input data and predicts, for each given input, which of two possible classes forms the output, making it a non-probabilistic binary linear classifier.

The idea behind SVMs is to map the original data points from the input space to a high dimensional feature space, or even infinite-dimensional feature space to simplify the classification problem. The mapping can be done by choosing a suitable kernel function. To map the input data into a higher dimension space where they are supposed to have a better distribution, kernel functions are implemented.

Then, an optimal separating hyper-plane in the high dimensional feature space is chosen. Consider a training dataset $\{x_i, y_i\}$, with $x_i \in R^d$ being the input vectors and $y_i \in \{+1, -1\}$ the class labels. SVMs map the d-dimensional input vector x from the input space to the d1-dimensional feature space using a function

$$\phi(.) : R^d \to R^f$$

The separating hyper-plane in the feature space is then defined as $W^T\phi(x) + b = 0$ with b $\in$ R and W is an unknown vector with the same dimension as $\phi(x)$. A data point x is assigned to the first class if $f(x) = sign(W^T\phi(x) + b))$ equals +1 or to the second class if $f(x)$ equals -1.

However, there were some overlapping values between the data in both classes, thus a perfect linear separation was impossible to conduct. Therefore, a restricted number of misclassification should be tolerated around the margin. The resulting optimization problem for SVMs, where the violation of the constraints is penalized, was written as:

$$\min \frac{1}{2} W^T W + C \sum_{i=1}^{N} \varepsilon_i \text{ subject to } y_i(W^T\phi(x_i) + b) \geq 1 - \varepsilon_i \text{ and } \varepsilon_i \geq 0$$

where C is a positive regularization constant. The trade-off between a large margin and misclassification error were defined by the regulation constant in the cost function. For non-separable data, an upper bound of the misclassification error was controlled using slack variable ε by the soft-margin SVM. The value of ε_i indicated the distance of x_i with respect to the decision boundary.

Equivalently, with Lagrange multipliers $\alpha_i \geq 0$ for the first set of constraints can be used to write the optimization problem for SVMs in the dual space. By solving a quadratic programming problem, the solution for the Lagrange multiplier can be obtained. Finally, the SVM classifier takes the form:

$$f(x) = sign\left(\sum_{i=1}^{\#SV} \alpha_i y_i K(x, x_i) + b\right)$$

where #SV represents the number of support vectors and the kernel function K(.,.).

Furthermore, called the kernel function $K(x, x_i) = \phi(x)^T \phi(x_i)$ is positively definite. In the optimization problem, only K(.,.) which is related to $\phi(.)$ is used. This enables SVMs to work in a high dimensional (or infinite-dimensional) feature space, without actually performing calculations in this space. To base oneself on the characteristic of features, we propose to use the Radial Basic Function as kernel function to map the original space which comprises considered features to new space within reduction of dimensions.

$$f(x) = \sum_{i=1}^{m} \alpha_i \cdot \exp\left(-\gamma \|x_i - x\|^2\right) + C$$

where x is input data and C, γ, α are constants

Two major parameters of the RBF applied in SVM, C and γ, have to be set appropriately. Parameter C is the cost of the penalty. The choice of value for parameter C influences the classification outcome. If C is too large, then the classification accuracy rate is very high in the training stage, but very low in the testing stage. If C is too small, then the classification accuracy rate is unsatisfactory, making the model useless. Parameter γ has a much stronger impact than parameter C on classification outcomes, because its value influences the partitioning outcome in the feature space. An excessive value for parameter γ leads to over-fitting, while a disproportionately small value results in under-fitting.

90.3 Results and Discussions

Our proposed method is evaluated on mammogram database Mini-MIAS. This database includes 322 digital mammograms from 161 patients. Every image in database always has extra-information or ground truth from the radiologists about characteristic of background tissue, type of abnormality present, severity of abnormality, the coordinates of center and approximate radius (in pixels) of a circle enclosing the abnormality. Mini-MIAS database [16] is a kind of reduced type of database MIAS, the original MIAS database has been reduced to 200 micron pixel edge and clipped/padded so that every image has a size of 1024 × 1024 pixels. The total number of detected ROIs is about 2700 and we archive detection sensitivity is 93.47 % and the FPpI is 9.03 [11].

The selection of features and pre-determining the workspace in input layers to train with SVM lead to obtain the different results respectively to the proportional of inputs on the training set and test set. We implement to create the SVM model with RBF kernel function to train and test the data on the dataset.

To evaluate the performance of a CAD system, a Receiver Operating Characteristics (ROC) is used. A ROC curve is a plotting of sensitivity as a function of specificity at different values of the decision threshold on the neural network output. Higher ROC, approaching the perfection at the upper left hand corner, would indicate greater discrimination capacity.

Table 90.1 shows that the classifying level depends on the proportion of input data, training method, and chosen kernel function. Its parameter is an important step to classify the features of lesion. The best area under the ROC curve (AUC) is 0.9102 with BDIP feature and is shown in Fig. 90.2. For this case, the number of Support Vectors (SVs) is about 18.36 % of the total of training samples.

This obtained $A_z = 0.9102$ is quite sanguine and it is a turning-point to reduce false positive in breast cancer CAD system. In comparison with other author work [17, 18] result $A_z = 0.9$, our result is quite better. It is also much greater than value 0.87 in our previous result [11]. This indicates that the method we proposed has the potential to be further investigated.

Table 90.1 Area under the ROC curve (AUC) among different extracted features

Proportion	Feature	AUC
40:60	FO	0.6935
	BDIP	0.9102
	GLCM	0.7839
30:70	FO	0.7932
	BDIP	0.8156
	GLCM	0.7278

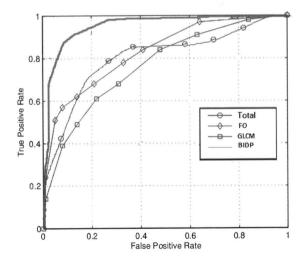

Fig. 90.2 ROCs correspond to different features with ratio 40:60 train and test set

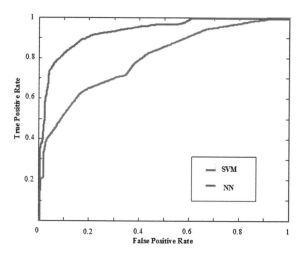

Fig. 90.3 Classification using BDIP feature corresponding to SVM and NN

The explicit evidence argues that all of above reasons are important leading to get the good accuracy for classification step. We also use all of features in the dataset with SVM and Neural Network (NN). The ROC curve which is shown in Fig. 90.3 expresses that the great advantage of Support Vector Machine to Neural Network as the same feature and same method to implement kernel function. In other words, within the implicit separation (overlapping) and the large number of input data, SVM provides the higher accuracy and more plausible than NN.

90.4 Conclusions

This research presents the new approaching to reduce false positive in breast cancer CAD system using SVM and BDIP feature.

The selection of texture features to train, the ratio of input data, the kernel function and its parameter (C, γ) are three main factors effected on our result. Experimental results show that BDIP is used for detection with AUC is 0.9102, and the number of SVs is approximately 18.36 % of the total number of training examples.

In the future, different textural feature sets and different feature selection methods will be used also in order to improve the performance of ROI classification and false positive reduction. Classification performance of several classifiers will also be compared to find out the optimum correct classification rate.

References

1. Bray F, McCarron P, Parkin DM (2004) The changing global patterns of female breast cancer incidence and mortality. Breast Cancer Res 6:229–239
2. Eurostat (2002) Health statistics atlas on mortality in the European Union. Official J Eur Union
3. http://globocan.iarc.fr/factsheet.asp
4. Buseman S, Mouchawar J, Calonge N, Byers T (2003) Mammography screening matters for young women with breast carcinoma. Cancer 97(2):352–358
5. Birdwell RL, Ikeda DM, O'Shaughnessy KD, Sickles EA (2001) Mammographic characteristics of 115 missed cancers later detected with screening mammography and the potential utility of computer-aided detection. Radiology 219:192–202
6. Brem RF, Rapelyea JA, Zisman G, Hoffmeister JW, DeSimio MP (2005) Evaluation of breast cancer with a computer-aided detection system by mammographic appearance and histopathology. Cancer 104(5):931–935
7. Cheng HD, Cai XP, Chen XW, Hu LM, Lou XL (2003) Computer-aided detection and classification of microcalcifications in mammograms: a survey. Pattern Recogn 36(12):2967–2991
8. Nishikawa RM, Kallergi M (2006) Computer-aided detection, in its present form, is not an effective aid for screening mammography. Med Phys 33:811–814
9. Taylor P, Champness J, Given-Wilson R, Johnston K, Potts H (2005) Impact of computer-aided detection prompts on the sensitivity and specificity of screening mammography. Health Techn Assess 9(6):1–58
10. Oliver A (2006) A new approach to the classification of mammographic masses and normal breast tissue. Proc Int Conf Pattern Recognit 4:707–710
11. Nguyen VD, Nguyen DT, Nguyen HL, Bui DH, Nguyen TD (2012) Automatic identification of massive lesions in digitalized mammograms. In: Proceeding of the fourth international conference on communications and electronics
12. Bevk M, Kononenko I (2002) A statistical approach to texture description of medical images: a preliminary study. In: Proceedings of the 15th IEEE symposium on computer-based medical systems, 239–244
13. Haralick RM, Shanmugam K, Dinstein I (1973) Textural features for image classification. In: IEEE Transaction on Systems, Man and Cybernetics, vol 3. pp 610–621
14. Nguyen TD, Thanh QT, Duc TM, Quynh TN, Hoang TM (2011) SVM classifier based face detection system using BDIP and BVLC moments. In: Conference on advanced technologies for communication (ATC2011), pp 264–267
15. Boser BE, Guyon IM, Vapnik VN (1992) A training algorithm for optimal margin classifiers. In: Proceedings of the 5th annual ACM workshop on computational learning theory, pp 144–152
16. http://peipa.essex.ac.uk/info/mias.html
17. Tourassi GD, Eltonsy NH, Graham JH et al (2005) Feature and knowledge based analysis for reduction of false positives in the computerized detection of masses in screening mammography. In: IEEE Conference Engineering in Medicine and Biology and Society, pp 6524–6527
18. Llad X, Oliver A, Freixenet J, Mart R, Mart J (2009) A textural approach for mass false positive reduction in mammography. Comput Med Imaging Graph 33(6):415–422

Chapter 91
Research on Distributed Synchronous CAD Collaborative Design System

Chen Li

Abstract The paper explores the key problems in CAD collaborative design of distributed synchronization. According to the characteristics of AutoCAD, the transmission of real-time operation command is replaced by modified underlying database, which improves the transmission speed of concurrent collaboration and reduces errors of real-time transmission. The paper presents the structure of the whole collaborative design system and expounds some key techniques of it, including the interface, data transmission, conflict elimination, fault disposal, etc.

Keywords Distribute collaborative design · Object database · AutoCAD · Conflict elimination · Fault disposal

91.1 Introduction

Distributed collaborative design, as the name indicates, means the product is designed collaboratively by experts distributed in different places [1]. It can be divided into asynchronous interaction and synchronous interaction. The former means designers in different places cooperate at different times, while the latter means designers in different places work simultaneously. Collaboration of designers, who specialize in different fields and work for the same project, is indispensable for CAD design. Currently, most collaborated ways of designers are limited to some simple ways such as online chatting, document transmission, and consultative meeting, which are time-consuming and indirect. Therefore, conflicts among designers may arise and deadline may be postponed. However, synchronous interaction is helpful in resolving conflicts and improving efficiency.

C. Li (✉)
School of Information Science and Engineering, Shandong Normal University, Jinan, China
e-mail: chli@163.com

On the research of synchronized collaborative design system, document [2] presents a distributed collaborative working environment based on J2EE platform, while document [3] proposes a distributed Concurrent and collaborative design platform architecture based on SOA, but neither take into account the conflict, fault and other possible issues of collaborative design; document [4] puts forward a cooperative design model of AutoCAD based on operational semantics, but the establishment of a state transition table of operation is complicated. In this paper, according to the characteristic of AutoCAD, this paper perfects collaborative design by replacing the transmission of operation command with the simple modification of underlying database, using objects component of AutoCAD through VBA, which will implement the graphic information real-time transmission of AutoCAD database and improve the transmission speed of Concurrent collaboration.

91.2 Relative Theory

91.2.1 AtiveX

Automation ActiveX is a technical approach proposed by Microsoft, which attempts to provide a common development platform, a viable "method" for all the interactions between applications. This method is based on the "object", including a number of the object read-write properties, methods of operation and the possible accidents in interactions. Many programming languages can use ActiveX technology methods, such as C, VC, VB and so on. Starting from AutoCAD 2000, Autodesk companies use hierarchy to organize the object data structure, the root of which is AutoCAD application object itself, and this level contains an object—the ActiveX object [5].

91.2.2 Vba

VBA(Visual Basic for Application), as a secondary development tool of AutoCAD, combines AutoCAD and Visual Basic functions, which can quickly create programs that meet user requirements and greatly improve user productivity. VBA develops and adopts ActiveX technology, enabling users to programmatically manipulate AutoCAD from AutoCAD internal or external, and share data with other Windows programs more easily [6].

91.2.3 Object Database

The object database of AutoCAD is based on *. dwg file format archiving. *. dwg file is actually an object database, which can derive data from any two-dimensional entity. Using VBA programming, we can go directly into the underlying database to access and change the object data in a database, so as to realize a direct query and modification of graphic element. Raw data can be inputted into general databases, but CAD is modified through a series of commands and user interface, thus securing correspondent records of database in the course of drawing. It is very easy to retrieve, because as the underlying CAD software, in addition to common database data structure, it is not only rich in geometry data structure, but also rich in non-graphical data structure, even user-defined data structure, which provides great convenience for User Programming [5].

DXF (Drawing eXchange Format) is used to represent the global information tag data contained in specific version of AutoCAD drawing file. Tag data means that in front of each data element, there is an integer called Group codes. The value of Group code indicates the data type of subsequent elements, illuminating the implication of the data elements for a given object (or record) type. In fact, all of the information in the graphics file can be represented by the DXF file format. The following Table 91.1 shows the group code content of an arc, and Table 91.2 is the DXF group code content of a specific arc:

Extended object database: DWG database allows users to extend the object data; that is, in addition to the original attributes of the object defined by CAD, we can add user-defined information to the database. In VBA, each object in object database as is viewed as an ActiveX object, and most of the database content can be expressed with the properties of the object. The contents of the object database can be directly read in AutoLisp.

91.3 Realization of System

91.3.1 Construction Design

In order to better implementation of distributed synchronous collaborative design, the structure of system adopts client–server model. The interface program on each client machine has a copy, while the shared information and information management component are only on the server. The data transferred between client and server includes the operation command of the shared information and the results of return. The user's operation needs to be sent between the clients, and results of operations are self-generated by the client application. The overall structure is shown as Fig. 91.1:

As is shown, the server is divided into two parts, the collaborative management module and the CAD management module. The collaborative management module is responsible for collaborative information (such as personnel information, etc.), connection with client, response to requests, and real-time management of the synchronized collaboration(such as the release of information, conflict resolution, fault recovery, etc.).The CAD management module is responsible for

Table 91.1 DXF group code significance of the arc

Arc Group codes

Group codes	Description
100	Subclass marker (AcDbCircle)
39	Thickness (optional; default = 0)
10	Center point (in OCS) DXFTM:X value; APP:3D point
20,30	DXF:Y and Z values of center point (in OCS)
40	Radius
100	Subclass marker (AcDbArc)
50	Start angle
51	End angle
210	Extrusion direction (optional; default = 0,0,1) DXF:X value; APP:3D vector
220,230	DXF:Y and Z values of extrusion direction (optional)

Table 91.2 DXF group code content of a specific arc in CAD

Object database list

Contents of database	Contents of symbol table
Begin...	Begin...
(−1. <the name of graphic element:4006ae60>)	(0. Layer)
(0. ARC)	(2. 0)
(330. <the name of graphic element:4006acf8>)	(70. 0)
(5. 7C)	(62.7)
(100. AcDbEntity)	(6. Continous)
(67. 0)	End...
(410. Model)	
(8. 0)	
(100. AcDbCircle)	
(10 3.73213 27.0247 0.0)	
(40. 8.67465)	
(210. 0.0 0.0 1.0)	
(100. AcDbArc)	
(50. 4.26366)	
(51. 0.557501)	
End...	

sending and receiving messages, updating collaborative database information and saving log in time.

The client has its own CAD system. The collaborative management module is responsible for the communication with the server, conflict resolution, fault recovery, etc. CAD management module is used to observe the change of designer's operation and send a message to the server, which is in turn forwarded to other collaborative users. On the other hand it receives the messages from the server about other user's operation, updates the interface of user, and additionally, it updates the local database and saves the log, etc.

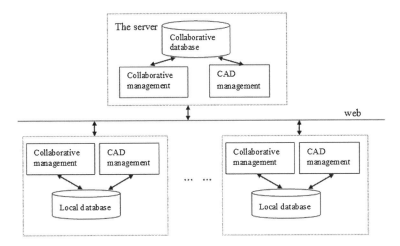

Fig. 91.1 The overall structure

91.3.2 The Implementation of Specific Technology

91.3.2.1 The Synchronous Display of Collaborative Interface

At the beginning, the server verifies the authority of users who apply for collaboration and then records the information of every user. Then the server receives the contents of the shared database and sends them to other designers after making a backup. In the collaborative design, the server updates the data in time to make sure that if there are new designers to participate or connection failures of an client machine and other errors occurs, collaborative contents are accessible. For each designer, the collaboration means inserting the other designers' contents in the local machine by making a copy. In AutoCAD the establishment of each pixel is identified by a unique handle. As a result, the handles of the same graphic element in the two machines are different. Therefore, it is necessary to record the handle of corresponding source graphic element of the copy. In other words, graphic elements can be distinguished by adding handles to the use-defined data structure in the object database.

In order to achieve the data consistency of the various terminals, the copy in other designers' machines must clearly record the graphic element handle in the source graphic so that the graphic element can be accurately located when modified in different machines and the source graphic can be located and modified according to the recorded handle. So on the basis of original database user-defined data, properties must be added by extending object database, such as the designer's name, the graphic's name and the handle, etc.

Some of the source program of adding extension object database

Private Sub SetobjectXdata(object As AcadEntity, appname As string, peoplename As string,drawname As string,handle As string)

```
Dim xdtype(0 to 3) as integer
Dim xddata(0 to 3) as variant
xdtype(0) = 1001
xddata(0) = Appname
xdtype(1) = 1000
xddata(1) = "1 = " & peoplename//the designer's name
xdtype(2) = 1000
xddata(2) = "2 = " & drawname//the graphic's name
xdtype(3) = 1000
xddata(3) = "3 = " & handle//the handle of the graphic element
object.SetXData XDataType, XData
……
End Sub
```

91.3.2.2 Data Transmission

For a large graphic file or multiple designers, it will slow down the sharing speed if the graphics have been re-passed for each updating [7]. In AutoCAD, the command can be transferred directly. But for the convenience of users, the command in AutoCAD can be carried out in various ways, such as menu selection, button selection or command line input, even some operations directly through the mouse operation(such as graphic element selection, the choice of point, movement, etc.). So to get a complete command is very difficult. From the perspective of the database, no matter what command it is, to the change of the database, it can be divided into three categories: records addition, records modification and records deletion(For instance, copying a graphic element only means adding a record to the database). Therefore, the designers' operations of the graphic element are divided into three categories: creation, modification and deletion.

If a new graphic element is created, its related properties (that is, the related records in the database) are transmitted to the server, which transmits the message to other designers according to the user information. The client makes a copy on the basis of the received data and records the source handle of the graphic element.

If a graphic element is modified, a reactor will be attached to each graphic element, which can transmit to the server the record of the modified graphic element in the database. Then the server transmitted the data to other designers, who will modify the corresponding record according to the received data and update the user interface so as to achieve a real-time synchronization.

Deletion of a graphic element is similar to modification, first, the attached reactor transmits the handle of the deleted graphic element to the server, which sends the data to other designers, who afterwards delete the corresponding record according to the received data and update the user interface.

So in each update, only a few data are transmitted, which will improve the speed of real-time display and avoid problems such as data inconsistencies caused by data loss in the large amounts of data transmission. In addition, to ensure accurate data reception, a message may be sent back after the data is received to prove that the data has been successfully transmitted. A time limit can be set so that if the message is not received within it the server will re-transmit the data.

During the collaboration, if one designer modifies a graphic element, the data should be transmitted to the server and then be rapidly sent to other designers. VBA uses event to replace the reactor. It adds function to the event of the whole graphic file rather than each graphic element. The VBA functions as follows:

Private Sub AcadDocument_ObjectAdded(ByVal Object As Object)
//when adding a graphic element return the object
Private Sub AcadDocument_ObjectModified(ByVal Object As Object)
//when modifying a graphic element return the object
Private Sub AcadDocument_ObjectErased(ByVal ObjectID As Long)
//when deleting a graphic element return its ID number

Based on the return value the graphic element which has been modified can be easily found and processed according to the object database.

Sending and receiving the data can be realized by calling an ActiveX control in VB, which is the Winsock control used in network communication. Windows Sockets specification provides a simple API function to the program developers, whose program can call the Windows Sockets API function to realize the communication. The Windows Sockets can use underlying network communication protocol and Operating System call to implement the work of communication. Windows Sockets also applies to multi-threaded Windows process.

91.3.2.3 Conflict Resolution

In the course of collaborative design, many designers are operating at the same time, which is likely to cause conflicts [8], for instance, data inconsistency, when two designers on different parts operate the same graphic element's copy at the same time. So the concurrency control is essential. The token is used to resolve the conflict [9].

The algorithm is as follows:

1. The designer selects the graphic element which he wants to modify, then sends the application to the server.
2. The server takes the token of this graphic element to the designer and takes a lock operation to the other copy of the graphic element.
3. If the server does not take the token back, it means that another designer is modifying the graphic element; the applicants can only wait for the return of the token. The token may be sent to the designer who first applies.

91.4 Fault Disposal

The collaboration may not be properly implemented because of the system fault including software and hardware failures or designer's operation mistake. So the data may be destroyed. Therefore recovery mechanism of system is essential, which can reduce the damage of fault to a minimum.

The fault of collaboration is divided into two categories [9]: one is the machine of a designer suddenly crashes or powers off, the other is the communication fault of the whole collaboration. Fault recovery is based on running log. Running log is a file to record the operation information of system periodically. When the fault occurs, the recovery mechanism of system recovers the system on the basis of running log. The operate information of system is recorded as running record, which contains operation object's identifier, the new value of the object and the old value of the object, etc. After the graphic element is created, modified or deleted, the update of the object database requires that the corresponding operation record be written in the log file for the fault recovery.

When single machine fault occurs, it can be recovered with local running log. If the local log is destroyed, it can be recovered with the running log in the server.

The communication fault is divided into two categories: one is transmission error, while the other is network-disconnection. The transmission error means that the data is not transmitted successfully due to the network speed or network congestion. If the server doesn't receive the message in a time limit that the client has received the data, the server will resend the data. If the client does not answer after the data have been sent to a maximum frequency, it is believed that the network is faulty or the machine is malfunctioned. The network-disconnection means that a number of the communicating machines are completely disconnected. The server counts the number of the clients who have responded, if the number is not more than half of that of all collaborative machines, the server will judge that the network disconnection occurs. The server notifies the communicating clients to stop collaboration, and saves the present information and data of the collaboration. The client stops the collaboration when it disconnects with the server, saves the data of the collaboration, which is useful to the recovery of the collaboration.

91.5 Conclusion

The paper is primarily about the research on distributed synchronous CAD collaborative design system. First it describes the overall structure. Then it expounds the realization of the system from three aspects: how to collaborate, which sets a format for the data to transmit depending on the particularities of AutoCAD, how to resolve the conflict with the token, and how to recover with the log when fault occurs. At last the key code is provided.

References

1. Gao ShM, He FZH (2004) Survey of Distributed and Collaborative Design. J Comput Aided Des Comput Graph 2:149–157
2. Li AJ, Yin JW, Chen G (2006) Study and development web-based distributed collaborative working environment. Appl Res Comput 23:22–23
3. Yu JQ, Cha JZh, Lu YP et al (2009) Research on the distributed concurrent and collaborative design architecture based on soa. J Beijing Jiaotong Univ 33:69–72
4. Wang Ch, Zhang ShSh, Chen Ch (2006) Operational Semantics Based Cooperative Design of AutoCAD. Comput Appl Softw 23:8–9
5. Chen BX, Feng W (2002) VisualLISP programming—techniques and examples. Post and Telecom Press, Beijing
6. Zhang F, Zheng LK, Wang HJ (2004) Wonderful example of the development of vba tutorial. TsingHua University Press, Beijing
7. Wang YP, Guo XX, Pan X, Lei Y (2003) Data management computer-aided cooperative design. J Comput Aided Des Comput Graph 15:1415–1421
8. Mao Y, Chen TX (2011) Study of real-time collaborative design platform based on AutoCAD. Machinery 38:39–42
9. Xue AR, Bao PD (2000) Design of database-based collaborative cad system. J JiangSu Univ Sci Technol 21:71–73

Chapter 92
Enterprise Evolution with Molecular Computation

Xiuting Li, Laisheng Xiang and Xiyu Liu

Abstract Enterprise life cycle theory is the most direct business growth study of enterprise development. This theory divides SMEs' (small and medium-size enterprises) life into different stages, and do research respectively in each stage on the growth of them. It holds that companies are like biological organisms, they also have the growth from birth to death, from gloom to doom. It makes an analog of SMEs' stages development combined with the core concept of membrane computing and the knowledge of biology. It is on a living point of view to analyze the growth of an enterprise, but also a continuation of the theoretical research on bionic-evolution theory. The discussion on how to extend the life of the enterprise and how to make it grow as longevity enterprise is of profound practical effect to the cultivation of domestic life-oriented enterprises.

Keywords Enterprise life cycle · Bionic-evolution theory · Membrane computing

92.1 Introduction

The question is weather the enterprise has life characteristics or not. Weather there exists some sort of periodic law of enterprises' life. If the answer is yes, then in the process of the evolution of enterprise life, what will be the stages like? And what factors and forces determine the whole growth from the creation to bigger and then

---

X. Li · L. Xiang (✉) · X. Liu
Management Science and Engineering, Shandong Normal University, Shandong, China
e-mail: sunnysddy@gmail.com

X. Li
e-mail: sunnysddy@126.com

X. Liu
e-mail: sdxyliu@163.com

die? And how to extend their life time and make them keep growing? Such questions or topics have been discussed for a long time and complex theories are all around, and this is enterprise life cycle theory.

The enterprise evolutionary theory compares the change trajectories during enterprise growth to the biological evolution which "objects of natural selection, survival of the fittest". And enterprises also reflect some characteristics of evolution in the process of interaction with market environment. For example, the performance of enterprise growth is the growth of the size and scope, which is similar to biological cells' growth and division. Some advantageous features adapt the market environment and then been strengthened, which is similar to the superior individuals can get rapid growth in biology. Furthermore, Nelson and Winter [1] likened the biosphere genes to enterprise practice.

Membrane computing is a new branch of natural computing which imitates the organizational characteristics. Combining membrane computing with life cycle theory, we suppose to simulate the enterprise development stages through the basic rules. We call it enterprise cytology, and this is a further study of bionics and bionic-evolution theory.

92.2 Enterprise Bionics and Enterprise Life Cycle

Enterprise bionics study of biological evolution is to study the organizational structure of enterprise from a biology perspective. The modern biology theory reveals that the natural life system has three basic characteristics: metabolism, self-replication and mutation. Enterprise bionics commentators also believe that the enterprise also has these life characteristics. Specifically, enterprises also need constant metabolism, and get continuous resources from outside. While their internal operational mechanism need to combines the personnel, capital, material, technology, information and other resources together. Then after various cycle processes, these all can be absorbed as companies' internal elements. In this process, consumption of inputs meanwhile produces outputs. Once this metabolic process stops, the enterprise life will stop. Secondly, companies are self-replicating mechanism. The production and reproduction of the enterprise itself is a self-replication process. The technical level and the quality of personnel can be improved, and the size also can get extended during the process. The extended enterprise both has the characteristics of the original enterprise, also new renewable and copy power. Thirdly, the enterprise may come across mutation. Changes in economic policy, in raw materials supply channels, in the thinking of employees, in the competitive situation, technology development, the success of technological innovation, changes of the users' needs, and so on, may cause a qualitative change in operating conditions of enterprises.

Just like describing a person, we also can say there's childhood, youth, middle age, old age in a firm cycle. Enterprise life cycle theory is a kind of reference to describe its development. In its surviving time, and according some standards, enterprise life can be divided into several stages. Through studying the characteristics of each stage, you can find the development law in the process of firm existence. The purpose is trying to find a specific form to adapt its development stages and promote them keep living continually, so that companies can find a relatively better pattern to keep their development ability. Through giving full play to the characteristics and advantages in each life cycle stage to extend the life cycle of enterprises and thereby help them to realize their sustainable development.

Different scholars give various expressions. Now the enterprise life cycle theory has become a relatively mature theoretical system. There are four branches: cycle stage theory, bionic-evolution theory, periodic cycle theory and attribution theory. Bionic-evolution theory is the first branch and the representative of this theory is Winter (1984). This theory holds that enterprise seems like any natural biological livings, there exists metabolism, mutation, self-replicating and others. The second branch is cycle stage theory and the representatives of the theory are Greiner and Adizes (1989). It pays attention on the characteristics of all development stages. The third is periodic cycle theory, and Ken Baskin is the main contributor. This theory starts from the specific factors which decide the enterprise life cycle, tries to figure out the "magic bullet" to extend the corporate life cycle. It is very practical. The fourth branch is attribution theory, and the scholar Peter M. Senge can be on behalf of it. This theory chooses its competitors as reference, and combines the advantages of them, explores methods that keep enterprises achieve sustained growth.

Enterprise evolution theory holds that the growth of enterprise is through the three core mechanism of biological evolution, that is diversity, genetic, and natural selection. It stresses that the organization, innovation, path-dependent are of importance to the evolution of business. Nelson considered that the three core mechanism carried the enterprise develop forward. The market environment offered some limitation, which closely related to the enterprise survival and growth rate. Bionic-evolution theory explores the enterprise life cycle in a biological point of view. It opens a new field of vision. However we need to point out that the enterprise as a labor organization has essential difference with nature life. In our study we combined molecular computation to extend the connotation of this theory in order that to give some new ideas to enterprise development.

92.3 Molecular Computation of Membrane Computing

Molecular computing is a generic term for any computational scheme which uses individual atoms or molecules as a means of solving computational problems. Molecular computing is most frequently associated with DNA computing, because that has made the most progress, but it can also refer to quantum computing or membrane computing. Membrane computing is an area that seeks to discover new computational models from the study of the cellular membranes. It not so much the task of creating a cellular model but to derive a computational mechanism from processes that are know to proceed in a cell. The various types of membrane systems have been formalized as P systems.

Petre and Petre [2] studied a class of P systems, the multi-sets of symbol objects can be packaged and transported from one area to another area. This kind of membrane only makes protective effect on the transport objects, so that the objects do not be affected by the rules when pass through the other regions. This method is very similar to the material transport with vesicles. First, vesicles wrap the mature protein, and then Golgi vesicles continue to use the transport mechanism, and forwarding them to different target membranes.

In a P systems, V is the list of alphabets, μ is the membrane structure labeled $\{1, 2, \cdots, m\}$. We mark the skin membrane with 0, and the other membranes with $\{1, 2, \cdots, m\}$. For each membrane i, we introduce a special symbol $@_j$, which is used to mark the destination membrane. The process of P systems gemmation:

$$[_0 \cdots [_i \cdots, w_1 @_j w_2, \cdots]_i \cdots]_0 \Rightarrow [_0 \cdots [_i \cdots]_i (_{i,j} w_1 w_2)_{i,j} \cdots]_0 \quad (92.1)$$

where $i \in \{1, \cdots, m\}$, $j \in \{0, 1, \cdots, m\}$, $j \neq i, h, f, m \in V^*$, $n_{1,2,3} = n'_{1,2,3} + n''_{1,2,3}$.

When $@_j$ is removed from object strings $w_1 @_j w_2$, a transport membrane will generate outside membrane i. The new generation membrane is used with two subscript parentheses, the first subscript is on behalf of the starting membrane, and the second is the mark of the target membrane, which is determined by $@_j$. In a membrane, different objects with $@_j$ will be packaged in different transport membranes, otherwise, packaged together if j is the same. Through gemmation, each vesicle transports its objects to the destination membrane, and then melts with specified membranes. This operation is denoted by the following form:

$$[_0 \cdots (_{i,j} w)_{i,j} [_j \cdots]_j \cdots]_0 \Rightarrow [_0 \cdots [_j \cdots, w, \cdots]_j \cdots]_0 \quad (92.2)$$

where $i \in \{1, \cdots, m\}$, $j \in \{0, 1, \cdots, m\}$, $j \neq i, w \in V^*$.

At the end of reaction, the objects of transporter membrane will become part of the target membrane. If the target is the skin, that is $i = 0$, the vesicles will melt with skin membrane and the objects go out into the environment. This system can be used to analog extracellular secretion of biological processes. The operation is described as follows:

$$[_0 \cdots (_{i,0} w)_{i,0} \cdots]_0 \Rightarrow [_0 \cdots]_0 w \quad (92.3)$$

Many big macromolecules can not get into a cell even with carrier protein because of its large size, but they can form vesicles across the cell membranes into the interior. This kind of transport includes exocytose and endocytosis. Exocytose is about to discharge macromolecules from a cell (such as secretions discharged from the Golgi) and endocytosis is about to transport macromolecules into an organelle. In endocytosis, the transport of molecules is involved and constituted by a series of operations and a number of carrier molecules. First, a wide variety of

Fig. 92.1 Process of exocytosis and endocytosis

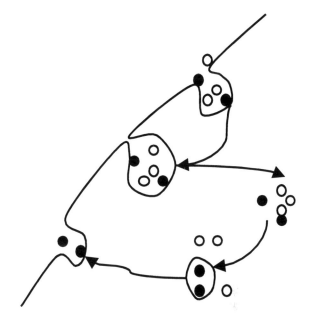

molecules transport into the cell in the promotion of certain chemical substances, such as with the matrix, receptors and clathrin. Then, the released matrix and clathrin participate in the new substances transportation process. Meanwhile, part of the substance in the vesicles is released into the cytoplasm, but the most to be transported into the interior. After the transportation, vesicles will blend with the cell membranes and release the redundancy molecular excreted outside (Fig. 92.1).

92.4 Life Cycle of Enterprise with P Systems

Membrane Computing looks at the whole cell structure and functioning as a computing device. Multi-sets of objects placed inside the regions delimited by the membranes. Sets of evolution rules associated with the regions, which allow the system to produce new objects starting from existing ones, and to move objects from one region to another. The processes of gemmation and transportation of objects between membranes may be used to illustrate some economic systems development of enterprises.

Within an enterprise, the transport of human resource, capital and material is formulized as:

$$[_0 \cdots [_i \cdots, h^{n_1} f^{n_2} m^{n_3} @_j, \cdots]_i \cdots]_0 \Rightarrow [_0 \cdots [_i \cdots, h^{n'_1} f^{n'_2} m^{n'_3}, \cdots]_i \left(_{i,j} h^{n''_1} f^{n''_2} m^{n''_3}\right)_{i,j} \cdots]_0$$

where, $i \in \{1, \cdots, m\}, j \in \{0, 1, \cdots, m\}, j \neq i, h, f, m \in V^*$. $n_{1,2,3}, n'_{1,2,3}, n''_{1,2,3}$ are the number of resources, usually $n_{1,2,3} = n'_{1,2,3} + n''_{1,2,3}$. The resources are transported from one mechanism to another in order to realize the optimal allocation of resources. Some extra or invalid resources need to eliminate to the environment, and can be achieved with vesicles. For example, sometimes machines need to update, and layoffs with internal mechanism adjustment. At this time, some of the resources $h^{n_1} f^{n_2} m^{n_3}$ need to be transported outside the membrane.

$$\left[0 \cdots \left({}_{i,o} h^{n_1} f^{n_2} m^{n_3} \right)_{i,o} \cdots \right]_0 \Rightarrow \left[0 \cdots h^{n'_1} f^{n'_2} m^{n'_3} \cdots \right]_0 h^{n''_1} f^{n''_2} m^{n''_3} \quad (92.4)$$

Through the division of enterprise life cycle is different, the researchers' expositions on enterprise development and survival agree with each other. They hold that enterprises roughly own the same pattern, and the corporate life cycle curve has a similar shape. The enterprise is divided into four stages, namely: the start-up period, growth, maturity, a period of recession. Figure 92.2 describes the whole life stages.

The concept of environment is more complex, it mainly refers to: customers and market requirements; social culture and value orientation; place, time and background of strategy implementation; guidance of government policy and regulations, etc. In the permission of proper environment, any prepared objects in the effect of e $\rightarrow E_0$ create an enterprise. Since from born to grow bigger, all kinds of resources (employees, capital, equipments...) gradually gather into the enterprise with the rule $u_i \rightarrow v_j$. Through $u_i \rightarrow_j v$, products and services export to the market. Meanwhile some uncertain factors come inside and outside, and because of this the enterprise get into a stable period. In the cycle of enterprise's developing and being stronger, the rule $u \rightarrow v_j$ may let the vision or the core values change, which may change the enterprise's developing direction. Chin operation of business is a kind of firm expansion, and it also expresses the accurate copy of enterprise genes. This progress can be displayed with $u_i \rightarrow [u_1]_j [u_2]_k$, and at the same time accompanies the duplication of DNA, so that guarantee the inheritance of core values. Rule $u_i \rightarrow_i u_j$ represents the division of enterprise cells in order to generate a child cell. That is to say with this rule we can create sub companies to expand our market occupancy. To improve the feasibility of enterprise strategy, the enterprise needs to tamp the quality of entrepreneurs, to cultivate them with international view and global angles. And then, it can make a good team with strong cohesive force. Only then, the enterprise will get a sustainable development. If in the development process, there's continuous output with no supply in the rule $u_i \rightarrow_j v$, the company is going to die. And the changes of policies or wrong choices of strategies, the vision will be difficult to realize, so, in the effect of rule $E_0 \rightarrow e$, the result is business failures or bankrupt. Therefore, to survive the enterprise, the entrepreneurs need to integrate various resources, to create proper environment and to construct competitive teams.

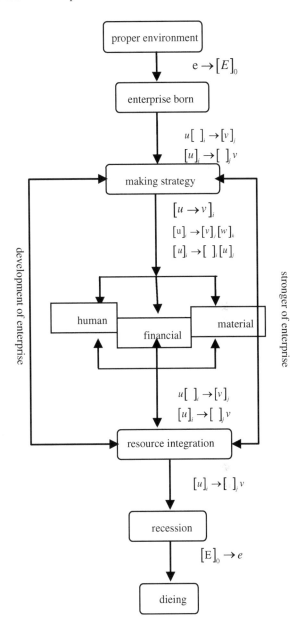

Fig. 92.2 Life cycle of enterprise with basic rules

92.5 Enterprise DNA for Longevity

From the perspective of computer genes, evolution is actually the process under the conditions of resource scarcity, and decided by the internal hierarchical relationship with the enterprise entity. It is also the process that the old enterprises

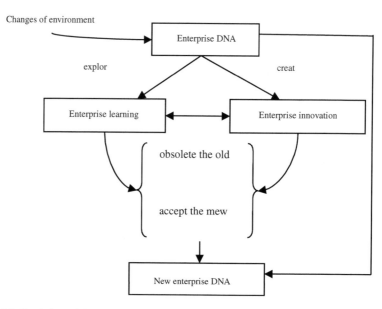

Fig. 92.3 Evolution of the enterprise DNA

genes change to the new one. There's enterprise DNA in an enterprise vision, and it guarantees the accurate replication and transmission of core values. In biology, the strongest fittest. Enterprise DNA via compare and select to produce the more suitable one, so that enterprise can get eternal youth vitality, and realize sustainable development.

The reason why enterprise genes change is because of changes in the corporate environment. When the environment changes, the enterprise need to find new suitable genes. This search process can be obtained by searching for the original genes or create new ones. The process of search and create is through enterprise learning and enterprise innovation. After comparison and selection, the new DNA can be accepted. Though accepting, there needs to continually be tested by the market. Once the enterprise get profit, the new DNA is what we need, and then we achieve the evolution of the enterprise. Evolution of the enterprise can be abstracted in Fig. 92.3.

92.6 Conclusion

It should also be noted that the life cycle is likely to be mutually overlap, probably because of tangled problems, the current stage may backward a lot; or stride over to next stage because of healthy development. The same problems may appear in not only one stage, just the importance is different.

Enterprise life cycle theory makes an investigation from the perspective of enterprise survival and development with life. The theory regards enterprises as living organisms, and dynamically evaluates the characteristics and strategies of the enterprise in different growth stages, and reveals the rules of enterprise growth. So it is advantageous for the enterprise managers to adopt a proper implementation, or changing the structure of the life cycle, delaying the arrival of the aging stage. Firms with longevity and health are not simply to escape the cycle of enterprise life, but comply with the rules and take suit strategies in order to avoid endangers or traps. To alter according to changes, while breakthrough the growth limitation and inject new nutrition into the enterprise continuously, then the enterprise life will be on cycle from recession to freshmen. It is the realization of enterprise's longevity and sustainable growth.

Acknowledgments This paper was finally supported by National Natural Science Foundation of China (61170038), Shandong Province Natural Science Foundation (ZR2011FM001), Humanities and Social Sciences Project of Ministry of Education (12YJA630152), Shandong Province Social Science Foundation (11CGLJ22), Project of Shandong Province Higher Educational Science and Technology Program (J12LN22).

References

1. Nelson RR, Winter SG (1982) An evolutionary theory of economic change. The Belknap Press of Harvard University Press, Cambridge, MA
2. Petre I, Petre L (1999) Mobile ambients and P systems. J Univers Comput Sci 5(9):588–598
3. Păun G, Rozenberg G, Salomaa A (2009) Handbook of membrane computing. Oxford University Press, Oxford
4. Păun G (2002) Membrane computing. An introduction. Springer, Berlin
5. Alhazov A, Freund R, Oswald M (2005) Tissue P systems with antiport rules and small numbers of symbols and cells. Lect Notes Comput Sci 3572:100–111
6. The P Systems Web Page. http://ppage.psystems.eu/
7. Mihalydeak T, Csajbok Z (2012) Membranes with local environments. In: 13th international conference on membrane computing, CMC13, Budapest, August 28–31, pp 311–322
8. Bin Y (2010) The theory of evolution for company reproduction. Zhejiang People's Publishing House, Hangzhou

Chapter 93
Research and Implementation of Auxiliary System for Waken-up Craniotomy

Liu Yu, Feng Wu, Hongmin Bai and Weimin Wang

Abstract Waken-up craniotomy is often used when space occupying lesion in brain functional region is cut off by manual intervention. The executive process is so complicated that it is difficult to acquire a desirable and reliable effect. This paper proposes a method that combines medical science, wireless sensor network, computing technology and virtual display mode together to aid this surgical procedure. After our work, a semi-automatic auxiliary system for waken-up craniotomy is built up. The myodynamia variation state of a patient in waken-up craniotomy can be tested by it and a doctor can be alerted inreal time by a virtual display mode reliably.

Keywords Waken-up craniotomy · Auxiliary system · Myodynamia testing

---

Project supported by the National Science Foundation of China (No.81201014).

L. Yu (✉)
Huangpu Branch of the First Affiliated Hospital, Sun Yat-sen University, Guangzhou, China
e-mail: jiil8912@yahoo.com.cn

F. Wu
School of Software Engineering, South China University of Technology, Guangzhou, China
e-mail: 1141952871@qq.com

H. Bai · W. Wang
Neurosurgery of Guangzhou Military Region General Hospital, Guangzhou, China
e-mail: 18664614266@163.com

W. Wang
e-mail: gzwangwmo@163.com

93.1 Introduction

Locating the maximum cutting off a space of lesions when space occupying lesion in brain functional region is cut off has been bothering neurosurgeon for many years until appearing waken-up craniotomy [1, 2].

A patient is waken up in operation by man-made from pre-operation CT MRI locating, language expression or limb exercise behaviour assessment for him in waken-up craniotomy. Now several approaches are often used in waken-up operation and tell a patient movement so that maximum space of lesions can be cut off and normal brain tissue in the area can be reserve as possible.

The shortages of waken-up craniotomy now are subjective to watch patient's behaviour and liable to a clinic or an anesthetist. This paper proposes a scheme of an auxiliary system for waken-up craniotomy, which combines medical science, wireless sensor network [3, 4] and computing technology together and provides corresponding functions more reliable than man-made.

In Sect. 93.1 introduces the background and meaning of this paper. In Sect. 93.2 presents method and scheme for waken-up craniotomy. Implementation, experiment and result are shown in Sect. 93.3. And conclusion is made in Sect. 93.4.

93.2 Method and Scheme

93.2.1 Method

Myodynamia sensor, sensor node and monitoring terminal are used and combined together as shown in Fig. 93.1. Tell a patient by a way he could understand what he should do with his right hand fingers wearing one or two myodynamia sensors, e.g. nip rubber ball repeatedly. Collect the signal and submitted it to a sensor node for data fusion in the system. The signal is submitted further to the medical monitoring intelligent terminal via Wi-Fi interface and the data are compared, analyzed and displayed with a predetermined color pattern.

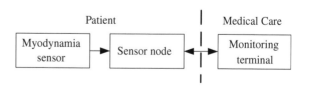

Fig. 93.1 Auxiliary system of waken-up craniotomy (ASWC)

Table 93.1 Algorithm of f_{ip}

Input: a threshold f_t and instantaneous values array arr consist of f_i
Output: peak value f_{ip}

Find the first value arr_{i_s} which is bigger or equal than f_t, if it is not exist i_s is -1;
if $i\_s > 0$ then
    Find the first value arr_{i_e} which is smaller than f_t and
$i\_e > i\_s$, if it is not exist i_e is -1;
    if $i\_e > 0$ then
    $f_{ip} = max\{arr_i(i\_s \leq i < i\_e)\}$
    end if
end if
note: i_s and i_e are the index of array arr

93.2.2 Scheme

Take 100 male and 100 female patients from a cerebropathy center first and test their myodynamia of right hand fingertip by wearing one or two myodynamia sensors to fingers and nipping rubber ball repeatedly. Then computing statistically in group. Two distributing curves for male and female got respectively as basic reference standards (BRS), e.g. Gaussian distribution $N(\mu, \sigma^2)$.

After assessing a patient's physical activities before operating, test myodynamia of a patient in operation and compare the preoperative and intraoperative distal myodynamia of the patient, shown as the formula (93.1).

$$\Delta = f_{ip}/f_{0p} \qquad (93.1)$$

Where Δ is the ratio of myodynamia peak values f_{ip} and f_{0p}, which are the distal myodynamia peak values measured at one pulsation, the former is intraoperative and the latter is preoperative. Sample n times during one pulsation at a interval, e.g. 100 ms, $i = 1, 2, 3 \ldots n$, and a threshold f_t is set, the detail will be seen as Table 93.1.

93.3 Implementation

The scheme implementation of this paper includes equipment selection, function implementation and experiments. The details are described as below.

93.3.1 Equipment Selecting

GT-305 type pinch force sensor from Japan JKY/GT-300 is selected as the distal myodynamia sensor used in surgery. The output of a sensor will be submitted to

Fig. 93.2 Implementation of ASWC

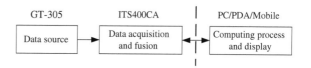

the sensor node ITS400CA with some data channels from Crossbow Technology Company. The monitoring terminal is an ordinary PC, PDA or mobile intelligent terminal. Implementation of ASWC shown as Fig. 93.2.

93.3.1.1 Data Acquisition and Fusion

GT-305 is put on strong fingers (e.g. thumb or/and middle finger) of right hand, following the prompts from a doctor or a voice system, a patient nips the rubber ball according to a rhythm (e.g. one time per second). GT-305 output pulsating signal and ITS400CA collects the data pulsation signals and fuse them. In order to acquiring a peak value during a pulsation, sample n times and compare it with a threshold f_t and submit it to a monitoring terminal.

The instantaneous value f_i of pulsation signal is summarized from pt_i (thumb finger) and pm_i (middle finger) respectively, $i = 1, 2, 3, \ldots, n$, and f_i is acquired as (93.2).

$$f_i = k_t pt_i + k_m pm_i \tag{93.2}$$

Where, k_t represents a weight coefficient of pt_i, k_m is a weight coefficient of pm_i.

93.3.1.2 Computing and Display

Calculating and comparing are down based on (93.2) and (93.1). Threshold range "normal", "slight" and "serious" are define from f_{0p}. Myodynamia of a patient is from a value near zero to a maximum value and then return to a value near zero and f_{ip} is the maximum value in one pulsation. The Algorithm of f_{ip} is shown as Table 93.1.

Supposing array arr is consist of f_i in a waken-up craniotomy and recorded, a threshold f_t that is smaller than most peak values (e.g. 8 *kgf*). First, find index i_s when $arr_{i\_s} \geq f_t$ and the first index i_e when $arr_{i\_e} < f_t$ and $i\_e > i\_s$. Then select the maximum value between arr_{i_s} and arr_{i_e} as peak value f_{ip} and find next peak value by the *arr* start from i_e, else we cannot get a peak value.

93.3.1.3 Boundary Conditions

During an operation, if the monitoring terminal extracts no data beyond a specified T_{max}, the possible reasons are that a patient does not follow a hinting scheduled, or the patient's function region has been seriously influenced by the surgery. Therefore, a calculation cycle T_n of a monitoring terminal usually is $T_n \leq T_{max}$.

The instantaneous value f_i get from the sensor node may beyond a specified F_{max} that a patient cannot make, the most possible reason is a mistake by the sensor. For this, we just ignore it and select the last value as this value.

93.3.2 Experiment and Result

Software tools and interface are described first in experiment. Then pre-operation estimating, real-time monitoring, computing and result display be discussed respectively.

93.3.2.1 Platform and Interface

The implementation of auxiliary system scheme is on MFC, reading data from a file periodically to simulate a real system to receive data and process data on a monitoring terminal. A graphical interface displaying of data is shown as Fig. 93.3. The upper left of Fig. 93.3 shows the myodynamia data received from the sensor node at real time (horizontal ordinate represents time and vertical coordinate indicates myodynamia testing value), and the bottom left Fig. 93.3 shows a ratio of myodynamia testing values between pre and intra operating (horizontal ordinate represents time and vertical coordinate represents a ratio of myodynamia testing values). The right of Fig. 93.3 describes some result values of myodynamia, e.g. the range of normal myodynamia (a constant range), preoperative myodynamia (a constant forecasting) of a special patient, intraoperative myodynamia (a measured value) of the same patient and the icon of current status is turned on when it is, e.g. normal, alert or danger from left to right.

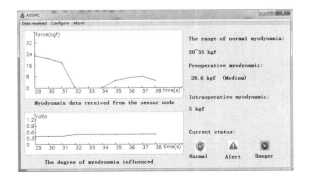

Fig. 93.3 Interface of ASWC

Table 93.2 A decision tree algorithm to P_{t1}

Input: data set S with class label "normal" and "slight"
Output: threshold P_{t1}

Order the values of S, get the values array $\{v_1, v_2, \ldots, v_{|s|}\}$, where vi is the value of S;
Set $gainRatio_{Max} = 0, P_{t1} = 0$;
for i from 1 to $|S|$-1
  $splitPoint = (vi + vi + 1)/2$;
  Use $splitPoint$ to split S into two subsets;
  Calculate the information gain ratio gr;
  if $gainRatioMax < gr$ **then**
    $P_{t1} = splitPoint$;
end if
end for

93.3.2.2 Pre-operation Estimating

Focusing on a patient, calculate according to formula (93.2) and Table 93.1, monitoring terminal gets f_{0p} and save it.

93.3.2.3 Computing and Showing

Myodynamia of 200 normal persons (half male and half female) is measured above and get the range $(\mu - 3\sigma, \mu + 3\sigma)$ of normal myodynamia of Gaussian distribution when the probability 99.7 % is cut off, with which can judge if myodynamia of a patient is normal range or not.

Get a ratio Δ when f_{ip} and f_{0p} get from (93.1). The three range "normal", "slight", "serious" are divide by thresholds P_{t1} and P_{t2} computing by a decision tree algorithm as Table 93.2. Color icon is on when ratio Δ is compared with thresholds, $\Delta \geq P_{t1}$ is normal and a green icon on. $P_{t2} \leq \Delta < P_{t1}$ is warning and an orange icon on. $\Delta < P_{t2}$ is seriously and a red icon on, shown as right corner of Fig. 93.3.

Suppose a dataset S and the size of S is $|S|$.

93.4 Conclusion

The idea is generated from seeing with the eyes of a medic in real-world operation and should be with good reference meaning on waken-up craniotomy. But the scheme here has no clinical test either and more than one aspects need to improve further, such as myodynamia measuring method, the implementation and analysis of the algorithm etc.

References

1. Hu L, Wei G, Li G (2005) Difficulties and countermeasure of operative nursing cooperation of tumour excision in cerebral function zone under intraoperative undergoing waken-up anesthesia. Chin J Nurs 40(10):793–794
2. Wang P, Chen X (2011) Research progress in cerebral function zone under intraoperative undergoing waken-up. J Ningxia Med Univ 33(2):195–198
3. Li L (2011) Analysis of data fusion in wireless sensor networks. In: International conference on Electronics, communications and control (ICECC). 9–11 September 2011, pp 2547–2549
4. Khaleghia B, Khamisa A, Karraya FO, Razavi SN (2013) Multisensor data fusion: a review of the state-of-the-art. Inf Fusion 14(1):28–44

Chapter 94
Investigation Performance on Electrocardiogram Signal Processing based on an Advanced Algorithm Combining Wavelet Packet Transform (WPT) and Hilbert-Huang Transform (HHT)*

Jin Bo, Xuewen Cao, Yuqing Wan, Yuanyu Yu, Pun Sio Hang, Peng Un Mak and Mang I Vai

Abstract The Electrocardiogram (ECG) is essential for the clinical diagnosis of cardiovascular disease. An advanced algorithm combining wavelet packet transformation (WPT) and Hilbert Huang transform (HHT) is presented for processing ECG (Electrocardiography) signal in this paper. First the WPT can resolve the ECG signal into a group of signals with narrow band. Then, the Empirical Mode Decomposition (EMD) process of Hilbert-Huang Transform (HHT) is applied on the narrow band signals. The unrelated IMFs of ECG signal are removed from result through a screening process. Finally, the Hilbert transform is employed to achieve the Hilbert spectrum and marginal spectrum. The results show the

---

The work was financially supported by The Science and Technology Development Fund of Macau under Grant 014/2007/A1, Grant 063/2009/A, and Grant 024/2009/A1, the National Natural Science Foundation of China under Grant 61201397 and University of Macau RG069/07-08S/MPU/FST.

J. Bo (✉) · X. Cao · Y. Yu · P. S. Hang · P. U. Mak · M. IVai
Department of Electrical and Computer Engineering, Faculty of Science and Technology, University of Macau, Taipa, Macau
e-mail: gfkbsncz@gmail.com

Y. Wan
Department of Computer and Information Science, Faculty of Science and Technology, University of Macau, Taipa, Macau

P. S. Hang · M. IVai
State Key Laboratory of Analog and Mixed-Signal VLSI, University of Macau, Taipa, Macau

effective performance of the algorithm combining WPT and HHT in reducing ECG noise and time–frequency analysis. By comparing with the original HHT, the proposed algorithm has the better performance on ECG signal processing.

Keywords ECG · WPT · EMD · HHT

94.1 Introduction

The Electrocardiogram (ECG) is a typical case of biomedical signal and can interpret the electrical activities over a period of time. The Electrocardiogram (ECG) detected and recorded by surface electrodes is essential for the clinical diagnosis of cardiovascular disease. Time series data sampled from biomedical signals are often considered linear and stationary arising from physical processes. But biomedical signals are considered nonlinear and nonstationary when signals are related to dynamic biological system. Due to nonlinear and nonstationary property of ECG signals, an adaptive processing method is required.

Time–frequency analysis is to describe a signal energy density in time and frequency domains simultaneously [1]. There are several common time–frequency analytic techniques such as Gabor-Wigner Transform, Wigner Distribution Function (WDF), Short-time Fourier Transform (STFT) and Wavelet Transform (WT). The Hilbert-Huang Transform (HHT) developed by Huang et al. is a new method to extract the features of nonlinear and nonstationary signals [2] and it is widely used in many fields. But in practical applications HHT has many deficiencies [3, 4]: First, IMFs undesired at the low-frequency section produced by EMD lead misinterpretation to the result easily. Second, depending on the analysed signal, the monocomponent property cannot be satisfied when the 1st IMF frequency range may be too wide. Third, signals containing low-energy components cannot be separated through the EMD operation.

In this paper, an advanced analysis method combining wavelet packet transform (WPT) and Hilbert-Huang transform (HHT) is applied on ECG signal. With this method, the deficiency of HHT can be solved to some extent.

94.2 Principle

94.2.1 Wavelet Packet Transform

Wavelet packet transform (WPT) is an extended multi-resolution signal processing method of wavelet transform (WT). The detail and approximation coefficients can be decomposed to create the full binary tree through WPT. More filters for input

Fig. 94.1 The wavelet packet decomposition process

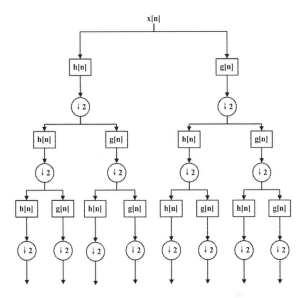

signal are needed to pass in WPT method than in the wavelet transform. Thus WPT can provide better local complete time–frequency analysis. The wavelet packet decomposition process can be shown as Fig. 94.1. 2n different sets of coefficients can be produced through WPT process and the signal can be decomposed into 2n narrow bands for n-level of decomposition [5].

The wavelet packet functions are defined through μ_0, μ_1, h, g as Eq. (94.1):

$$\begin{cases} \mu_{2n}(t) = \sum_{k \in Z} h_k \mu_0(2t-k) \\ \mu_{2n+1}(t) = \sum_{k \in Z} g_k \mu_0(2t-k) \end{cases} \quad (94.1)$$

Where $\{\mu_n(t)\}_{n \in z}$ are the orthogonal wavelet packets, h_k are low-pass filter coefficients, g_k are high-pass filter coefficients. When $n = 0$, the functions denote the scaling function: $\mu_0(t) = \phi(t)$ and wavelet function: $\mu_1(t) = \varphi(t)$

94.2.2 Hilbert-Huang Transform

Empirical mode decomposition (EMD) and Hilbert spectral analysis (HSA) these two approaches comprise the Hilbert-Huang transform (HHT) [2] which is a development method for processing nonstationary and nonlinear signals.

The first procedure of HHT is EMD which can decompose a signal to a series of intrinsic mode function (IMF) which needs to fulfill two constraints [2]. In EMD process, assume x(t) represents a non-linear and non-stationary input signal. Curve fitting technique is applied to achieve the upper and lower envelopes of the input signal. The difference between input signal $x(t)$ and the mean value of the upper and lower envelopes of input signal $x(t)$ is calculated repeatedly until the sifted signal satisfies IMF condition. The same procedure is applied to the residual result again and again until the residual is a mean trend or constant. The final result of EMD through above procedures indicates input signal $x(t)$ consists of a series of IMF (c_i) and a remainder (r_n), a constant or mean trend, which can be represented as Eq. (94.2).

$$x(t) = \sum_{i=1}^{n} c_i + r_n \tag{94.2}$$

The second procedure of HHT is Hilbert spectrum analysis. The input signal can be expressed as Eq. (94.3) in which $a_j(t)$ is instantaneous amplitude corresponding to j th IMF and $\omega_j(t)$ is instantaneous frequency corresponding to j th IMF after performing the Hilbert transform (HT) on each IMF:

$$x(t) \sum_{j=1}^{n} a_j(t) \exp\left(i \int \omega_j(t) dt \right) \tag{94.3}$$

Equation (94.3) can indicate that one signal can be represented in three-dimension by its instantaneous amplitude $a_j(t)$ and instantaneous frequency $\omega_j(t)$ as a function of time t. The marginal spectrum $h(\omega)$ which indicates the contribution of energy on each frequency value is defined as Eq. (94.4) in which the Hilbert spectrum $H(\omega, t)$ replacing $x(t)$ is considered as time–frequency distribution of amplitude:

$$h(\omega) = \int_{0}^{T} H(\omega, t) dt \tag{94.4}$$

94.2.3 Combining WPT and HHT

In the algorithm combing WPT and HHT, the ECG signal is separated into a set of narrow band signals through the WPT process in which Soft-Thresholding method [6] is selected firstly. Second, the EMD process of HHT is applied on the narrow band signals. Screening procedure is applied to remove IMFs which is unrelated. Last, the HT is utilized to achieve the Hilbert spectrum and marginal spectrum. The flow chart of the algorithm combining WPT and HHT is shown as Fig. 94.2.

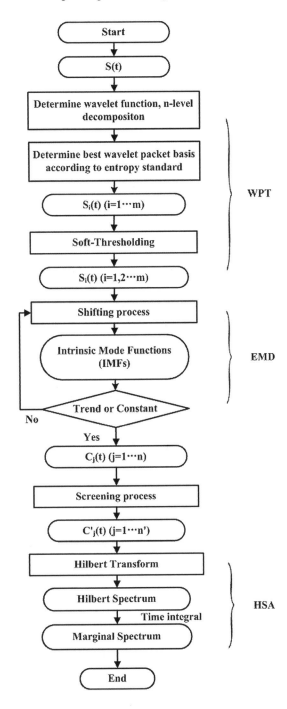

Fig. 94.2 The flow chart of the algorithm combing WPT and HHT

94.3 Application on ECG

The recording of Electrocardiogram (ECG) is vital for the clinical diagnosis of cardiovascular disease. But ECG signal which frequency range is from 0 ~ 100 Hz is very weak compared with the interference noise including Electromyography (EMG) signal interference which frequency range is 2–5 Hz, power line interference which frequency is 50 Hz, movement artifact which frequency range is below 7 Hz and baseline wander which frequency range is 0.15–0.3 Hz. Denoising is essential for extract features for clinical diagnosis.

94.3.1 Simulated ECG Denoising

For investigating the performance of the algorithm, the ECG signal from MIT-BIH standard database (see Fig. 94.3a) adding simulated white noise (SNR 15 dB), power line interference simulated a cosine function of 50 Hz and baseline wander simulated by a function of combining cosine function and sine function is used. As mentioned above, WPT process is prior to HHT. The Bior 5.5 wavelet, 3-level decomposition is selected. The HHT algorithm is also applied comparing with the WPT and HHT combination algorithm. The result is shown as Fig. 94.3. From Fig. 94.3c and d, no matter white noise, power line interference and baseline wander are reduced in both method but more noise is retained in through HHT method alone than through WPT and HHT. And significant information in original waveform is also retained by proposed method.

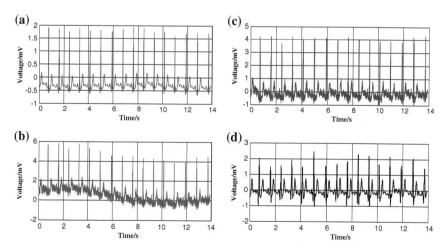

Fig. 94.3 **a** The clear ECG signal and the ECG signal with simulated noise; **c** the denoised ECG signal with HHT; **d** the denoised ECG signal with WPT and HHT

Table 94.1 Parameters for Denoise Performance

Signal	SNR	MSE	Correlation coefficient
$x_1(t)$	5 dB	2.83e-4	0.620
$x_1'(t)$	12.4 dB	3.25e-5	0.872
$x_2(t)$	10 dB	2.37e-4	0.690
$x_2'(t)$	16.8 dB	3.51e-5	0.916
$x_3(t)$	15 dB	2.25e-4	0.722
$x_3'(t)$	21.5 dB	2.99e-5	0.923

$x(t)$ is signal before denoising, $x'(t)$ is signal after denoising

By using simulated noisy signal, the performance of the algorithm of combining WPT and HHT is investigated. The result shown as Table 94.1 indicates the proposed algorithm is effective. SNR and Correlation Coefficient increase obviously while MSE decreases after denoising. Furthermore, practical ECG data is applied.

94.3.2 Real ECG Analysis

Data of ECG signal used is from MIT-BIH standard database. From MIT-BIH databases header file, we know that data file of 203.dat includes considerable noise including muscle artifact and baseline shifts. The EMD result with WPT preprocessing and without WPT preprocessing and is shown as Fig. 94.4. IMF1 and IMF2 which cannot satisfy monocomponent definition very well in Fig. 94.4a contain high frequency components obviously, while IMF1 and IMF2 in Fig. 94.4b do not have, which is because that WPT process can denoise and retain the low-energy component. Thus the EMD efficiency increases by WPT preprocessing.

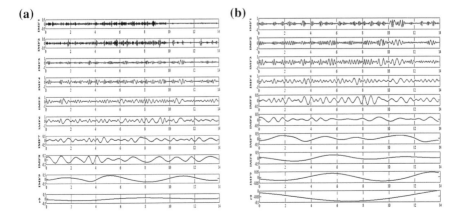

Fig. 94.4 The EMD result for (**a**) the algorithm without WPT (**b**) the algorithm with WPT

Before reconstruct the signal, a screening process through calculating correlation coefficient is applied after EMD process to remove the low frequency IMF and unrelated component. The results of denoising with WPT and without WPT are shown in Fig. 94.5. From Fig. 94.5a and b both two algorithms have denoise function, but HHT performs not well. The algorithm combining WPT and HHT not only can denoise well but also retain the specific waveform significant annotated in original waveform. The conclusion from Fig. 94.5 is that the algorithm combining WPT and HHT is more effective and better than HHT, which is consistent with simulated result.

The FFT spectrum of the original signal of 203.dat and the marginal spectrum which is through the proposed method are shown in Fig. 94.6. In Fig. 94.6a, FFT spectrum shows the energy mainly below 20 Hz of the ECG signal is disperse, which is affected by the noise. While in Fig. 94.6b the marginal spectrum shows the concentration of energy. The energy is more concentrate on the low frequency section, which is not only because noise reduction of the proposed algorithm and indicates the effectivity of the proposed algorithm but also because marginal spectrum represents the accumulation of amplitude corresponding to instantaneous frequency, which is different with definition of Fourier transform.

Equation (94.3) can represent the instantaneous amplitude, instantaneous frequency and time as a contour map. The distribution of amplitude of Hilbert-Huang spectrum is shown as Fig. 94.7 which is of 203.dat. In Fig. 94.7, though the main energy is concentrate on the low frequency section, the frequency of ECG signal

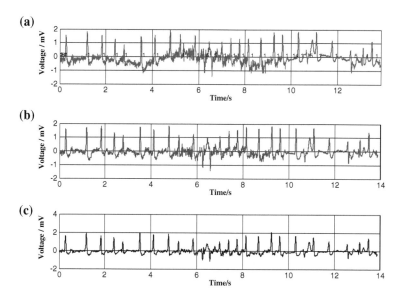

Fig. 94.5 Results of denoising. The original signal of 203.dat is in red line (**a**). The denoised ECG signal with HHT is in blue line (**b**). The denoised ECG signal with WPT and HHT is in black line (**c**)

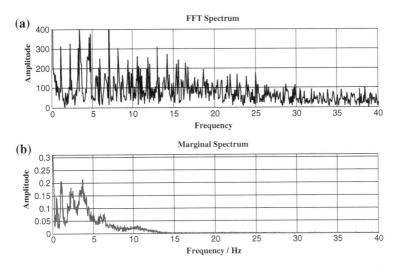

Fig. 94.6 **a** The FFT spectrum of the original ECG signal and **b** The marginal spectrum

varies in an abnormal range as time flows in Hilbert-Huang spectrum, which is an arrhythmia phenomenon that can be proved through transforming R–R interval signal to HRV signal to perform proposed method. The Hilbert-Huang Spectrum by proposed method can indicate the resolution is uniform for overall frequency part and reveal the instantaneous phenomenon in Fig. 94.7. The reason is that in proposed method the concept of time resolution and frequency resolution is not used, while the concept of instantaneous frequency is applied.

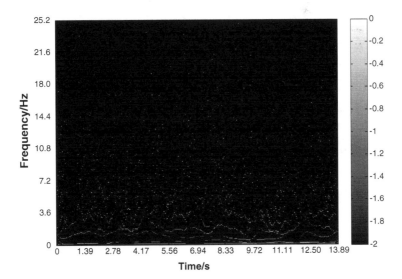

Fig. 94.7 The Hilbert-Huang Spectrum

94.4 Conclusion

In this paper, we have investigated the performance on ECG signal processing based on an advanced algorithm combing WPT and HHT. The result of application on ECG processing indicates the proposed method enhances the EMD efficiency and is effective on denoising ECG. In addition, the marginal spectrum of the proposed method can show the exact energy contribution corresponding to instantaneous frequency and Hilbert-Huang spectrum of the proposed method can provide clear uniform resolution and time–frequency distribution for extract features.

References

1. Cohen L (1995) Time-frequency analysis. Prentice Hall, New Jersey, p 299
2. Huang NE, Shen Z, Long SR, Wu MC, Shih HH, Zheng Q, Yen NC, Tung CC, Liu HH (1998) The empirical mode decomposition and Hilbert spectrum for nonlinear and nonstationary time series analysis. Proc R Soc London V454:903–995
3. Peng Z, Tse P, Chu F (2005) A comparison study of improved Hilbert–Huang transform and wavelet transform: application to fault diagnosis for rolling bearing. Mech Syst Signal Process 19:974–988
4. Peng ZK, Tse PW, Chu FL (2005) An improved Hilbert–Huang transform and its application in vibration signal analysis. J Sound Vib 286:187–205
5. Dequeiroz RL, Rao KR (1993) Time-varying lapped transforms and wavelet packets. IEEE Trans Signal Process 41:3293–3305
6. Donoho DL (1995) De-noising by soft-thresholding. IEEE Trans Inf Theory 41(3):613
7. Huang NE, Shen SSP (2005) Hilbert-huang transform and its applications. Interdiscip Math Sci 5:1–26
8. Rilling G, Flandrin P, Goncalves P (2003) On empirical mode decomposition and its algorithms. In: Proceedings IEEE-EURASIP workshop on nonlinear signal and image processing, Grado (I)
9. Flandrin P, Rilling G, Gonçalves P (2004) Empirical mode decomposition as a filterbank. IEEE Signal Proc Lett 11:112–114
10. Kopsinis Y McLauglin S (2008) Empirical mode decomposition based soft-thresholding. In: Proceedings 16th European signal processing conference (EUSIPCO), Lausanne, Switzerland, 25–29 Aug 2008, Available:CD-ROM
11. Kopsinis Y, McLauglin S, Empirical mode decomposition based denoising techniques. In: Proceedings 1st IAPR workshop cognitive information processing (CIP), Santorini, Greece, 9–10 Jun 2008, pp 42–47

Chapter 95
Study on Self-Adaptive Clinical Pathway Decision Support System Based on Case-Based Reasoning

Gang Qu, Zhe Liu, Shengnan Cui and Jiafu Tang

Abstract To regulate medical behavior, improve medical quality and reduce health-care costs, clinical pathway is served as a standard treating model for both reducing the sources and sticking to the principles of managing the quality, which has been adopted worldwide. Thus we introduce an artificial intelligence method to meet this need which complete origin system of self-adaptive clinical pathway based on some cases inducing, give the whole framework and procedures of working, realize several key managements. Take the classified files of clinical path and electrical medical records as the origin database. Meanwhile, regard the unimplemented clinical pathways and as new cases. Then the clinical pathway can be calculated by using the above self-adaptive system based on CBR. The results are of great importance when to examining the feasibility and effectiveness of the system, determine a flexible, self-adaptive clinical pathway in the treatment process.

Keywords Case-based reasoning (CBR) · Clinical pathway (CP) · Self-adaption · Decision

G. Qu (✉) · Z. Liu · J. Tang
School of Business Administration, Northeastern University, Shenyang 110819, China
e-mail: dlqugang@yahoo.com.cn

G. Qu
Xinhua Hospital Affiliated to Dalian University, Dalian 116000, China

Z. Liu
School of Medical Devices, Shenyang Pharmaceutical University, Shenyang 11016, China

S. Cui
School of Information Science and Engineering, Northeastern University, Shenyang 110819, China

95.1 Introduction

According to the definition of, foreign scholars like Coffey [3], Spath, Ibarra [2] as well as domestic scholars like Zhang Yin, Li Congdong. The clinical pathway is a method of organization and management which by medical experts and based on evidence-based medicine for the disease treatment, is to build a standard treatment mode and treatment programs, and is a integrated model for the clinical treatment. When implemented, clinical pathway is the guidance principles of the overall service planning documents with a sequence requirement and time list for the diagnosis and treatment of certain diseases. After that, the hospital can analyze and evaluate the differences of each patient, so that to specify individualized treatment plan. The fundamental purpose of the clinical pathway is to standardize medical behaviors, reduce variation, decrease costs, and improve health care quality and patient satisfaction, following the PDCA (Plan-Do-Check-Act-Cycle) circle of Deming.

During the latest 30 years, the clinical pathway has been widely used in the United States, Europe and some developed countries in Asia, such as Hong Kong, Macao and Taiwan regions. Clinical data shows that it has significant effects in improving the quality of medical services, standardizing medical behavior, reducing treatment costs and enhancing patient satisfaction. In the domestic, the clinical pathway has also done the corresponding experiment site work and had a certain effect since the concept first introduced in 1996. On December 8, 2009, the Ministry of Health of China points out that, Choosing 50 experiment sites at least in the nationwide, undertaking 22 specialty and 112 diseases Clinical pathway management pilot projects, having been an important part of the reform of public hospitals, clinical pathway management pilot project will officially launched in 2010, and level-III hospital will be the full implementation of "clinical pathway management modeled" on the design of industrial pipeline. However, it also encountered implementation difficulties, such as lacking of methodological guidance system, the rigidity of clinical pathway, not be adapted automatically when the patient each has different path mutation, leading to a reduction of the efficiency of the implementation.

Some scholars have done a series of relevant researches; Syed SRABIDI proposed a semantic Web model, this model not only achieves a synthesis the knowledge of heterogeneous and operational, but also proposes the service-oriented technical basis for the generation of specific patient clinical pathways. Based on Syed's [6] semantic model, Katrina and Syed [5] extracted the practice knowledge of clinical pathway, expressing the structure and the function in details.In the project of PARADIGMA [4] (Participative Approach to Disease Global Management), which has defined the clinical pathway, the clinical pathway has been divided into screening, diagnosis, treatment, etc. and generated a specific path in the designing of clinical pathway to the specific disease refinement. L. Ardissono et al. [1] defined different ways to complete some sorts of medical behavior under different context through the conditional rules of BDI Agent mode, combining with Web services integration technology and proposing context-aware self-adaptive medical workflow management system framework. Li Congdong [8] constructedthe models of knowledge reconstruction of task model, process model and method model from the perspective of knowledge management. By utilizing the organizational semiotics and theoretically Yang Hongqiao [9] extracts and expresses the clinical pathway knowledge. Among all the studies, they are either limited to the theory of implemetion or describe the clinical pathway from the structural point of view of the concept, conceptual relationship and the property of concept. However, in the real treatment, the clinical pathway is a complex process which requires the accumulation of abundant existing knowledge and needs to have the knowledge to analyze, optimize, as well as modify processing [7]. Therefore, put forward a case-based reasoning artificial intelligence modeling approach which is storing the existing experiences of clinical pathway in a case way, and select from the case base for similar cases according to the characteristics of the patient to apply, especially the variability of clinical pathway as well as complex diseases, and need to match the new medical records to the large number of cases in the case. Then check whether the matching path is feasible, if not, we need to negotiate to modify the new clinical pathway, and decide whether to use it as a new case after the treatment. According to this method, this paper presents the overall process and framework of the modeling, given the critical techniques and methods for modeling, and finally, verifies the availability and effectiveness of the system by the result.

95.2 System Modeling

95.2.1 Business Analysis

At present, The National Hospital (all level-III hospitals and parts of level II hospitals) carry out the management of the clinical pathway modeled on the design of industrial pipeline, 112 diseases have a standard flow chart ", But each patient's own situation has obvious or small differences, Such as patient age, time of onset and whether there are other medical history and complications. Therefore, implementation of clinical pathways in accordance with the "standard process" is bound to cause a corresponding variation, this variation is extremely complex, and the variation of positive and negative points, the negative variation refers to the planned activities were not carried on (or did not produce the results), Or delay in completion, such as discharged delay, CT scan delay. Positive variation means a planned activity or results in advance or completed, such as early discharge, CT check in advance, Variations can be divided into the patient/family variation, hospital/system variability, clinicians/service providers' variation. These variations caused by changes of the clinical pathway, should be given into records, and determined whether to put into the case library according to the probability of mutations and whether it is a typical case. The initial clinical case data base is cleaned and classified by the data from the and its change records and electronic medical records system. (See Fig. 95.1 data clearing and classification.)

Although the clinical path is unified formulate by the Ministry of Health, because of the various medical institutions, we need slightly readjustment, leading to the differences of software. In practical work, the design, application, management and maintenance of clinical pathway related to numerous staff. Play a leadership and supervisory role of staff in the formulation and implementation are hospital administrators, members of the Steering Group, and the department head; On the specific implementation of clinical pathway, including doctors, psychologists, nurses, pharmacists, surveyors, radiologists, nutritionists, therapists, anesthetists, operating room staff and logistical support staff, and even patients and their families are Jointly participated in the completion. Some of the above-mentioned persons need to collaborate together to complete the task, while others need to complete the task along undertake continued.

95.2.2 System Architecture

The proposed case-based reasoning self-adaptive clinical pathway Optimization decision support system is a management information system supported by three different database systems (electronic medical records database, case library of clinical pathway, and Optimization model library), shown in Fig. 95.2, in which the CBR core module is the core part of the whole system. In addition, Good human–computer interaction interface, making expertise a useful complement to the CBR technology, and help to achieve better application effect in the generation and management of actual clinical pathway.

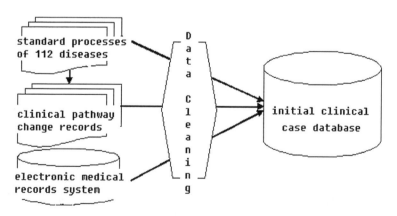

Fig. 95.1 The building of the clinical pathway case base

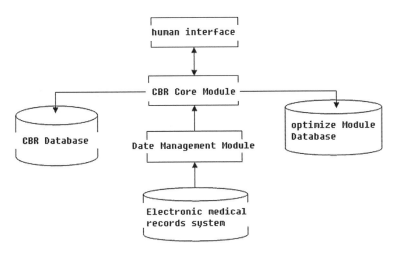

Fig. 95.2 Framework of the system based CBR

95.3 Implement of Key Technologies of CBR

CBR is a rapid and effective reasoning method in the field of Artificial Intelligence. As a cognitive similarity reasoning simulation, the basic assumptions of which is similar solutions solve similar problems, CBR essentially solve the problem of past depending on experience. By putting problem-feature sets and relevant solutions that describe past problems in case base, CBR gets the solution of the problem in case base when new problem occurs. See detail steps in the following. Figure 95.3 shows work flow of the clinical pathway system based on case reasoning. During the case search, if the new case can't get its matching case, CBR will find help in optimization model by establishing relevant mathematical model and optimize the case in order to obtain a new solution.

1. search: to search for similar cases based on several characteristics of the new problem;
2. reuse: to generate solutions from the sample of best examples;
3. revise: to evaluate and correct the obtained solutions;
4. save: to update the case base by analyzing and storing the current problems.

95.3.1 Case Presentation

Case presentation is to have the existed problems, characteristics of the problems and solutions to the problems presented in the form of case. As the most important step in the development of self-adaptive clinical pathway system, it directly affects

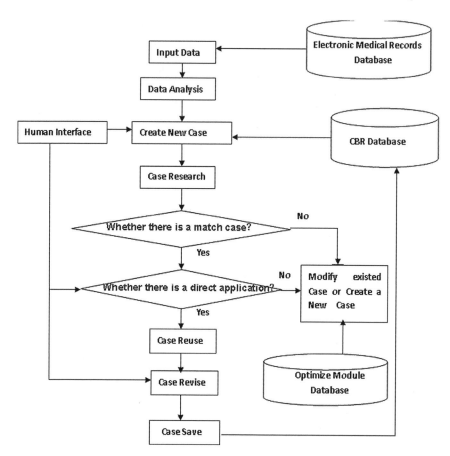

Fig. 95.3 Work flow chart of the system based CBR

quality and speed of case research, as well as the operation efficiency of the whole system. As a result, case presentation in the system should try to cover the most effective information and to highlight key features of the problem as economical as possible. A case which involves case presentation and problem solutions includes characteristic types, characteristic attributes, characteristic values and additional comments as a complete CBR case description in the clinical pathway system. Characteristic types consist of departments, diseases, age, gender, attack time, attack season, hospitalized time, complications, PMH (past medical history) and drug allergic history. Table 95.1 gives a general presentation of case feature in clinical pathway system. Yet for different kinds of diseases, the characteristic types, characteristic attributes and characteristic value are disparate, which is also the embodiment of complexity and difficulty in construction of CBR clinical pathway.

Table 95.1 Case features of adaptive clinical pathway system

Characteristic types	Characteristic attributes	Characteristic values
Departments	Surgery, medical	Department numeration (e.g. respiration department)
Diseases	Single, complex	Disease numeration (e.g. appendicitis)
Age	Old, middle, young	Successive numerical value (e.g. 26, 34 etc.)
Gender	Male, female	Boole numerical value (e.g. 0,1)
Attack time	Long, medium, short	Successive numerical value (e.g. 2, 7 etc.)
Attack season	Cold, warm	Discrete numeration (e.g. 0,1,2,3)
Hospitalized time	Holiday, non-holiday	Date 2010-9-8
Comorbidity	Yes, no	Comorbidity type coding (e.g. diabetes)
Complications	Yes, no	Complication type coding (e.g. haemorrhagia)
PMH	Yes, no	Disease numeration (e.g. heart disease)
Drug allergic history	Yes, no	Drug numeration (e.g. penicillin allergies)

95.3.2 Case Research

Case reasoning is divided into four steps, research, matching (which is the core of case reasoning), reuse and maintenance. In the source cases researched by case reasoning system, if its feature set is similar to the target case, the solutions of both cases are considered to be parallel. And the judgment is dependent on matching, which is generally divided into the following three steps: (1) to calculate the similarity between the corresponding properties of the source cases and the target case; (2) to calculate the ensemble similarity between source cases and the target case; (3) to sort the source cases on ensemble similarity and to select source case with the highest similarity to provide decision support for the target case. The steps are as follows:

Step 1. According to the actual situation of the case to be solved, we do the initial search. We select same department from the disease case library for preliminary classification, and then reduce research space by choosing the same disease;

Step 2. We refine research by measuring the similarity between case to be solved and the historical case using the definition of similarity indicators. And then, based on the similarity, we select the most relative representation cases. This paper solves case similarity using the traditional most neighboring method. The following is the calculation model on case matching based on most neighboring function: EMBED Eq. (3). We assume case set, the attribute set of case I is, and the similarity between the source case and the target caseis.n is the number of case attributes, is weight for attribute j, and represents the similarity between attributes j of source case and target case, which is defined as, among which is numerical area of feature j. The difficult point is to determine the weight of each characteristic in a certain case when using most neighboring method to seek for similarity S.

If weight of disease case is not properly assigned, the research quality of the case is hard to be guaranteed. Therefore, this paper uses the AHP (The analytic hierarchy process, hereinafter referred to as AHP) and ranking method (determining the weights according to expert opinions) to give the initial solutions to characteristics weights, and then optimize through application of taboo.

95.3.3 Rase Reuse, Revise and Maintenance

The reuse of the case is to solve new problems regarding the case with old-case-solving experience. In the clinical pathway cases, when the system access to case with similarity larger than a certain threshold, which implies higher similarity between the new case and old cases and can confirm details in the clinical pathway, application is started. If similarity is below a threshold value, the old case needs to be modified in order to adapt to the current new case. The modified case should be temporarily put into current database, once they are accumulated to a certain degree, they have to be evaluated by experts who will decide whether they are stored or not. And another situation is there is no result after search. In this kind of extreme cases, particular case should be analyzed particularly. Considering whether it's because of the case is too special or the case base has already need to be maintained, one can design corresponding clinical pathway according to the actual condition based on the former one, if not we need to check case validity, including case research accuracy, case redundancy, case coverage and times to be researched, etc.

95.4 Prototype System Operation Results and Analysis

Prototype system based on CBR self-adaptive clinical pathway gets its application from three-structure JAVA Spring and MySQL database, which now have completed the study of 22 professional 112 clinical disease path formulated by Medical Administrative Department of the Ministry of Health, designed the cases database, and gives the Clinical case test. The practice shows that adaptive clinical path management system can further improve the efficiency of medical services. In the future, the Average length of stay in hospital and the waiting time of surgery is expected to be shorten, while improving patient satisfaction with health care.

Since launched a clinical pathway management, our hospital has conducted nearly 1000 cases of seven single disease in Gynecology and obstetrics planned. We obtained the clinical pathway forms of planned cesarean of these cases and detailed records in electronic database to do data cleaning and sorting. Put these cleaned cases of them as the CRB case base, and then stratified sampling cases from non-use clinical pathway cases in 2011 (a year has 12 months and we monthly random select eight cases), then we got a total of 96 *7 patients as a test

Table 2 CBR adaptive clinical path prototype system test results

Disease name	Test cases	CBR cases	Test cases fall in the different fit interval			
			(60–70) %	(70–80) %	(80–90) %	(90–100) %
Adenomyosis	96	716	3	16	35	42
Benign ovarian tumors	96	805	4	9	44	39
Tubal pregnancy	96	665	8	11	37	40
Uterine leiomyoma	96	813	5	14	46	31
Premature rupture of membranes line vaginal delivery	96	733	6	17	48	28
Natural labor vaginal delivery	96	718	9	11	39	37
Planned cesarean	96	829	3	7	30	56

case to test this system. What is more, we also shrink the search space in choice of same departments and diseases (single, complex), then we match the cases on nine attributes, including age, PMH (heart disease, diabetes), symptoms, genetic diseases, drug allergy history, complications, hospitalization time (whether on holidays), hospital season and specific diseases. The number of test cases falled in different fit interval are as follows Table 95.2.

From above test results, as we found a few lower fitness cases, the data should be analyzed and readjusted appropriately, and after evaluation, temporarily accumulating in temporary database, statistical analysis and combining the expert opinion, then decide whether there is a need to put it into the CBR case base. The setting of system threshold also needs to be further studied. And a large amount of repetitive tests are demanded in searching for the precise critical range.

95.5 Conclusion

This paper applies method based on case reasoning in clinical pathway system of medical field and provides a new attempt and beneficial exploration for clinical path system. But to establish self-adaptive clinical system is a complicated systematic engineering, and there still a lot of work to be completed. At present, the index weight, the threshold value and process of cases with lower similarity have to rely on expert experience. We need to further study algorithm in the field of artificial intelligence in order to quantitatively and automatically screening every patient's attribute types, set the index weight and threshold, automatic completion of the expansion of rule base and maintenance of the case base. All we have to do is to further improve building method of self-adaptive clinical pathway based on reasoning.

References

1. Ardissono L, Di Leva A, Petrone G et al (2006) Adaptive medical workflow management for a context-dependent home healthcare assistance service. Electron Notes Theor Comput Sci 146:59–68
2. Barra V, Laoffon T et al (1997) Clinical pathways in the peri-operative setting. Nursing Case Manage 2(3):97–106
3. Coeffy RJ et al (1992) An introduction to critical paths. Qual Manage Health Care 1(1):45–54
4. Di Leva A, Reyneri C (2004) The PARADIGMA project: an ontology based approach for cooperative work in the medical domain. Proc EMOI-INTEROP conference
5. Hurley KF, Abidi SSR (2007) Ontology engineering to model clinical pathways: towards the computerization and execution of clinical pathways. In: Proceedings of the twentieth IEEE international symposium computer-based medical systems, pp 536–541
6. Li CD (2004). Study of knowledge reconfiguration for clinical pathway implementation. Ph.D. thesis, Tianjin University, Management Science and Engineering
7. Li H, Liu ZX, Men F (2010) Study on method of single disease cost prediction based on clinical pathway and CBR. Ind Eng Manage 15(2):105–110
8. Abidi SSR, Chen H (2006) Adaptable personalized care planning via a semantic web framework. In Proceedings of the 20th international congress of the European federation for medical informatics. IOP Press, Maastricht
9. Yang HQ, Li SZ, Zhao JP, Li WZ (2009) Study of clinical pathway based on organizational semiotics methods. Comput Eng Des 30(13):3189–3192

Chapter 96
Wireless Body Sensor Networks with Cloud Computing Capability for Pervasive Healthcare: Research Directions and Possible Solutions

Xiaoya Xu and Miao Zhong

Abstract In pervasive healthcare services, the efficient management of the large number of monitored data from various wireless body sensor networks (WBSNs) in terms of processing, storing and analysis is an important problem. Now, cloud computing is becoming a promising technology to provide a flexible stack of massive computing, storage and software services in a scalable and virtualized manner at low cost. In this article, we try to investigate and overcome these issues associated with WBSN-cloud integration (abbr. bCloud) platform. For this purpose, we design a novel system architecture for the general bCloud platform, and then propose the methodologies for quality of service (QoS) improvement, including three directions: reliable and energy efficient routing protocols for WBSNs, effective QoS-aware novel resource allocation model for the bCloud platform, and efficient data mining for extracting behavioral regularity from WBSN data. The proposed methodologies to design bCloud platform will facilitate the better pervasive healthcare.

Keywords Pervasive healthcare · Cloud computing · Data mining · Wireless body sensor networks

---

X. Xu
Guangdong Jidian Polytechinc, 510515 Guangzhou, China
e-mail: xiaoyaxu33@gmail.com

M. Zhong (✉)
Guangdong University of Education, 510303 Guangzhou, China
e-mail: miao_zhong@126.com

96.1 Introduction

Due to the recent developments of several technological advances and new concepts, such as wireless body sensor networks (WBSNs) [1, 2] and low-power wireless communications, pervasive health monitoring and management services are increasing dramatically [3]. WBSNs are typically placed strategically on the human body as tiny patches or hidden in users' clothes or even implanted in the human body. They enable real-time collection of vital signs (e.g., body temperature, heart rate, blood pressure, and electrocardiogram (ECG)), physical activity (e.g., body posture), and environmental data (e.g., location, temperature, and humidity) unobtrusively during normal daily activities of a patient for the purpose of preventing terminal illness, monitoring the progression of chronic disease, assessing post-operative care and enhancing emergency services, especially for elderly and physically challenged.

However, the efficient management of the large number of monitored data collected from various WBSNs is an important issue for its large scale adoption in pervasive healthcare services [4]. Since WBSNs are limited in memory, energy, computation, and communication capabilities, they require a powerful and scalable high performance computing and massive storage infrastructure for real-time processing and storing of the data as well as on-line and off-line analysis of the processed information under context (i.e. temporal, spatial and vital sign parameters) using inherently complex models to extract knowledge about the health condition of patients. Now, cloud computing is becoming a promising technology to provide a flexible stack of massive computing, storage and software services in a scalable and virtualized manner at low cost. Because of its elasticity and scalability, cloud computing can potentially provide huge cost savings, flexible high-throughput, and ease of use of WBSN services [5].

The integration of WBSNs and cloud computing can facilitate to build an intelligent, autonomous, cost-effective, scalable and data driven pervasive healthcare services platform to realize the long-term monitoring, analysis, sharing, forecasting and management of health status at any time and any place. Nevertheless, the research regarding the WBSN-cloud integration (bCloud) platform is still in its infancy, and several technical challenges remain to be addressed to maximize the opportunities. Current researches [6–8] related to bCloud platform focus on architectural design to realize a health monitoring and analysis system. The problems with current methods limit their long-term effectiveness to support reliable transmission of vital sign data, real-time seamless access and efficient processing of monitored data to derive meaningful results, and context-aware patient-centric decision making at a large scale. Fortunately, the continuous development of many related domains, such as machine-to-machine communications [9], cyber-physical systems [10, 11], and internet of things, will promote the integration of WBSNs and cloud computing. In this article, we try to investigate and overcome the technical challenges associated with the bCloud platform for enabling a new generation of advanced, cost-effective and scalable pervasive healthcare services and application.

96.2 Literature Review

In this section, we in brief explore the previous work related to integration of WBSNs and cloud, routing protocols for WBSNs, resource management for bCloud, and data mining techniques for analyzing WBSN data.

Previous works on WBSN-integrated cloud platform: Recently, the integration of WBSNs and cloud computing is getting much attention due to its immense potential. Most of the current works [12] related to bCloud platform focus on architectural design to realize a health monitoring and analysis system. For example, Pandey et al. [8] proposed an autonomic system that integrates body sensor network, mobile computing and cloud computing for collecting, disseminating and analyzing health data. They mainly focused on cloud-based architectural design for ECG data analysis and its benefits in terms of cost and scalability. Figure 96.1 shows some of the biosensors that are developed in the UbiMon project.

Related work on routing protocols for WBSNs: The protocols developed in the projects target single-hop communication only with no or limited focus on multi-hop communication that is required for many applications. Most of these researchers considered the famous IEEE 802.15.4 for single-hop WBSN communication [13]. Others such as [14] considered either TDMA or CSMA or the combination of both methods. These protocols do not address many issues including reliability, patient's mobility and multi-hop communication. The proposed protocols nevertheless resolve some of the issues in WBSNs. However

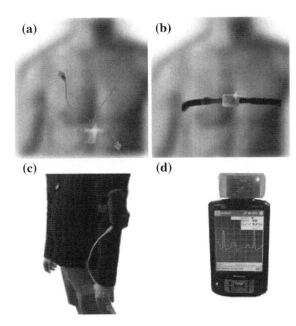

Fig. 96.1 a ECG sensor, b ECG strap (*center*), c SpO2 sensor, and the portable base station

there are many issues including network topology selection, node's mobility, data aggregation, quality of service (QoS), and energy efficient routing that must be technically addressed. Also, the QoS issues in particular are very important to be addressed for the bCloud platform.

Current researches of resource allocation model for a bCloud platform: Few studies have been conducted related to effective resource allocation to support various WBSN services such as pre-processing, storing, sharing, prioritizing, visualizing, and analysis of monitored data as well as acquiring context-awareness. Viswanathan et al. [15] proposed an autonomic resource provisioning framework that can harness under-utilized computing resources in the vicinity (e.g., laptops, tablets, PDAs, DVRs, medical terminals) to support real-time processing of vital signs and to acquire context awareness from WBSN data. However, to the best of our knowledge, there are few researches regarding efficient resource allocation in a bCloud platform to ensure QoS guarantee for WBSN services.

Existing works on discovering interesting knowledge from WBSN data based on data mining techniques: Finding such interesting knowledge from WBSN data by using pattern matching [16] or activity recognition [17] algorithms may not be suitable, mainly because of the involvement of large volume of WBSN data, and the requirement of testing and training phases, as most of the activity recognition algorithms rely on classification technique, respectively. Recently data mining techniques are being utilized in discovering interesting knowledge from the WBSN data [18]. Ali et al. [19] has developed a software architecture to find routine behavior based on patient's activi3ty pattern. It uses a frequent pattern mining [20] technique to obtain frequent activity patterns which enables the observation of the inherent structure present in a patient's daily activity. Gu et al. [21] exploited the notion of emerging patterns to identify the significant changes between the classes of data for a smooth and efficient recognition of daily living activity.

96.3 System Architecture of a General bCloud Platform

Figure 96.2 depicts the system architecture of a general bCloud platform. The system is comprised of five main components: body sensors, mobile device, cloud servers, users, and display terminals, such as Television (TV), personal computer or smart phones. In the data acquisition end, vital signals such as body temperature, electrocardiograph (ECG), and blood pressure (BP), are collected from WBSNs. The collected monitored data are transmitted to the mobile device via Bluetooth and then to the cloud server via Internet or 3G. Cloud servers provide powerful virtual machine (VM) resources, such as the CPU, memory, GPU and network bandwidth on demand, for faster management of these data.

Such integrated system thus provide various WBSN services such as real-time pre-processing, storing, sharing, prioritizing, visualizing, analyzing, summarizing and searching of monitored data as well as acquiring context-awareness to different users such as hospitals, clinics, researchers, or even patients ubiquitously by a variety of interfaces such as personal computer, TV and mobile phones. It can also allow sharing of monitoring data to authorized social networks or medical communities to search for personalized trends and group patterns, letting insights into disease evolution, the rehabilitation process, and the effects of drug therapy.

The bCloud platform has significant potential to enable several new, essential, value-added pervasive healthcare applications. These applications include, but are not limited to, context-aware or location-based mobile healthcare such as elderly monitoring; access to patients electronic health records; tracking progression of diseases, intelligent emergency management using location maps; analysis and sharing of monitored data from home, hospitals, field trips and even major events. While attempts have been made to integrate WBSN and cloud computing to

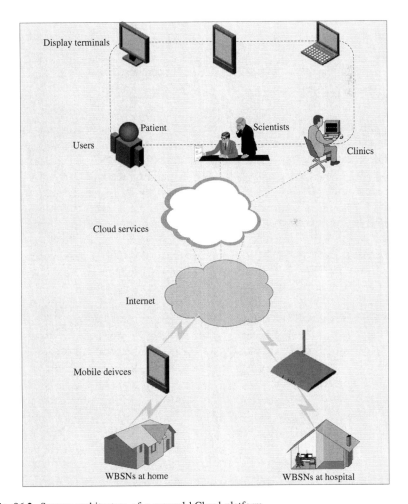

Fig. 96.2 System architecture of a general bCloud platform

improve pervasive healthcare services, existing work had their limitations to develop a clinically-effective system for this purpose, and so the potential of this integrated technology remains fully unutilized. In this article, we identify several key issues that we believe need to be addressed carefully for enabling an advanced, cost-effective and scalable pervasive healthcare services and applications.

96.4 Research Directions and Possible Solutions

We propose the methodologies including three aspects: developing routing protocols to support efficient transmission of WBSN data to cloud, cloud resource provisioning to facilitate seamless access and processing of WBSN data, and effective data mining techniques in the cloud for patient-centric decision making.

96.4.1 Reliable and Energy Efficient Routing Protocols for WBSNs

One of our objectives is to consider reliable routing protocols for WBSNs that must support multi-hop communication and provide low end-to-end delay, low packet drop rate, and low energy consumption. Because the patients' condition change continuously and may cause massive mobility, the new routing protocols can provide numerous methods to solve the fast mobility issues. To start with, we may investigate proactive, reactive, and hybrid routing protocols for WBSNs and particularly focus on temperature, cluster-based, and cross layer routing solutions. In temperature routing, we study the effects of tissue heating on the human body and their consequences during multi-hop communication. One of the approaches to reduce tissue heating is to minimize the transmission power and traffic rate. Another approach is to always avoid high temperature node when forwarding the data packets. The TARA adapted the same approach but it has a high packet drop rate and low reliability. We may propose alternative solutions that can select the least temperature route (not necessarily the next hop) to forward the data packets and provide low packet loss and high reliability. For sparse WBSNs, we investigate the use of clusters as done in LEACH. Although the conventional LEACH aggregates data from cluster heads, it is extremely unreliable for WBSNs. We propose cross-layer solutions to solve this problem. Much of the research work on cross-layer routing solutions considered IEEE 802.15.4 standard at medium access control (MAC) and physical layers. However, as discussed earlier, the IEEE 802.15.4 is not suitable for WBSNs due to many problems including limited data rata and high energy consumption. Our cross-layer routing protocol will partially consider the new IEEE 802.15.6 MAC protocol. Because the IEEE 802.15.4 MAC protocol is solely designed for WBSNs, adding an efficient routing protocol at the network layer will increase the network performance by connecting the nodes that are not in the non-line of sight. This may ultimately decrease the packet drop rate and average energy consumption. In addition, we compare the proposed routing protocols with other conventional protocols such as TARA, LEACH, and CICADA for different application scenarios and come up with useful suggestions and guidelines. Because the proposed protocols can decrease the packet drop rate and end-to-end delay, they must be able to ensure efficient data transmission to the bCloud platform.

96.4.2 Effective QoS-Aware Novel Resource Allocation Model for bCloud Platform

We hope to find a scalable, dynamic, energy efficient and cost effective VM resource allocation mechanism in order to support a high standard of QoS for various WBSN services in a bCloud platform. The basic concern of a VM allocation is that a physical machine must have enough capacity for hosting the VMs. To reduce the hosting cost, the number of active physical machines needs be minimized. To save energy or power consumption, most power-efficient physical machines need to be selected. To avoid frequent VM migration, certain amount of CPU capacity needs to be preserved as backup resource for handling workload burst. To reduce the response time, the delay of the services needs to be controlled. According to above considerations, we use two methods to solve the VM resource allocation problem. The first method is to design a linear programming (LP) model of quantitatively optimizing VM allocation using cost objectives and constraints on the resource utilization condition, CPU utilization, energy consumption and delay of services.

The second approach to solve the VM resource allocation problem is to use different heuristics. We study existing heuristics and modifythem to fit our situation. Then, by using appropriate heuristics, we generate candidate allocation schemes and choose the best scheme for real VM allocation. In addition, we may allocate each VM to a host that provides the least increase of power consumption due to this allocation. This allows leveraging the heterogeneity of resources by choosing the most power-efficient servers first.

We also need to determine the optimal threshold value of the constraints in the above methods. For this, we may use an iterative approach similar to the bisection method that enables us to find the optimal value of the constraints after a number of repeated experiments. The VM resource allocation process is performed in a single step using the peak load demands of each workload. Based on the workload demand, the process can dynamically change virtual machine capacities. However, migration of VMs may be required between physical servers. Thus, when a new service requirement arrives, the system can use the proposed VM allocation algorithm to find the appropriate physical servers. If VM migration is required because of an overloaded state, the system can also adopt the same VM allocation algorithm for selecting new physical servers.

96.4.3 Efficient Data Mining for Extracting Behavioural Regularity from WBSN Data

The body sensors can measure metrics on several parameters such as blood pressure, body temperature and heart rate. The proposed data mining technique RegMiner is used to identify the set of patterns that occur at a regular interval among different parameters in body sensor data. As an example, if the blood pressure of a patient falls and the heart rate decreases at most mornings, the RegMiner is able to identify this {*low blood pressure, low heart rate*} pattern as a regular/periodical event with a one day period for that particular patient. Similarly, if a patient experiences high body temperature almost once a week, the RegMiner can find the {*high body temperature*} as a regularly occurring pattern with the period of one week for that particular patient. The discovered patterns are then analyzed and used to extract important inherent knowledge about the change behavior of these parameter values.

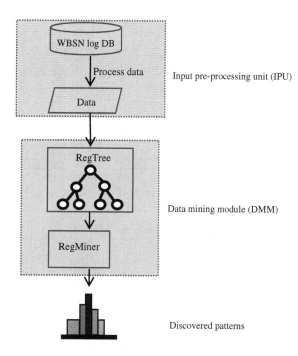

Fig. 96.3 RegMiner model overview

The major phases of the data mining module would be studying the body sensor data, pre-processing the sensor data, extracting the occurrence regularity knowledge from data, and presenting the knowledge in a prescribed manner. The overall methodology of this module is proposed in Fig. 96.3.

96.5 Conclusions

WBSNs, a specific class of wireless sensor networks, are emerging as a noteworthy technology capable of pervasive continuous monitoring of temporal, spatial and vital sign data of a patient for the purpose of managing chronic conditions and detecting health emergencies. However, the integration of WBSNs and cloud computing impose several technical challenges that have not yet received enough attention from the research community. Some of these challenges are reliable transmission of vital sign data to cloud, dynamic resource allocation to facilitate seamless access and processing of WBSN data, and effective data mining techniques in the cloud for context-aware patient-centric decision making. In this article, we design a novel system architecture for the general bCloud platform, and then propose the methodologies to solve the current challenges and issues. These methodologies can facilitate the pervasive healthcare.

References

1. Chen M, Gonzalez S, Vasilakos A, Cao H, Leung V (2011) Body area networks: a survey. ACM/Springer Mob Netw Appl 16(2):171–193
2. Chen M, Wan J, Li F (2012) Machine-to-machine communications: architectures, standards, and applications. KSII Trans Int Inform Syst 6(2):480–497
3. Chen M, Gonzalez S, Zhang Q, Li M, Leung V (2010) A 2G-RFID based E-healthcare System. IEEE Wireless Commun Mag 17(1):37–43
4. Ullah S, Kwak K (2010) An ultra low-power and traffic-adaptive medium access control protocol for wireless body area network, J Med Syst
5. Chatman C (2010) How cloud computing is changing the face of health care information technology. J Health Care Compliance 12(3):37–70
6. Doukas C, Maglogiannis I (2011) Managing wearable sensor data through cloud computing. In: Proceedings of 2011 IEEE third international conference on cloud computing technology and science (CloudCom), pp 440–445
7. Liu J, Wang Q, Wan J, Xiong J, Zeng B (2013) Towards key issues of disaster aid based on wireless body area networks. KSII Trans Int Inform Syst 7(5):1014–1035
8. Pandeya S, Voorsluys W, Niua S, Khandokerb A, Buyyaa R (2012) An autonomic cloud environment for hosting ECG data analysis services. Future Gener Comput Syst 28:147–154
9. Wan J, Chen M, Xia F, Li D, Zhou K (2013) From machine-to-machine communications towards cyber-physical systems. Comput Sci Inform Syst. doi: 10.2298/CSIS120326018W
10. Wan J, Yan H, Li D, Zhou K, Zeng L (2013) Cyber-physical systems for optimal energy management scheme of autonomous electric vehicle. Comput J. doi: 10.1093/comjnl/bxt043

11. Suo H, Wan J, Huang L, Zou C (2012) Issues and challenges of wireless sensor networks localization in emerging applications. In: Proceedings of 2012 international conference on computer science and electronic engineering. Hangzhou, pp 447–451
12. Perumal B, Rajasekaran P, Ramalingam H (2012) WSN-integrated cloud for automated telemedicine (ATM) based e-Healthcare applications. In: Proceedings of the 4th international conference on bioinformatics and biomedical technology, vol 29, Singapore
13. Li C, Li H, Kohno R (2009) Performance evaluation of IEEE 802.15.4 for wireless body area network (WBAN). In: Proceedings of IEEE international conference on ICC workshops. Dresden, pp 1–5
14. Ullah S, Higgins H, Islam S, Khan P, Kwak K (2009) On PHY and MAC performance in body sensor networks. EURASIP J Wireless Commun Netw
15. Viswanathan H, Chen B, Pompili D (2012) Research challenges in computation, communication, and context awareness for ubiquitous healthcare. IEEE Commun Mag 50(5):92–99
16. Minnen D, Starner T, Ward J, Lukowicz P, Troster G (2005) Recognizing and discovering human actions from on-body sensor data. In: Proceedings of the IEEE international conference on multimedia and expo (ICME 2005), pp 1545–1548
17. Suman M, Prathyusha K (2012) A body sensor network data repository with a different mining technique. Int J Eng Sci Adv Technol 2(1):105–109
18. Rashidi P, Cook D (2010) Mining sensor streams for discovering human activity patterns over time. In: Proceedings of the 2010 IEEE international conference on data mining, pp 431–440
19. Ali R, ElHelw M, Atallah L, Lo B, Yang G (2008) Pattern mining for routine behavior discovery in pervasive healthcare environments. In: Proceedings of the 5th international conference on information technology and application in biomedicine. Shenzhen, pp 241–244
20. Han J, Pei J, Yin Y. (2000) Mining frequent patterns without candidate generation. In: Proceedings 2000 ACM SIGMOD international conference on management of data, pp 1–12
21. Gu T, Wang L, Wu Z, Tao X, Lu J (2011) A pattern mining approach to sensor-based human activity recognition. IEEE Trans Knowl Data Eng 23(9):1359–1372

Chapter 97
Robust Predictive Control of Singular Systems with Structured Feedback Uncertainty

Xiaohua Liu and Rong Gao

Abstract The problem of output feedback robust model predictive control is presented for the singular systems with structured feedback uncertainties which is described into linear fractional model. When the system states are immeasurable, the sufficient conditions for the existence of output feedback controller are obtained by linear matrix inequalities. The infinite time domain "min-max" optimization problem is converted into convex optimization problem. The robust stability of the closed-loop singular systems is guaranteed by the initial feasible solution of the optimization problem.The regularity and the impulse-free of singular systems are also held. A simulation example shows the effectiveness of the method.

Keywords Robust predictive control · Singular systems · Uncertainty · Output feedback · Linear matrix inequalities

97.1 Introduction

Singular system is more general system than normal state space system, this kind of model plays an important role in dealing with multiple targets, multi-level and dynamic and static combination of large-scale systems. In recent years, the research of singular system is paid close attention [1].On the other hand, robust predictive control which fuses robust control for treatment of uncertainties and predictive control roll optimizing thoughts, has the broad practicability [2–5]. Thus, the research about robust predictive control of singular system has important theoretical and applied value [6, 7].

X. Liu (✉) · R. Gao
School of Mathematics and Information, Ludong University, Yantai 264025 Shandong, People's Republic of China
e-mail: xhliu_yt@sina.com

Zhang [6] first studied the problem of robust predictive control based on state feedback and proposed a robust predictive control algorithm for a class of uncertain singular systems using LMI method, the robust stability of the closed-loop system is also ensured. In the actual control proceeding, the states may not be measured directly, so it is difficult to use state feedback control law to control the system. Sometimes even if the state of the system can be directly measured, considering the cost of implementing control and reliability of system, it is more suited to select output feedback control method if it can achieve the performance required by closed-loop system, the output variables can measured directly, and have definite physical meaning in most cases, so output feedback is a kind of common feedback mode which is easy to realize in technology. Liu [7] given the sufficient condition of the existence of the output feedback robust predictive control law and analyses the asymptotical stability and feasibility of the closed-loop system. But Ref. [6, 7] only considered the parametric uncertainties. A lot of practical systems not only have parametric uncertainties, but also have dynamic uncertainties, we use linear fractional model to describe systems which have the two kinds of uncertainties at the same time, and this description has more practical significance [2]. The systems described by linear fractional model are called structured feedback uncertain systems. By using multi-Lyapunov function approach, Lee [8] presents an output feedback robust model predictive control algorithm for normal system with structured feedback uncertainty.

In consideration of singular system with structured feedback uncertainty described by linear fractional model, this paper studies output feedback robust predictive control of the system. Based on the idea of variable transformation and LMI methods, the nonlinear inequalities with output feedback controller gain matrixes are decoupled, and the infinite time domain "min-max" optimization problems are converted into convex optimization problems, a group of piecewise output feedback control sequence are identified at the same time, the sufficient conditions for the existence of this controller are derived. And then, the robust stability and the regular and the impulse-free of singular system are analysed. A simulation example shows the effectiveness of the method.

97.2 Problem Formulations

97.2.1 Linear Fractional Model

The general form of linear fractional model is shown in Fig. 97.1.

Where linear time-invariant system P(s) contains all the known linear time-invariant part, such as the controller, the system nominal model, sensors, actuators, etc. al. The input vector u contains the entire external signal in the system, y signifies the entire output signal generated by the system, $\triangle$ which is a structured description of uncertainty, has the following form

Fig. 97.1 Linear fractional model

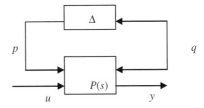

$$\Delta = diag\{\Delta_1, \ldots, \Delta_r\}$$

Where Δ_i, $i = 1, 2 \cdots, r$ reflects a particular uncertainty, for example, the ignored dynamic characteristics, nonlinearity, uncertain parameters etc.

97.2.2 Linear Fractional Model of Singular System

Consider a singular system described by

$$E\dot{x}(t) = \tilde{A}x(t) + \tilde{B}u(t)$$
$$y(t) = \tilde{C}x(t), \quad (97.1)$$

Where $\tilde{A}, \tilde{B}, \tilde{C}$ are respectively uncertainty matrixes dependent on uncertain parameters, they have the following representation

$$\tilde{A} = A + E_1 \Delta_1 F_1, \tilde{B} = B + E_2 \Delta_2 F_2$$
$$\tilde{C} = C + E_3 \Delta_3 F_3$$

A, B, C are real constant matrixes of appropriate dimension, which describe the nominal model of the system. $\Delta_1, \Delta_2, \Delta_3$ are respectively matrixes of uncertain parameters, which reflect parameter uncertainty of the system model.

$E_1, E_2, E_3, F_1, F_2, F_3$ are respectively constant matrixes of appropriate dimension, they reflect the influence the uncertain parameters to the system model, that is to say they reflect the structure of the model uncertainty. Although the uncertain parameters of the model are unknown, but it can be assumed that they are mutative in a bounded area. Specially, by multiplying appropriate scale matrixes to correlated coefficient matrixes, the ranges of uncertainty matrixes can be standardized. That is $\|\Delta_i\| \leq 1$, $i = 1, 2, 3$, where norms are taken as the maximum singular value of matrixes.

Linear fractional model of singular system described by

$$\begin{aligned} E\dot{x}(t) &= Ax(t) + Bu(t) + B_p p(t), \\ y(t) &= Cx(t) + C_q u(t) \\ q(t) &= C_p x(t) + D_{qu} u(t) \\ p(t) &= \Delta q(t) \end{aligned} \qquad (97.2)$$

where $x(t) \in R^n$ is the state, $u(t) \in R^m$ is the control input, $y(t) \in R^p$ is the system output. $p(t), q(t)$ are input and output vectors of uncertain block. E is singular matrix, satisfying $rank(E) = r < n$; uncertain matrix Δ is a block diagonal matrix, which has the following form

$$\Delta = diag\{\Delta_1, \cdots, \Delta_r\},$$

where,

$$\Delta_i : R^{n_i} \to R^{n_i} \|\Delta_i(t)\|_2 \equiv \bar{\sigma}(\Delta_i(t)) \le 1, i = 1, \cdots, r, \qquad (97.3)$$

B_p, C_p, C_q, D_{qu} are matrixes of appropriate dimension.

Associated with the structured feedback uncertainty singular system (97.2), we consider the min–max optimization problem with

$$\min_{u(kT+\tau,kT), \tau \ge 0} \max_{\Delta} J_k, \qquad (97.4)$$

$J_k = \int_0^\infty (x(kT+\tau,kT)^T Q x(kT+\tau,kT) + u(kT+\tau,kT)^T R u(kT+\tau,kT)) d\tau$,
$Q > 0, R > 0$ are symmetric weighting matrices, T is sampling period, $x(kT) = x(kT,kT)$ is the state of sampling time kT, $x(kT+\tau,kT)$ is the state predictive value of sampling time $kT + \tau$ at time kT, $u(kT+\tau,kT)$ is the control action for sampling instant $kT + \tau$ obtained by an optimization problem over the infinite prediction horizon.

Consider the following output feedback controller with whole dimensions

$$\begin{cases} E\dot{\hat{x}}(t) = A_c \hat{x}(t) + B_c y(t) \\ u(t) = C_c \hat{x}(t), \hat{x}(0) = x(0) \end{cases}, \qquad (97.5)$$

Where $\hat{x}(t) \in R^n$ is the states vector of controller, A_c, B_c, C_c are pending controller coefficient matrixes.

Substituting (97.5) into (97.2), we obtain generalized closed-loop system

$$\bar{E}\dot{\bar{x}}(t) = (\bar{A} + \bar{B}\Delta\bar{D})\bar{x}(t), \qquad (97.6)$$

where $\bar{x}(t) = \begin{bmatrix} x(t) \\ \hat{x}(t) \end{bmatrix}, \bar{A} = \begin{bmatrix} A & BC_c \\ B_c C & A_c + B_c C_q C_c \end{bmatrix}, \bar{B} = \begin{bmatrix} B_p \\ 0 \end{bmatrix},$

$\bar{D} = \begin{bmatrix} C_p & D_{qu} C_c \end{bmatrix}, \bar{E} = diag\{E, E\}$

The corresponding closed-loop system performance index is

$$\min_{u(kT+\tau,kT),\tau\geq 0} \max_{\Delta} J_k, \quad (97.7)$$

$$J_k = \int_0^\infty (\bar{x}(kT+\tau,kT))^T \begin{bmatrix} R & 0 \\ 0 & C_c^T Q C_c \end{bmatrix} \bar{x}(kT+\tau,kT) d\tau$$

$$= \int_0^\infty \bar{x}(kT+\tau,kT)^T \bar{C}^T \bar{C} \bar{x}(kT+\tau,kT) d\tau$$

where $\bar{x}(kT+\tau,kT) = \begin{bmatrix} x(kT+\tau,kT) \\ \hat{x}(kT+\tau,kT) \end{bmatrix}$, $\bar{C} = \begin{bmatrix} R^{1/2} & 0 \\ 0 & Q^{1/2} C_c \end{bmatrix}$

The object of output feedback RMPC for the structured feedback uncertain singular system (97.2) can be described as: at each sampling time kT, we solve the optimization problem (97.7) in order to identify output feedback controller coefficient matrixes $\{A_c, B_c, C_c\}$, make uncertain singular systems (97.2) asymptotically stable when the feasible conditions satisfied.

97.3 Output Feedback Robust Predictive Control

97.3.1 Approximately Output Feedback Robust Predictive Control

The key to design output feedback robust model predictive controller is solving the optimization problem (97.7), because of the existence of structured uncertainty Δ. Considering the following Lyapunov function

$$V(\bar{x}(t)) = \bar{x}(t)^T \bar{E}^T P \bar{x}(t), \quad (97.8)$$

With P satisfying

$$\bar{E}^T P = P^T \bar{E} \geq 0. \quad (97.9)$$

where matrix $\bar{E} \in R^{2n\times 2n}$, and $rank(\bar{E}) = 2r \leq 2n$. Suppose $\bar{E} = \begin{bmatrix} I_{2r} & 0 \\ 0 & 0 \end{bmatrix}$, $P \in R^{2n\times 2n}$, P is invertible matrix, and let $P = \begin{bmatrix} P_{11} & P_{12} \\ P_{21} & P_{22} \end{bmatrix}$, where $P_{11} \in R^{2r\times 2r}, P_{11}^T = P_{11}, P_{21} \in R^{(2n-2r)\times 2r}, P_{22} \in R^{(2n-2r)\times(2n-2r)}$.

At sampling time kT, suppose that V satisfies

$$\frac{d}{d\tau} V(\bar{x}(kT+\tau,kT)) \leq -\bar{x}(kT+\tau,kT)^T \bar{C}^T \bar{C} \bar{x}(kT+\tau,kT). \quad (97.10)$$

To ensure that the performance index is finite, we suppose that $\bar{x}(\infty, kT) = 0$, then $V(\bar{x}(\infty, kT)) = 0$, by integrating both sides of (97.10) from $\tau = 0$ to ∞, we can obtain: $\max_\Delta J_k \leq V(\bar{x}(kT))$. Obviously, $V(\bar{x}(kT))$ is the super mum of $\max_\Delta J_k$. So, minimizing $\max_\Delta J_k$ in the optimization problem (97.7) can be transformed into minimizing $V(\bar{x}(kT))$.

Theorem 1 For the structured feedback uncertain singular system (97.2) with output feedback control structure (97.5), at sampling time kT, if the inequality constraint (97.10) is satisfied, then the closed-loop optimization problem (97.7) can be transformed into the optimization problem of the following inequality.

$$\min_{\gamma, W, \bar{W}, \bar{A}, \bar{B}, \bar{C}, \bar{D}} \gamma, \tag{97.11}$$

$$\begin{bmatrix} \gamma & \bar{x}(kT)^T V_1 \\ V_1^T \bar{x}(kT) & W \end{bmatrix} \geq 0, \tag{97.12}$$

$$\begin{bmatrix} \bar{W}^T \bar{A}^T + \bar{A}\bar{W} & \bar{B} & \bar{W}^T \bar{D}^T & \bar{W}^T \bar{C}^T \\ \bar{B}^T & -\frac{1}{\varepsilon}I & 0 & 0 \\ \bar{D}\bar{W} & 0 & -\varepsilon I & 0 \\ \bar{C}\bar{W} & 0 & 0 & -\gamma I \end{bmatrix} < 0. \tag{97.13}$$

where $\bar{W} = \gamma P^{-1}$.

Proof. Minimizing $V(\bar{x}(t)) = \bar{x}(t)^T \bar{E}^T P \bar{x}(t)$ is equal to

$$\min_{\gamma, P} \gamma \tag{97.14}$$
$$s.t\, \bar{x}(t)^T \bar{E}^T P \bar{x}(t) \leq \gamma,$$

Multiply P^{-T}, P^{-1} both sides of (97.9), and let $Z = P^{-T}$, we obtain

$$ZE^T = EZ^T, \tag{97.15}$$

Form Lemma 2, $P = Z^{-T} = (EV_1 W V_1^T + SV_2^T)^{-T} = U_1 \hat{W} U_1^T E + U_2 \hat{S}$, where $\hat{W} = \Sigma_r^{-1} W^{-1} \Sigma_r^{-1}, \hat{S} = U_2^T (EV_1 W V_1^T + SV_2^T)^{-T}$, and $U_1^T E = U_1^T U \begin{bmatrix} \Sigma_r & 0 \\ 0 & 0 \end{bmatrix} V^T = \Sigma_r V_1^T$, $U_2^T E = 0$, then $\bar{x}(kT)^T E^T P \bar{x}(kT) = \bar{x}(kT)^T E^T U_1 \hat{W} U_1^T E \bar{x}(kT) = \bar{x}(kT)^T V_1 W^{-1} V_1^T \bar{x}(kT) \leq \gamma$.

By using the Schur complement lemma, linear matrix inequality (97.12) is proofed.

By the state equation (97.6) and (97.10), we get

$$[\bar{A} + \bar{B}\Delta\bar{D}]^T P + P^T[\bar{A} + \bar{B}\Delta\bar{D}] + \bar{C}^T \bar{C} \leq 0, \tag{97.16}$$

Pre- and post-multiplying both sides of (97.16) by P^{-T}, P^{-1}, respectively, and let $\bar{W} = \gamma P^{-1}$, we obtain

$$\bar{W}^T\bar{A}^T + \bar{A}\bar{W} + \frac{1}{\gamma}\bar{W}^T\bar{C}^T\bar{C}\bar{W} + \bar{W}^T\bar{D}^T\Delta^T\bar{B}^T + \bar{B}\Delta\bar{D}\bar{W} < 0,$$

Form Lemma 1, it is noted that there exist a constant $\varepsilon > 0$, such that

$$\bar{W}^T\bar{A}^T + \bar{A}\bar{W} + \frac{1}{\gamma}\bar{W}^T\bar{C}^T\bar{C}\bar{W} + \varepsilon\bar{B}\bar{B}^T + \varepsilon^{-1}\bar{W}^T\bar{D}^T\bar{D}\bar{W} < 0.$$

By using the Schur complement lemma, the up formula is equivalent to (97.13). The proof of the theorem is completed.

97.3.2 Strict Output Feedback Robust Predictive Control

In inequality (97.13), the coefficient matrixes A_c, B_c, C_c are coupled together with other variables by the nonlinear way, so, they are not determined directly. In the following, using the thought of variables transformation [11] to decouple it, we can translate (97.13) into linear matrix inequality.

Firstly, resolving the matrixes $\bar{W}, \bar{W}^{-1}$ as following

$$\bar{W} = \begin{bmatrix} \bar{W}_{11} & \bar{W}_{12} \\ \bar{W}_{21} & \bar{W}_{22} \end{bmatrix}, \bar{W}^{-1} = \begin{bmatrix} \bar{P}_{11} & \bar{P}_{12} \\ \bar{P}_{21} & \bar{P}_{22} \end{bmatrix}.$$

Where $\bar{P}_{11}, \bar{W}_{11} \in R^{2r \times 2r}$ are symmetric matrixes. By $\bar{W}\bar{W}^{-1} = I$, we get
$$\bar{W}\begin{bmatrix} \bar{P}_{11} \\ \bar{P}_{21} \end{bmatrix} = \begin{bmatrix} I \\ 0 \end{bmatrix},$$
then, we obtain

$$\bar{W}\begin{bmatrix} \bar{P}_{11} & I \\ \bar{P}_{21} & 0 \end{bmatrix} = \begin{bmatrix} I & \bar{W}_{11} \\ 0 & \bar{W}_{21} \end{bmatrix}.$$

Suppose $\Psi = \begin{bmatrix} \bar{P}_{11} & I \\ \bar{P}_{21} & 0 \end{bmatrix}, \zeta = \begin{bmatrix} I & \bar{W}_{11} \\ 0 & \bar{W}_{21} \end{bmatrix}$, then $\bar{W}\psi = \zeta$. Though simple matrix operation, we get

$$\psi^T\bar{W}\zeta = \zeta^T\psi = \begin{bmatrix} \bar{P}_{11} & I_{2r} \\ I_{2r} & \bar{W}_{11} \end{bmatrix}.$$

Pre- and post- multiplying both side of (97.9) by Ψ^T, Ψ, respectively, then (97.9) is equivalent

$$\begin{bmatrix} I_{2r} & 0 \\ 0 & I_{2r}^T \end{bmatrix}\begin{bmatrix} \frac{1}{\gamma}\bar{W}_{11} & I \\ I & \gamma\bar{P}_{11} \end{bmatrix} = \begin{bmatrix} \frac{1}{\gamma}\bar{W}_{11}^T & I \\ I & \gamma\bar{P}_{11}^T \end{bmatrix}\begin{bmatrix} I_{2r}^T & 0 \\ 0 & I_{2r} \end{bmatrix}, \quad (97.17)$$

$$\bar{W}_{11}^T \bar{P}_{11} = I_{2r} - \bar{W}_{21}^T \bar{P}_{21}. \tag{97.18}$$

Let

$$\begin{cases} \hat{A} = \bar{P}_{11} A \bar{W}_{11} + \bar{P}_{21} A_c \bar{W}_{21} + \hat{B} C \bar{W}_{11} + \hat{B} C_q \hat{C} + \bar{P}_{11} B \hat{C} \\ \hat{B} = \bar{P}_{21} B_c \\ \hat{C} = C_c \bar{W}_{21}^T \end{cases}, \tag{97.19}$$

where positive definite matrix $\bar{P}_{11}, \bar{W}_{11}$ and invertible matrix $\bar{P}_{21}, \bar{W}_{21}$ are given, then matrix A_c, B_c and C_c can be determined by $\hat{A}, \hat{B}, \hat{C}$.

Theorem 2 For the structured uncertain singular system (97.2) and performance index (97.7), at sampling time kT, if there exist a output feedback robust model predictive controller (97.5), such that the upper bound of performance index is minimum, then the following LMI problem exist optimization solution $\hat{A}, \hat{B}, \hat{C}, \bar{P}_{11}, \bar{W}_{11}$, and the coefficient matrix A_c, B_c, C_c of output feedback controller are given by (97.19).

$$\min_{\gamma, \varepsilon, \lambda, W, \hat{A}, \hat{B}, \hat{C}, \bar{P}_{11}, \bar{W}_{11}} \gamma + \varepsilon + \lambda, \tag{97.20}$$

$$\begin{bmatrix} \gamma & \bar{x}(kT)^T V_1 \\ V_1^T \bar{x}(kT) & W \end{bmatrix} \geq 0, \tag{97.21}$$

$$\begin{bmatrix} \lambda & 1 \\ 1 & \varepsilon \end{bmatrix} \geq 0, \tag{97.22}$$

$$\begin{bmatrix} H_{11} & H_{12} \\ H_{12}^T & H_{22} \end{bmatrix} < 0. \tag{97.23}$$

Where $H_{11} = \begin{bmatrix} H_{11}^1 & A^T + \hat{A} \\ A + \hat{A}^T & H_{11}^2 \end{bmatrix}$, $H_{12} = \begin{bmatrix} \bar{P}_{11} B_p & C_p^T & R^{1/2} & 0 \\ B_p & \bar{W}_{11} C_p^T + \hat{C}^T D_{qu}^T & \bar{W}_{11} R^{1/2} & \hat{C}^T Q^{1/2} \end{bmatrix}$,

$H_{22} = diag\{-\lambda I, -\varepsilon I, -\gamma I, -\gamma I\}, H_{11}^1 = \bar{P}_{11} A + A^T \bar{P}_{11} + \hat{B} C + C^T \hat{B}^T$

$H_{11}^2 = A \bar{W}_{11} + \bar{W}_{11} A^T + B \hat{C} + \hat{C}^T B^T$

97.4 Robust Stability Analyses

According to robust predictive controller design method proposed by theorem 2, we can give the coefficient matrix A_c, B_c, C_c of output feedback controller at the time kT, when k from 0 to ∞, a subsection continuous feedback sequence $\{A_c^k, B_c^k, C_c^k\}$ can be obtained. By lemma 3, if the solution is feasible at sampling time, then the solution of the optimization problem (97.20)–(97.23) is feasible at any time. Putting the control sequence $\{A_c^k, B_c^k, C_c^k\}$ into system (97.2), the closed-loop system can be expressed as

$$\bar{E}_k \dot{\bar{x}}(t) = (\bar{A}_k + \bar{B}_k \Delta \bar{D}_k)\bar{x}(t), \ t \in [kT, (k+1)T], k \geq 0. \tag{97.24}$$

Theorem 3 If the optimization problem (97.20)–(97.23) has the feasible solution at the initial time, then the closed-loop system (97.24) is asymptotic stable, and holds the regular, impulse-free, where the parameter of the controller $\{A_c^k, B_c^k, C_c^k\}$ are determined by (97.19).

97.5 Simulation Examples

Consider the following uncertain singular system

$$E\dot{x}(t) = \begin{bmatrix} 1 & 0.1 \\ 0 & 0.1 - 0.01\alpha(t) \end{bmatrix} x(t) + \begin{bmatrix} 1 \\ -0.2 \end{bmatrix} u(t)$$

$$y(t) = [1 \ 0] x(t)$$

Where $\alpha(t)$ is uncertain parameters and satisfies $0.1 \leq \alpha(t) \leq 10$.
Let $\Delta(t) = \frac{\alpha(t) - 5.05}{4.95}$, then follows $|\Delta(t)| \leq 1$. The system described by structured feedback uncertainty is

$$A = \begin{bmatrix} 1 & 0.1 \\ 0 & 0.0495 \end{bmatrix}, B = \begin{bmatrix} 1 \\ -0.2 \end{bmatrix}, B_p = \begin{bmatrix} 0 \\ -0.1 \end{bmatrix},$$

$$C = [1 \ 0], C_p = [0 \ 0.495], C_q = [0 \ 0], D_{qu} = \begin{bmatrix} 0 \\ 0 \end{bmatrix}.$$

If initial state $x(0) = [-49.5]^T$, and also let $R = I, Q = I$, sampling period according $T = 0.5s$, by theorem 1, using the *gevp* of LMI tool-box to solve inequality (97.20–97.23), and by (97.18), (97.19), we obtain the coefficient matrix of output feedback controller are

$$A_c = \begin{bmatrix} 0.8147 & -0.1270 \\ -0.9058 & 0.9134 \end{bmatrix}, B_c = \begin{bmatrix} 0.6324 \\ -0.0975 \end{bmatrix}, C_c = [0.2785 \ 0.5469].$$

Substituting A_c, B_c, C_c into (97.5), we obtain the control signal, the output path, the state path, which are shown in Fig. 97.2 and Fig. 97.3 respectively. The simulation results indicate that when the system states are not completely measured, using the method proposed in this note can make the states of the structured feedback uncertain singular system gradually towards zero, and the system is asymptotically stable.

Fig. 97.2 The control input

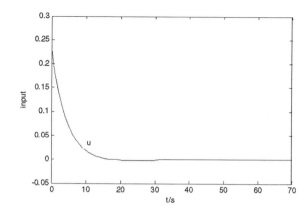

Fig. 97.3 The states of closed-loop system

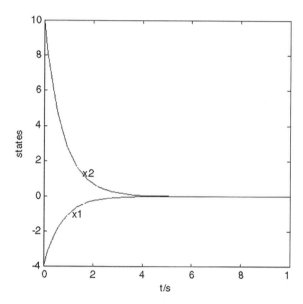

97.6 Conclusions

This paper considers singular system with structured feedback uncertainty described by linear fractional model, when the system contains parametric and dynamic uncertainties meanwhile. The output feedback robust predictive control is investigated based on the idea of variable transformation and LMI methods. The robust stability and the regular and the impulse-free of generalized closed-loop system are guaranteed. Finally, we present a simulation example to show the effectiveness of the algorithm proposed in the paper.

Acknowledgments This work is supported by National Nature Science Foundation under Grant 61174097.

References

1. Marija D, Marko S (2009) Singular systems, state feedback problem. Linear Algebra Appl 4(24):1267–1292
2. Kothare MV, Balakrishnan V, Morari M (1996) Robust constrained model predictive control using linear matrix inequalities. Automatica 32(10):1361–1379
3. Kouvaritakis B, Rossiter JA, Schuurmans J (2000) Efficient robust predictive control. IEEE Trans Autom Control 45(8):1545–154
4. Lee YI, Kouvaritakis B (2006) Constrained robust model predictive control based on periodic invariance. Automatica 42(12):2175–2181
5. Francesco A, Cuzzola J, Geromel C, Manfred M (2002) An improved approach for constrained robust model predictive control. Automatica 38(7):1183–1189
6. Zhang L, Huang B (2004) Robust model predictive control of singular systems. IEEE Trans Autom Control 49(6):1000–1006
7. Liu XH, Wang LJ (2009) Robust model predictive control for singular systems via dynamic output feedback. Control Decision 24(9):1371–1376
8. Lee SM, Park JH (2007) Output feedback model predictive control for LPV systems using parameter dependent Lyapunov function. Appl Math Comput 190(1):671–676

Chapter 98
Image Enhancement Methods for a Customized Videokeratography System Designed for Animals with Small Eyes

Bin Chen, Shan Ling, Hongfei Cen, Wenfu Xu, Kee Chea-su, Yongjin Zhou and Lei Wang

Abstract We built a Placido's disc videokeratographic system intended for eye examination of small animals. To derive the corneal topology and other corneal biometric parameters we rely on precise extraction of Placido ring patterns. However, since the images from CCD are noisy, image enhancement is necessary as a pre-processing procedure in order to prevent further noise magnification during the corneal surface topography reconstruction. In this study, two popular image enhancement methods, namely Gabor Filtering (GF) and Multiscale Vessel Enhancement Filtering (MVEF), are quantitatively evaluated in the context of image enhancement before corneal reconstruction. The two methods were tested on 21 images of steel balls with different diameters. Both methods have been

B. Chen · S. Ling · Y. Zhou (✉) · L. Wang
Shenzhen Institutes of Advanced Technology, Chinese Academy of Sciences, Shenzhen, People's Republic of China
e-mail: yj.zhou@siat.ac.cn

B. Chen · W. Xu
Harbin Institute of Technology Shenzhen Graduate School, Shenzhen, People's Republic of China

S. Ling
School of Geosciences and Info-Physics, Central South University, Changsha, People's Republic of China

H. Cen
Peking University Shenzhen Hospital, Shenzhen 518036, People's Republic of China

K. Chea-su
School of Optometry, Hong Kong Polytechnic University, Hong Kong, People's Republic of China

Y. Zhou · L. Wang
The Shenzhen Key Laboratory for Low-cost Healthcare, Shenzhen, People's Republic of China

Y. Zhou
Interdisciplinary Division of Biomedical Engineering, The Hong Kong Polytechnic University, Hong Kong, People's Republic of China

demonstrated to be useful for Placido ring extraction; however, the GF method showed better performance on images of steel balls with smaller diameter. Compared to the GF method, the MVEF method performed better on images of steel balls with larger diameter. The result of the present work implies that the two methods should be used cooperatively.

Keywords Videokeratography · Gabor filtering · Multiscale vessel enhancement filtering

98.1 Introduction

The study of human corneal surface topography is usually predicated on the study of animal cornea surface topography model. Previous researches [1–3] showed that almost all the astigmatism of animals that induced by sphericity and astigmatic lens are corneal-originated, and more detailed information of cornea should be provided to make further study of astigmatism mechanism. Generally, static measurements for corneal surface topography could be evaluated based on a Placido disc pattern in the image data obtained using videokeratography System. In such a system, a set of concentric rings formed in a bowl can be projected on the anterior surface of the cornea and its reflection is imaged onto a CCD [4]. For the previous study of animal corneal, the system designed by the size of human eyes was directly used for the estimation of animal cornea surface topography [5–11], which caused some limitations to the measurement results. Recently, a new videokeratography system was designed specifically for small animals' eyes, which improved techniques for accurate estimations of corneal surface topography.

The recognition and location of placid-rings in videokeratoscopic images are essential in the process of estimating corneal topography. However, due to the presence of strong interference from eyelashes and instabilities in tear film under the limits of the instrumentation, the acquired videokeratoscopic images may contain a mass of noises, which leads to poorer estimates of corneal topography [12]. Thus, it is necessary to implement a reliable image enhancement operation as a pre-processing step for accurate measurement of corneal topography. Gabor Filtering (GF) [13–18] and Multiscale Vessel Enhancement Filtering (MVEF) [19, 20] are both popular enhancement methods for alternating textures, and this study makes a comparison to evaluate their performance in a customized videokeratography system designed for animals with small eyes.

98.2 Methods

98.2.1 Gabor Filtering

A 2D Gabor filter is modulated by a Gaussian kernel, consists of a complex sinusoidal plane wave. It is sensitive to wavelength and orientation, which makes it suitable for applications such as texture segmentation [15, 21–23], fingerprint image enhancement [24], and edge detection [25].

The 2D Gabor filter can be defined as [12],

$$f[n, m; \theta, \lambda, \sigma_n, \sigma_m] = \exp\left(-\frac{1}{2}\left\{\frac{R_1^2}{\sigma_n^2} + \frac{R_2^2}{\sigma_m^2}\right\}\right) \exp\left(i\frac{2\pi R_1}{\lambda}\right) \quad (98.1)$$

where $R_1 = n\cos\theta + m\sin\theta$ and $R_2 = -n\sin\theta + m\cos\theta$. λ and θ are the wavelength and orientation of the sinusoidal plane wave, respectively. σ_n and σ_m are the standard deviations of the Gaussian envelope along the n- and m-axes, respectively.

98.2.2 Multiscale Vessel Enhancement Filtering

The MVEF method was proposed by Alejandro F. Frangi in 1998. Inspired by former reasearcher, Frangi used all the eigenvalues of the Hessian to determine locally the likelihood that a vessel was present. For the 2D images, the vesselness function could be defined as,

$$V_o(\sigma) = \begin{cases} 0 \text{ if } \lambda_2 > 0, \\ \exp\left(-\frac{R_B^2}{2\beta^2}\right)\left(1 - \exp\left(\frac{S^2}{2c^2}\right)\right) \end{cases} \quad (98.2)$$

where λ_2 is one of the eigenvalues, the other is $\lambda_1 \cdot |\lambda_1| < |\lambda_2|$, $R_B = |\lambda_1|/|\lambda_2|$, and $S = \sqrt{\lambda_1^2 + \lambda_2^2} \cdot \beta$ and c are thresholds which control the sensitivity of the line filter to the measure R_B and S.

For the linear structure, based on the scale space theory, we get the maximum output of the filter when σ matches the real thickness of vessel. MVEF can get several V_o on different scale σ, in which the maximal V_o will be the output.

98.2.3 Experimental Procedure

A Placido disc based videokeratography system was custom made for small animals' eyes. The system was made up of a dome (80 mm in radius) with an inner aperture of 12 mm diameter to house a telecentric imaging system. The dome surface has 16 bright rings interspaced with 15 dark rings concentric to the inner aperture, illuminated by white LEDs arranged for evenness of illumination (see Fig. 98.1a). To align the center of Placido rings with the subject's pupil center, four infrared LEDs were installed at the outer perimeter of the dome to illuminate the pupil. These LEDs can be switched off independently once a good alignment was achieved (Fig. 98.1b). Another four red LEDs were installed near the inner aperture, served as central fixation targets to attract chick's attention and can also be switched off independently. Once the image was aligned and sharply focused, the alignment LEDs were switched off and a series of images were captured in multiple-shot mode (frame rate up to 53 frame per second) using the software (AVT FirePackage version 3.0) provided by the CCD camera (Guppy AVT F-046, Edmund Optics, NJ, USA).

The diameters of curvature was obtained with a set of four standard chromium steel balls (Grade 25, AISI 52100) of known diameters that cover the range of corneal diameters in young chicks ('2.0, '3.0, '4.0, '5.0 mm'; Amazon.com, USA). The steel ball was fixed on a platform and its surface was cleaned with alcohol and dried with cotton rod before measurement. Twenty-one images were used in the study, including seven images of steel ball with diameter of 2.0 mm, five with diameter of 3.0 mm, four with diameter of 4.0 mm and five with diameter of 5.0 mm. A user interface written in Matlab software (Version 7.12, MathWorks, Inc., Massachusetts, USA) had been serving for the whole research.

To reduce the difficulty and increase the efficiency of image process, images were cropped to keep a region of interest (ROI) only. Only nine innermost rings were used for evaluation since that the bottom part of cornea with large diameters may not get imaged properly due to a flaw in mounting design for the steel balls. The flowchart of image processing in this study was shown in Fig. 98.2.

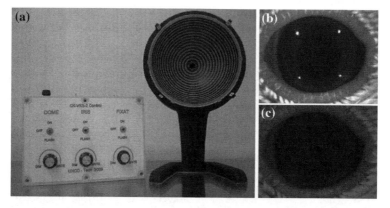

Fig. 98.1 a Setup of the videokeratography system which composed of a measuring dome and a control panel. **b** The alignment of the Placido rings with the pupil was assisted with the four LEDs. **c** Image used for analysis was taken with the alignment LEDs turned off

98 Image Enhancement Methods

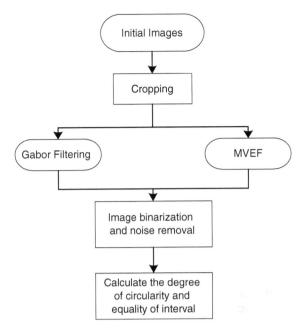

Fig. 98.2 The flowchart of the proposed strategy for experiment

Each image was first processed using the two methods respectively and then binarized with threshold value obtained by using Hui-Fuang Ng's method [26, 27]. Subsequently, a morphological opening operation was applied on the binarized image and regions with areas smaller than an appropriate threshold would be removed as noises. Finally, widths of rings were thinned to one pixel to reduce the computation. Two criteria, degree of circularity (DOC) and equality of interval (EOI), were designed in this paper to assess the two image enhancement methods. The mean radius of the jth ring was determined first as:

$$R_j = \sum_{i=1}^{n_j} \sqrt{(x_i - x_0)^2 + (y_i - y_0)^2} / n_j \qquad (98.3)$$

where (x_0, y_0) represented the centroid of the concentric circles, n_j was the pixel number of the jth ring. So the variance of radii on jth ring was:

$$V_j = \sum_{i=1}^{n_j} \left[\sqrt{(x_i - x_0)^2 + (y_i - y_0)^2} - R_j \right] / n_j \qquad (98.4)$$

Then the degree of circularity (DOC) could be given by:

$$\text{DOC} = 1 - \sum_{j=1}^{m} \frac{V_j}{m} \qquad (98.5)$$

where m represented the number of rings. The mean value of distances between each ring and its adjacent rings could be represented as:

$$D = \sum_{j=1}^{m-1} \frac{R_{j+1} - R_j}{m-1} \qquad (98.6)$$

Finally, the equality of interval (EOI) could be determined as:

$$\text{EOI} = 1 - \sum_{j=1}^{m-1} \left[(R_{j+1} - R_j) - D \right]^2 / (m-1) \qquad (98.7)$$

Both EOI and DOC take 1 as the ideal value, and larger value indicated better performance.

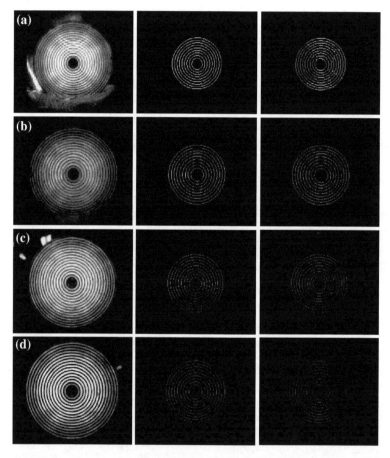

Fig. 98.3 Ring extraction results of four representative videokeratography images using GF or MVEF method, where (a)-(d) represent images of steel balls with diameter of 2.0, 3.0, 4.0 and 5.0 mm respectively. Initial images of steel ball with various diameters are shown in the first column and images of ring extraction using GF and MVEF method are shown in the second and third columns respectively

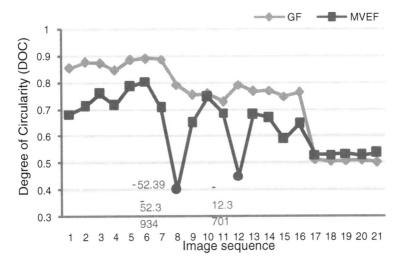

Fig. 98.4 Calculated results of DOC of images obtained by GF and MVEF

98.3 Results and Discussion

Ring extraction results of four representative videokeratography images are shown in Fig. 98.3. The initial images of steel balls with various diameters are shown in the first column, and their results of ring extraction using GF and MVEF are shown in the second and third column respectively.

It can be seen from Fig. 98.4 that GF method performs better than MVEF method on the first sixteen images of steel balls with small diameters ('2.0, '3.0,

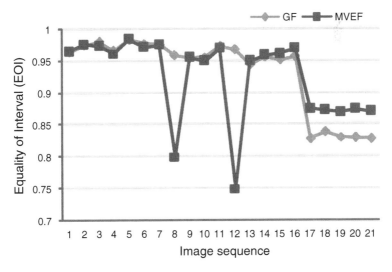

Fig. 98.5 Calculated results of EOI of images obtained by GF and MVEF methods

and '4.0 mm', respectively) in term of DOC, especially in image #8 and image #12 whose DOC values obtained by MVEF are much smaller than GF. But for the last five images of steel balls with big diameters ('5.0 mm'), MVEF method does better than GF. Calculated results of EOI of images obtained by GF and MVEF methods are displayed in Fig. 98.5. Numeral differences of EOI between the two methods are much smaller than those of DOC shown in Fig. 98.4. But similar with DOC, the EOI obtained by MVEF method in image #8 and #12 also have pretty smaller values than those of GF method.

The computation costs for both methods were also computed. GF required 5.5 ± 3.4 s and MVEF required 0.2 ± 0.1 s respectively. MVEF had shown significant advantage in terms of computation cost in all sizes of steel balls.

98.4 Conclusion

For a customized Placido disc videokeratography system, which is built for small animals' eyes, both GF method and MVEF method are used to enhance images before ring extractions. Experiments showed that the GF method performed better on images of steel balls with smaller diameters, but the deviation decreased sharply when it was used to process images of steel balls with larger diameters. MVEF method performed better for steel balls with larger diameters. In addition, MVEF ran much faster than GF method. Therefore, two methods could be used in a cooperative strategy according to the size of tested animal's eyes and the needs of processing speed.

Acknowledgments This work is supported in part by grants from National Natural Science Foundation of China (NSFC: 81171402, 61103165), the next generation communication technology Major project of National S&T(2013ZX03005013), Guangdong Innovative Research Team Program (GIRTF-LCHT, No. 2011S013), Low-cost Healthcare Programs of Chinese Academy of Sciences and International Science and Technology Cooperation Program of Guangdong Province (2012B050200004) and Shenzhen Key Laboratory for Low-cost Healthcare (CXB201005260056A).

References

1. Kee CS, Deng Li (2008) Astigmatism associated with experimentally induced myopia or hyperopia in chickens. Invest Ophthalmol Vis Sci 49(3): 858–867
2. Kee CS, Huang LF, Qiao-Grider Y (2003) Astigmatism in infant monkeys reared with cylindrical lenses. Vision Res 43(26):2721–2739
3. Schmid K, Wildsoet CF (1997) Natural and imposed astigmatism and their relation to emmetropization in the chick. Exp Eye Res 64(5):837–847
4. Alonso-Caneiro D, Iskander DR, Collins MJ (2008) Computationally efficient interference detection in videokeratoscopy images. In: 2008 IEEE 10th Workshop on Multimedia Signal Processing, pp 486–490 Oct 2008

5. Zhong X, Ge J, Smith EL 3rd (2004) Compensation for experimentally induced hyperopic anisometropia in adolescent monkeys. Invest Ophthalmol Vis Sci 45(10):3373–3379
6. Paulino LV, Paulino E, Barros RA, Salles AG, Rehder JR (2005) Corneal topographic alteration after radiofrequency application to an animal model. Arq Bras Oftalmolog 68(4):451–456
7. Norton TT, Amedo AO, Siegwart JT Jr (2006) Darkness causes myopia in visually experienced tree shrews. Invest Ophthalmol Vis Sci 47(11):4700–4707
8. Hanuch OE, Agrawal VB, Bassage S, delCerro M, Aquavella JV (1998) Myopic picosecond laser keratomileusis with the neodymium-yttrium lithium fluoride laser in the cat cornea. Ophthalmology 105(1):142–149
9. Busin M, Yau CW, Yamaguchi T, McDonald MB, Kaufman HE (1986) The effect of collagen cross-linkage inhibitors on rabbit corneas after radial keratotomy. Invest Ophthalmol Vis Sci 27(6):1001–1005
10. Carrington SD, Woodward EG (1984) Woodward, The topography of the anterior surface of the cat's cornea. Curr Eye Res 3(6):823–826
11. Oshita T, Hayashi S, Inoue T, Hayashi A, Maeda N, Kusaka S, Ohji M, Fujikado T, Tano Y (2001) Topographic analysis of astigmatism induced by scleral shortening in pig eyes. Graefe's Arch Clin Exp Ophthalmol 239(5):382–386
12. Alonso-Caneiro D, Iskander DR, Collins MJ (2008) Estimating Corneal Surface Topography in Videokeratoscopy in the Presence of Strong Signal Interference. IEEE Trans Biomed Eng 55(10):2381–2387
13. Gabor D (1946) Theory of communication. Part 1: The analysis of information. J Ins Electr Eng 93(26):429–441
14. Daugman JG (1988) Complete discrete 2-D Gabor transforms by neural networks for image analysis and compression. IEEE Trans Acoust Speech Signal Process 36(7):1169–1179
15. Dunn D, Higgins WE (1995) Optimal Gabor filters for texture segmentation. IEEE Trans Image Process 4(7):947–964
16. Dunn D, Higgins WE, Wakeley J (1994) Texture segmentation using 2-D Gabor elementary functions. IEEE Trans Pattern Anal Mach Intell 16(2):130–149
17. Zhou Y, Zheng Y-P (2009) Enhancement of muscle fibers in ultrasound images using gabor filters. In: Ultrasonics Symposium (IUS), 2009 IEEE International, pp 2296–2299
18. Zhou Yongjin, Zheng Yong-ping (2011) Longitudinal enhancement of the hyperechoic regions in ultrasonography of muscles using a gabor filter bank approach: a preparation for semi-automatic muscle fiber orientation estimation. Ultrasound Med Biol 37(4):665–673
19. Frangi AF, Wiro JN, Koen LV, Max AV (1998) Multiscale vessel enhancement filtering. Lect Notes Comput Sci, vol 1496, pp 130–137
20. Wink O, Niessen WJ, Viergever MA (2004) Multiscale vessel tracking. IEEE Trans Med Imagin 23(1):130–133
21. Weldon TP, Higgins WE, Dunn DF (1996) Gabor filter design for multiple texture segmentation. Opt Eng 10(35):2852–2863
22. Jain AK, Farrokhnia F (1991) Unsupervised texture segmentation using Gabor filters. Pattern Recogn 24(12):1167–1186
23. Teuner A, Pichler O, Hosticka BJ (1995) Unsupervised texture segmentation of images using tuned matched gabor filters. IEEE Trans Image Process 4(6):863–870
24. Yang J, Liu L, Jiang T, Fan Y (2003) A modified Gabor filter design method for fingerprint image enhancement. Pattern Recogn Lett 24(12):1805–1817
25. Mehrotra R, Namuduri KR, Ranganathan N (1992) Gabor filter-based edge detection. Pattern Recogn 25(12):1479–1494
26. Ng H-F (2006) Automatic thresholding for defect detection. Pattern Recogn Lett 27(14):1644–1649
27. Otsu N (1979) A threshold selection method from gray-level histograms. IEEE Trans Syst Man Cybern 9(1):62–66

Chapter 99
Cloning and Expression of Catechol 2,3-dioxygenase from *Achromobacter Xylosoxidans* LHB21

Shuang Yu, Naiyu Chi and QingFang Zhang

Abstract *Achromobacter xylosoxidans* LHB21 isolated from a cold oil-contaminated site could utilize alkanes from pentadecane (C_{15}) to dotriacontane (C_{32}) as the sole carbon source and energy. The C23O gene was cloned and sequenced. Nucleotide sequence analysis of the C23O gene revealed a 924 base pairs open reading frame (ORF) initiating at ATG and terminating at TGA which predicted a protein of 35.16 kDa containing 307 amino acid residues. By comparison, the C23O of *A. xylosoxidans* LHB21 showed 44–100 % identity in amino acid sequence with other C23Os. The C23O gene was overexpressed in *E. coli* BL21(DE3) and the gene product was identified by SDS-PAGE and Western blotting.

Keywords Catechol 2,3-dioxygenase · *Achromobacter xylosoxidans* LHB21 · Cloning · Overexpression

99.1 Introduction

Polycyclic aromatic compounds (PAHs) are ubiquitous environmental pollutants that have been found to have toxic, mutagenic, and carcinogenic properties [1]. The key step in the degradation of PAHs is the opening of the stable aromatic ring.

S. Yu · N. Chi · Q. Zhang (✉)
School of Life Science and Biotechnology, Dalian University, Liaoning Marine Microbial Engineering and Technology Center, Dalian, China
e-mail: zqf7566@126.com

S. Yu
e-mail: yushuang119@yahoo.cn

N. Chi
e-mail: cny7566@126.com

Catechol itself is an intermediate in the microbial degradation of many different PAHs. Ring cleavage of catechol, catalyzed by C23O, which plays an important role in the environment protection [2]. In this study, a psychrophilic oil degrading bacterium, designated LHB21, was isolated from soil and identified as *Achromobacter xylosoxidans*. The C23O gene from *A. xylosoxidans* LHB21 was cloned and overexpressed in *E. coli*. As far as we know, this is the first reported of a C23O gene cloned from a psychrophilic bacterium and successfully expressed. The gene product was characterized by sodium dodecyl sulfate–polyacrylamide gel electrophoresis and western blotting. Furthermore, characterization of the C23O sequence enabled the construction of phylogenetic trees to evaluate the evolution of enzymes whose possible catalytic and structural roles are proposed.

99.2 Materials and Methods

99.2.1 Strains, Plasmids and Growth Conditions

Bacterial strains and plasmids used in this study are described in Table 99.1 *A. xylosoxidans* LHB21, a psychrophilic oil-degrading bacterium, was isolated from oil-contaminated soil. *E. coli* JM109 and pMD-19 simple T vector were used for cloning and sequencing, and *E. coli* BL21(DE3) and pET-32a(+) for expression. *E. coli* cells were cultivated in either Luria–Bertani (LB) medium or SOC medium [3] at 37 °C. Recombinants were selected on LB agar plates containing 100 μg/ml ampicillin.

Table 99.1 Strains and plasmids used in this study

Strain or plasmid	Relevant characteristics	Source or reference
Bacterial strains		
A. xylosoxidans LHB21	Oil-degrading isolate	This study
E.coli JM109	recA1, endA1, gyrA96, thi-1, hsdR17, supE44, relA1, Δ(lac-proAB)/F'[traD36, proAB +, lac Iq, lacZ ΔM15].	TaKaRa
E.coli BL21(DE3)	Ap^r, cloning vector	TaKaRa
pMD 19-T Simple Vector	Ap^r, Expression vector	TaKaRa
pET-32a(+)	Ap^r, Expression vector	Zhong et al. [19]
pDSFL17	Ap^r, pMD 19-T Simple Vector derivative carrying 924 bp C23O	This study
pDSFL01	Ap^r, pET-32a (+) derivative carrying 924 bp C23O	This study

99.2.2 Primers, Enzymes and Kits

Primers used in this study (Table 99.2) were designed based upon the conserved regions of C23O genes from organisms or vectors which produce C23O. Nco I and Hind III restriction endonucleases, PrimeSTAR HS DNA Polymerase, MiniBEST Bacterial Genomic DNA Extraction Kit Ver.2.0, Plasmid Purification Kit Ver.2.0, Agarose Gel DNA Purification Kit Ver.2.0, DNA Fragment Purification Kit Ver.2.0, DNA A-Tailing Kit and DNA Ligation Kit were purchased from Takara Biotech Co. Ltd (Dalian, China).

99.2.3 DNA Gene Cloning, Sequencing and Sequence Analysis

The C23O gene was cloned via three steps of nested PCR based on the conserved regions of homologous genes. Step One: The target gene was amplified with primers F/R. Step Two: PCR products from the first PCR reaction were subjected to a second PCR run however with three new set of primers F/YR3, YF3/YR3 and YF3/R2, respectively. Step Three: PCR products from step two were overlapped with primers F0/R0 which incorporated NcoI I and Hind III sites into their respective 5 ends. Subsequently, the PCR product dealed with TaKaRa DNA A-Tailing Kit was directionally cloned into the pMD19-T Simple Vector. The resulting plasmids were transformed into *E.coli* JM109. Positive clones was selected after cultivated on LB ampicillin-agar plates overnight at 37 °C.

For sequencing, plasmids DNA was prepared with TaKaRa Plasmid Purification Kit Ver.2.0. Sequencing of both strands of C23O gene was performed with ABI 3730xl Sequencer and BigDye Terminator v3.1 Cycle Sequencing Kit. Similarity searches was carried out with the Genebank database. Multiple sequence alignment was generated by Clustal X software Instead of simply listing headings of different levels we recommend that every. Phylogenetic tree was constructed using the neighbor-joining method with MEGA 3.1 program.

Table 99.2 Primers used in this study

Name	Sequence (5' → 3')	Orientation
F	ATGAACAAAGGTGTAATGCGAC	Sense
R	TCAGGTCAGCACGGTCATGAA	Antisens
YF2	TGTTCACCAAGGTGCTCGG.	Sense
YR2	GGTCGAAGAAGTAGATGGTC	Antisens
YF3	GCCTCCATCATGTGTCCTTC	Sense
YR3	TGTGTCGGTCATGGAGATCA	Antisens
R02	TCAGGTCAGCACGGTCATGAATCGTTCGTTGAGAAT	Antisens
F0	CCATGGCTATGAACAAAGGTGTAATGCGAC	Sense
R0	AAGCTTTCAGGTCAGCACGGTCATGAA	Antisens

99.2.4 Overexpression of C23O Gene in E. coli

The cloned C23O gene was digested with Nco I/Hind III and subcloned into the Nco I/Hind III site of pET-32a(+) to construct pDSFL01. The positive clones were verified by sequencing with primers T7/T7t. *E. coli* BL21(DE3) was transformed with pDSFL01 for expression, and with pET-32a(+) carrying no C23O gene as negative control. The transformants were cultivated in 2 ml of LB medium supplemented with 100 lg/ml ampicillin overnight at 37 °C. A 100 μl aliquot of the pre-culture was transferred to 6 ml fresh LB medium and further incubated to an OD_{600} of 0.55–0.7. Induction was brought about at 30 °C for 3 h by addition of isopropyl-β-D-thiogalactopyranoside (IPTG) to a final concentration of 1.0 mM. Then, cells were harvested by centrifugation and stored frozen at −25 °C.

99.2.5 SDS-PAGE and Western Blotting

Total cell extracts were prepared by resuspending *E. coli* cells in PBS buffer, followed by sonication and centrifugation. Proteins of total cellular were subjected to 5 × SDS sample buffer and heated at 95 °C for 10 min prior to subsequent analyses by SDS-PAGE. SDS-PAGE was carried out with 10 % polyacrylamide gel and Tris/glycine buffer, pH 8.3. After electrophoresis, SDS-PAGE gel was stained with Coomassie brilliant blue R250 and destained in ethanol/acetic acid/water (10:5:85) solution.

For Western blotting, the proteins were transferred to a PVDF membrane by electroblotting in transfer buffer for 80 min. The membrane was blocked in blocking buffer containing 1.5 % BSA at 4 °C overnight, and then incubated with penta-his antibody at proper dilution for 1 h. After washing, the blotting membrane were incubated with HRP-Rabbit anti mouse IgG, washed and visualized with TrueBlue peroxidase substrate.

99.3 Results

99.3.1 Cloning of the C23O Gene and Sequencing

The C23O gene was successfully amplified from start codon to stop codon via three steps of nested PCR using genomic DNA as template. The yield of PCR product and correct size was verified by the agarose gel electrophoresis (Fig. 99.1). Dealed with TaKaRa DNA A-Tailing Kit, the PCR product was ligated to pMD 19-T Simple Vector and transformed into *E.coli* JM109. Positive clones was selected and the plasmid DNA was extracted. Recombinant plasmid pDSFL17

Fig. 99.1 Agarose gel electrophoresis of PCR product. Lane 1, DL2, 000 DNA marker (bp); lane 2, PCR product

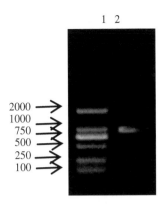

carrying C23O gene between NcoI I and Hind III was used as template to determine the sequence of C23O gene with BcaNEST sequencing primers RV-M and M13-47. These results are in agreement with our nucleotide sequence.

99.3.2 Sequence Analysis of the C23O Gene

Analysis of the nucleotide sequence revealed that the C23O gene encodes an ORF of 924 bp initiating at ATG and terminating at TGA. The C23O gene exhibited 57 % G + C content. As would be predicted from the high G + C content of the C23O gene, its codon usage is highly biased (72.1 %) in favour of G or C in the wobble base. The ORF predicted a polypeptide of 307 amino acids with a calculated molecular weight of 35.16 kDa. Homology searches with C23O sequence suggested that it exhibited 100 % identity with that from *P. putida* [4], and no less than 90 % identity with those from Pseudomonas sp. S-47 [5], *Pseudomonas sp.* OX1 [6] and *A. xylosoxidans* kf701 [7], But the identity was less than 45 % as compared to the corresponding enzymes of *B. cepacia* [8] and *Burkholderia sp.* 383 (YP_373719) (Table 99.3).

Alignment of the amino acid sequence of the C23O from *A. xylosoxidans* LHB21 with those of C23Os from *P. putida* KF715 [9], *P. putida* mt-2 [10], P. putida MT4 [11] and *Pseudomonas sp.*S-47 [5]revealed one hundred and fifty-nine amino acid residues were conserved, these conserved amino acid residues may be of catalytically and structurally importance. To explore the phylogenetic relationship among various extradiol dioxygenases, phylogenetic trees were constructed. The C23Os from *A. xylosoxidans* LHB21 and *P. putida* belong to the same branch on phylogenetic trees shown in Fig. 99.2. The C23Os were divided into two groups the members of each group exhibit greater homology among one another than to members of the other group. Group 1 belonged to the gamma subclass of Proteobacteria. Group 2 in belonged to the beta subclass of Proteobacteria.

Table 99.3 Identity of C23O from *A. xylosoxidans* LHB21 with other reported C23Os

Organism	Identity (%)	Accession no.	E-value
P. putida	100 %	NP_542866	0.0
Pseudomonas sp. S-47	99 %	AAF36683	0.0
Pseudomonas sp. OX1	95 %	CAD43168	6e-174
A. xylosoxidans kf701	92 %		1e-175
Burkholderia sp. 383	44 %	YP_373719	1e-69
B. cepacia AA1	43 %	AAB88079	3e-73

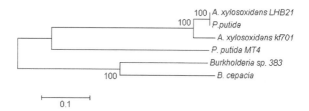

Fig. 99.2 Phylogenetic tree based on a distance matrix analysis of the C23O sequences. The numbers indicated at the nodes are bootstrap values calculated from 1000 replications with neighbor-joining method. The scale bar indicates 0.1 substitutions per amino acid site

99.3.3 Expression and Enzyme Assay of C23O

The C23O reading frame was cloned in-frame with pET-32a(+) reading frame and under transcriptional control of the IPTG-inducible T7 promoter in expression vector pET-32a(+). Crude lysate prepared from *E. coli* BL21(DE3) harboring pDSFL01 exhibited C23O specific activity of 32 U/mg protein. Analysis of the crude lysate by SDS-PAGE indicated an overexpressed protein band of 51.6 kDa which was the expected size of the C23O protein with an N-terminal His6-tag (Fig. 99.3). The fusion protein including soluble and insoluble was not detected in lanes 2, 3 and 4 comparing with lanes 5, 6 and 7, in which the band of the fusion protein was quite apparent, indicating that the protein had an overexpression in *E. coli* BL21(DE3). Western blotting using Penta-His Antibody followed by HRP-Rabbit Anti-Mouse IgG and TrueBlue Peroxidase as substrate validated the presence of the His-tag in the overexpressed protein (Fig. 99.4).

99.4 Discussion

In the oil degradation, C23O enzymatic activity from *A. xylosoxidans* LHB21 was detected. So, according to the high similarity of homologous genes, we successfully cloned the C23O gene from *A. xylosoxidans* LHB21 with primers designed base on the conserved regions of genes encoding C23Os, designated *xylE*, from

99 Cloning and Expression of Catechol 2,3-dioxygenase

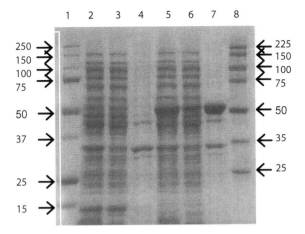

Fig. 99.3 SDS-PAGE analysis of overexpressed C23O from *E. coli* on a 10 % gel. Lanes 1 and 8 are Precision Plus Protein Standards and perfect protein marker(kDa), repectively; lanes 2, 3 and 4 are total proteins, soluble proteins and insoluble proteins of the *E. coli* BL21(DE3) harboring pET-32a(+) as control, respectively; lanes 5, 6 and 7 are total proteins, soluble proteins and insoluble proteins of *E. coli* BL21(DE3) harboring pDSFL01, respectively

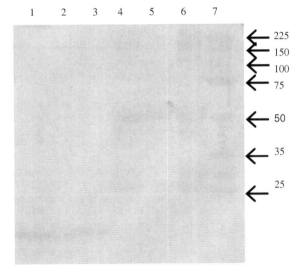

Fig. 99.4 Western blotting analysis of the expression of C23O proteins. Penta-His Antibody and HRP-Rabbit Anti-Mouse IgG were used. Lanes 1, 2 and 3 are total proteins, soluble proteins and insoluble proteins of the *E. coli* BL21(DE3) harboring pET-32a(+) as control, repectively; lanes 4, 5 and 6 are total proteins, soluble proteins and insoluble proteins of *E. coli* BL21 (DE3) harboring pDSFL01, respectively; lane 7 is perfect protein marker (kDa)

cloning vector pX1918G and pX1918GT [12], Suicide vector pMO90 [13], *Burkholderia* suicide vector pMo130 and Burkholderia replicative vector pMo168 [14] and *Pseudomonas sp.* S-47 [15]. Due to nonspecific amplication, we employed nested PCR to amplify the target gene.

For expression, two bases C and T were inserted before the C23O ORF to keep in-frame with pET-32a(+) reading frame. The C23O enzyme expressed in *E. coli* was the same as the one from *A. xylosoxidans* LHB21 in physical, chemical, and kinetic properties including subunit molecular weight, tetrameric structure, Fe2 + cofactor, amino acid composition, N-terminal sequence, substrate specificity, differing only in specific activity and iron content [7, 16].

The C23O protein is a member of the extradiol dioxygenase family. Comparison of the amino acid sequence of C23O with other extradiol-type dioxygenase whose structures have been characterized revealed that the amino acid residues were highly conserved (Fig. 99.2). Among the conserved amino acid residues His_{199}, His_{246} and Tyr_{255}, may be important for catalytic activities and His_{153}, His_{218} and Glu_{265} for metal binding ligands. One of the conserved histidine residues (His_{199}) seems to have important roles in the catalytic cycle. [5,11]. These residues are candidates for further site-directed mutagenesis experiments. The C23O is a homotetramers of four identical subunits, each with a non-heme ferrous ion of high spin state as a sole cofactor in the active site and 307 amino acids [17, 18]. The active site ferrous ion of this enzyme is easily oxidized to inactive the ferric form by various oxidizing agents, and could be reactivated by incubation with reducing agents [10]. In this study, the protein encoded by C23O gene we cloned from the isolate is only a subunit of the C23O tetramer.

References

1. Ahn Y, Saseverino J, Sayler GS (1999) Analysis of polycyclic aromatic hydrocarbon–degrading bacteria isolated from contaminated soils. Biodegradation 10:149–157
2. Parales RE, Ontl TA and Gibson DT (1997) Cloning and sequence analysis of a catechol 2,3-dioxygenase gene from the nitrobenzene-degrading strain comamonas sp JS765. J Ind Microbiol Biotechnol 19:385–391
3. Sun QY, Ding LW, He LL, Sun YB, Shao JL, Luo M and Xu ZF (2009) Culture of Escherichia coli in SOC medium improves the cloning efficiency of toxic protein genes. Anal Biochem 394:144–146
4. Greated A, Lambertsen L, Williams PA and Thomas CM (2002) Complete sequence of the IncP-9 TOL plasmid pWW0 from pseudomonas putida. Environ Microbiol 4:856–871
5. Noh SJ, Kim Y, Min KH Karegoudar TB and Kim CK (2000) Cloning and nucleotide sequence analysis of xylE gene responsible for meta-cleavage of 4-chlorocatechol from *Pseudomonas sp. S-47*. Mol Cells 10:475–479
6. Viggiani A, Siani L, Notomista E, Birolo L, Pucci P and Di Donato A (2004) The role of the conserved residues His-246, His-199, and Tyr-255 in the catalysis of catechol 2,3-dioxygenase from pseudomonas stutzeri OX1. J Biol Chem 279:48630–48639
7. Moon J, Min KR, Kim CK, Min KH and Kim Y (1996) Characterization of the gene encoding catechol 2,3-dioxygenase of *Alcaligenes sp. KF711*, overexpression, enzyme purification, and nucleotide sequencing 332:248–254
8. Ma Y, Herson DS (2000) The catechol 2,3-dioxygenase gene and toluene monooxygenase genes from *Burkholderia sp. AA1*, an isolate capable of degrading aliphatic hydrocarbons and toluene, J Ind Microbiol Biotechnol 25:127–131
9. Lee J, Oh J, Min KR, Kim CK (1996) Structure of catechol 2,3-dioxygenase gene encoded in chromosomal DNA of pseudomonas putida KF715. Biochem Biophys Res Commun 224:831–836

10. Bertini I, Briganti F, Scozzafava A (1994) Aliphatic and aromatic inhibitors binding to the active site of catechol 2,3-dioxygenase from pseudomonas putida mt-2. FEBS Lett 343:56–60
11. Takeo M, Prabu SK, Kitamura C, Hirai M, Takahashi H, Kato D, Negro S (2006) Characterization of alkylphenol degradation gene cluster in pseudomonas putida MT4 and evidence of oxidation of alkylphenols and alkylcatechols with medium-length alkyl chain, J Biosci Bioeng 102:352–361
12. Schweizer HP, Hoang TT (1995) An improved system for gene replacement and xylE fusion analysis in pseudomonas aeruginosa. Gene 158:15–22
13. Jones-Carson J, Laughlin J, Hamad MA, Stewart AL, Voskuil MI and Vazquez-Torres A (2008) Inactivation of [Fe-S] metalloproteins mediates nitric oxide-dependent killing of Burkholderia mallei, PLoS ONE, 3
14. Hamad MA, Zajdowicz SL, Holmes RK and Voskuil MI (2009) An allelic exchange system for compliant genetic manipulation of the select agents Burkholderia pseudomallei and Burkholderia mallei. Gene 430:123–131
15. Park DW, Kim Y, Lee SM, Ka Jo and Kim CK (2000) Cloning and sequence analysis of the xylL gene responsible for 4CBA-dihydrodiol dehydrogenase from *pseudomonas sp. S-47*, J Microbiol 38:275–280
16. Kobayashi T, Ishida T, Horiike K, Takahara Y, Numao N, Nakazawa T and Nozaki M (1995) Overexpression of pseudomonas putida catechol 2,3-dioxygenase with high specific activity by genetically engineered *escherichia coli*. J Biochem 117:614–622
17. Takeo M, Nishimura M, Shirai M, Takahashi H and Negro S (2007) Purification and characterization of catechol 2,3-dioxygenase from the aniline degradation pathway of acinetobacter sp. YAA and its mutant enzyme, which resists substrate inhibition. Biosci Biotechnol Biochem 71:1668–1675
18. Dai L, Ji CN, Gao DC and Wang J (2001) Modeling and analysis of the structure of the thermostable catechol 2,3-dioxygenase from Bacillus Stearothermophilus. J Biomol Struct Dyn 19:75–82

Chapter 100
Design of Trust Model Based on Behavior in Cloud Computing Environment

Yong Sheng Zhang, Ming Tian, Shen Juan Lv and Yan Dong Zhang

Abstract This paper studies the characteristics of cloud computing environment, based on the traditional access control management technology, proposes a reference model for access control management in the cloud computing, designs a model based on trust grade of behaviors and role control, its basic thought is through entity behaviors, or the results which entity's behaviors produced, and integrated calculation processing generates the entity of credible value, with this as basis determines or changes entity of trust grade, as to change the entity of role and authority, to reach the purpose of supervision and protection about single entity or even the whole cloud system.

Keywords Cloud computing · Role control · Trust · Behavior

100.1 Introduction

Cloud computing as a new information service model, although brings new security risks and challenges, its core demands are still the confidentiality of the data and applications, integrity, availability, and privacy protection, which is no

Y. Zhang · M. Tian (✉) · S. Lv · Y. Zhang
School of Information Science and Engineering, Shandong Provincial Key Laboratory for Novel Distributed Computer Software Technology, Shandong Normal University, Jinan 250014, China
e-mail: Tiancius@163.com

Y. Zhang
e-mail: zhangys@sdnu.edu.cn

S. Lv
e-mail: lvshenjuan2011@163.com

Y. Zhang
e-mail: 903874269@qq.com

essential difference between Information service of traditional IT security [1]. And the key technologies to meet these security requirements are access control technology. The following part will overview the existing mainstream access control [2].

100.1.1 Discretionary Access Control

Discretionary Access Control (DAC) [3] is on the basis of confirmed the main identity, corresponding to their identity and permissions for authorization. The basic idea of DAC is that the object owner decides the other permissions for that object, the owner can also grant the permission to other entity.

100.1.2 Mandatory Access Control

Mandatory Access Control (MAC) [4] is based on subject and object security properties to decide whether have the right of an access authorization. MAC's basic idea is that each subject and object has a security attribute label on their behalf. The security attributes of the subject reflect the main access permission levels, the security attributes of the object reflect the sensitivity of the object. MAC by comparing to the subject and object security attributes to determine whether users can gain access right.

100.1.3 Role-Based Access Control

Role-Based Access Control (RBAC) [5] establishes roles sets between user sets and permission sets, permission granted is a 2-step process. First of all, rights management sets' different roles depending on the application system of the organization, and establishes a mapping relationship between the roles and permissions: "role → right subset", in this relationship, the role becomes the owner of a subset of permissions. Second, different rights management according to the subject corresponds to the role assigned to it, which established a mapping relationship between the subject and the role: "object → role". In this relationship, the subject is the role of the consumer. Through the above 2 steps, RBAC can develop a mapping relationship between the subject and right: "subject → role → right subset" [6].

100.2 Design of a Trust Model Based on Behavior

100.2.1 The Definition of Trust

The so-called trust, it is easy to have some understanding, it is difficult to have a clear definition, particularly in the areas of information technology, quantitative description of the trust if you need to be, the social sciences, general definition of the nature of trust cannot be used directly [7]. Different people's understanding of trust are varied, this paper's definition of trust is as follows: if entity B strictly does what entity A desires B to act, then A trusts B [8]. Trust is differentiated, this paper uses trust value to measure trust degree, trust can step over from no trust to full trust, trust value from 0 to 1, of which 0 corresponds to no trust, 1 corresponds to full trust [9].

100.2.2 Design of Trust Model

This paper designs a model based on behaviors of trust grade and role control, its basic thought is through entity behaviors, or the results which entity's behaviors produced, and integrated calculation processing generates the entity of credible value, with this as basis determines or changes entity of trust grade, as to change the entity of role and authority, to reach the purpose of supervision and protection about single entity or even the whole cloud system. The basic principle of this model is shown in Fig. 100.1.

This model in the cloud server sets up a Trust Center to unified management entity's trust level. Users log on to the server after the authentication is completed, the Trust Center will look at the user's current level of trust. If the trust level is lower than the minimum service level (Minimum service levels, namely, trust level is very low, but still providing the critical level of service, if levels of trust still declines, it can reach the level of denial service, the server rejects the user's request) cloud server will deny access to cloud resources. In actual operation, when a user's last trust level is reduced to the minimum service level and denial of

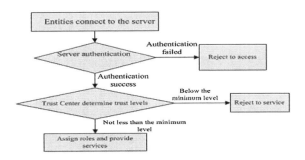

Fig. 100.1 The basic principle diagram

service level will receive a warning and downgrade cause notifications, if he has a question, can contact the managers. If the confidence level is classified as a service level, Trust Center will notify the system to provide appropriate services. Users in using cloud services, cloud system will monitor and audit user's behavior, such as entity attempts unauthorized operations, entity does DOS attacks and so on, will be recorded, through the analysis and calculations, change the trust value for the user, and have the potential to affect the levels of trust, and change user role properties, permissions will also be reassigned. The core of this model is through the entity's behavior can acquire the trust value and the change of levels of trust, thus affects user rights.

100.3 Calculation of Trust Value

100.3.1 The Acquirement of User's Behavior Evidence

Trusted value in this paper is based on the entity's behavior, or that is a result of user behavior. The result of user's behavior is a cloud service using entities in the process of using the cloud service provider resources, cloud services providers can base directly on the hardware and software testing and other methods, quantitative assessment of cloud-based services using entity overall trust value, it has the characteristics of objective and subjective, but it does not have a trust trait by itself. The results of user's behavior in some studies, also referred to as user behavior evidence, that can be directly obtained under testing of software and hardware to quantitatively evaluate the overall behavior of the underlying value. From a hardware perspective, the cloud service provider has the right to complete control of cloud resources, but the purpose of cloud services provider and the commercial confidentiality and privacy requirements of users make cloud service providers shall not be sniffing the content of user data, really great big data in the cloud is unlikely to carry out a detailed investigation. Therefore, the monitoring of user behavior rely primarily on statistical characteristics of mining from the massive network traffic behavior.

100.3.2 Trust Level of Behavior

1. The form of percentage. For example, in order to detect whether someone using cloud services to a DOS attack, we need to list the characteristics of DOS attack, and examine the proportion of conforming to attack characteristic of an entity's behavior. 0 represents that the condition does not meet the DOS attack, this trust is completely trust. Vice versa, the more in accordance with the conditions, the less credible percentage and the lower the levels of trust.

2. Boolean type. For example, when a user logs on, the user name is correct or not, that only two results: exist, the trust level of the project is 1, do not exist, trust level is 0. in other words, there will be only two levels of trust.
3. Specific value in a range. For example, the number of scanning port is not less than zero, which is a specific number, generally the less number of scans, the higher trust level for the project. In different situations, which are divided into different levels of trust. Take the number of scanning port for example, zero is the full trust level, marked 4, one-three is a trusted level 3, four-six is an unclear trust level 2, seven-nine is a alert trust level, more than nine times is a mistrust level, which is divided into 5 levels. Trust value is a number, so we need a normalization method to obtain each of the trust levels of the corresponding trust value. Assuming the result of original behavior according to actual needs B_i is assigned into L_i trust degree, and current behavior result is R_i, then the B_i's trust value:

$$t_i = \frac{r_i - 1}{L_i - 1} \tag{100.1}$$

The entity behaviors which need to study are recorded as $B_1, B_2, B_3..., B_n$, the result of each behavior B_i is assigned L credit ratings. The behavior result recorded at present is $r_i(r_i \in [0, L_i - 1])$. The weight coefficients of every behavior B_i is $w_i(w_i \in [0,1]$且$\sum_{i=1}^{n} w_i = 1)$, The entity's trust value which is called T can be calculated by the formula 100.2 as follows.

$$T = \sum_{i=1}^{n} w_i t_i = \sum_{i=1}^{n} w_i \frac{r_i - 1}{L_i - 1} w_i \in [0, 1] \cap \sum_{i=1}^{n} w_i = 1 \tag{100.2}$$

$$r_i \in [0, L_i - 1] \; L_i \in N_0 \cap L_i \geq 2$$

The method which is used to determine the weight coefficient (w_i) of various behaviors can be got through the level analysis (AHP). We assume N behavioral evidences which need to be investigated and collected, they are $B_1, B_2, B_3......B_n$, for the N evidences, we use comparison method to compare the importance of N characteristics and introduce 9 points in the comparison, 9 points can be represented 1–9, and its meaning is shown in Table 100.1.

Compares between any two factors, we can obtain judgment matrix of order N like formula 100.3.

$$\begin{array}{c} B_1 \\ B_2 \\ \vdots \\ B_N \end{array} \begin{bmatrix} B_1 & B_2 & \cdots & B_N \\ P_{11} & P_{12} & \cdots & P_{1N} \\ P_{21} & P_{22} & \cdots & P_{2N} \\ \vdots & \vdots & \vdots & \vdots \\ P_{N1} & P_{N2} & \cdots & P_{NN} \end{bmatrix} \tag{100.3}$$

Table 100.1 9 Point scale and meaning in the analytic hierarchy process

Scale	Meaning
1	Said two factors compared with and they have the same importance
3	Said two factors compared with and one factor is more important than another factor slightly
5	Said two factors compared with and one factor is more important than another factor
7	Said two factors compared with and one factor is more important than another factor
9	Said two factors compared with and one factor is more important than another factor extremely
2, 4	An intermediate value of the above two Classifying (1 and 3, 3 and 5)
6, 8	An intermediate value of the above two Classifying (5 and 7, 7 and 9)
Reciprocal	The importance of corresponding exchange order to compare two factors

Standardize matrix P as formula 100.4.

Add matrix $\bar{p}$ by row, we can get formula 100.5.

$$\bar{P} = \begin{bmatrix} \frac{p_{11}}{\sum_{i=1}^{N} p_{i1}} & \frac{p_{12}}{\sum_{i=1}^{N} p_{i2}} & \cdots & \frac{p_{1N}}{\sum_{i=1}^{N} p_{iN}} \\ \frac{p_{21}}{\sum_{i=1}^{N} p_{i1}} & \frac{p_{22}}{\sum_{i=1}^{N} p_{i2}} & \cdots & \frac{p_{2N}}{\sum_{i=1}^{N} p_{iN}} \\ \vdots & \vdots & \cdots & \vdots \\ \frac{p_{N1}}{\sum_{i=1}^{N} p_{i1}} & \frac{p_{N2}}{\sum_{i=1}^{N} p_{i2}} & \cdots & \frac{p_{NN}}{\sum_{i=1}^{N} p_{iN}} \end{bmatrix} = \begin{bmatrix} p'_{11} & p'_{12} & \cdots & p'_{1N} \\ p'_{21} & p'_{22} & \cdots & p'_{2N} \\ \vdots & \vdots & \cdots & \vdots \\ p'_{N1} & p'_{N2} & \cdots & p'_{NN} \end{bmatrix} \qquad (100.4)$$

$$\left[\sum_{j=1}^{N} p'_{1j} \quad \sum_{j=1}^{N} p'_{2j} \quad \cdots \quad \sum_{j=1}^{N} p'_{Nj} \right]^{T} \qquad (100.5)$$

And then standardize the result above to obtain weight like formula 100.6.

$$W = (w_1, w_2, \cdots, w_N)^T = \left[\frac{\sum_{j=1}^{N} p'_{1j}}{N} \quad \frac{\sum_{j=1}^{N} p'_{2j}}{N} \quad \cdots \quad \frac{\sum_{j=1}^{N} p'_{Nj}}{N} \right]^T \qquad (100.6)$$

For these weights, we also should verify the consistency, and order $\lambda_{\max}$, CR, CI are equal to the following values as formula 100.7.

$$\lambda_{\max} = \frac{1}{N} \sum_{\text{row sum}} \frac{P \times W}{W} \quad CI = \frac{\lambda_{\max} - N}{N-1} \quad CR = \frac{CI}{IR} \qquad (100.7)$$

RI is the mean random consistency index, Saaty gives the value of RI for the 1–9 order of judgment matrix in Table 100.2.

If CR < 0.1, through the consistency check, W is the weight of evidence related to the performance characteristics. Otherwise, if CR ≥ 0.1, we have to construct judgment matrix, calculate weight, and conduct consistency test again until CR < 0.1.

Table 100.2 the mean random consistency index of 1 ~ 9 order matrix

1	2	3	4	5	6	7	8	9
0	0	0.58	0.90	1.12	1.24	1.32	1.41	1.45

Examine the n entities behavior during time t and use Eq. 100.2, we can get credible value. The credible value is very sensitive to the entity behavior's change, when the investigation time is short, it can reflect the state of entity better. When the investigation time is long, Long-term behavior of entities can be monitored.

100.4 Conclusion

This paper begins with an analysis of the characteristics of current cloud computing environment, summarizes the existing popular access control policy, and proposes an access control model based on behavior and roles, its basic thought is through entity behaviors, or the results which entity's behaviors produced, and integrated calculation processing generates the entity of credible value, with this as basis determines or changes entity of trust grade, as to change the entity of role and authority, to reach the purpose of supervision and protection about single entity or even the whole cloud system. It is a complement to the existing access control model of cloud computing.

Acknowledgments This research was supported by Natural Science Foundation of Shandong Province of China under Grant No. ZR2011FM019, and Postgraduate Education Innovation Projects of Shandong Province of China under Grant No.SDYY11117. It was also supported by the Project of Shandong Province Higher Educational Science and Technology Program under Grant No. J12LN61. In addition, the authors would like to thank the reviewers for their valuable comments and suggestions.

References

1. Feng D, Zhang M, Zhang Y, Xu Z (2011) Study on cloud computing security. J Softw 22(1):71–83
2. Chakraborty S, Ray I (2006) TrustBAC-integrating trust relationships into the RRAC model for access control in open systems. In: Proceedings of the ACM symposium on access control models and technologies. ACM, New York, pp 49–58
3. Wei LK, Jazabek S (1998) A generic discretionary access control system for reuse frameworks. In: Proceedings of the 22nd international computer soltware and applications conference. IEEE, Piscataway, pp 356–361
4. Fen Y, Hen Zhen, Liu J et al (2009) A mandatory access control model with enhanced flexibility multimedia information networking and security. In: Proceedings of the inernational conference on digital object identifier 2009. IEEE, Piscataway, pp 120–124
5. Sejong O, Seog P (2003) Tank-role-based acceas control model. Inf Syst 28(6):533–536

6. Balachandra RK, Ramakrishna PV, Rakshit A (2009) Cloud security issues. In: IEEE international conference on services computing, pp 512–520
7. Li W, Ping L, Pan X (2010) Use trust management module to achieve effective security mechanisms in cloud environment. In: Proceedings of the ICEIE 2010, pp 14–19
8. Zhang G, Kang J, Li H (2007) Research on subjective trust management model based on cloud model. J Syst Simul 19(14):3310–3317
9. Hur J, Noh DK (2011) Attribute-based access control with efficient revocation in data outsourcing systemsdd. IEEE Trans Parallel Distrib Syst 22(7):1214–1221

Chapter 101
The Study of Community–Family Remote Health Supervisory System Based on IOT

Dongxin Lu and Wei Li

Abstract With the accelerating pace of modern life, people can't get efficacious healthy guardianship, especially for this kind of sudden onset and requiring long-term guardianship disease, for example, cardiovascular disease. Along with the demand of people on the quality of life and medical care raise, imbalanced use and coverage of medical resources problems have become increasingly prominent. Realization of remote ECG monitoring and diagnosis service using the advanced technology of IOT, to minimize the risk of cardiovascular disease is brought to the patients and sub-health, improving people's health and quality of life. In this paper, based on the concept of the IOT, we put forward the system of community health services and discuss the significance of remote health care service to the community health service center.

Keywords IOT · ECG · Telemedicine

101.1 Background

101.1.1 Introduction of IOT

The Internet of Things refers to uniquely identifiable objects and their virtual representations in an Internet-like structure. The term Internet of Things was first used by Ashton [1]. The concept of the Internet of Things first became popular through the Auto-ID Center and related market analysts publications [2]. Radio-frequency

---

D. Lu (✉) · W. Li (✉)
Software College, Nanchang University, Nanchang, China
e-mail: lu.dongxin@zte.com.cn

W. Li
e-mail: Jane_liwei@qq.com

identification (RFID) is often seen as a prerequisite for the Internet of Things. If all objects and people in daily life were equipped with radio tags, they could be identified and inventoried by computers [3, 4]. However, unique identification of things may be achieved through other means such as barcodes or 2D-codes as well.

Equipping all objects in the world with minuscule identifying devices could be transformative of daily life [5, 6]. For instance, business may no longer run out of stock or generate waste products, as involved parties would know which products are required and consumed [6]. One's ability to interact with objects could be altered remotely based on immediate or present needs, in accordance with existing end-user agreements [3].

Ashton's original definition of IOT was: "Today computers—and, therefore, the Internet—are almost wholly dependent on human beings for information. Nearly all of the roughly 50 petabytes (a petabyte is 1,024 terabytes) of data available on the Internet were first captured and created by human beings—by typing, pressing a record button, taking a digital picture or scanning a bar code. Conventional diagrams of the Internet... leave out the most numerous and important routers of all—people. The problem is, people have limited time, attention and accuracy—all of which means they are not very good at capturing data about things in the real world. And that's a big deal. We're physical, and so is our environment... You can't eat bits, burn them to stay warm or put them in your gas tank. Ideas and information are important, but things matter much more. Yet today's information technology is so dependent on data originated by people that our computers know more about ideas than things. If we had computers that knew everything there was to know about things—using data they gathered without any help from us—we would be able to track and count everything, and greatly reduce waste, loss and cost. We would know when things needed replacing, repairing or recalling, and whether they were fresh or past their best. The Internet of Things has the potential to change the world, just as the Internet did. Maybe even more so..." [7].

101.1.2 The Application of IOT

In recent years, people have been paid more and more attention to the health care, gradually from the diagnosis and treatment to prevention [8]. Therefore, daily heath care service is becoming more and more urgent.

In the long-term care and prevention of all diseases, cardiovascular disease is the most serious situation. The patients of cardiovascular disease in our country show an obvious increasing trend. According to incomplete estimates, the patients with cardiovascular diseases in China have reached 200,000,000. Currently there have been many prevention and treatment for cardiovascular disease on the portable ECG device in the market. Meanwhile, the hospital also has a lot of ECG workstation to treat patients with cardiovascular disease.

However, the use of portable ECG device and ECG workstation does not really solve the majority of patients with cardiovascular disease difficult problems: first, the portable device can only localized in use, the doctor couldn't obtain ECG waveform acquisition to the patient; secondly, ECG workstation is only suitable for use in hospital. It's bulky, expensive and not suitable for general use.

In China, family health care is still in the initial stage. Along with the need to improve overall health level of medical services, community hospitals will gradually become the main provider of medical health service [9]. By adopting the technology of the IOT in the community health service center, the quality and efficiency of medical service can be rapidly improved. Through the RFID sensing technology, electronic health records, remote disease detection application and so on, we can monitor physiological index of community patients, upload related data to community physicians. Thus, patients can get lower costs; doctors can reduce the intensity of the work. As long as it is connected with the network, you can contact doctors at any time.

101.2 The Design of Community–Family Remote Health Supervisory System

The main functions of the system include information management, cost settlement, diagnosis, monitoring and health education. Among them, one of the most important functions is diagnosis module system. Diagnosis module is divided into the user's local monitoring and remote monitoring of the community. The functional module is responsible for collecting physiological parameters, monitoring human physiological state and assessing the current physiological state. Through the monitoring, analysis, judging the information of patients, we can get the diagnosis reports and record them to electronic medical records of individual. Patients can query for themselves' medical records later. The information management module mainly realizes the equipment management, user management and database management. Health education module has a wide range of service object, which not only can give the medical staff to provide continuing education opportunities and improve medical staff medical level, but also to the general patients and healthy people to provide a learning opportunity to enhance the ability of medical knowledge, health care and disease prevention for all. In addition, cost settlement module generates the entire fee that system operates costing.

The basic function design of Community–Family Remote Health Supervisory System is as Fig. 101.1.

The system includes the mobile phone client software, PC client software, the server and network platform. The portable ECG device is for monitoring ECG waveform information; mobile phone client software and PC client software are for the diagnosis and management information; the server is to store patient electronic medical records and various physiological signals; network platform is

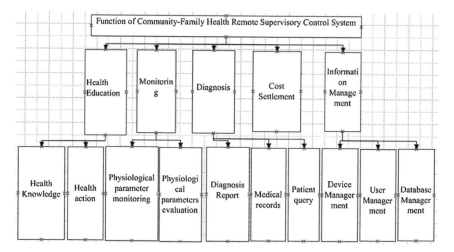

Fig. 101.1 The basic function design of Community–Family Remote Health Supervisory System

used for health education and cost settlement. The overall structure of Community–Family Remote Health Supervisory System is as shown in Fig. 101.2.

Usually, the family of patients through the portable device collects the physical signal, such as ECG and so on, then send the signals through the intelligent mobile phone to the community health service center server. The server will store all electronic health records. Medical professionals or health administrators can view the information through the PC client software, statistics and analysis. Any changes can be recorded into the patient's electronic medical record. Qualified health service unit can also be access to the community hospital database via the Internet, providing health services. The design of community–family remote health supervisory system is shown as Fig. 101.3.

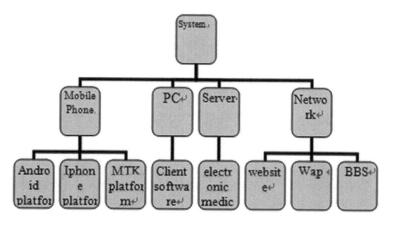

Fig. 101.2 The overall structure of Community–Family Remote Health Supervisory System

101 The Study of Community–Family Remote Health Supervisory System

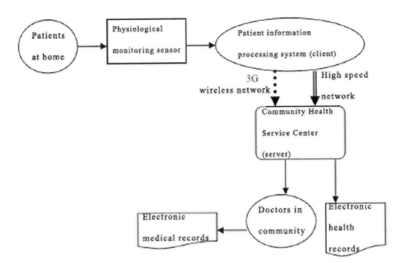

Fig. 101.3 The Design of Community–Family Remote Health Supervisory System

The network design of community medical service center is as shown in Fig. 101.4.

Users login the system through intelligent mobile phone at home, through the portable ECG device to collect a variety of physiological parameters. These parameters are stored in a local database and backup database. In the visual interface users can see health analysis report, health behavior guide users. At the same time, user information will be uploaded to the database of community hospital, for medical experts online/offline diagnosis.

The service architecture of system is shown as Fig. 101.5.

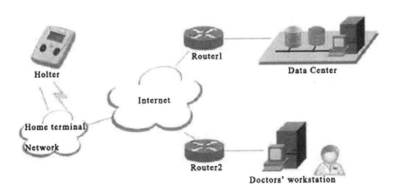

Fig. 101.4 The network design of community medical service center

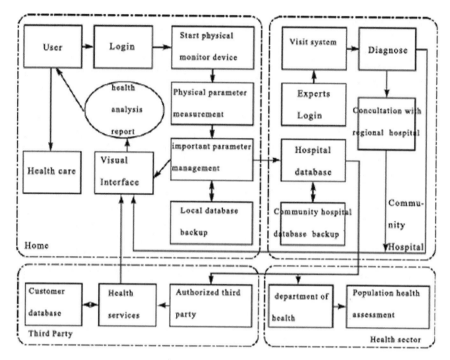

Fig. 101.5 The service architecture of system

101.3 The Core Technology of the System

101.3.1 RFID

101.3.1.1 RFID Card

We use remote sensing RFID card to store the patient ID, address, contact information and so on. The electronic health record number, insurance information are also inside the card. As long as the patients carrying RFID card to enter the community hospital, the system can automatically recognize the identity. RFID card can also integrate electronic medical records. For the patients who transferred to the hospital, the only thing that the medical staff needs to do is scanning the card. Then they can quickly understand the condition and treatment, such as injection drug name, specification, etc.. All of this information is available through the RFID reader, which reduces unnecessary manual input, avoiding error.

101.3.1.2 ID Card

The ID card is mainly used as the identity, rights management and staff daily management. Take an example, the authorization of electronic medical records.

101.3.2 Network Model

Patients can use the intelligent mobile phone integrated with the client application via the 3G network; They can also use the portable ECG Device + computer + high-speed broadband network, to realize the high speed real-time transmission of physiological monitoring data.

The community medical service center network uses the wireless local area network (WLAN) + a pair or an optical high-speed star Ethernet. This network architecture in the precondition of ensuring data high speed transmission can reduce the network cabling, network mobility, flexibility increase. RFID reading device is mainly uses the way of wireless transmission of information to the computer. With the higher medical institutions network connected by optical fiber high speed and high bandwidth, is designed to fit the data of medical imaging, high transmission of large amount of information of the patient information etc....

101.3.3 Information Acquisition and Processing

In the community health service center information processing involves basic patients' personal information, information of physiology and medicine, medical image information, electronic medical records. In the part of patients with remote detection involves the transmission of physiological data. The deployment of RFID relates to the front induction data collection, processing etc. In many types of information, which are collected through application, will be uniformed data format. The final integration is in the HIS platform which is promoted by the Ministry of health, to facilitate unified process and realize the data share and formats.

101.4 Some Issues

101.4.1 The Secure of Patients' Information

In order to protect patient privacy and information security, make sure only the ones who have corresponding authority can check patients' electronic medical records and health information by doctor grading, classification authority.

101.4.2 Costs

The positioning of the system is to provide quality affordable medical and health services. We can offer a variety of services for patients with voluntary choice. For example, remote disease and health monitoring can use service monthly settlement; lease physiological detection equipment; electronic health records and electronic medical records are provided for free of charge.

101.4.3 The Standard of Technology

In the community medical service, we must pay attention to system standard, convenient function expansion and modification. Taking into account the interworking problem with the medical insurance system and the medical unit system, we should unified data format. The final integration is on the HIS platform which is in promotion by the Ministry of health. We also should be in accordance with the technical specifications of the existing medical information system.

101.5 Conclusion

In this paper, we propose an application of community–family remote health supervisory system based on IOT. Though continuous monitoring of physiological parameters of healthy population or patients, we can display the parameters by the pictures, establish a long-term human physiological information database. So we can make corresponding health plans for individuals or groups. Through the Internet platform, we can provide the prevention and treatment of customized solutions for patients. Better understanding the fluctuation characteristics of human physiological parameters of heart can help the doctor provide timely and effective intervention and treatment. Thus we reduce the occurrence even eliminate the risk status. The system can effectively delay the complications and strengthen the treatment process before the malignant complications occurs, achieving the treatments best. The system has wide applicability that it can be applied to aspects of EEG, respiratory, fatal monitoring etc. The system not only has great economic benefits, but also has good social benefits. From the microcosmic view, the cardiovascular patients can get a convenient way for medical treatment by modern communication technology, greatly improved the treatment experience. From the macro point of view, the system will expand the telecom technology from communication and entertainment business into the field of medical and health. At the same time, valuable clinical data collected by network and IT technology, will promote the development of medical technology in China and make great contribution to the improve of people's health level.

References

1. Ashton K (2009) That 'Internet of Things' Thing, in the real world things matter more than ideas. RFID J 22
2. Analyst Geoff Johnson interviewed by Sue Bushell in Computerworld, on 24 July 2000 ("M-commerce key to ubiquitous internet")
3. Magrassi AbP, Berg T (2002) A world of smart objects. Gartner research report R-17-2243, 12 August 2002 [1]
4. Commission of the European Communities (18 June 2009). "(Internet of Things—An action plan for Europe" (PDF). COM(2009) 278 final
5. Magrassi P, Panarella A, Deighton N, Johnson G (2001) Computers to acquire control of the physical world. Gartner research report T-14-0301, 28 September 2001
6. Casaleggio Associati Ab (2011) The evolution of internet of things
7. Ashton K (1989) That 'Internet of Things' Thing. In: RFID Journal, 22 July 2009. Retrieved 8 April 2011
8. Li K, Lu J (2011) The application of IOT technology to community-family health care [J]. Microcontrollers Embed Syst 6:P63-65
9. Zeng Q (2012) The analyst and design of an application in community health service center based on IOT [J]. Microcomput Appl 28(1):P23–P25

Chapter 102
Consistent Metric Learning for Outcomes of Different Measurement Tools of Cervical Spondylosis: Towards Better Therapeutic Effectiveness Evaluation

Gang Zhang, Ying Huang, Yingchun Zhong and Wuwei Wang

Abstract Various measuring tools have been developed to evaluate the therapeutic effectiveness of neck pain caused by cervical spondylosis (CS). However, due to different evaluation bias of these tools, it has been observed empirically that there may be some inconsistency between the outcomes of different measuring tools, leading to great challenges to precisely evaluate therapeutic effectiveness. We propose to apply a supervised metric learning algorithm to learn a metric integrating the concerned outcomes of measuring tools with least inconsistency according to the training set. Through a pair-wise constraints metric learning algorithm, the metric is expressed as a parameterized transformation. We evaluate the learnt metric and the original outcomes with three well-known learning models on the clinical data from a multi-center clinical study on acupuncture for neck pain caused by CS. The result shows that the learned integrated metric has better performance than the original outcomes.

Keywords Cervical spondylosis · Metric learning · Pair-wise constraints · Therapeutic effectiveness evaluation

---

G. Zhang · Y. Huang (✉) · Y. Zhong · W. Wang
School of Automation, Guangdong University of Technology, Guangzhou 510006, China
e-mail: huang_ying@yeah.net

G. Zhang
e-mail: ipx@gdut.edu.cn

Y. Zhong
e-mail: 736759143@qq.com

W. Wang
e-mail: 704643960@qq.com

102.1 Introduction

Cervical spondylosis (CS) is a very common health disorder. The main complaint of CS is chronic neck pain which is reported by approximate 30–50 % from the patients [1]. In the clinical treatment of CS, an important measure is how much the degree of neck pain is alleviated.

To evaluate the effectiveness of the treatments for CS, questionnaires based on the patient-reported outcome (PRO) [2] measuring method were developed and applied in clinical practice and trials, in which the Northwick Park Questionnaire (NPQ) [3, 4], McGill Pain Questionnaire (MPQ) [5] and SF-36 quality of life questionnaire [6] are widely recognized and applied in various studies. However, there may be some substantial inconsistency between these methods, which would lead to some confusion on evaluating the treatment effectiveness [7]. Broadly speaking, the inconsistency of these methods would directly lead to two general problems. On one hand, it is difficult to evaluate whether the treatment is effective to a specific diagnostic sub-type based on a simple combination use of these measuring tools. Since potential conflict outcomes would make the doctor confused of the status of the patient. On the other hand, in a data analysis view, it is not practical to build a consistent model to describe relationship between CS diagnostic sub-types and their corresponding effectiveness by a specific treatment or treatment combination. Hence a derived combination of existing measures that maximizes the consistency between different outcomes is important to provide a comprehensive view of effectiveness of different treatments.

The inconsistency between these PROs has been observed as different changing trends between certain therapy stages of the same patient. For example, a patient's NPQ and MPQ scores increase during before treatment (stage-1) to in the middle of the treatment (stage-2), while his SF-36 scores decrease during the same period. In this example, increment of NPQ and MPQ scores indicated that a patient felt more painful in stage-2 than stage-1, but decrement of SF-36 indicated that a patient felt his quality of life was going down. Doctors may be confused about the therapeutic effectiveness when these results were reported. Moreover, due to the inconsistency of data would greatly affect the performance of machine learning model, it prevent us from obtaining an effective therapeutic effectiveness evaluation model. Medically speaking, an effective treatment would make the patient feel less painful, leading to the decrement of NPQ and MPQ. But in practice there are cases that after some treatment the NPQ of a patient decreases while MPQ increases, or vice visa. In these cases, the doctor may be confused of the real effect of the treatment to the patient.

Since these PROs are widely used in CS therapeutic effectiveness evaluation and much previous theoretical work has been done on them, we owe the inconsistency to patients' subjectiveness and background noise, as well as the lack of consideration of different importance of PROs with respect to different types of therapy [8]. To tackle these problems so as to minimize the inconsistency between different PROs, the following ideas can be considered. The first is building a

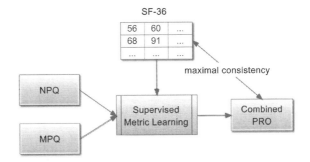

Fig. 102.1 The roadmap of this paper

machine that can tell the doctor at any time which measure is "true". The second is deriving a combined measure based on the existing measures that can reveal the true state of the patient. In this paper, we follow the second idea which is more reasonable and easier to implement than the first one.

Generally speaking, we propose to apply metric learning [9] to obtain a transformation from input space to some feature space with lower dimensionality, where the inconsistency between PROs is reduced to a certain degree or even disappeared. In our work the transformation is expressed as a matrix to be applied to PRO change matrix of each patient. We apply a supervised metric learning with some training data labelled by domain experts. Three PROs are concerned in this work, i.e. NPQ, MPQ and SF-36. The first two PROs are measures of neck pain, and SF-36 is a set of measures indicating the quality of life. We learn a weight vector that combines NPQ and MPQ together supervised by the corresponding SF-36 scores. The road map of this paper can be sketched as Fig. 102.1.

The rest of this paper is organized as follows: Sect. 102.2 reviews some important work closely related to this paper. Section 102.3 presents the metric learning algorithm of PROs and the evaluation framework of therapeutic effectiveness with the learned metric of PROs. Section 102.4 reports the evaluation result of the proposed algorithm with comparison to some baseline methods. Finally we conclude the paper in Sect. 102.5.

102.2 Related Work

We briefly review some work closely related to this paper. Machine learning technology has been applied in therapeutic effectiveness evaluation in Traditional Chinese Medicine. In a recent related work [7], Zhang et al. proposed a machine learning method to reduce the inconsistency between concerned PROs for CS treatment. They proposed to use a KCCA based method to find a nonlinear transformation in kernel space so as to maximize the correlation between three concerned PROs. They solved the correlation maximization problem as a quadratic optimization problem. Although their method can find an optimal transformation through a close form expression, it is time consuming since in their method it has to calculate two matrix-inverse problems in the whole sample space. Hence it doesn't work for large scale dataset.

The inconsistency of different measures also appears in the fields other than TCM therapeutic effectiveness evaluation. In the application research of machine learning, there was some study on the non-metric distance functions derived from real datasets, especially in psychological data or questionnaire data, which is potentially equivalent to the problem addressed here. Laub et al. [10] reviewed some important work in tackling the non-metric problem. They proposed a metric decomposition method to divide a non-metric into two parts, each of which is metric, and then apply a weighting scheme to combine two parts together. Their methods can be extended to combine more than two parts of metrics with different weights.

Another work should be emphasized here is a distance metric learning method with locality constraints, proposed by Lu et al. in [11]. In their work, they proposed a metric learning method that preserves the locality of the training samples. They jointly modelled the metric/kernel over the data along with the underlying manifold, and showed that for some parameterized forms of the underlying manifold model, the model parameters and transform matrix can be estimated effectively. Their work is closely related to our metric learning framework for PROs. Intuitively saying, we want to get rid of the cross-PRO inconsistency by modifying the original ones as least as possible and keep the consistency with SF-36.

Metric learning has been applied to get rid of the non-metric property of data sets. Non-metric data referred to those that can't be perfectly embedded into a Euclidean space, which often appears in psychological data [12]. The work presented in this paper can be viewed as a special application study in metric learning for subjective data.

102.3 The Method

102.3.1 Problem Definition

Before going further, we give a formal definition of the problem to be solved in this paper. Our general goal is to find a measure combined from two PROs, namely NPQ and MPQ, reflecting the "true" therapeutic effect of CS treatment, supervised by the SF-36 scores. The target dataset is the clinical data from a multi-center clinical study on acupuncture for neck pain caused by CS. Each patient has a unique record in the dataset. Each record contains 5 NPQ and MPQ fields together with 4×8 SF-36 fields. For NPQ and MPQ, the 5 fields stand for the scores of five check points, namely before treatment, a month after treatment starts, at the finish of treatment, a month after treatment and three months after treatment, respectively. For SF-36, there are 8 fields for each check point, i.e. PF, RP, BP, GH, VT, SF, RE and MH. Only 4 check points of SF-36 have been recorded.

The problem is to learn a parameterized metric such that it combines NPQ and MPQ scores of each check point together and the combined score is consistent with the corresponding SF-36. Formally, let $D = (NPQ, MPQ, SF36)$ be a set of records of PRO scores, we want to find a 10-ary vector w^* such that:

$$w^* = \arg\min_w \sum_i Con(w * (NPQ_i, MPQ_i), SF36_i) + \Omega(w) \quad (102.1)$$

In Eq. (102.1), $w * (NPQ_i, MPQ_i)$ calculates the weighted combination of corresponding fields of NPQ and MPQ and the result is a 5-ary vector. $\Omega(w)$ is a regularization term that controls the model complexity. The function $Con(A, B)$ quantifies the inconsistency between vectors A and B. We follow the definition used in our previous work [13] in this paper:

$$Con(A, B) = \frac{\sum_i \left| \frac{A_{i+1} - A_i}{A_i} - \frac{B_{i+1} - B_i}{B_i} \right|}{|A|} \quad (102.2)$$

Equation (102.2) sums up the difference between changing ratios of measures A and B. If the changing trends of A and B are exactly consistent, $Con(A, B)$ would be 0.

There are also two important issues to be addressed here. The first is that there are 8 subfields in each record of SF-36 that cannot be directly processed within our framework. To do with this, we propose two strategies denoted as SF-A and SF-B. For SF-A, the mean of 8 subfields is calculated as a representative score of SF-36. For SF-B, we use the average changing ratio of 8 subfields in Eq. (102.2). Either strategy would loss some information of SF-36 measures. If no additional prior knowledge of such subfields, these two strategies would be reasonable choices, as indicated in our previous work [7, 8, 13]. The second is that there are 4 check points SF-36 but 5 for NPQ and MPQ. We simply add a check point for SF-36 to come up with those of NPQ and MPQ by averaging the scores of two nearest check points.

102.3.2 Supervised Metric Learning

Now the problem is how to find the optimal w^*. We formularize this optimization problem as a locality preserved metric learning problem based on the methodology proposed in [11]. First of all, since the cardinalities of A and B are the same, note that $Con(A, B)$ is a parameterized metric governed by w. For the whole dataset, denote the Gram matrix with respect to the combined measure as k, we have $K_{ij} = Con(w * (NPQ_i, MPQ_i), w * (NPQ_j, MPQ_j))$. And denote the Gram matrix with respect to NPQ and MPQ as K_N and K_M, similar to the definition of k.

As shown in Eq. (102.1), an optimal w is required to maximize the consistency between SF-36 and the combined measure. At the same time, we also want the combined measure to be similar to the original PROs, which obeys the principle of

Occam's Razor [11]. To do this, we impose the distribution difference between the learned combined measure and the original PROs. We adopt the LogDet matrix divergence for difference evaluation. Thus the optimization problem in Eq. (102.1) can be further written as:

$$w^* = \arg\min_w LD(K, K_S) + \alpha LD(K, K_N) + \beta LD(K, K_M) \qquad (102.3)$$

The function $LD(X, Y)$ calculates the LogDet divergence between matrix X and Y. The parameters α and β control the trade-off of between the consistency with SF-36 and the locality of original measures, as shown in Fig. 102.2.

Equation (102.3) cannot be solved analytically. Following [11]'s idea, we can solve the problem through a local optimization style algorithm. From [14] we know $LD(X, Y)$ is convex in X. Notice that α and β are positive, and the optimization target is a convex combination of convex functions. Hence the optimal w can be reached through an iterative procedure, as follow.

(1) Input D, α and β, randomly initial w
(2) Calculate K, K_N, K_M, K_S
(3) Calculate $LD(K, K_N)$, $LD(K, K_M)$, $L(K, K_S)$
(4) Evaluate and record Eq. (102.3), if convergent then exit
(5) Gradient descendent update w, w, $w_{new} = wold - grad(w)$
(6) Goto step (102.2).

In Step (5), a gradient descendent process has been applied to update w. Because LD is convex, gradient descendent search can converge to the optimal solution. We set the stop criteria as the different between two iterations is smaller than a pre-set threshold. Note that we do not impose a normalization constraint on w, i.e. $\sum_i w_i = 1$. The reason is that the *Con* function only concerns the ratio of measures. In fact w weights NPQ and MPQ to combine them into a single measure. Only the changing trend is considered in the optimization procedure. Hence w can be bounded by any value.

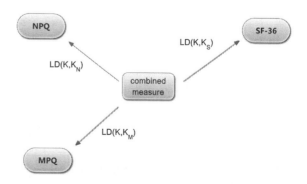

Fig. 102.2 The relationship between the combined measure and the concerned PROs

102.4 Evaluation

The proposed method is implemented in Matlab 2011b. And SeDuMi 1.3 is used to solve the optimization problem. Similar to our previous work, two learning models for therapeutic effectiveness evaluation are implemented using WEKA 3.4. To use WEKA in Matlab environment, we also use Spider as a middle layer which allows the direct usage of WEKA in Matlab environment.

The dataset for evaluation comes from a multi-center clinical study on acupuncture for neck pain caused by cervical spondylosis. Totally there are 1018 records in the evaluation dataset. Each record contains 5 NPQ fields, 5 MPQ fields and 4×8 SF-36 fields. We use the dataset to evaluate the combination weight vector w in two settings, i.e. SF-A and SF-B. The proposed method is run 10 times for each setting and the mean is recorded as the optimal solution.

Two experiments have been conducted. The first experiment is to reveal the influence of dataset size to the target. The motivation for setting this experiment is to show that whether the proposed method can find a w for large unseen data given a limited-size dataset. The second experiment is to answer whether the combined measure is able to improve the performance of current therapeutic effectiveness evaluation models.

For the first experiment, we randomly select some records from the whole dataset to evaluate w. Figure 102.3 plots the selected ratios and the consistency of equal size test set. In this experiment, the size of the test set is set to half of the whole record set, which makes the quantity of inconsistency comparable in Fig. 102.3.

From Fig. 102.3 we can see that by increasing the size of training set, the quantity of inconsistency measured by the left part of Eq. (102.3) decreases, which shows the proposed method works. The optimal w can be learned from a small set of records and then applies to unseen data records

In the second experiment, the combined measure is used in a therapeutic effectiveness evaluation model. Following [13]'s setting, we compare the original PROs, the KCCA measure [7] and the combined measure in three evaluation model, namely Kernel Decision Tree (KDT), SVM and KNN. The result is shown in Table 102.1.

Fig. 102.3 The relationship between the size of training set and the total inconsistency

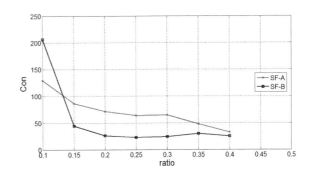

Table 102.1 Therapeutic evaluation results of KDT, SVM and KNN with different

	KDT (%)	SVM (%)	KNN (%)
Original	71.2	74.6	72.9
KCCA	73.6	**76.4**	77.3
Metric learning	**79.4**	75.8	**80.1**

The best result of each column is highlighted. From Table 102.1 it can be seen that the measure learned through the proposed method achieves competitive results. Meanwhile, we can also see that the learned measures achieves better results that the original one, which is consistent with our previous viewpoints.

102.5 Conclusion

We have proposed a metric learning framework to reduce the inconsistency between three PROs widely used in therapeutic effectiveness of CS treatment. The proposed method learns a weight vector to combine NPQ and MPQ into single measure that maximizes the consistency with SF-36. The proposed method provides a new way for the doctors to diagnose more precisely, and most important it can get rid of some non-metric ingredients of the concerned PROs, leading to a more effective evaluation model. The experiment shows the effectiveness of the proposed method. Future work includes the analysis of more PROs and the integration of existing evaluation models.

Acknowledgments This work is supported by the 2012 College Student Career and Innovation Training Plan Project (1184512043), the 2011 Higher Education Research Fund of GDUT (2011YZ09) and Science and Technology Planning Project of Haizhu District, Guangzhou (2011-YL-05).

References

1. Hogg-Johnson S, van der Velde G, Carroll LJ, Holm LW, Cassidy JD, Guzman J et al (2008) The burden and determinants of neck pain in the general population: results of the bone and joint decade 2000–2010 task force on neck pain and its associated disorders. Spine 33(4 Suppl):S39–S51
2. Zhao L, Chan K (2005) Patient-reported outcomes (PROs): an approach to evaluate treatment efficacy of Chinese medicine or integrative medicine. Chin J Integr Med 11(2):151–153
3. Vernon H, Mior S (1994) The Northwick Park Neck Pain Questionnaire, devised to measure neck pain and disability. Br J Rheumatol 33(12):1203–1204
4. Chiu TTW, Hui-Chan CWY, Chein G (2005) A randomized clinical trial of TENS and exercise for patients with chronic neck pain. Clin Rehabil 19(8):850–860
5. Melzack R (1975) The McGill Pain Questionnaire: Major properties and scoring methods. Pain 1:277–299

6. Willich SN, Reinhold T, Selim D, Jena S, Brinkhaus B, Witt CM (2006) Cost-effectiveness of acupuncture treatment in patients with chronic neck pain. Pain 125:107–113
7. Zhang G, Fang J, Liang Z, Fu W, Liu J, Xu N (2011) Therapeutic effectiveness evaluation algorithm based on KCCA for neck pain caused by different diagnostic sub-types of cervical spondylosis. In: 2011 4th International conference on biomedical engineering and informatics, BMEI 2011, October 15, 2011–October 17, 2011. vol. 4 of Proceedings - 2011 4th international conference on biomedical engineering and informatics, BMEI 2011. IEEE Computer Society. p. 1794–1798
8. Di Z, Zhang HL, Zhang G, Liang ZH, Jiang L, Liu JH, et al. A clinical outcome evaluation model with local sample selection: A study on efficacy of acupuncture for cervical spondylosis. In: 2011 IEEE international conference onbioinformatics and biomedicine workshops, BIBMW 2011, November 12, 2011–November 15, 2011. 2011 IEEE international conference on bioinformatics and biomedicine workshops, BIBMW 2011. IEEE Computer Society. p. 829–833
9. Yang L, Jin R (2006) Distance metric learning: a comprehensive survey. Department of computer science and engineering, Michigan State University
10. Laub J, Muller KR (2004) Feature discovery in non-metric pairwise data. J Mach Learn Res 5:801–818
11. Lu Z, Jain P, Dhillon IS (2009) Geometry-aware metric learning. In: Proceedings of the 26th annual international conference on machine learning. ICML'09. New York, NY, USA. ACM, pp 673–680
12. Zhang Y, Zhou ZH (2009) Non-metric label propagation. In: Boutilier C, (ed). IJCAI pp 1357–1362
13. Liang Z, Zhang G, Xu S, Ou A, Fang J, Xu N, et al (2011) A kernel-decision tree based algorithm for outcome prediction on acupuncture for neck pain: A new method for interim analysis. In: BIBM Workshops. IEEE pp 760–764
14. Davis JV, Kulis B, Jain P, Sra S, Dhillon IS (2007) Information-theoretic metric learning. In: Proceedings of the 24th international conference on machine learning. ICML'07. New York, NY, USA: ACM pp 209–216

Chapter 103
Design and Creation of a Universal Model of Educational Process with the Support of Petri Nets

Zoltán Balogh, Milan Turčáni and Martin Magdin

Abstract The paper deals with the design and realization of the model of educational processes by means of Petri nets in the managerial educational environment (LMS-MOODLE). It focuses on the effectiveness and employability of such tool for the creation of models. Based on the created educational models in Petri nets we are able to verify and simulate individual processes, which are carried out during the passage of the student through the e-course in LMS. The realized model can serve as a prototype for the creation of other electronic courses in the virtual educational environment. We can make oneself certain of effectiveness of the created model by evaluating the obtained relevant data from the questionnaire filled in by the students after finishing the passage through the e-course, but also from the modified log files of observed e-courses. We can thus find certain rules of behaviour of applicants in the e-course by means of the usage analysis and compare them with the process models created by us. By means of such comparisons we shall be able to eliminate all interfering elements from process models of e-courses, thus making the other created e-courses more effective and more attractive.

Keywords Evaluation · Educational process · Modelling · LMS · Petri nets · Universal model

---

Z. Balogh (✉) · M. Turčáni · M. Magdin
Department of Informatics, Faculty of Natural Sciences, Constantine the Philosopher University in Nitra, Tr. A. Hlinku 1, 94974 Nitra, Slovakia
e-mail: zbalogh@ukf.sk

M. Turčáni
e-mail: mturcani@ukf.sk

M. Magdin
e-mail: mmagdin@ukf.sk

103.1 Introduction

E-learning has become an increasingly popular learning approach in universities due to the rapid growth of web-based technologies. E-learning implementation at universities is a long-lasting and complicated process. This process has to overcome a wide range of internal and external factors influencing e-learning effectiveness and content quality resulting in stakeholders' satisfaction and acceptance of web-based learning [1].

The Internet and related web technologies do offer great solutions for presenting, publishing and sharing learning content and information, as is the case in many other areas. Special software called Learning Management System (LMS) is generally used in most institutions providing web-based learning [2]. Most universities combine a form of learning using one of a number of commercial or free LMS. They decided to use products such as Claroline, Fle3, ILIAS, MS Class Server, WebCT, Eden, Enterprise Knowledge Platform, LearningSpace, eAmos, eDoceo, Uniforms, uLern, Oracle iLearnin, NETOPIL School and Moodle [3].

Information and knowledge society, in which we are active, is built on the knowledge and experiences applied in the cooperation networks. For the description of these actions are frequently used process models. Implementation and administration of any processes requires their description of solution, inspection, observation, optimization, and first of all their simple verbalization, while their expression of logics is very important [4]. The asset of process modelling using Petri nets is their formal description, which is complemented by a figurative graphic depiction. This way, the precise and exact specification of the process is ensured, thus contributing to the elimination of unequivocalities, indefinitesses and contradictions. Besides the figurative graphic expression, Petri nets have substantially defined mathematical fundaments, which can be employed in various software tools for the specification and analysis of computer solved processes [5].

Higher education institutions, and more and more frequently also lower grade schools, use e-learning support of education, for the most part ensured by means of LMS (Learning Management System). Moodle, currently one of the most widespread systems of this kind, was used also for the creation of e-learning courses at the workplace of the authors of this article. The created e-courses in the LMS Moodle environment have a unified structure, which was approved of in advance by the representatives of each partner organization [5]. E-course is thus composed of initial information (characteristics of the course, list of mentors and warranters, input questionnaire…), lectures (study materials, self-tests, assignments…) and final part (output questionnaire, final test, or assignment). E-courses are complemented by figures as well as icons logically dividing individual parts of the lecture. Main study materials (book) are complemented by automatically interconnected dictionaries with terms, or a video-recording. Fast navigation in e-courses was ensured by the incorporation of complementary modules. It is possible to get from each section into the beginning of the e-course by clicking on the message "back to the beginning of the course". Upon creating navigation, elementary knowledge of the language HTML was satisfactory [6].

103.2 Materials and Methods

Based on the modelling of educational processes in the LMS environment it is possible to create e-courses for the support of educational process. The aim of the system for the management of education (LMS) is to direct the communication as to the knowledge and abilities of the learner, thus modifying the amount and complexity of the submitted materials to the learner. The concept of the theory of management clearly presents the transition from combinatory procedures to the chains of sequential and optimized processes (strategy of partial assessment of the picture of student's instruction, and based on that, accommodation of further explanation is comparable with the dual principle of identification and adaptive management). When modelling educational process it is inevitable to come out of its interactive understanding, of mutual social interactions of the participants of educational process. The consequently created universal model of educational process includes then wider environs, input factors, the process itself, as well as its products (immediate results and long-term effects).

Interactions upon instruction between the student and the information system managing the education represent a complex process, for which it is suitable to employ Petri nets. Our aim of research in the area of modelling was to create a new methodology of teaching subjects with the use of the Petri nets' structures. The consequence of the whole modelling, its purpose and at the same time also expected (marked) asset is shortening of the sequentiality and increasing of the demonstrativeness of educational processes in individual subjects, which results in an increased level of knowledge of students, and upheaval of the level of various final works of students in the given area.

103.2.1 Petri Nets

Petri Net is abstract model which is created on paper "Communication with Automata" in order to express information flow of system which Carl Adam Petri is operated with parallel and asynchronous [7–9]. This net can be regarded as similar with flowchart and automata which is located between finite state automata and turning machine. Benefit of Petri Net is able to display concurrency and synchronized event and is able to display visuality as well as convenient to understand. A lot of logical studies as well as development tools with Petri Net have been developing till now. Major application part of Petri Net is modeling. However it's not possible to study some appearances at various studying fields, these appearances can be studied through models and also can be modeling through a tool such as Petri Net [10]. Modeling constituent of Petri Net is composed with transition, place, arcs and token [11]. Transition displays to happen accident, action or behavior and questionnaire area for real world or process, accident and work of system can be indicated. Transition is displayed with bar.

Fig. 103.1 Basic component of PN

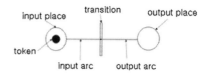

Fig. 103.2 Enabled and fire of PN

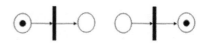

Place displays preliminary condition to happen transition at system or further condition after transition. Enter place indicates preliminary condition, input data, desired sources and conditions and output place indicates further condition, output data, released resources and conclusion. Place can be displayed as cycle. There should be transition between place and place nearby another place at Petri Net. It means that the place shouldn't be closed each other. Relationship between place and transition is displayed through arc. Arc is displayed as directional arrow and indicates relationship with place which effects to or after accident happening. Token is located at the place and indicates sufficiency rate and then displays as dot(•) [12] (Fig. 103.1).

When input places of a transition have the required number of tokens, the transition is enabled (firable). An enabled transition may fire (event happens) taking a specified number of tokens from each input place and depositing a specified number of tokens in each of its output place (Fig. 103.2).

Petri Net is defined as PN = {P, T, A, W, M0} where P = {p1, p2,..., pm} is a finite set of places. T = {t1, t2,..., tK} is a finite set of transitions. A: {P*T} U {T*P} is a finite set of arcs. W is Weight function and M0 is initial marking. Petri Net which doesn't have the initial marking can be displayed as N = (P, T, A, W). Marking is a number of token at the place and describes active behavior progress through transaction of marking according to timing. Arc can be classified with weight and arc, k is added up can be interpreted as a set of parallel arc. There are Ordinary PN, Timed PN, Generalized PN, Colored PN, Extended PN and etc. at Petri Net [13–15].

103.2.2 Design of the Universal E-course Model

The aim of the research activity of authors of this article in the area of modelling of educational processes was to create a functioning model of management of communication of a student in the employed LMS system, by means of well-known procedures of creation of models in Petri nets. Partial results of creation of the universal model were described in publications by Balogh et al. [4]. The intention was to create a universal model of e-course in LMS, depicting activities of a pedagogue and a learner in the e-course, according to which e-courses could be created in any subjects. Our ambition was that the created model reflected the needs of both the students and the pedagogue, and that it was sufficiently modular and was not too complicated, but understandable and compendious. For the description of the management of man's communication with the computer it is suitable to use graphic tools [16] allowing for suitably describing and expressing the interaction.

For the graphic support of modelling we had to choose suitable software means, which would reflect our needs. It was just the software product HPSim, which is available cost free (freeware) for research and educational purposes.

When creating the e-course model itself, we reflected all aspects of creation of e-courses. A proper e-learning course should contain the following fundamental parts for the creation of the explanatory part of e-materials [17]:

- Introduction,
- Aims of study,
- Time schedule and guide to the study material,
- Explanatory text complemented with resolved exercises, partial questions, tests, etc.,
- Correspondence tasks,
- Summary,
- Final tests,
- Vocabulary of terms,
- Literature, important references, annexes, etc.,

When designing the model of educational process several technical problems can appear, such as overlapping of edges. Overlapping of edges is one of the many problems at interpreting the model in Petri nets, but in many cases it is unavoidable. This problem can be resolved by the marking of individual edges using different colours (Fig. 103.3). Divergency of colours helps at identification of various flows of processes and also to the understanding of the model functionality. Then, it is possible to divide the model into individual sectors, thus designating their individual components. This helps identification of the function of the given component, i.e. naming of points and passages.

In the model were used also inhibitory and testing edges, deterministic types of passages, points with the determined capacity as well as various IF–THEN rules. The process model of e-course solved in LMS includes also other parts such as points awarding, continuous assessment of the student, and overall final evaluation (exam) of the student.

The benefit of educational process modelling using Petri nets is its formal description, which is complemented by a visual graphic depiction. This allows for a precise and exact specification of the process, which facilitates elimination of ambiguity, vagueness and contradictions. Besides the visual graphic expression, Petri nets have also square defined mathematical fundaments which can suitably be used in various software tools for the specification and analysis of computer-

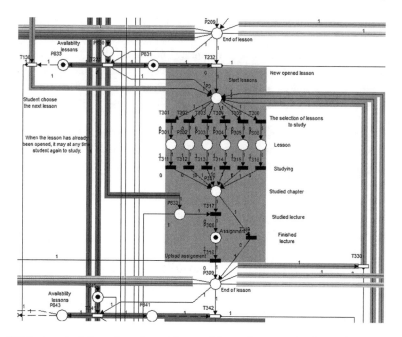

Fig. 103.3 A part of the universal model created in petri nets: student's passing through the lecture

solved company processes. For the description of educational processes, such as passing through the study material in e-learning education, it is appropriate to use mathematic and graphic methods, where mostly serial machines are profitably used. However, they have certain limitations. The issue can be solved by means of Petri nets, thanks to their precise and exact specification [5, 18, 19].

Integration of adaptation into the process of education using Web-Based education brings us an opportunity of individual access to the study. It offers the students a possibility to take decisions about the part to follow after. Thanks to that the student is able to choose the way to continue in the study, which forms a certain feeling of freedom upon studying and creates an opportunity for a nonlinear transition through the instruction system. One of the main assets of the adaptive access is widening of the accessibility of information for the user. Since available information are scattered in the hyper-space, a risk of loss of orientation of the user arises and finding out the sought information need not necessarily be always simple. The task of the adaptive system is then to help the user upon mediation of the sought information. This goal is reached through an accommodation of the contents and functionality of the system depending on the level of knowledge on the user. From the point of view of adaptive techniques it is recommended to use in adaptive e-courses the strategy of direct management. At creating e-courses one should not forget the recommendations well-known for years: the content of education should be divided into smaller fragments, at the end of which the question should follow, by which we verify the understanding of the particular fragment. In spite of complexity of the creation of models of educational activities and their implementation into the educational process, there is a presumption that the given problems will not discourage authors of e-courses and pedagogues employing the created e-courses from further utilization of this progressive technology. It is possible already today to observe the success in research and tracking of suitable adaptive educational activities. At creating materials authors start to deal with not only technical improvement of the systems in the area of Web-Based education, but they lay a more pronounced impact on the implementation of educational and psychological concepts into the designing of electronic aspects of education, such as learning curves, curves of reviewing and forgetting. Even that an ideal system, which would fully come nearer to each student, is surely a utopia, by means of well-designed models using Petri nets we can closely approach the perfect personalization of education.

103.3 Evaluation of Results of Modelled Educational Processes with the Use of Standard Statistic Methods

Referring to the evaluation of electronic courses using statistical methods was the practical outcome and partial aim. By means of the model created in Petri nets and described in the previous publications [4, 20], several courses have been created, where all aspects of functional model were reflected. The quality and success of e-learning support of the study does not rest in the quantity of created courses (usually en block entered into a certain template). The success of the e-learning support of the study is built on the prerequisites such as systematic planning, premeditated creation of the design, evaluation and implementation of the system into the practice and its adequate utilization in the practice, in which education is actively supported and stimulated. In order that the e-learning system was successful, it is inevitable that it be an asset for all participating components, not only for the learners, but also for pedagogues, support staff as well as the institution.

By the modelling of educational processes by means of Petri nets we created such model, by means of which we are able to direct the instruction according to the knowledge and abilities of the learner, thus changing the amount and difficulty of the submitted materials to the learner. By means of the created universal model we are able to prepare specialized e-courses evaluated by means of standard statistical methods.

From the point of view of e-courses the following terms were used: web page—study material, label, glossary—help, forum, assignment—upload a single file and quiz. The dictionary was set in the mode of the so-called automatic linking of words in all study materials (except for the final quiz, where the linking is blocked). In order to increase the lucidity of the e-course also the modules of third parties were used, book and feedback to be particular, which should have been additionally installed into the system.

103.3.1 Methods of Research

Our aim was to assess the quality of e-courses using various approaches. The following frequently used research methods were used.

103.3.1.1 Input Questionnaire

It serves for the acquisition of unanonymous pieces of information on the statistic sample, such as age, employer, experience, etc.

103.3.1.2 Output Questionnaire

It provides feedback on the quality of the content, tests, employed means, procedures, methods and effectiveness of the study, as well as the attitude of quizees to e-learning. Responses in the surveys realized in the form of an unanonymous questionnaire use to be rather subjective. This is one of the reasons of the decision not to rely only on the answers of quizees, but also to find another, more objective view of the passed e-course. We can learn from the output questionnaire of how the users studied, what was their navigation in the course like (transfer between the modules), which materials they accessed (or how frequently they accessed them), etc. By means of similar findings we are able to create the model of the user's behaviour in the particular course.

103.3.1.3 Usage Analysis

The system usage analysis helps us understand the behaviour of students in the virtual educational environs (LMS).

Usage analysis (with the focus on terminal users) represents an important source of information. It is possible to obtain very interesting and useful information from the Log files. Log file is an electronic file automatically generated by software. It includes information on the activities of users stored in a pre-defined format in advance. In order that the file could be analysed, minimum information is necessary such as: who, when, what and how did it do [21]. The sequence of data on the behaviour of users (in our case recorded during the study of participants), stored on a permanent medium [22], are in question.

Analysis of the log file is one of the systematic approaches of investigation and interpretation of data on behaviour. Its aim is to find patterns of behaviour of users and their interactions with a PC [22]. The analysis serves at formulating association rules of users' behaviour in an e-course, as well as at the formulation of the rules of sequence and multiplicity of accesses to electronic sources. It is an important tool allowing for making the behaviour of terminal users more transparent. This helps us to understand better the behaviour of students in the electronic educational environs.

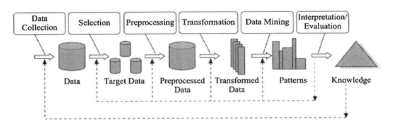

Fig. 103.4 Procedure of data mining [26]

At data preparation, recommendations accruing from the series of experiments are taken into account. Good quality data, however, are the prerequisite for a serious analysis. If there is "garbage" at the input, output will also, regardless of which method to extract knowledge use. This applies more in the area of web log mining, where the log file requires thoroughful preparation of data.

Log file analysis is one of the methods of "data mining" (Fig. 103.4). Data mining is a process used for large volumes of data and for an identification of hidden, unexpected patterns or relationships. Data mining foresees further orientation and behaviour. Data mining disposes the data basis of hidden patterns, searches for predictable information, which could have been overlooked by professionals, since they were out of the range of their original expectations. In our case, the log file is formed by the LMS Moodle system automatically. It stores all information on the events in the course. In order that the data be analyzed, it is necessary to modify them in advance, remove invalid items, convert the system time, create categories of events, etc. In the data modified in this way, it is possible to find the model of behaviour of the user in the particular course. We can monitor, for example, its navigation, accessed materials, or time spent in the course. However, we cannot mine from these data whether the material, which had been visited by him, was really read and understood by the learner [23–28].

Research question could be formulated as follows: Do there exist any contradictions between the answers in the questionnaire survey and real behaviour of students in e-course? By comparing the answers and outcomes of the analysis of users we can find out the real process in the participants' studies, or interpret the difference between the answers and the real behaviour [5, 29–32].

103.4 Results and Discussion

The data obtained either from the questionnaire, or mainly from the modified log files of e-courses, were assessed using the method of usage analysis, where certain rules of behaviour of e-course applicants were observed.

The created course was thus used to a greater degree for the communication between the participants and also as a tool for the distribution of assignments and collection of elaborated tasks, which form a condition for the awarding of credits necessary for the career rise.

Among the most frequent passages of students from the main page into other ones, were depicting of all assignments, depicting of all users and depicting of all tests (assignment view all, User view all, Quiz view all). Study materials were used much less frequently than expected, which means that students did not visit them. It is, however, possible that they just printed them at the first visit. On the contrary, students actively used tests, which turned up a good preparation for final exams. It was frequently seen that they repeated self-tests until they reached 100 % evaluation. The results of self-tests were displayed for all participants for a certain period of time. They could compare with one another, which partly provoked their competitiveness. By obtaining the relevant data from the feedback, i.e. the questionnaire, but mainly from the modified log files of e-courses, we can find certain rules of behaviour of applicants in the course by means of usage analysis. Then, the found rules can be visualized in the web graph.

By means of similar analyses we shall be able to gradually eliminate all interfering elements from the process models of e-courses created by means of Petri nets, and make more effective and attractive also other e-course, so that we could reach the highest possible effectiveness upon e-learning studies of applicants.

103.5 Conclusion

The article deals with the possibilities of modelling education processes using Petri nets. Based on the principles of modelling a universal model of electronic course, by means of which real electronic courses have been designed, was created. The advantage of the employed method of modelling is the consequential simulation of individual statuses of a student's passing through the e-course and simulation of mutual interaction between the student and the pedagogue within the e-course. Evaluation of e-courses based on standard statistic methods was also important in order to be able to find out correctness and validity of the designed model.

By means of suitable analytical methods we shall be able to remove undesirable effects from process models of electronic courses created using Petri nets, thus approaching the ideal (universal) model, which could serve as a prototype for the creation of other electronic courses in various LMS.

References

1. Drlik M, Skalka J (2011) Virtual faculty development using top-down implementation strategy and adapted EES model. Procedia Soc Behav Sci 28:616
2. Cavus N (2008) Education technologies of the information age: course management systems. Extend, vol 28, No. 2

3. Cápay M, Tomanová J (2010) Enhancing the quality of administration, teaching and testing of computer science using learning management system. WSEAS Trans Inf Sci Appl 7(9):1126–1136
4. Balogh Z et al (2012) Creating model educational processes using petri nets implemented in the LMS, 2012. In: Efficiency and responsibility in education 2012 : 9th international conference, FEM CULS Prague 7–8 June 2012. Czech University of Life Sciences, Prague, pp 7–16
5. Balogh Z, Turčáni M, Burianová M (2010) Modelling web-based educational activities within the combined forms of education with the support of applied informatics with an e-learning support. In: Proceeding of the 7th international conference efficiency and responsibility in education (ERIE 2010). Czech University of Life Sciences, Praha, pp 14–23
6. Cápay M, Balogh Z, Burianová M (2009) Using of e-learning in teaching of non-medical health personnel. Bratislava : EKONÓM, Inovačný proces v e-learningu 2009, Ekonomická univerzita v Bratislave, ISBN 978-80-225-2724-8
7. Yang S-M (1985) A study on modeling with petri net. The thesis of master degree, Hanyang university
8. Oh G-R (1983) Petri net and its variants. J KISS 2(2):137–144
9. http://icat.snu.ac.kr:3000/discrete_event/index.html
10. Bae S-H (2003) A study on an intrusion detection using colored petri nets. The thesis of master degree, Dongguk University
11. Jo C-H (2004) An effectiveness analysis on logistics information system using M&S. The thesis of master degree, National Defense University
12. http://www.ee.duke.edu/~kst/
13. Chang W-C, Lin HW, Shin TK, Yang H-C (2005) SCORM learning sequence modeling with petri nets in cooperative learning. Learn Technol Newsl 7(1):28–33
14. Chang W-C (2006) Applying SCORM in cooperative learning. J Comput 17(3)
15. Lin HW, Chang W-C, Yee G, Shin TK, Wang CC, Yang H-C (2005) Applying petri nets to model SCORM learning sequence specification in cooperative learning. IEEE 1:203–208
16. Markl J (2003) HPSim 1.1—uživatelská příručka, Ostrava: VŠB-Technická univerzita
17. Balogh Z, Turčáni M (2009) Modelling and simulation of education of natural science subjects with e-learning support. Information and communication technology in natural science education. Probl Educ 21st Century16:8–16
18. Magdin M, Cápay M, Mesárošová M (2011) Usage of interactive video in educational process to determine mental level and literacy of a learner. In: 14th international conference on interactive collaborative learning, ICL 2011—11th international conference Virtual University, VU'11, pp 510
19. Brečka P, Magdin M, Koprda Š (2011) Two-state regulation in MATLAB for the comparison of some parameters (damage, power consumption) by PSD regulation. Lecture notes in electrical engineering, vol 121. LNEE, pp 369–376
20. Balogh Z, Koprda Š (2012) Modelling of control in educational process by LMS. DIVAI 2012. In: 9th international scientific conference on distance learning in applied informatics : conference proceedings. Štúrovo, Hotel Thermal, 2–4 May 2012, Nitra: UKF, 2012, pp 43–51
21. Borghuis MGM (1997) User feedback from electronic subscriptions: the possibilities of logfile analysis. Libr Acquisition Pract Theor 21(1997):373–380
22. Hulshof CD (2005) Log file analysis. Encycl Soc Meas 2005:577–583
23. Munk M, Kapusta J, Švec P (2009) Data pre-processing dependency for web usage mining based on sequence rule analysis. In: IADIS European conference on data mining, Algarve, pp 179–181
24. Munk M, Kapusta J, Švec P, Turčáni M (2010) Data advance preparation factors affecting results of sequence rule analysis in web log mining. E a M: Ekonomie a Manage 13(4):143–160
25. Škorpil V, Šťastný J (2008) Comparison of learning algorithms. In: 24th biennial symposium on communications. Kingston, Canada, pp 231–234

26. Alsultanny YA (2011) Comparison between data mining algorithms implementation. In: Digital information and communication technology and its application, Part II, CCIS 167, pp 629–641
27. Klocoková D, Munk M (2011) Usage analysis in the web-based distance learning environment in a foreign language education: case study. Procedia Soc Behav Sci 15:993–997 (ISSN 1877-0428)
28. Klocoková D (2011) Integration of heuristics elements in the web-based environment: experimental evaluation and usage analysis. Procedia Soc Behav Sci 15:1010–1014 (ISSN 1877-0428)
29. Cápay M, Mesárošová M, Balogh Z,(2011) Analysis of students' behaviour in e-learning system. In: Proceedings of the 22nd EAEEIE annual conference (EAEEIE 2011), pp 35–40
30. Cápay M, Balogh Z, Boledovičová M, Mesárošová M,(2011) Interpretation of questionnaire survey results in comparison with usage analysis in e-learning system for healthcare. In: DICTAP 2011, Part II, CCIS 167, pp 504–516
31. Balogh Z, Munk M, Turčáni M,(2011) Analysis of students' behaviour in the web-based distance learning environment, 2011. In: Recent researches in circuits, systems, communications and computers : proceedings of the 2nd European conference of computer science (ECCS '11).WSEAS Press Puerto De La Cruz, ISBN 978-1-61804-056-5, pp 339–344
32. Balogh Z, Munk M, Cápay M, Turčáni M (2010) Usage analysis in e-learning system for healthcare, 2010. In: The 4th international conference on application of information and communication technologies AICT2010, Tashkent, IEEE, 2010, pp 131–136

Chapter 104
The Application of MPC-GEP in Classification Rule Mining

Min Yao, Zhepeng Xu and Zenhong Wu

Abstract Gene Expression Programming algorithm Based on Multi-Phenotype Chromosomes (MPC-GEP) makes it possible for single chromosome to be decoded into multiple expression trees, that is to say, it will contain multiple possible solutions so that the possibility for population to involve optimal solution will be increased. In this paper, MPC-GEP algorithm will be introduced and then be applied to classification rule mining. The experiment results show that compared with classification method based on GEP, MPC-GEP algorithm can improve the efficiency and the reliability of classification rule mining.

Keywords Gene expression programming (GEP) · MPC-GEP · Classification rule mining

104.1 Introduction

Gene Expression Programming (GEP) is a kind of new genetic evolutionary algorithm inherited from Genetic Algorithm (GA) and Genetic Programming (GP). GEP has been widely used in many areas such as regression analysis, classification rule mining and time series analysis [1–3].

Gene Expression Programming based on Multi-Phenotype Chromosomes (called MPC-GEP) makes each multi-gene chromosome correspond to multiple expression trees, that is, it contains multiple possible solutions so that the

M. Yao (✉) · Z. Xu (✉) · Z. Wu
College of Computer Science and Technology, Zhejiang University, Hangzhou 310027, People's Republic of China
e-mail: myao@zju.edu.cn

Z. Xu
e-mail: 21121212@zju.edu.cn

possibility for population to involve optimal solution will be increased. Compared with traditional gene expression programming algorithms, for populations with same number of individuals, MPC-GEP can acquire the best individual with fewer iterations and shorter time.

Data classification is an important issue in data mining. This paper firstly introduces a new gene expression programming algorithm based on Multi-Phenotype Chromosomes (called MPC-GEP), then introduces the application of MPC-GEP algorithm in classification rule mining and compares the result with classification algorithm based on GEP.

104.2 MPC-GEP

MPC-GEP algorithm is based on GEP and uses more efficient encoded mode so that it can improve the expression space remarkably [4, 5]. The basic and main difference between MPC-GEP and GEP is that in traditional GEP algorithm, each chromosome corresponds to one expression tree (called ET) and the size of population is as same as the number of possible solutions contained in the population; Populations in MPC-GEP consist of multi-phenotype chromosomes and each chromosome corresponds to multiple expression trees whose quantity grows exponentially along with the number of genes in chromosome. That means, for populations consist of multi-phenotype chromosomes, the possible solutions in such populations may be several times as much as the number of chromosomes. Hence, when population evolves to a certain stage, the probability for MPC-GEP of getting optimum solution will so much larger than traditional GEP algorithm. In other words, for same problem, compared with GEP MPC-GEP can acquire the final solution with more simple chromosomes and in shorter time.

In GEP, there are one or more genes in one chromosome and each gene consists of linear operator string with fixed length. Although the length is fixed, every gene can be decoded into expression trees with different size and shape. In MPC-GEP, there are also one or more genes in one chromosome, but the gene series will no longer be divided into head and tail. Each bit of gene series could be functional operator or terminal operator, MPC-GEP has simpler encoded mode and easier implementation of genetic manipulation. In MPC-GEP, the process gene series converting into expression tree can be seen as prefix expression translation process, that is, see the gene code as prefix expression and translate from front to back. If it still does not form a complete expression when reaching the end of the gene series, then fill it with a random terminal operator.

In GEP algorithm, chromosomes connect the gene transferred sub-trees with each other by using connection function to form expression tree for each chromosome, that is to say, each chromosome in GEP corresponds to one expression tree. In MPC-GEP, any number of sub-trees in Multi-Phenotype Chromosomes can be constructed into an expression tree by connection function. Assume that the number of genes in chromosome is g, then i $(1 \leq i \leq g)$ genes can be constructed into an expression tree.

Each chromosome transferring expression tree corresponds to a dominant of the chromosome; we define the dominant number of a chromosome as the chromosome's expression value. Obviously the expression value is as same as the number of expression trees corresponding to chromosome. Apparently, the expression value of chromosomes in traditional GEP is 1. In MPC-GEP, it is easy to prove that the expression value of chromosomes is $2^g - 1$. Here, g represents the number of genes in one chromosome.

104.3 Classification Rule Mining

Till now there have been many kinds of classification rule mining methods. Although these methods have different principles, they have their own characteristics when solving classification rule mining problems. Here, the basic theory and algorithm of MPC-GEP's application in classification rule mining problems is focused.

104.3.1 Basic GEP Classification Method

Ferreira first use GEP to solve classification problems in paper [6]. The chromosomes of GEP can be translated into mathematic expressions and the principles can be expressed by mathematic expressions. According to calculation, the expression trees transformed from chromosomes of GEP will return floating numbers. Ferreira compares the calculation results of expression trees, the output of chromosomes, with certain threshold R. If the output of chromosome is bigger than R, then transform the output into 1 otherwise 0. In this way, with the output of 0 or 1, the chromosome can correspond to two categories.

In classification rule mining, the algorithm can use simple adaptive functions to make the number of rightly classified samples correspond to the fitness value of the chromosome. Here, right classification includes two cases: positive samples whose outputs are 1s and negative samples whose outputs are 0s. At this time, the adaptive function could be like this:

$$F_i = n = TP_i + TF_i \tag{104.1}$$

Here, F_i is the number i fitness value of chromosome, n is the number of rightly classified chromosomes, TP_i is the positive samples rightly classified and TF_i is the negative samples rightly classified.

GEP can easily solve two-category classification problem by way of 0/1 rounding threshold. For classification problem which have more than two categories, it can be solved by way of transformed the n-category problem into n independent two-category problems. Assuming that there are n categories: $\{C_1, C_2, \ldots, C_n\}$, it can be transformed into n independent two-category problems, i.e.

$$C_i \text{ versus } \{C_1, C_{i-1}, C_{i+1}, \ldots, C_n\}$$

For the problem above with n independent two-category, evolve n classification models respectively using GEP and combine these n models, then it will arrive at the classification rule of n-category problem.

104.3.2 Improved GEP Classification Method

The basic GEP classification method is brief and neat, but adaptive function showed in Eq. (104.1) may cause local optimum and thus not be able to evolve appropriate classification rule model when the number of samples is small.

To solve unbalanced data classification problem, Ferreira brought up the sensitivity/specificity adaptive function. This function considers the distribution problem of samples. In two-category classification problem, divide the possible outputs of single sample into four categories:

1. True Positive (called *TP*), sample which belongs to this category and is judged to be in this category.
2. True Negative (called *TN*), sample which does not belong to this category and is judged to not be in this category.
3. False Positive (called *FP*), sample which does not belong to this category but is judged to be in this category.
4. False Negative (called *FN*), sample which belongs to this category but is judged to not be in this category.

According to such four kinds of samples, the sensitivity function and specificity function will be designed like this:

$$\text{Sensitivity} = TP/(TP + FN) \qquad (104.2)$$

$$\text{Specificity} = TN/(TN + FP) \qquad (104.3)$$

The adaptive function will be:

$$F = M \times \text{Sensitivity} \times \text{Specificity} \qquad (104.4)$$

Here, M is a default constant and it limits the fitness value of individual to a reasonable extent. According to the equation above, the fitness value of individual is limited to 0 to M. When taking M, it is the most ideal situation, that is to say, the rule can totally and rightly classify the dataset. This kind of fitness function is very useful when meeting highly unbalance datasets such as datasets with excessive positive samples or negative samples.

Besides, with the help of Kishore's thought in GP classification rule mining [8], Zhou et al. [7] brought up another way to improve GEP. The improvement mainly reflects in encoded mode and the design of fitness function.

The encoding of chromosomes is single-gene organization and without head–tail structure, the genetic manipulation of chromosomes will be simpler. At the same time, it extends the formula length of chromosomes which can be transformed so that complex problems will be solved by simpler chromosome encoding.

Fitness function use consistency gain function, it can also efficiently solve the problem of data unbalance division. Consistency gain considers the ratio of positive and negative samples in training set. For rule R the definition of consistency gain is:

$$consig_R = \left(\frac{p}{p+n} - \frac{P}{p+N}\right) * \frac{P+N}{N} \quad (104.5)$$

Here, p and n are the number of positive and negative samples in the range of rule R, P and N are the number of positive and negative samples in training set. The fitness function is:

$$compl_R = p/P \quad (104.6)$$

$$fitness_R = consig_R {}^* \exp(compl_R - 1) \quad (104.7)$$

The exponential function in fitness function above makes the rule incline to consistency gain. Such fitness function has simple design and can limit the fitness value of chromosomes in the range of [0, 1].

In the classification method brought up by Chi Zhou, rather than using 0/1 rounding threshold strategy, it directly evaluate the output of expressions. If the return value is bigger than 0, then it is considered that this sample belongs to target category, otherwise, does not belong to it.

104.3.3 MPC-GEP Applied to Classfication Rule Mining

In the past two sections, we introduced basic GEP classification method and the improvement method related. In this section, the application of MPC-GEP in classification rule mining will be introduced in detail and the experiment result will be compared with which obtained from Zhou's GEP classification algorithm.

(1) Set of Terminal Operators and Functional Operators
   The MPC-GEP's set of functional operators includes common arithmetic operators, that is {+, −, *, /}, at the same time, the conditional operator *if* is also included. Function *if* includes three parameters:

$$if(x, y, z) = \text{if}(x > 0) \text{ then } y, \text{ else } z \quad (104.8)$$

When using function *if*, MPC-GEP can deal with piecewise continuous functions, and it is quite useful in daily life classification problems.

For the design of terminal operator, the characteristics of classified data should be considered in detail. In MPC-GEP algorithm, the set of terminal operators firstly contains the features of classified data, that is, when having n features of classified data, there are n operators corresponding to. In theory, features in set of terminal operators can express any constant. To avoid redundant expression, constants {1, 2, 3} have been added into the set of terminal operators. According to these three constants and the functional operators, algorithm can generate any rational number.

(2) Adaptive Function

Adaptive function is the standard to judge an individual, whether an algorithm can solve a problem or not largely depends on the design of adaptive function. In classification rule mining, the simplest adaptive function uses the number of samples whose individuals are correctly classified. Such function has simple design but has bad performance when the positive and negative samples divide asymmetrically.

For two-category classification rule problems, let *TP* be the true positive samples, *TN* be the true negative samples judged by rule. *FP* is the false positive samples and *FN* is the false negative samples judged by rule. The adaptive function is defined as follow:

$$F_i = \frac{TP_i}{TP_i + FN_i} \times \frac{TN_i}{TN_i + FP_i} \qquad (104.9)$$

This adaptive function can well handle the dataset with asymmetric divided samples, such as Balance Scale dataset [9].

(3) Conflict Solution

For classification problems of n-category, MPC-GEP eventually evolves n classification models and combines these n models to form the final rule. When judging the category of cases by the classification rule, the most ideal situation is that there is only one classification model judged to be positive while all of others negative and in this way could the classification be classified. That is to say, the classification rule could be effective when the output of the case has been calculated and judged to be positive by one of those models. However, it will fail to classify correctly and cause the classification conflict when the positive outputs come from more than one models. Except for the conflict above, there is another situation which will cause the incorrect classification, that is, outputs of n models are all negative so that the case has not been classified into any category. Both two situations will cause the failure of classification rule. MPC-GEP has strategies to deal with such two failures. When evolving models from each two-category problem, if the precision of current population has reached the default precision, the two chromosomes with highest fitness value will be chosen to be classification rules and the chromosome with less fitness value will be the backup. That is to say, each category corresponds to two classification models that one is the backup. While classifying the cases, only the model with high fitness value will be used to detect and the backup will play a role when classification rule failed. For the first situation that more than one model has the positive outputs, the case has been judged to belong to multiple categories, such as m categories. At this time, the corresponding backups will be useful and if the output is negative, then the case does not belong to this category; if the case is still judged to belong to multiple categories, then the model with highest fitness value in classification models corresponding to this n-category will be effective. For the second situation that the case has not been classified into any category, the algorithm will set a default category at the beginning and use the backup model to identify the case. If the case has been classified by the backup into one of the categories, it will be effective; if the case belongs to multiple categories, then the strategy in situation one will be adopted; if the case still does not belong to any category, and then it will be judged to belong to the default category.

(4) Genetic Operator

Genetic operator is the basic condition to generate genetic diversity. As same as which of traditional GEP, genetic operator of MPC-GEP also contains mutation, transposition and recombination.

The mutation of chromosomes transforms the each symbol of gene series into random character according to the probability set up. Every chromosome in population will perform mutation operation.

The algorithm contains three transposition operators: transposition of insertion sequence, transposition of root IS and transposition of the entire genes. Firstly, the algorithm chooses the chromosome to perform transposition operation according to the set probability. Transposition of insertion sequence chooses a section from the chosen chromosome randomly and then copies the section to a random position in the chromosome without the position of head. To ensure the length of gene will not change, some characters will be removed from the tail of gene series. Transposition of root IS chooses a random section in gene and copies it to the head of the chosen gene. Similarly, to ensure the length of gene without being changed, some redundant characters will be removed from the end of gene. Transposition of entire genes is aimed at multi-gene chromosomes. It chooses a gene randomly and moves it to the beginning of the chromosome.

Recombination operator also contains three categories: one-point recombination, two-point recombination and gene recombination. Algorithm randomly chooses two chromosomes from population with the probability set before. In one-point recombination, at the position randomly chose in chromosome the two chosen chromosomes will be divided into two parts. The head part of one chromosome will be combined with the tail part of the other one to form a new chromosome and then the rest parts will be combined to form another new chromosome. In two-point recombination, according to the two random positions chose from a chromosome, implement two times of one-point recombination on two chromosomes. Gene recombination operator is aimed at multi-gene chromosomes. It chooses one gene from a chromosome randomly and exchanges the two chosen genes from two chromosomes to form two new chromosomes.

From what has been discussed above, the algorithm for classification mining based on MPC-GEP may be described ad following.
Input: Dataset to be classified and the associated parameters.
Output: Classification results and classification rule.
Method:

(a) Initiate the population;
(b) Calculate fitness value: Translate the chromosomes into multiple expression trees and calculate the fitness value according to the transferred expression, dataset and fitness function.
(c) Meet the precision or not? If it is a YES, choose the individual with highest fitness value to be the classification model and the individual with second highest fitness value to be the backup and then end the algorithm; otherwise, continue;
(d) Choose the individuals to be copied to next generation and the ones to be processed by genetic operators according to the individuals' fitness values and the chosen strategy;
(e) Implement three genetic operators: mutation, transposition (of insertion sequence, root IS and gene) and recombination (of one-point, two-point and gene);
(f) Compose new population by the individuals copied from d) and the new individuals formed by genetic operators, and then go to b);

For n-category classification problems, to divide into n independent two-category classification problems, the algorithm has to implement n times to evolve n rule models. When meeting the conflicts, it will be handled by the way mentioned before. For each category, the classification rule is as following:

If $(R_i(x) > 0$ Then x belong to Class$_i$ Else x not belong to Class$_i$

Here, x is the test samples, R_i is the rule model evolved from Class$_i$. At last, integrate the n models to form the classification rule of n-category classification problem.

104.4 Experimental Consequence and Analysis

The datasets is from the multiple standard datasets in UCI repository of Machine Learning Databases [9]. It includes 10 datasets such as Balance Scale, Breast Cancer, Iris, etc.

Each dataset has been divided into 5 parts, every part will examine the classification precision of the model trained and evolved from other 4 parts. The final classification precision is the average of the examined precisions from all five parts.

The functional operator set is $\{+, -, *, /, \text{if}\}$. The terminal operator set includes all features of input data and constants $\{1, 2, 3\}$ are also added in.

For all two-category problems divided from datasets, the algorithm will stop after 1,000 times of iteration or there appears individual whose fitness value is 1 which means the individual can classify samples absolutely correctly. For each dataset, the algorithm will run 5 times independently and the classification precision takes the highest one.

In paper [7], Zhou et al. used GEP to solve classification rule mining problems, and compared the GEP classification performance with traditional method including C4.5 and C4.5 rule learning algorithm which are used separately for generating decision tree and classification rule. In their experiment, to comparing with GP algorithm based on tree structure, the length of gene in GEP is as same as the maximum number of nodes in GP tree.

Here, we use MPC-GEP to solve classification rule mining problems, and the comparison of classification precision with the result of Zhou et al. shows in Table 104.1. In this table, every precision is the highest in 5 times of running. It can be seen from Table 104.1, there are 3 datasets whose precisions are a little bit lower than GEP, 6 datasets whose precisions are higher than GEP (showed in boldface), 1 dataset who has the same precision as GEP. Therefore, MPC-GEP is much better than C4.5, C4.5 rule classification and GP in classification precision, and a litter better than GEP.

Table 104.1 Comparison of classification precision

Dataset	C4.5 (%)	C4.5 rule (%)	GEP (%)	GP (%)	MPC-GEP (%)
Balance Scale	78.7	77.3	100.0	100.0	100.0
Breast Cancer	94.7	95.6	95.9	96.8	96.1
Glass	65.7	65.8	67.2	56.1	67.9
Heart Disease	77.7	80.6	77.8	77.4	77.6
Ionosphere	91.1	90.0	88.9	91.2	91.1
Iris	93.9	94.6	95.3	93.3	96.8
Lung Cancer	44.3	38.6	52.4	59.5	53.1
Pima Indian	74.8	75.4	72.9	71.0	72.7
Wine	91.6	91.6	92.1	91.6	92.3
Zoo	92.0	91.0	95.1	95.0	94.9

Here, Balance Scale dataset is used to model psychological experimental results. It contains three categories: B, L, R and four characteristics corresponding to four terminal operators: {A, B, C, D}. The final classification rule is showed as follow:

$$\text{If } \left(\frac{A}{D} * B - C\right) > 0, \text{Then Class = L}$$

$$\text{Else If } \left(1 - 7.0 * \left(\frac{C * D}{A} - B\right)\right) > 0, \text{ThenClass = B}$$

$$\text{Else If } \left(\frac{D}{B} * C - A\right) > 0, \text{ThenClass = R}$$

As showed in Table 104.1, the precision of MPC-GEP on Balance Scale dataset is 100 %, much better than 78.7 and 77.3 % of C4.5 and C4.5 rule. Although the number of category B is little, because of the consideration of data asymmetric distribution problem, MPC-GEP can have excellent classification precision. Besides, comparing with the complex decision tree and classification rule generated by C4.5 and C4.5, classification rule generated by MPC-GEP is simpler and more precise.

104.5 Conclusions

The most basic and important characteristic of Gene expression programming algorithm based on Multi-Phenotype Chromosomes (MPC-GEP) is that the multi-gene chromosomes can be transformed into multiple expression trees. In classification rule mining area, each multi-gene chromosome contains multiple classification models. Classification Models contained in population will be several times as much as the size of population, so the algorithm can get the possible solutions several times as much as GEP, and evolve optimum individuals faster.

MPC-GEP uses the basic thought of GEP, that is, for two-category classification, a best individual will be evolved to be the classification rule; for n-category classification, it will be divided into several two-category classification problems to obtain multiple classification models and then, the combination of the models will be the final classification rule. For two kinds of conflicts, MPC-GEP has ways to deal with them. The experiment results show that, compared with GEP, MPC-GEP is better to solve classification rule mining problems.

Acknowledgments This paper is the partial achievement of project 2013CB329504 supported by National key basic research and development program (973 program), project 61272261 supported by National natural science foundation of China, and project Y1110152 supported by the Natural Science Fund of Zhejiang Province.

References

1. Dehkordi PK, Kyoumarsi F (2013) Using gene expression programming in automatic text summarization. Middle East J Sci Res 13(8):1070–1086
2. Azamathulla HM, Jarrett RD (2013) Use of gene-expression programming to estimate manning's roughness coefficient for high gradient streams. Water Resour Manage 27(3):715–729
3. Hosseini SSS, Gandomi AH (2012) Short-term load forecasting of power systems by gene expression programming. Neural Comput Appl 21(2):377–389
4. Jing Peng, Changjie Tand, Chang-An Yuan, Ming-Fang Zhu, Shao-Jie Qiao (2005) M-GEP: A new evolution algorithm based on multi-layer chromosomes gene expression programming (In Chinese). Chin J Comput 28(9):775–785
5. Zenhong Wu, Min Yao (2009) A new GEP algorithm based on multi-phenotype chromosomes. In proceedings of WCSE 2009:204–209
6. Ferreira C (2012) Gene expression programming: mathematical modeling by an artificial Intelligence. Angra do Heroismo, Portugal
7. Zhou C, Nelson PC, Xiao W, Tirpak TM (2002) Discovery of classification rules by using gene expression programming. In: Proceedings of the international conference on artificial intelligence (IC-AI′02), 1355–1361, Las Vegas, USA, 24–27 June 2002
8. Kishore JK, Patnaik LM, Mani V, Agrawal VK (2000) Application of genetic programming for multicategory pattern classification. IEEE Trans Evol Comput 4:242–258
9. Murphy PM, Aha DW (1994) UCI repository of Machine Learning Databases. http://www.ics.uci.edu/~mlearn/MLRepository.html. University of California, Department of Information and Computer Science, Irvine CA

Chapter 105
Effects of Informationization on Strategic Plan of Regional Universities

Guilin Chen, Shenghui Zhao and Chunyan Yu

Abstract Making strategic plan of universities has a crucial influence on the development of universities. In this paper, we analyzed the influence of informationization on the goals and styles of universities, and discussed some problems of collecting teaching resource and implementing strategic plan for achieving the goal of universities. According to concrete conditions of regional universities, we proposed some recommendations, such that facing up the varieties and challenges result from informationization, seizing the opportunities of informatization, and promoting the fast development of universities.

Keywords University and college strategic plan · Informationization · Leap-forward development · Information technology

105.1 Introduction

With the rapid development of emerging computing technologies, such as Internet, Cloud Computing and Internet of Things, the classical industrial society is transforming to the information society. The emergence for all kinds of novel economical mode and applying model of network, such as e-Commerce, Micro-blogging, Facebook, and so on, are promoting the process of globalization and internationalization and the changes for traditional study, work and even inter-personal mode change. At the age of full of challenge and opportunities, universities are facing the huge innovation and competitive pressure. For most universities, especially the new university and colleges, they must turn traditional development patterns to new development patterns, and provide individualized

G. Chen (✉) · S. Zhao · C. Yu
School of Computing and Information Engineering, Chuzhou University, Chuzhou, China
e-mail: glchen@ah.edu.cn

educational service to students, which is the requirement of this information age [1]. Furthermore, the globalization and popularization of higher education lead to a fiercer competition among universities. In particular, the new university and colleges are confronted with the issues that how to obtain various superiority educational resources and how to surpass the competitors in virtue of the resources.

Stratagem determines success or failure. The essential function of stratagem is to coordinate various relationships between organizations and environment. For improving the universities and colleges to adapt the rapid changing environment and with their coordinated development better, it is necessary to make strategic planning for themselves. In recent years, owing to new challenges, more and more universities and colleges begin to realize the importance of strategic planning. Especially, some well-known universities pay attention to their strategic plan. For example, Oxford University has made their 2005–2009, 2008–2009 and 2012–2013 planning. Also, Oxford University put forward the requirements that they will review and have a self-criticism the university and department plan, and redesigns the plan triennially [2, 3]. A strategic plan of a university or college always includes the development background, development goals, and development plans, etc. Daniel James Rowley and Herbert Sherman considered that strategic of universities and colleges are composed of three main dimensions, which are resource, academy philosophy and risk [4]. Daniel etc. also pointed out, when the universities and colleges will make their strategic plan and the corresponding supporting and guaranteeing strategy, they must take all background factors into consideration which effect their development, such as society requirement, themselves basic conditions and so on.

Informationization has become a basic feature and the greatest factor of today's society, its influence on universities and colleges is revolutionary, from development pattern, talent-training objectives, teaching content, teaching methods, as well as guaranteeing strategy and sustentative conditions. Furthermore, information technology facilitates the change of relationships among organization, operation and management, all students and teachers [5]. Certainly, the revolutions are both opportunity and challenge. The influence of resulted by informationization should be understand and deal with rightly and wholly while universities and colleges make their strategic development plan. When Oxford University made their 2005–2009 plan, they also made the development plan of information technology. Meanwhile, they emphasized that information and communication technology were the key for a university to obtain continuance success and achieve its strategic aim, and also are important for its each member [6]. In this paper, we mainly analyze its influence on the development goal and various resources of universities and colleges, and discuss how to consider informationization factor when new universities and colleges make their development plan.

105.2 Influence of Informationization on the Development Goals of Universities

Development goals have a great influence on universities and colleges. A general perception is that development goal of university and college is an important factor of universities culture, which represents their ideals, ambitions and pursuits and has a strong guidance and encouragement role on all aspects for universities and colleges. Meanwhile, development goal is one of three main aspects of universities and colleges strategic planning, which include the choice of university pattern, position of academic research and objectives of talents cultivation.

105.2.1 Informationization Changes the Traditional University Pattern

Determining development pattern is the principal task for universities and colleges. In the western countries, universities and colleges are always sorted into five types traditionally, which include the Research Universities, the Teaching Universities, the Small Universities, Community Colleges and the Specialty Universities. However, with the coming of information age, popularization of new technologies breakthroughs the walls of the traditional universities and colleges, which leads to an unprencedented level of openness and results to some new open universities and open student, courses, teachers [7, 8]. More importantly, in the information age, it is wrong that teachers just impart knowledge and students just receive knowledge passively [9]. In order to adapt to the social change and new learning requirement, universities and colleges need to redesign their targets and specifications of talent-training, and reform traditional teaching approaches [10]. Most universities and colleges have changed their organizational structures, technologies and courses in some degree. As shown in Fig. 105.1, Daniel etc. proposed sixteen patterns of universities and colleges of the information age according to their resource and philosophy [4].

From the Fig. 105.1, we can find that the strategic pattern of universities has been changed greatly in the information age. Although these patterns may not be suit for Chinese universities and colleges, and can not follow them hidebound, some reforming concepts and developing ideas have a very good enlightenment and use for reference to us. When making orientation and development pattern of universities and colleges, they should not be limited by several traditional patterns, such as Research Universities, Teaching Universities, and Research & Teaching Universities etc. They should employ one of them, or employ an integrate pattern by combining several of them, according to their philosophy, ideas, possessing of resources, region environment, talent demand and competition situation etc. Many new universities and colleges can orient themselves as Teaching University according to traditional university pattern. Meanwhile, they also orient themselves

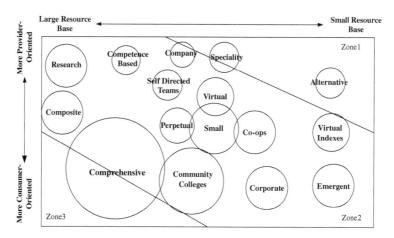

Fig. 105.1 Strategic positioning of information age colleges and universities

as Applied-oriented University or College according to the market requirement. Farther, the orientation can be detailed concretely at the applied aims. For example, Chuzhou University presented "Constructing high level applied undergraduate university", "Developing emphases the engineering specialty group supporting by information technology", which represents their concrete orientation in the applied way. In the implementation process, this orientation can be pluralistic. For example, universities can orient some majors to train special applied technicians by taking talent-training pattern of some famous special universities. Meanwhile, they also can provide perpetual education in e-learning for students based on taking talent-training pattern of virtual universities. And even, they also can orient some majors as research subjects. In fact, German University of Applied Sciences is a typical example for integrating several university patterns.

105.2.2 Informationization Changes the University Academic Research Pattern

Academic research is one of three main functions of universities and colleges, also is the main difference between the traditional sense of research universities and other universities. Research universities often have abundant resources to carry out many basic pure science research activities. With the improvement of the information technology, academic research is no longer the patent of research universities. Meanwhile, the boundary between research universities and other universities is increasingly becoming blurred. The boundary between basic science and applied science is no longer clear [11]. For example, research results of fundamental subjects, such as mathematics, physics, from research universities, can be transformed into applied technology by companies. On the other hand, in the information age, more and more companies cooperate with universities and colleges laboratories directly, which expand the connotation of traditional research concept.

Furthermore, information technology makes teaching and research blend into each other more and more. At present, more and more research ideas are becoming the content of curriculum system of postgraduate and even undergraduate [2]. Some research results have become the straight contents of theory or practice in undergraduate courses. The selected topics of diploma project which are from kinds of teachers' research projects, is at least 20 % proportion in 2011. That is from computer science and technology of Chuzhou University. But in 2012, the proportion rose to nearly 35 %. On the other hand, students can learn and do some academic research expediently by Internet and mobile intelligent terminal, do not go to the library and elsewhere owing to rich information resources, which is convenient for more students to dive into academic research.

This development trend also has a certain influence on research orientation and development of universities. For the traditional research universities, superiority resources, which belonged to themselves originally, will be lose in the competition power if they still do some traditional pure academic researches rather than envisage the new research direction and content brought by the information technology. For the applied-oriented universities, teaching-oriented universities, and community colleges, especially new colleges, they should pay more attention to the opportunities brought by informationization. When they make their goal of academic research, they should adjust their position and orientation of academic research audaciously, and aim a higher goal in a specific field such as applied technology in accordance with new strategic industry according to their foundation conditions. They are entirely possible to promote their academic status greatly in this ever-changing age. Contrarily, if they still strutting or shambling along the traditional ways, they may be miss development opportunities.

105.2.3 Informationization Changes the Talents Demands

Talents training objectives are another important content of strategic planning of universities and colleges. In 2005, Oxford University proposed to serve the region, the country and the international world by its achievements of researches, qualities of graduates, activities with enterprises, policy guidance and continuing education in its 5 year development plan [2]. In fact, training high-quality graduates for society has been an important aim of almost all universities and colleges.

In the information age, talent demands happens a certain change. Many institutions demand comprehensive talents, who can not only discover and use information rationally but also can appropriately integrate information technology and professional technical. Comprehensive talents have an obvious difference with the traditional creative talents. Generally speaking, impacts of IT on the aim of talent cultivation is mainly embody the following several aspects. First, with the development of information technology, information abilities or computing thinking [14] has been the obligatory and basic quality of graduates. For most applied-oriented universities and colleges, their graduates are consumer-oriented. So, they must adjust the standards of talent cultivation according to the change of talent demands. Secondly, many traditional specialties have been advanced rapidly by information technology. The ability of combining information technology and professional technical has been the significant components of graduate professional ability. Thirdly, owing to information spreading rapidly, the "hot effect" of part of hot specialties has been expanded, and the hot fields period has been shorten. Fourth, because of the influence of information technology, some traditional neglected cold specialty may be paid more attention again. The demands of market are various. The Long Tail theory thinks the hot fields attracted 80 % attention. But, all these are being changed at this information age. The neglected 20 % fields may be created tremendous market benefits [12]. Similarly, the neglected majors in the end of Long Tail also have their market space. Therefore, universities should not blindly pursue the so-called hot majors when they make their major planning. Contrarily, a university needs to analyze market demands calmly, and seizes various opportunities and takes a leading development of the neglected specialties.

Different universities or colleges have different competence standards of graduates. Graduates of the famous research universities are provider-oriented, and they are leading elite. For many Chinese universities and colleges, especially the new universities and colleges, their graduates are consumer-oriented, and they are practical and technical talents. So, they must meet the demands of information age, and must have the ability of studying, living and working in this information age. In the early 1990s, some countries considered information literacy as a basic ability of students, for example, University of California, Berkeley proposed that information literacy should be integrated with general education [13]. In "Action Scheme for Invigorating Education Towards the twenty-first Century", our country also proposed to improve the information literacy of students. However, many universities, especially some new universities and colleges do not arrange information literacy into their cultivation objectives definitely, and not integrate it with professional ability. In the practical teaching, it is also ignored factually.

Therefore, when making talents training objectives of applied-oriented universities and colleges, cognition of information ability should be improved based on the demands of society and market, especially the ability of using information technology to solve major problems, should be joined into talents training standards. Furthermore, corresponding content system and guarantee strategy should be made and executed according to the talents training standards.

105.3 Informationization Improves Resources Possession Condition and Service Efficiency

Making strategic development planning is important, however, it is more important to actualize the strategic development planning. Resources are the foundation of all activities. Various activities of universities and colleges cause their goals being implemented by raising, scheduling and employing recourses. Generally speaking, during actualizing strategic development planning, it is inevitable to involve resources raised, scheduled and reassigned, which provide the support and guarantee for realizing the strategic aim of universities and colleges by regulating resources. However, a university or a college always own limited resources, which can not meet its development requirements. Therefore, any efforts, which can enhance the efficiency of using resources or enlarge possess of resources, are necessary. For the universities and colleges, which have very limited resources, implementing fine management and some leading stratagems with low-cost is even more practical significance [4].

The basic characteristics of informationization are sharing, openness and collaboration etc. Owing to the characters, a university can increase the efficiency of resource by informationization and expand the approaches for obtaining resource. Information technology provides a foundation for implementing low-cost leading strategic, as well as establishing the administration structure adapting to current universities institution, actualizing scientific, meticulous and personalized management. In other words, informationization provides more options, opportunities and ways for universities and colleges to make their supporting and guaranteeing strategy around their development goal.

105.3.1 Informationization Provides New Ways for Universities and Colleges to Attract Talented Persons

Talent resource is the most important resource. It is pivotal to achieve their strategic planning success or failure for universities and colleges that if they can establish a ranks of teachers to adapt their development goal. Traditionally, the shortage of high-level teachers is the most difficult problem for most universities. The development of information technology provides more opportunities and possibilities of communicating among people. All kinds of digital exchange platforms and social networks, such as Skype, QQ, Facebook, etc., allow people to communicate directly without the limit of time and space. Recurring to this digitized platform, universities and colleges can attract high-level experts and scholars by some flexible ways. They can share talented persons remotely by elasticity and on demand to make their talented persons resources better. For example, supported by Internet, a renowned scholar of well-known university can instruct other universities youthful scholars to carry out academic researches, and offer networks courses for other universities students. In fact, in recent years, the fast-growing open network courses are the excellent examples and explanation.

105.3.2 Informationization Enriches Teaching and Academic Research Resources

In modern society, the data becomes more and more important. The data is namely resource and wealth. For universities and colleges, various teaching resources library and academic databases has become one of the most important resource. Now, owing to information environment, many resources, which are impossible to gain by general universities and colleges in past, are easy to gain. For example, many Chinese universities and colleges are difficult to access scholarly literatures published by famous institutions in past, such as ACM, IEEE, and Springer etc. But now, teachers of general universities and colleges can search and obtain kinds of the most recent literatures fast and expediently by the Internet just as teachers of famous universities. Furthermore, researchers can share some expensive equipments & facilities, and communicate with famous experts directly by the Internet.

105.3.3 Informationization Provides More Opportunities and Approach for Universities and Colleges to Cooperate with Other Universities and Colleges

Informationization makes them became more open, and promote the communication among them as well. Academic exchange and education cooperation become easier in information age. Some general teaching-oriented and applied-oriented universities and colleges can do some basic science research by cooperating with some research universities. Contrarily, the research universities can also develop some new research fields and spaces by cooperating with applied-oriented universities or corporations. For the universities and colleges with limited resource, they can solve the problem partly by sharing resource and cooperating with other universities and colleges.

105.3.4 Informationization Provides More Approaches for Practical Teaching

Traditionally, due to the limit of teaching resources, some applied-oriented universities and colleges are very difficult to get involved the majors, which have greater technicality and specialty. At present, based on information technology, many expensive equipments & facilities can be share in virtual approaches or remote shared. Certainly, benefits provided by informationization are so much more than these. Generally speaking, informationization provides more spaces and approaches for practical teaching.

105.3.5 Informatization Provides the Basis of Scientific, Meticulous and Personalized in the Modern University Management

Till to now, the meanings of modern university still have many different understanding. Most people believe that the modern university should make full use of people's personality and potential, which is benefit to the whole society. Moreover, the administration structure of the modern university provides the supports for those. Similarly, people have a different understanding for the administration structure of the modern university. However, scientific, meticulous and personalized characters are necessary for the management [14]. Such management must be established based on collection and fast exact analysis of the basic data. That analysis can also provide support for strategic decision, all of which can not be achieved by the traditional management ways, but by the means of information technology. Therefore, the informationization is becoming the foundation of scientific, meticulous and personalized in the modern university management.

Therefore, the colleges and universities should put into full play to the role of information technology when they make strategic development planning. Colleges enrich the ways of access to resources by information technology. Information technology provides the management for achieving the scientific, meticulous and personalized architecture. The management supports for the colleges development goal.

105.4 Informationzation Brings the Leap Development Opportunities to Universities and Colleges

Informationization causes an important society transformation, as well as brings many development opportunities. If the colleges and universities wants to surmount competitor and get advantages, it must achieve leap-forward development. They should pay enough attention to be able to seize the opportunities of informationization, which can make them to develop rapidly only if they seize the opportunities.

Yang Morrison has summarized the development rules of many famous enterprises in his book "The Second Curve" [15], and proposed The Second Curve Theory. He defined The First Curve as the enterprise life cycle of carrying out traditional business in a familiar corporate climate, and defined The Second Curve as the thoroughly and irreversible transformation, or the new enterprise life cycle, which is experienced by a enterprise when facing the new technologies, new consumers, and new markets. The basic characteristics of The Second Curve are various changes, such as society, market, individual and enterprise etc. An enterprise can achieve leap-forward development during the change. Though The Second Curve Theory is used to describe the enterprise development, it also fit the universities and colleges development. Universities and colleges can also achieve leap-forward development by searching development opportunities in this ever-changing age.

As previously mentioned, the basic characteristic of this age is informationization. So, we also can say the rapid change is the basic feature of this age. According to The Second Curve Theory, the change brings universities and colleges many great challenges as well as many development opportunities. At present, informationization is still at the developing stage, its development will be sure to cause the reposition among universities and colleges. If the opportunities are seized, new universities and colleges will achieve a leap-forward development.

Certainly, some preconditions are necessary for seizing the opportunities, and one of the most fundamental preconditions is the faith of achieving rapid development. So, new idea, magnificent goal and constant innovation are very important for universities and colleges. Meanwhile, universities and colleges must reform their organizational structure and resource management decidedly, which could not meet the development goal. As a result, they can take a lead on institutional innovation. Secondly opportunities should be seized. When an opportunity is coming, they should take aggressive action and make a breakthrough by integrating low-cost strategy with difference strategy. Meanwhile, they should catch up and surpass competitors by concentrating on some main breakthroughs.

Because the main function of universities and colleges is cultivating talents, some persons believe that leap-forward development of universities and colleges should not be advocated. Otherwise, the quality of talent cultivating will be descending. But as the article mentioned before, universities and colleges are facing unprecedented competition in this ever-changing age. The fierce competition must generate some winners, and who must achieve leap-forward development. Certainly, they have their own patterns of development, which are different with ordinary companies. So, it can not be expected that universities and colleges can achieve spanning development in the short period of 3 or 5 years.

105.5 Conclusion

The importance and influence of information technology on universities and colleges have been commonly accepted. However, due to some problems on economics and management, many universities and colleges just understand and concern some specific technology of informationization, and just take it as a mean or a method. Few universities in China, especially new universities and colleges consider and treat it strategically. Many of them just symbolically treat it without any specific measures. On the other hand, as the main changing factor, informationization brings universities and colleges the most challenge and opportunity in this age. Meanwhile, new winners and losers will be generated. So, informationization should be considered and pay much attention strategically when they making their development strategic planning.

References

1. Duderstadt JJ, Trans. Liu T et al (2005) University of the 21st century. Beijing University Press, Beijing, pp 31–57
2. University of Oxford (2005) Corporate plan 2005–6 to 2009–10. Oxford University Gazette, Oxford, p 6
3. University of Oxford (2008) Strategic plan 2008–9 to 2012–13. Oxford University Gazette, Oxford, p 6
4. Rowley DJ, Sherman H (2006) From strategy to change: implementing the plan in higher education based on resource. vol 6, Guangxi Normal University Press, Guilin, pp 18–21, pp 24–31
5. Duderstadt JJ, Womack FW (2006) The Future of the public university in America. Beijing University Press, Beijing, pp 53–54
6. University of Oxford Information and communications technology strategic plan 2005–06 to 2009–10. http://www.ict.ox.ac.uk/strategy/plan
7. Oblinger DG (2010) Innovation: rethinking the future of higher education. EDUCAUSE Rev 45(1):4–6
8. Wiley D (2010) Openness as catalyst for an educational reformation. EDUCAUSE Rev 45(4):14–20
9. Brown JS, Duguid P (1995) Universities in the digital age. http://www2.parc.com/ops/members/brown/papers/university.html
10. Egol M (2006) The future of higher education. Educause Rev 7–8:72–73
11. Trow M (2011) Some consequences of the new information and communication technologies for higher education. http://ishi.lib.berkeley.edu/cshe/
12. Anderson C, Trans. Qiao J (2006) The Long Tail. China Citic Press, Beijing, pp 69–84
13. Schudson M, Smelser NJ (2007) General education in the 21st Century. http://cshe.berkeley.edu/research/gec/. p 4
14. Jeannette M (2006) Wing. Comput Thinking. Commun ACM 49(3):33–35
15. Yizu G (2009) University governance structure: the cornerstone of modern university system. Educ Res (6):22–26
16. Morrison Y (1997) The second curve. Tuanjie Press, Beijing

Chapter 106
A Survey on Wireless Camera Sensor Networks

Xiaolan Liu

Abstract Recently, with the development of low-power and low-complexity hardware such as camera sensors, wireless camera sensor networks have been widely used in the novel field, e.g., smart home and medical. Wireless camera sensor networks can provide richer information such as image and picture during a monitored environment. However, the large amount of image data produced by the camera sensors requires exploring new means for data storage, processing and communication. In this paper, we first introduce the concepts and characteristics of the wireless camera sensor networks and discuss the applications of wireless camera sensor networks. Moreover, we present the architectures involved in the wireless camera sensor networks, along with their algorithms and protocols. Finally, we discuss other research issues briefly.

Keywords Wireless camera sensor networks · Smart home and medical · Education · Coverage · Architectures · Security · Characteristics

106.1 Introduction

During the past few years, wireless sensor networks (WSNs) have gained fast development and become increasingly popular in many different application fields [1]. With the development of low-power and low-complexity hardware such as camera sensors, wireless camera sensor networks (WCSNs) have been widely used in the novel field, e.g., smart home and medical [2].

Unlike simple wireless sensor networks, the WCSNs are more complex, because cameras generate much more information such as image and picture and

X. Liu (✉)
Department of Computer Science and Engineering, Chuzhou University, Chuzhou, People's Republic of China
e-mail: 729041187@qq.com

cameras are directional devices, which are low power devices called camera sensors and integrate processor, memory, power supply, radio, an actuator, wireless transceiver. However, the large amount of image data produced by the camera sensors requires exploring new means for data storage, processing and communication. In this paper we provide an overview of the current research directions, characteristics, architectures, and potential applications for wireless camera sensor networks.

The rest of this paper is organized as follows. Section 106.2 introduces characteristics of wireless camera sensor networks, which are different from the other sensor networks. Section 106.3 describes several specific applications of wireless camera sensor networks in various fields. Section 106.4 present system architectures involved in the wireless camera sensor networks, along with their algorithms and protocols. Section 106.5 discusses other research issues by stressing topics such as barrier coverage, security, privacy, and data compression. Conclusions are given in Sect. 106.6.

106.2 Characteristics

Compared to traditional wireless sensor networks, one of the main differences of wireless camera sensor networks lies in the nature of direction and image capturing. Therefore, wireless camera sensor networks have unique characteristics. In [2], these novel characteristics of wireless camera sensor networks are described.

106.2.1 Resource Constraints

Wireless camera sensor networks consist of camera nodes which can perceive, compute, communicate and store. Since these devices are battery-operated, the lifetime of camera sensors is limited by their energy consumption. For camera sensors, minimizing energy is a primary challenge. Thereby optimizing energy usage is therefore an important topic, and many research issues are left to be solved, e.g., a survey of energy optimization is provided in [3], where Xi fang presents strategizing surveillance for resource-constrained event monitoring.

106.2.2 Camera Collaboration

Due to the different angles of the camera node, they can only capture one side of the target image. Hence, camera nodes need to merge on image data during monitored fields [4]. Additionally, different from traditional sensor networks, the detecting range of a camera sensor note has the characteristics of the sector [5].

Through collaboration, camera sensors capture image from a different perspective, the aforementioned mean enhances understanding of monitored environment.

106.2.3 Local Processing

Wireless camera sensor networks offer images and videos, which contain large amounts of data. Thus, we need to tackle the difficulty of processing raw data, under resource (e.g., energy and bandwidth) constraints of wireless camera sensor networks. Besides, also wireless camera sensor networks generate redundant information. Before transferring information, camera sensor notes need to deal with image data from uninteresting scenes [6]. Hence, it is necessary to develop local processing for the raw data gathered from monitored areas.

106.2.4 Location

In wireless camera sensor networks, most of the image information requires locations of the camera sensor nodes. Thus, location is a significant issue. In literature, there are several localization methods. These works mainly focused on interactions among the camera sensor nodes to be located. Global positioning system (GPS) can be used for some specific areas independently, but GPS devices do not work in some domain with obstacle. To address the above issues, Yuan He [1] proposes LISTEN, an irrelevant localization algorithm for wireless camera sensor networks.

106.3 Applications

With the rapid development of wireless camera sensor networks, their range of applications becomes more and more widely. Wireless camera sensor networks will not only enhance existing traditional sensor networks applications such as target tracking, traffic surveillance, and environmental monitoring, but they will expand some new application areas as illustrated in the Fig. 106.1. In the following sections, we describe some important applications. These can be grouped into the following domains:

- Healthcare domain.
- Smart environment domain.
- Surveillance domain.
- Virtual reality domain.

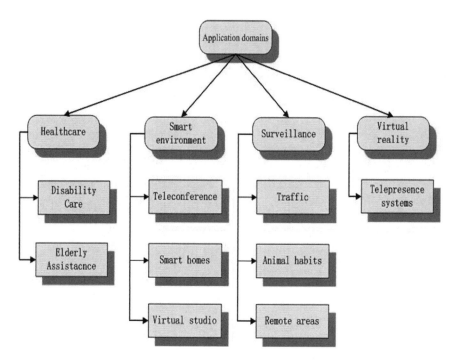

Fig. 106.1 Wireless camera sensor networks application

106.3.1 Healthcare Domain

In the healthcare field, there are some important applications of wireless camera sensor networks, (e.g., elderly and handicapped person). Camera sensor notes can monitor patients' behavior to identify the causes of illnesses and transmit information to the healthcare center, where intelligent decisions will be made for collected information, such as unusual behavior or an emergency situation. Based on the above methods, most patients can benefit from the wireless camera sensor networks.

Another potential application relates to personal healthcare. Camera sensor notes can track people daily activities, provide suggestions for enhancing their lifestyle and preventing disease. Thus, the WCSNs create convenient environments for healthful people and disabilities. In the future, there will be more intelligent applications for camera sensors in the medical field. In this text, we will not elaborate in detail.

106.3.2 Smart Environment Domain

Thanks to wireless camera sensor networks, we can enjoy the comfort and intelligent life, whether at home, in the office or a teleconference. Currently, the applications for wireless camera sensor networks are mainly reflected in the following aspects: intelligent curtains, automatic switches, heating equipments, monitoring devices, and alarm systems [7].

106.3.3 Surveillance Domain

Surveillance has become a necessity for animal habitats, remote and inaccessible areas, traffic domains and many other public places. In these applications, wireless camera sensor notes obtain important image data from monitored sites, then process timely. Meanwhile, the processed data represent the state of the environment and provide appropriate information. Based on the above methods, we can better comprehend, manage and manipulation the external environment.

106.3.4 Virtual Reality Domain

The systems for virtual reality allow users to visit some interesting areas which are monitored by wireless camera sensor networks. Such as museums, virgin forest or exhibition rooms can be covered by camera sensor notes. In these areas, the users can choose to view monitored surrounding from different views [8].

In future, there will be more applications for wireless camera sensor networks. Currently, more and more college education focused on practical operation in the field of education. The traditional way is to allow students to practice operating equipment, observe data, and deliver your assignments to the teacher; it is not only time-consuming but also inefficient. In order to improve the efficiency of guiding students, we can make use of wireless camera sensor networks for teaching. Additionally, student attendance, counseling and laboratory building also require more wireless camera module incorporation.

106.4 Architecture

The architecture of wireless camera sensor networks are composed of the following layers: sensor layer, access gateway layers, internet layer, middleware and application layer. In the context, the functionalities of the various layers are discussed briefly in the following. As illustrated in Fig. 106.2. First of all, we introduce the concept of camera sensor related to hardware platform, hardware architecture, hardware management, and date acquisition. Secondly, we provide an overview of access gateway layer related to date storage and real-time data processing. Furthermore, we discuss data processing include object location, object tracking, date fusion and object detection. Next, internet layer which provides communication protocol and networking processing are discussed. Finally, Middleware as a system software is described.

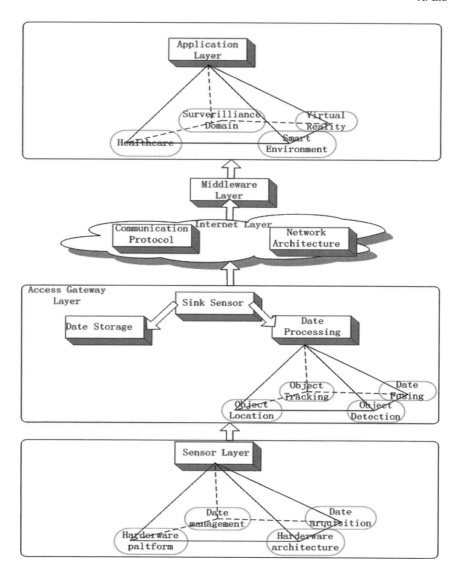

Fig. 106.2 The architecture of wireless camera sensor network

106.4.1 Sensor Layer

Wireless camera sensor network consists of image sensor nodes with computing, storage, communication capability. Thus, the network collects image information (e.g., video, image) from the surrounding environment through camera sensor notes, which transfer the image information to the sink notes by multi hop.

Furthermore, the sink notes monitor environment effectively by analyzing the collected data.

As camera sensor notes can monitor, acquire and process large amounts of information from the environment. Energy consumption is very high compared with the traditional sensors. Because of energy and bandwidth constraints, so improve the ability of information processing is necessary. Currently, Intel has developed several prototypes that constitute important application platform [6]. In addition, we reduce the energy consumption through sensor management policies, which can control the state (active or sleep) of camera sensor notes.

106.4.2 Access Gateway Layer

Camera sensor notes transmit image data to a wireless gateway through a multi-hop path. The gateway is connected to a storage module, which is in charge of storing image data timely. In addition, camera sensor notes need to transmit the image data to the network and need real-time data processing for reducing the burden on the network. Likewise, data processing mainly takes care of target location, tracking, detection and date fusion. Their functionalities are summarized as follows:

- Target location: In wireless camera sensor networks, the precise location of camera nodes is crucial prerequisite for the application. Especially in the areas where person are not suitable to visit. GPS is a good way to obtain location information. However, some factors limit the application of GPS, such as expensive cost, large volume, and high energy consumption. Currently, the main research work is concentrated in node localization with mobile beacon.
- Target tracking and detection: In wireless camera sensor networks, there are a very wide range of applications fort target detection and tracking. Target tracking requires real-time data processing. The basic methods for target tracking include template matching [9]. Target detection may control state of camera sensor notes. Target detection is mostly based on pattern recognition algorithms [10].
- Date fusion: To avoid transmitting large amounts of raw image data, Hence, it is necessary to fuse all image data from different camera sensor notes. Moreover, date fusion can reduce the communication volume and the energy consumption. In the future, algorithms for data fusion need to be developed.

106.4.3 Internet Layer

Like the internet architecture of tradition wireless sensor networks, the architecture of the WCSNs is also based on the same architecture in which every camera sensor has the same processing capability. The same architecture is not suited to process

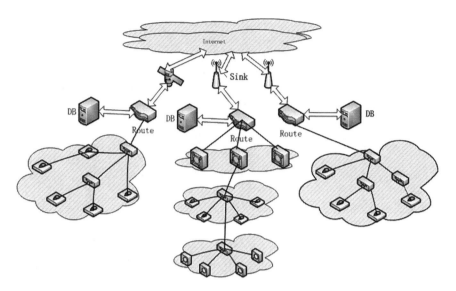

Fig. 106.3 The internet architecture of wireless camera sensor networks

image data. In Fig. 106.3, we introduce the different architecture for WCSNs, where three different camera sensor networks are discussed. The left section presents single network structure of the identical camera sensors, the middle section presents single network structure of the distinct camera notes; the right section presents a multi-level network structure, with the distinct camera notes [6].

Additionally, the Internet network layer provides variable quality of service (QoS) depending on communication protocols. The QoS is the key factor of designing wireless camera sensor networks, which mainly contain reliability, latency, and jitter. Since the traditional communication protocols are mostly focused on energy efficiency in the low data rate communications. Thence, the traditional communication protocols cannot be suitable in camera sensor networks [6]. In literature, there are several works on communication protocols.

106.4.4 Middleware

As a link connected with hardware devices and applications, the middleware provides standardized APIs that are portable over different platforms and hides the details of different technologies. In order to meet different application requirements, the middleware includes rich querying languages and specific algorithms. For example, we can make use of image processing algorithms which contain data filtering and data aggregation in the middleware. As a crucial role, the middleware is gaining more and more attention in the last years.

106.5 Other Issues

Apart from the above mentioned characteristics, there are some additional directions that need to be introduced in wireless camera sensor networks. This section discusses other issues in this field. These can be grouped into the following two domains: coverage and security.

106.5.1 Coverage

In recent years, coverage has caught the attention of the research community in the WCSNs. Previous researches mainly focused on scalar sensor networks. However, the coverage of camera sensors is more complicated than the traditional sensor networks. Existing researches have proposed techniques to solve the coverage. In [11], the algorithm which is called Distributed Belt-Barrier construction algorithm is proposed. It can enhance the Quality of Monitor of WCSNs by lessening bandwidth. To achieve comprehensive monitoring purpose, the [12] introduces a barrier-coverage algorithm. In the near future, it is expected there will be more researches in the field.

106.5.2 Security

With the application of wireless camera sensor networks in fields of military and security, network security attracts massive attention. In this domain, we mainly introduce two key issues: privacy and trust, camera sensor notes get a lot of private information from people's daily lives. As information can be transmitted to the network, the privacy of the people will be exposed to a dangerous environment. It is clear that this problem is a source of concern for many people with the widespread use of camera sensor networks. In the domain of trust, although it has been of great concern, there is no unified definition. Thus, it is a different problem to the establishment of safety control standards [13].

106.6 Conclusion

In this survey article, we provided an overview of camera sensor networks, and pointed out the unique characteristics which are different from tradition sensor networks. In the field, we discussed the state of current research on wireless camera sensor networks, and listed the main application areas. Such as healthcare, smart environment, surveillance, virtual reality domains were surveyed.

Meanwhile, we presented system architecture in detail, along with their algorithms and protocols. Furthermore, we discussed other research issues which contain coverage and security. In the near future, more problems still need to be investigated. Finally, we hope that this survey may help researchers to understand this field of wireless camera sensor network.

Acknowledgments This research was supported by the Natural Science Research Projects of Chuzhou University under Grant 2012kj005B, as well as the Natural Science Foundation Projects form Education Department of Anhui Province under Grant KJ2011ZD06. The authors would like to thank the Professor Jiang Xiaohong and the Professor Chen Guilin for their valuable comments.

References

1. He Y, Liu Y, Member S, Shen X, Mo L (2013) Noninteractive localization of wireless camera sensors with mobile beacon. IEEE Trans Mobile Comput 12:333–345
2. Balasubramaniam S, Kangasharju J (2013) Realizing the internet of nano things: challenges, solutions, and applications. IEEE Comput Soc 46:62–68
3. Fang X, Yang D, Xue G (2012) Strategizing surveillance for resource-constrained event monitoring. Proc IEEE INGOCOM 2012:244–252
4. Liu L, Zhang X, Ma H (2009) Dynamic node collaboration for mobile target tracking in wireless camera sensor networks. IEEE INFOCOM Proc 2009
5. Ma H, Yang M, Li D (2012) Minimum camera barrier coverage in wireless camera sensor networks. IEEE INFOCOM Proc 2012:217–225
6. Akyildiz IF, Melodia T, Chowdhury KR (2007) A survey on wireless multimedia sensor networks. Comput Netw 51:921–960
7. Atzori L, Iera A, Morabito G (2010) The internet of things: a survey. Comput Netw 54:2787–2805
8. Schreer O, Kauff P, Sikora T (2005) 3D video communication. Wiley, New York
9. Soro S, Heinzelman W (2009) A survey of visual sensor networks. Adv Multimedia Volume
10. Lipton A, Fujiyoshi H, Patil R (1998) Moving target classification and tracking from real-time video. IEEE Image Underst Workshop
11. Cheng C-F, Tsai K-T (2012) Belt-barrier construction algorithm for WVSNs. IEEE Wireless Commun Netw Conf 2012:3155–3160
12. Chang C-Y, Hsiao C-Y, Chang C-T (2012) The k-barrier coverage mechanism in wireless visual sensor networks. IEEE Wireless Commun Netw Conf 2012:2318–2322
13. Miorandi D, Sicari S, De Pellegrini F, Chlamtac I (2012) Internet of things: vision, applications and research challenges. Ad Hoc Netw 10:1497–1516

Chapter 107
A Modified Hexagon-Based Search Algorithm for Fast Block Matching Motion Estimation

Yun Cheng, Tiebin Wu and Minlei Xiao

Abstract Hexagon-based Search (HEXBS) is one of the most famous and efficient fast block matching motion estimation algorithms. Based on the directional characteristic of SAD distribution and the center-biased characteristic of motion vector, a modified hexagon-based search algorithm for block matching motion estimation, MHEXBS, was proposed in this paper. MHEXBS uses small hexagon-based search pattern to refine the motion vector, and large hexagon-based search pattern to locate the best matching block with large motion vector approximately. Although the proposed MHEXBS may also be trapped in local minima, those experimental results demonstrate that the computational complexity of MHEXBS decreased about 99.01–99.53 % compared with that of FS, or about 14.77–53.75 % compared with that of HEXBS, while it caused little, if any, loss in encoding efficiency. MHEXBS is especially efficient for those video series with simple and slow motion characteristics.

Keywords Motion estimation · Search · Pattern · Hexagon

107.1 Introduction

The technique of block-matching motion estimation and compensation can improve the encoding efficiency greatly by eliminating the temporal redundant information between successive frames and it was adopted by many video coding

Y. Cheng · T. Wu
Department of Communication and Control Engineering, Hunan University of Humanities, Science and Technology, Hunan, China

M. Xiao (✉)
Department of Computer Science and Technology, Hunan University of Humanities, Science and Technology, Loudi 417000, China
e-mail: chy8370002@gmail.com

standards such as MPEG-1/2/4, H.261, H.263 and H.264/AVC etc. [1, 2]. The most basic block-matching motion estimation algorithm is FS (Full Search). Although FS can find the best matching block by exhaustively testing all the candidate blocks within the search window, its computation is too heavy: experimental results show that the time of motion estimation consumed by FS in H.264/AVC is about 60–80 % of the total encoding time. In order to speed up the process of motion estimation, many researchers have been working hard for many years and have proposed many kinds of fast block-matching motion estimation algorithms [3–4].

Most of those fast block matching motion estimation algorithms find the best matching block by adopting some specific search patters. For example, J. Jain et al. used "+" pattern in TDLs (Two-Diamond Logarithmic Search) [3]; TSS (Three-Step Search), NTTS (New Three-Step Search) [5], 4SS (Four Step Search) [6], and BBGDS (Block-Based Gradient Descent Search) [7] adopt square pattern to find the best matching blocks; DS (Diamond Search) uses diamond pattern[8]; C. Tian et al. used parallelogram pattern in their fast motion algorithm [9]; C. Zhu et al. used hexagon search pattern in HEXBS (Hexagon-Based Search) [10]; L. P. Chau et al. used octagon search pattern in OCTBS (Octagon-Based Search) [11] etc. Some improved fast block matching motion estimation algorithms usually use two different search patterns, for example, M. Ghanbari used "X" and "+" pattern in CSA (Cross Search Algorithm) [12]; S. Shin et al. used "X" and diamond pattern in CBHS (Center-Biased Hybrid Search) [13]; C. Cheung et al. used cross and diamond pattern in CDS (Cross Diamond Search) [14] and its improved algorithms [15, 16]; H. C. Tourapis et al. used diamond and square patterns in their fast motion estimation [17]; etc.

Among all those fast block matching motion estimation algorithms, HEXBS is one of the most famous and efficient one. So it is very important to research deeply on the HEXBS algorithm.

Based on the analysis of the HEXBS algorithm, we proposed MHEXBS (Modified Hexagon-Based Search) algorithm for block matching motion estimation in this paper.

The remainder of this paper is organized as follows. In Sect. 107.2, we briefly analyze the HEXBS algorithm. The proposed MHEXBS algorithm is described in Sect. 107.3. Simulation results are presented in Sect. 107.4. Finally, conclusions are given in Sect. 107.5.

107.2 Analysis of the HEXBS Algorithm

The HEXBS (Hexagon-Based Search) is one of the most famous and efficient fast block matching motion estimation algorithm being proposed by C. Zhu, X. Lin and L. P. Chau in [10]. S. Zhu et al. pointed out in [9] that over 50 % of the motion vectors are enclosed in a circular area with a radius of two pixels and centered on the position of zero motion as illustrated in Fig. 107.1.

Fig. 107.1 Motion vectors distribution

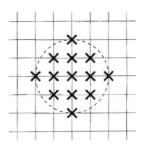

The HEXBS algorithm employs two search patterns as illustrated in Fig. 107.2. The first pattern, called large hexagon-based search pattern (LHEXBSP), comprises seven checking points from which six points surround the center one to compose a bigger hexagon shape. The second pattern consisting of five checking points forms a smaller hexagon shape, called small hexagon-based search pattern (SHEXBSP). In the searching process of the HEXBS algorithm, LHEXBSP is repeatedly used until the step in which the minimum block distortion (MBD) occurs at the search center. Then the search pattern is switched from LHEXBSP to SHEXBSP as reaching to the final search stage. Among the five checking points in SHEXBSP, the position yielding the MBD (Minimum Block Distortion) provides the motion vector of the best matching block.

By analyzing the HEXBS algorithm, we can found that it has the following limitations:

(1) It doesn't utilize the motion information of the adjacent blocks, so it will take a long time to find the best matching block which has large motion.
(2) It doesn't utilize the center-biased characteristic of motion vectors, so it will take eleven search points to find the best matching block with zero motion, and in this case, the idea search points is only five.
(3) Based on the assumption that the block displacement of real-world video sequences would be mainly in horizontal and vertical directions, the HEXBS algorithm will take a very long time to find the best matching block with large motion vector in the diagonal directions, sometimes it may be trapped in the local minimum block.

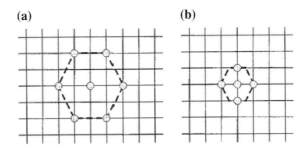

Fig. 107.2 Two search patterns are employed in the proposed HEXBS algorithm. **a** Large hexagon based search pattern **b** Small hexagon based search pattern

In short, the efficiency of the HEXBS algorithm can be improved. So we proposed a modified hexagon-based algorithm, MHEXBS, which is still based on the hexagon-based search patterns.

107.3 The Modified Hexagon-Based Search Algorithm

107.3.1 MHEXBS Patterns

It is well know that the form and size of the search pattern used in the motion estimation algorithm will affect directly the speed and performance of the video encoder. Better search patterns can reduce the searching points remarkably without being trapped into the local minimum point. Considering the block displacement of natural video sequences may be mainly in horizontal and vertical directions and most of the best matching blocks' motion vectors are small or even zero, a small hexagon-based search pattern, SHEXBSP (as shown in Fig. 107.2b), is used in the proposed MHEXBS algorithm at the beginning of the block-matching motion estimation, and if the best matching point is located in the search center, the process of block-matching motion estimation will be terminated immediately. Then in order to find the best matching block perhaps with large motion vector, a large hexagon-based search pattern, LHEXBSP (as shown in Fig. 107.2a), is adopted.

In the searching process of block-matching motion estimation, SHEXBSP is adopted to refine the motion vectors and it is necessary no matter how the motion vector being small or large, while LHEXBSP is used to locate the best matching block with large motion vector approximately and it can be skipped if the motion vector is zero.

107.3.2 Description of the Proposed MHEXBS Algorithm

The proposed MHEXBS algorithm mainly comprises two stages. In the first stage, in order to reduce the search points for the best matching block with large motion vector, we use the median motion value of the adjacent blocks (as shown in Fig. 107.3.) to predict the motion vector of the current block. The median prediction is expressed as formula (107.1).

Fig. 107.3 Reference block location for predicting motion vector

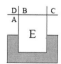

$$pred\_mv = median(mv\_A, mv\_B, mv\_C) \tag{107.1}$$

- If A and D are outside the picture, their values are assumed to be zero.
- If D, B, C are outside the picture, the prediction is equal to A.
- If C is outside the picture or still not available due to the order of vector data, C is replaced by D.
- If A, B, C and D are outside the picture, the prediction is equal to the value of the co-located block in the previous frame.

In the second stage, the proposed MHEXBS algorithm adopts SHEXBSP and LHEXBSP adaptively according to video series with different motion vectors. Based on the assumption that most of the macro blocks in a natural video would be quasi-stationary or stationary, the MHEXBS algorithm uses SHEXBSP at the first search step. If the best matching block locates at the search center, the MHEXBS algorithm needs only five search points to find it out. Otherwise, in order to judge whether the best matching motion vector would be large, the MHEXBS algorithm employs LHEXBSP at the next search step. If the new MBD point located in SHEXBSP, that indicates the best matching motion vector would be small, SHEXBSP is repeatedly used until the step in which the MBD point occurs at the search center. Otherwise, do the same as the beginning.

The MHEXBS algorithm is summarized as follows.

Preparation: Use formula (107.1) to predict the initial motion vector of the current block, and set the initial search center point according to the predicted value.

Step1: Test the five checking points of SHEXBSP. If the MBD point located at the search center, go to **step5**; otherwise, go to **step2**.

Step2: The new MBD point found in the previous search step is re-positioned as the search center. Test the rest two or three checking points of SHEXBSP. If the MBD point located at the search center, go to **step5**; otherwise, go to **step3**.

Step3: The new MBD point found in the previous search step is re-positioned as the search center. Test the six or the rest of the three checking points of the LHEXBSP. If the new MBD point still located at the search center, go to **step4**; otherwise, recursively repeat this step.

Step4: The new MBD point found in the previous search step is re-positioned as the search center point. Test the two or three checking points of SHEXBSP. If the MBD point located at the center position, go to **step5**; otherwise, recursively repeat this step.

Step5: Stop searching. The center point is the final solution of the motion vector which points to the best matching block.

Table 107.1 Comparison of search points near the initial search center for HEXBS and MHEXBS

The best matching point is located in the				
	Center	Circular area with a radius of 1 pixel	Circular area with a radius of $\sqrt{2}$ pixels	Circular area with a radius of 2 pixels
HEXBS	11	11	17	15.5
MHEXBS	5	8	15	15

Table 107.2 ASP of different search algorithm

Video series	QP	FS	HEXBS	MHEXBS
Akiyo	4	1089	11.009	5.092
	10	1089	11.010	5.095
	16	1089	11.012	5.331
	22	1089	11.028	7.798
	28	1089	11.023	9.274
News	4	1089	11.194	5.647
	10	1089	11.187	5.677
	16	1089	11.211	6.039
	22	1089	11.209	7.314
	28	1089	11.198	8.684
Mobile	4	1089	11.313	7.979
	10	1089	11.331	8.011
	16	1089	11.324	8.060
	22	1089	11.334	8.137
	28	1089	11.369	8.202
Foreman	4	1089	12.599	10.026
	10	1089	12.247	9.532
	16	1089	12.187	9.560
	22	1089	12.209	10.002
	28	1089	12.352	10.738

107.3.3 Analysis of the Proposed MHEXBS Algorithm

For block matching motion estimation, computational complexity could be measured by average number of search points for each motion vector. According to the statistical distribution law of motion vectors in different video series, assume that the best matching point is located in the circle area as shown in Fig. 107.1, the search points needed for HEXBS and MHEXBS are listed in Table 107.1. The search points required for those best matching blocks which are located in the circular area with a radius of two pixels is variable. For example, in horizontal direction, the search points required for the best matching point is fourteen, while in the vertical direction, the search points required for the best matching blocks is seventeen. So the average search points for the best matching blocks which are located in the circular area with a radius of two pixels is fifteen point five.

From Table 107.1, we can observe that the search points required for MHEXBS is always less than that of HEXBS, and the reduced search points is about zero point five to six.

107.4 Simulation Results

Table 107.2, Fig. 107.4.

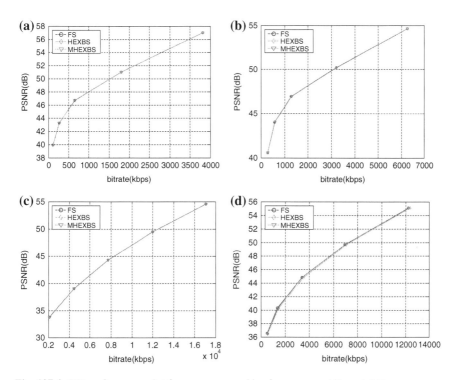

Fig. 107.4 RD performance plot for sequences **a** akiyo **b** news **c** mobile and **d** Foreman

107.5 Conclusions

Based on the directional characteristic of SAD distribution and the center-biased characteristic of motion vector, a modified hexagon-based search algorithm for block matching motion estimation, MHEXBS, was proposed in this paper. MHEXBS uses small hexagon-based search pattern to refine the motion vector, and large hexagon-based search pattern to locate the best matching block with large motion vector approximately. Although the proposed MHEXBS may also be trapped in local minima, those experimental results demonstrate that the computational complexity of MHEXBS decreased about 99.01–99.53 % compared with that of FS, or about 14.77–53.75 % compared with that of HEXBS, while it caused little, if any, loss in encoding efficiency. MHEXBS is especially efficient for those video series with simple and slow motion characteristics.

Acknowledgments This work was financially supported by the Research Foundation of Education Committee of Hunan Province, China (09A046, 11C0701), the Hunan Provincial Natural Science Foundation of China (12JJ2040), the Construct Program of the Key Discipline in Hunan Province, China, the Aid program for Science and Technology Innovative Research Team in Higher Educational Institute of Hunan Province, and the Planned Science and Technology Project of Loudi City, Hunan Province, China.

References

1. Rao KR, Hwang JJ (1996) Techniques and standards for image, video and audio coding. Prentice Hall, Englewood Cliffs
2. Thmomas Wiegand and Gary Sullivan. Joint Video Team (JVT) of ISO/IEC MPEG and ITU-T VCEG. Draft ITU-T Recommendation and Final Draft International Standard of Joint Video Specification (ITU-T Rec. H.264|ISO/IEC 14496-10 AVC), document JVT-G050d35.doc, 7th Meeting: Pattaya, Thailand, 2003 March
3. Jain J, Jain A (1981) Displacement measurement and its application in interframe image coding. IEEE Trans Commun 29:1799–1808
4. Ng KH, Po LM, Wong KM, Ting CW, Cheung KW (2009) A search patterns switching algorithm for block motion estimation. IEEE Trans Circuits Syst Video Technol 19(5):753–759
5. Li R, Zeng B et al (1994) A new three-step search algorithm for block motion estimation. IEEE Trans Circuits Syst Video Technol 4:438–442
6. Po LM, Ma WC (1996) A novel four-step search algorithm for fast block motion estimation. IEEE Trans Circuits Syst Video Technol 6:313–317
7. Liu LK, Feig E (1996) A block-based gradient descent search algorithm for block motion estimation in video coding. IEEE Trans Circuits Syst Video Technol 6:419–423
8. Zhu S, Ma KK (2000) A new diamond search algorithm for fast block-matching motion estimation. IEEE Trans. Image Processing 9:287–290
9. Tian C, Shen C et al (2004) A fast motion estimation algorithm based on context-adaptive parallelogram search pattern. LNCS 3311:175–186
10. Ce Z, Xiao L et al (2002) Hexagon-based search pattern for fast block motion estimation. IEEE Trans. Circuits Syst video technol 5:349–355
11. Chau LP, Zhu C (2003) A fast octagon-based search algorithm for motion estimation. Sig Process 83:671–675
12. Ghanbari M (1990) The cross-search algorithm for motion estimation. IEEE Trans Commun 38:950–953
13. Shin S-C, Hyunki Baik, et al (2000) A center-biased hybrid search method using plus search pattern for block motion estimation. In: IEEE international symposium on circuits and systems, vol IV. Geneva, Switzerland, pp 309–312, May, 2000
14. Cheung C-H, Po L-M (2002) A novel cross-diamond search algorithm for fast block motion estimation. IEEE Trans Circuit Syst video Technol 12:1168–1177
15. Cheung C-H, Po L-M (2002) A novel small-cross-diamond search algorithm for fast video coding and videoconferencing applications. IEEE ICIP I:681–684

16. Lam C-W, Po L-M et al (2003) A new cross-diamond search algorithm for fast block matching motion estimation. In: IEEE International Conference on Neural Networks & Signal Processing, pp 1262-1265, Nanjing, China
17. Tourapis HC, Tourapis A (2003) Fast motion estimation within H.264 codec. ICME
18. Jeong CU, Ikenaga T, Goto S (2008) An extended small diamond search algorithm for fast block motion estimation. In: Proceedings of the 23rd international technical conference on circus/systems, computaters and communications, Shimonoseki City, Yamaguchi Prefecture, Japan, pp 1037–1040, 6–9 July
19. Joint Video Team (JVT) (2012) Test Model JM18.4. http://iphome.hhi.de/suehring/tml/download/. Accessed Aug 2012

Chapter 108
Protection of Xi Lei Powder to Intestinal Mucosa in Enema-Microstructure Observation by TEM and Light Microscope

Feng Zhang, DuanYing Cai and Juan Xu

Abstract Nowadays, enema injuries are only confirmed by symptoms in clinic and there is no protection related. In this article, light microscope and transmission electron microscope were used to observe microstructure changes of rabbits' intestinal mucous membrane injured by enema of various pH, which helped to identify whether Xi Lei powder can be used to protect intestinal mucosa injuries. The results showed Xi Lei powder was quite effective in protecting intestinal mucosa by microstructure observation through TEM and light microscope.

Keywords Edema solutions · Xi Lei powder · Transmission electron microscope (TEM) · Microstructure · Light microscope

108.1 Introduction

The most common complications of enema include functional disorder of intestine and electrolytic disturbances, and acid and alkaline solutions led to more severe injuries than neutral solutions [1–3]. It's a pity that physician can only judge by patients' complains and clinical symptoms like dysfunction of intestine, without definite diagnostic criteria for the intestinal damages. The only thing we can do to the damages is waiting for the process of spontaneous healing. Xi Lei powder known as one of the traditional Chinese medicines is quite effective in relieving inflammation reaction. So with the purpose of exploring its protective roles to the

---

F. Zhang · D. Cai (✉) · J. Xu
School of Nursing Nantong University, 19 QiXiu Road, Nantong, Jiangsu, People's Republic of China
e-mail: caiduanying@ntu.edu.cn

F. Zhang
e-mail: zhangfeng820909@163.com

intestinal mucosa, we mixed Xi Lei powder into the enema solutions of various pH and observed the degree of congestion and edema of intestinal mucosa through light microscope and changes of cellular ultrastructures through TEM.

108.2 Method

We selected healthy adult (1.8–3 kg) Chinese rabbits provided by the animal experiment center of Nantong University, and randomized them into four groups administrated with different enema solutions (Table 108.1). Enema solution was maintained at about 40 °C, with 15 ml administered to the subjects through a 20 ml syringe. The enema procedure lasted for about 5 min. The depth of anal canal was about 7 cm. The rabbits completed their defecation within 3–4 h after enema. Then, 1 and 5 mm samples, for TEM (JEM-1230 Transmission Electron Microscope, JEOL Ltd., Japan)and microscopic examination (Nikon ys-100 Optical Microscope, Guangzhou), were obtained from the following three parts: rectum (15 cm away from the anus), distal part of colon (50 cm away from the anus), and proximal part of colon (25 cm away from the cecum). The experiments were approved by the Authorized Ethics Committee of experimental animals of Nantong University. The intestinal mucosal damage grades are classified by Chiu's methods [4]. The data was analyzed by SPSS15.0.

108.3 Results

108.3.1 Intestinal Mucous Membrane Changes Through Light Microscope

Injuries can be seen in four groups (Table 108.2, according to Chiu's injury classification) (Figs. 108.1, 108.2, 108.3, 108.4).

Table 108.1 Groups and enema solutions

Groups	n	Components of enema solution	pH
Group A (vinegar group)	20	75 ml vinegar + 75 ml normal sodium	2.76
Group B (vinegar + Xi Li Powder group)	20	75 ml vinegar + 75 ml normal sodium + 1.5 g Xi Lei powder	4.12
Group C (soapsuds group)	20	150 ml 0.2 % soapsuds	9.78
Group D (soapsuds + Xi Lei powder group)	20	150 ml 0.2 % soapsuds + 1.5 g Xi Lei powder	9.52

Table 108.2 Chiu's classification methods of intestinal mucosa injury in different sites of each group (n)

Classification	Rectum (n = 20)						Distal part of colon (n = 20)						Proximal part of colon (n = 20)					
	0	1	2	3	4	5	0	1	2	3	4	5	0	1	2	3	4	5
Group A	0	0	0	1	6	13	0	0	3	4	7	6	14	5	1	0	0	0[a]
Group B	0	0	1	2	11	6[b]	0	2	6	9	1	2[c]	16	4	0	0	0	0[a]
Group C	0	0	0	3	7	10	0	0	2	5	8	5	13	5	2	0	0	0[a]
Group D	2	4	6	3	3	2[df]	2	5	8	2	3	0[eg]	16	3	1	0	0	0[a]

[a] classification of intestinal mucosa injury within each group, $P < 0.01$; [b] compare with rectum in group A, $P < 0.05$; [c] compare with distal part of colon in group A, $P < 0.01$; [d] compare with rectum in group C, $P < 0.01$; [e] compare with distal part of colon in group C, $P < 0.01$; [f] compare with rectum in group B, $P < 0.01$; [g] compare with distal part of colon in group B, $P < 0.05$

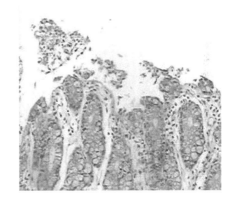

Fig. 108.1 The group A, neutrophils infiltrated in epithelial lamina and lamina propria. There were some ulcer due to the loss of cellula epithelialis and glands in lamina propria. (HE x100)

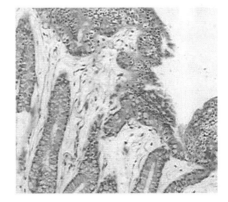

Fig. 108.2 The group B, congestion and hydrops appeared in interstitial portion. Small amounts of neutrophils infiltrated in epithelial lamina and partial surface epithelium is gone that led to superficial erosions. (HE x100)

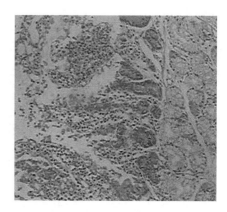

Fig. 108.3 The group C, there was neutrophil infiltration all around the visual field. There were multiple superficial erosions due to the loss of cellula epithelialis. Lots of Inflammatory cells combined with exfoliated cells. (HE x100)

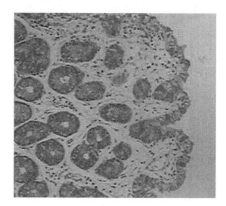

Fig. 108.4 The group D, the mucous membrane kept intact, slight mucosal edema and infiltration of few inflammatory cells can be found. Glands in lamina propria were morphologically normal with distinct structural layers. (HE x100)

108.3.2 Alteration for Ultramicrostructure of Intestinal Cells Through Electron Microscope

The cell injuries in groups A and C were critical, while intermediate damages appeared in group B. Almost no change or light injuries of ultramicrostructure were detected in group D. (Figs. 108.5, 108.6, 108.7, 108.8).

108.4 Discussion

Electronic microscope is a high accuracy electronic optical instrument for cell morphology, with the observation range of 0.1 nm [5]. Light microscopic observation range is 100–200 nm, which can observe the cell congestion and edema, intestinal mucosa structure integrity, inflammatory cells [6]. This study mainly used light microscopic to observe intestinal mucosa injuries caused by acidic and

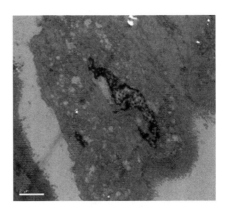

Fig. 108.5 The group A, chromatin margination and karyopyknosis (x8000)

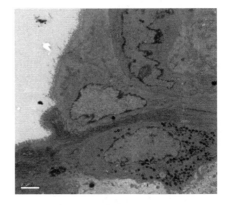

Fig. 108.6 The group B, endothelial cells linked tightly and arranged in-line (x6000)

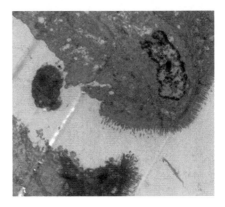

Fig. 108.7 The group C, necrosis and apoptosis of intestinal mucosal epithelium cells (x8000)

alkaline enema solutions, and the possible protection of Xi Lei Powder. The grade of damages and protective effect of Xi Lei Powder were determined by light microscopy. In addition, intestinal mucosal injuries begins from intestinal mucosal cell damage, however, there is no outcomes from optical microscope for the early

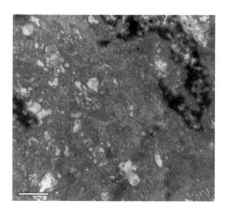

Fig. 108.8 The group D, there was edema of intestinal columnar ciliary epithelium cells, and swelling of mitochondrion and endoplasmic reticulum (x20000)

damages. Therefore, TEM was needed in the observation of changes for cell junction and cell microstructure, which helped to understand the degree of injury for intestinal mucosa membrane.

Xi Lei powder plays a pivotal role in detoxicating and invigorating the blood circulation, besides, they also inhibit the growth of bacteria. Animal experiments have indicated that Xi Lei powder promotes injurious healing by activating fibroblast division [7]. Besides, it was pointed out that Xi Lei powder could increase the mouse's pain threshold in 2 h after medication due to the effect of cyclooxygenase and lypoxygenase [8]. We found that the injuries of intestinal mucosa were lighter after enema by soapsuds or vinegar mixed with Xi Lei powder. This is attributed to the fact that Xi Lei powder attaches to the intestinal mucous membrane quickly when enema solution pours into the bowel. On one hand, Xi Lei powder plays an important role as a mechanical defense barrier. Thus, it decreases the injuries of acid and alkaline enema. On the other hand, it can reduce inflammatory cell aggregation and promote ulcerous agglutination.

It suggests us to pay attention to the intestinal injuries caused by enema. Additionally, it's necessary for us to unify the criteria of enema damages. Since outcome measures for enema injuries to the naked eyes are not so accurate, so we need to use TEM to observe the early damages of intestinal mucosa membrane by enema. Clinically, Xi Lei powder is the common Chinese medicine that is found to be effective. It has significant protective roles to intestinal mucosa when mixed into common enema solutions. We need further clinical researches before clinical application.

References

1. Akahashi M, Fukuda T (2011) Ileorectal fistula due to a rectal cancer—a case report. Int J Surg Case Rep 2:20–21
2. Mendoza J, Legido J, Rubio S et al (2007) Systematic review: adverse effects of sodium phosphate enema. Aliment Pharmacol Ther 26:9–20

3. Xu XJ, Zhang F, Sheng MY, Zhang JG (2010) Research on injuries to rabbit's intestinal mucosa caused by enema with different pH. J Nurses Train 25:2120–2122
4. Chiu CJ, McArdle AH, Brown R et al (1970) Intestinal mucosa lesion in low flow states.I. a morphological, hemodynamic, and metabolic reappraisal. Arch Surg 101:478–483
5. Duchamp M, Lachmann M, Boothroyd CB et al (2013) Compositional study of defects in microcrystalline silicon solar cells using spectral decomposition in the scanning transmission electron microscope. Appl Phys Lett 102 doi: 10.1063/1.4800569
6. Hanna REB, Moffett D, Brennan GP et al (2013) Fasciola hepatica: a light and electron microscope study of sustentacular tissue and heterophagy in the testis. Vet Parasitol 187:168–182
7. Liu DY, Zhao HM, Zhao N et al (2006) Pharmacological effects of Ba-Wei-Xi-Lei powder on ulcerative colitis in rats with enema application. Am J Chin Med 34:461–469
8. Dai JP (2008) Study on the mechanism and effective fractions of xilei san to promote mucosal ulcers healing. ph.d. dissertation, Department of Sitiology, Jiangsu University, China

Chapter 109
Study on the Theory Building of Relationship Between National Culture Benefit and Language Education Policy

Jingying Ma

Abstract The paper analyzes language education policy from the perspective of national culture benefit. The aim of paper is to answer some questions such as: what logical relations exist between national culture benefit and language education policy? What influences on each other? What is the theoretical basis while analyzing language education policy from the view of national culture benefit? Furthermore, the paper would structure theoretical frame of language education policy in order to maintain benefits of national culture and establish theoretical basis for the following text.

Keywords National cultural interests · National interests · Language educational policy · Soft power of language and culture · Strategic language planning concept

109.1 Introduction

Language education policy is assembled with language policy and education policy so that language policy should be understudied firstly. Language policy is also known as language planning, it is a planning and purpose program that nation manages language life. Language education policy means that the government establishes plans and measures in language education and teaching in order to realize the national language education. Language education policy is not only the reflection of language policy in education realms but also the plans and measures of education policy that aim at language teaching. As language education guidance, language education policy and language education have close relationship.

J. Ma (✉)
Beihua University Teacher's College, Jilin city, China
e-mail: automesh@gmail.com

Language education policy has the following characteristics: Firstly, language education policy is a measurement adopted by government which aims at the problems of national language education. Secondly, language education policy is the foundation and premise of the other education policy. Thirdly, language education policy is divided into dominant and recessive policy.

Language education policy and the development of state nation are closely linked; it has three functions for the development of nation. Firstly, it has guidance function. Secondly, it has harmonization function. Language education policy could harmonize and balance various relationships of language education. Thirdly, language education policy has control function.

Language is the vehicle of culture and it is the cultural root of a nation. In global competition, language superiority is often taken advantage of or exploited to propagate values and promote the soft power of a nation, thereby gaining or obtaining national cultural interests. Acquiring language superiority relies on the guidance of language educational policy, which, as a guiding document, promotes the development of language education. Therefore, the making of language educational policy and its execution or implementation has become a critical means for a nation to safeguard and also to realize its national cultural interests. The making of language educational policy and its implementation must be tightly linked to the development strategy of a nation, aiming highly in order to ensure the protection of or safeguarding of the national cultural interests of a nation and realization of these national cultural interests.

The goal of this dissertation lies in offering systematic knowledge of the inner logical relationship between language educational policy and national cultural interests, and providing reference for the strategic selection and language educational policy making of our nation. The central arguments that this dissertation tries to clarify are as follows: first, the national interests of a nation is the guidance of its language educational policy, and the language educational policy of a nation is beginning to play a more crucial role in terms of promoting.

109.2 Interaction Mechanism of National Culture Benefit and Language Education Policy

Language education is education of culture and value, language education policy is a culture education policy in nature. The influence of language education policy in language learners and people would reflect on the transform of national culture level and culture requirement which would change the national culture benefit. Moreover, the transform of national culture benefit could reflect on the language education policy. The relationship between national culture benefit and language education policy is dynamic changed that is bidirectional but not unidirectional. There is interaction mechanism between them. From the view of embryology, this section divides the interaction mechanism of national culture benefit and language education policy into three hierarchies: both are driving force, maintenance energy and guidance force.

109.2.1 Driving Force with Each Other in National Culture Benefit and Language Education Policy

Driving force is power to drive an object. Due to the carrier of exchange and basis of culture, language education policy is a tool to maintain culture benefit when the early days of the republic, and then national culture benefit drives the establishment and complement of language education policy.

109.2.2 Maintenance Energy with Each Other in National Culture Benefit and Language Education Policy

National culture benefit and language education policy are interaction and interdependent, even mutual maintenance and conglutination.

109.2.3 Guidance Force with Each Other in National Culture Benefit and Language Education Policy

National culture benefit guides the goal and value orientation of language education policy and the language education policy plays a guidance role in the trend of national culture benefit. There is mutual lead effect between them. National culture benefit guides the orientation of language education so that the benefits of national culture should be as the ultimate goal while the language education policy is formulated.

109.3 Theoretical Framework of Language Education Policy with the Ultimate Goal of National Culture Benefit

As a national education policy, language education policy belongs to national public policy. From the view of system elements, public policy system is a social politics system which is constituted by policy subject, policy object and policy environment according to the theory of policy system. As a public policy, language education policy consists of policy subject, policy object and policy environment.

The establishment of language education policy is the most critical in the whole process of language education policy. It is premise of the policy to reach the goal. The goal of language education policy is the premise and basis of policy analysis because that decides the value orientation of policy immediately. The paper builds theoretical frame of language education policy in order to maintain benefits of national culture according to the main point of policy system theory. The kernel goal of language education policy formulation is the advancement of soft power in language culture; the basic value orientation of language education policy is the strategic concept of language planning; the fundamental guarantee of language education policy to maintain benefits of national culture lies in the interaction coordination mechanism of the components of language education policy system.

109.4 Education Language Discourse Construction Control Field and Contemplation

Gravitational field of educational languages (vector field) is the functional coupling system formed by the interactions between the speech subject and the education objectives (demand orientations like education policy, cultivation purpose, specifications, etc.) and discourse audience under the control of special speech contexts. In terms of performance characteristics, due to the special characteristics of unfinished linearity of the constructed control field of educational languages, the expresser often fails to reflect every details of each factor and makes instant choices of expressing behaviors in the moment of expressing control. The running of thinking and decision making is instant, and the instant choice and decision can only depend on the suspension state of the partial unfinished linearity to make the quick planning and controlling. As a result, the generalized casualty of the objective "concluding" is realized time after time, and the repeated points and lines are fused and cared. This feature is mostly expressed in the speech acts like mono-directional speech control and multi-directional debate stress.

The proposal of the gravitational field of educational languages attaches emphasis on the functions and mechanisms of the nonlinearity, non-single-cause-or-consequence and synchronicity of human speech behavior. It directly exposes and pulls in the distance between the theories and practices of educational languages. The speech behaviors are combined with the expressing thoughts under the synchronicity of historical and social backgrounds, cultural conventions, vision and requirements, and hence formed an active controlling field. It exposes the general characteristics of controlling space of a certain speech behavior under certain times, and breaks through the traditional recognition mode of linear, single cause and consequence, stationary and abstract usage of educational languages. Diachronism is transformed into synchronicity, abstraction is transformed into corporeality, dispersibility is transformed into integrity, and static is transformed into dynamic. It opens up a whole new and wide development space for the vivid and diversified educational languages, and is doomed to bring a huge breakthrough to the pragmatics fields.

109.5 Conclusion

Above all, the language education policy has been deep analyzed in this paper, and the interaction mechanism between national culture benefit and language education policy has been analyzed from the view of embryology. It pointed out that national culture benefit and language education policy were driving force, maintenance energy and guidance energy with each other. On that basis, the theoretical framework has been constructed from three dimensions as the ultimate goal of national culture benefit. Dimension 1 discussed that the core objective position of language education policy was the enhancement of the soft power of language culture. Enhanced soft power of language culture should from both domestic and international level according to different internal and external function of nations. At the national level to enhance the recognition of the extent of the national language culture, to enhance the cohesion and charisma of national culture; at the international level to defend the sovereignty and security of national language culture and to promote the spread of language culture in external. The second dimension discussed that the basic value orientation of language education policy was the view of language strategy planning. Language strategic planning was guided by scientific development concept. All areas involved in language issues are fully integrated into the national language culture development strategic vision. Language strategy and planning in our country have been orientated under the global platform background and have got rid of the drawbacks of previous language planning concept of on-sided guide language education policy. The third dimension analyzed that the fundamental guarantee of language education policy to maintain national culture benefit was coordination mechanism of the inner components of language education policy system which included coordination between subject and object of policy and between policy subject object and environment.

References

1. Shi GS, Wang Zl (2002) The study of the instructional content and course series of the physical education programs of regular higher education in the province of Jiangsu (I): commentary on the Curricula. J Nanjing Inst Phys Educ (Soc Sci) 16(4):6–8
2. Wang L (2007) Reasonable consideration about the course reform of P.E.major of teachers' college. J Nanjing Inst Phys Educ(Soc Sci) 28(6):57–60
3. Liao M (2007) Investigation and analysis on current sports science achievement in University in Guangdong Province. J Nanjing Inst Phys Educ (Soc Sci) 15(5):72–74

4. Peng J-m (2005) Discussion on courses setting for P.E. major in four-year P.E. colleges. 28(4):522–524
5. Huang B (2001) The ways to deal with the present situation and the developmental goal of scientific research of P.E. in colleges and universities. J Nanjing Inst Phys Educ(Soc Sci)4:67–69
6. Li J-b, Bin SU (2006) Present condition and problem of common university's PE teachers at the beginning of 21 centuries in China. J Shandong Inst Phys Educ Sports 22(6):86–98
7. Sheng C, Zhao C (2010) Study on college sports scientific research comprehensive evaluation system in Beijing. J Capital Inst Phys Educ 22(6):19–28
8. Zhao Y, Lin Z, Lian B, Xu X (1994) Evaluating system of scientific research institutions of sport. J Beijing Univ Phys Educ 17(1):1–8
9. Lin Z (2005) Study on the conter-measure of reinforcing P.E. scientific research in colleges and universities. J Anhui Sports Sci 26(6):93–98

Chapter 110
Study on the Defect and Research About Discipline Speech Act Theory of Educator

Li Ying

Abstract The research of philosophy appears linguistic turns and raises the proposition of "the study of language is to study the ideas themselves". The effect of language on cognition performs in many aspects which are based on numerous facts and results of cognitive psychology. Despite the language influences cognition is confirmed in different languages or same language, the ultimate goal of language comprehension by means of language forms to create sense and reaches to the illocutionary act. Does language influence cognition and in turn affect the behavior? Is the behavior enslaved to language? In this regard, the discussion of speech act theory possesses ground breaking. Language, society and psychology are integrated while speech act as the axis which is the significance of speech act theory.

Keywords Speech act · Speech events · Perlocutionary act, · Discipline · Psychological effect

110.1 Introduction

There are lots of limitations from the structure of academic thoughts to specific problems, and then to the implement of research process which are based on the research of language influences cognition and language influences behavior. Those researches are throughout the relationships of language philosophy and language existent, the research of pragmatics and study of psycholinguistics on speech act.

L. Ying (✉)
Jinlin Medical college, Jilin, People's Republic of China
e-mail: automesh@gmail.com

110.1.1 The Theory of Speech Act Analyzes in the Sentence Level Rather Than the Discourse

The theory of speech act regards speech act as language act. In fact, the semantics of the sentence is restricted by the entire dialog.

110.1.1.1 The Speech Act of Speaker is Concerned and the Role of Recipient is Ignored

The function of language in social interaction cannot be explained due to that only the speech act of speaker is concerned and the role of recipient is ignored. There are non-direct multivariate relationships between the sentence structure and function. There are significances of connotation, style, emotion and even association in the utterance meaning except that the meanings of logic, cognition and extension content. Meanwhile, these cognitive differences between speaker and recipient exist inconformity. The inconformity would influence the take effect of speech act of speaker.

110.1.1.2 Speech Act Theory Does Not Discuss the Language Environment Systematically

Speech act theory does not touch the language environment systematically and could not elaborate the language environment exactly. The integrated language environment should do something satisfactorily and successfully which satisfy the speech act.

110.1.1.3 The Research Method Focuses on Description But Lacks of Empirical Study

The innovation of "speech is action" is raised by speech act theory; it emphasizes the perlocutionary act and the effects of speech on recipient. However, the theory does not clarify the problems such as: how does language influence cognition? What are ways and factors to affect cognition? How to do the take effect of language? Therefore, it lacks of empirical research according to the theory that real corpus should make the test to theoretical contracture. The analysis of few words is seen by readers.

110.2 Proposition of Discipline Speech Act Research

110.2.1 Logical Extension of Speech Act Research

As a concerned theory of language use, the speech act theory is the tremendous progress of language research which is influenced by language philosophy. However, under the guidance of new ideas of the language and cognition relations, the research of speech act should extend to the discussion between language and recognition, language and act, the relations of speech act effect. It seems to take the following positions in the further study:

(1) Research the speech act under fixed language environment
(2) Pay full attention to the mechanism of speech act.
(3) Comprehensive investigate the conditions to realize the illocutionary act.

110.2.2 Discipline Speech Act

Language is not only the communication tool but also instrument of labor in the education area. Parents, teachers and students all need the tool. The role of language is throughout the whole process of education. Language is the home of existence and also is the home of education.

110.2.3 Basic Conception of the Psychological Effects Research of Discipline Speech Act

The psychological effects of educators' discipline speech act are researched from cognition, emotion and behavior tendency. Cognition is evaluation of educatees to the discipline speech act of educators, which decides the attitude of educatees to educators and their discipline speech act. Emotion refers to the emotional experience of educatees while accept the discipline speech which includes properties and intensities of emotion and it restricts the harmony of the relationship between them. Behavior tendency refers to actions of educatees after accept the discipline speech of educators which is restricted by cognition and emotion of educatees. The relationships between them are complex.

110.3 Application of Flanders Interaction Analysis System in Classroom Teaching

Flanders Interaction Analysis System is an analyzing technique used to explore the essence of classroom teaching and the regularity of teaching. It is a innovation in the field of education, which provides a brand new research perspective in the interaction analysis of the classroom language.

With the help of SPSS, calculation is conducted towards the major parameters in the Flanders Interaction Analysis System in the unit of one minute. The dynamic graphs of each major parameter are drawn so as to observe the dynamic changes of each major parameter in the classroom teaching more systematically and more directly.

Figures 110.1 and 110.2 show case respectively the dynamic graphs of the ratio of teacher languages and student languages. We can have a clear and direct observation of the fluctuation and rhythm of the languages of teachers and students. Figure 110.1 show that the ratio of teacher languages is more than 80 % and forms 11 peaks. Figure 110.2 show that the chances for students to speaking in the class are abundant, with only two occasions without students' participation and no less than 3 min. Flanders Interaction Analysis System is one of the interaction analyses of classroom language. It captures the essence of the classroom teaching, and provides a new research perspective for the education study. It is a self-evaluating method for teaching. Teachers can videotape the classroom teaching, and keep records of the significance of the classroom language behaviors in the unit of 3 s according to the Flanders Interaction Analysis System. Then, attach values to them based on the understanding of the significances, so one can avoid the changes of the classroom situation due to the intervention of others.

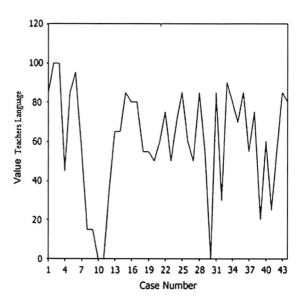

Fig. 110.1 The dynamic graphs of the ratio of teacher languages

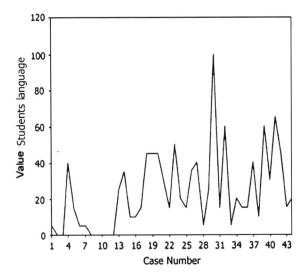

Fig. 110.2 The dynamic graphs of the ratio of student languages

110.4 Conclusions

In the specific research, the study methods and technology of cognitive psychology, psychometrics, education and development psychology are widely adopted. Such as the methods of typical assessment, semantic assignment, scenario simulation, confirmed semantics, structured questionnaires and interviews. In order to overcome the deficiencies of previous researches, the investigative and experimental study are combined. To improve the research level, the contents of discipline speech act are standardized evaluated and the occurred situations are controlled.

References

1. Huang B (2001) The ways to deal with the present situation and the developmental goal of scientific research of P.E. in colleges and universities. J Nanjing Inst Phys Educ (Soc Sci) 4:67–69
2. Jing-bo LI, Bin SU (2006) Present condition and problem of common university's PE teachers at the beginning of 21 centuries in China. J Shandong Inst Phys Educ Sports 22(6):86–98
3. Sheng C, Zhao C (2010) Study on college sports scientific research comprehensive evaluation system in Beijing. J Cap Inst Phys Educ 22(6):19–28
4. Zhao Y, Lin Z, Lian B, Xu X (1994) Evaluating system of scientific research institutions of sport. J Beijing Univ Phys Educ 17(1):1–8
5. Zuming L (2005) Study on the conter-measure of reinforcing P.E. scientific research in colleges and universities. J Anhui Sports Sci 26(6):93–98
6. Li W, Ren B (2000) Present problems under hot discussion of research on higher physical education in China. J Beijing Univ Phys Educ 23(1):89–92
7. Types and Cultivating Model of Chinese Physical Education (2001). J Beijing Teach Coll Phys Educ 13(1):74–78

Chapter 111
Study on the Nature of Education Information: The Education of Digital Virtual World

Zhang Junmei

Abstract The object of this research is the nature of education information in the view of pedagogy. The nature of information technology is a digital representation of the physical world that will build a digital virtual world. Information is the diffusion of information technology in the social life and builds a digital virtual world in all areas and levels such as work, life, study and entertainment space. The new changes of nature, research purposes, value orientation, study objects and research methods in education information are generated. Furthermore, a new research paradigm of education information is formed eventually.

Keywords The essence of e-education · Perspective of pedagogy · Perspective of technology

111.1 The Essence of E-Education; Perspective of Pedagogy; Perspective of Technology

In the technical perspective, E-education main concern educational software, educational information system, e-learning model issues. But we paid little attention to the principle of teaching learning theory and the being in the cyberspace. Therefore, the cause of E-education is the technical Perspective. Education is social activities which to influence awareness of the physical and mental development of people. Education is the study of how bring up people like to be independent, self-improvement, self-reliance. Education is social activities which to influence awareness of the physical and mental development of people. Education is the study of how bring up people like to be independent, self-improvement, self-reliance.

Z. Junmei (✉)
Beihua University Teacher's College, Jilin, People's republic of China
e-mail: kingmesh@gmail.com

E-education is the core conditions of how bring up by ICT. So, the research of E-education must move from the technical perspective to pedagogy. The essence of E-education is the development of student in the cyberspace. It includes three levels of study: First, to research being and moral issues in cyberspace by philosophy; Second, to research the theory of educational curriculum, teaching learning and evaluation by science; Third, to research the teaching model and evaluation model by technology. The main understandings of domestic educational technology researchers on the nature of education information are the following:

From the above discussions on the nature of education information, if we analyze the definitions according to the theories of socio-technical form, it could be grouped into two categories: one of the views defines the process of information technology that used in education, which is process inform; another view is a new education system that based on the usage of information technology, which is results form.

Therefore, the research view is focused on the information technology and its utilization methods but there is no further cognition of information technology and adults from the technology perspective to cognize the nature of information. The research perspective should be transformed and the education information and its nature should be re-recognized from education perspective so that could achieve the target that mentioned above.

111.2 Re-recognize of the Education Information Nature in Pedagogy

As a sub-domain in education, the cognition of education information nature must establish on the basis of cognition of education nature and rebuild the nature of education information from another view.

As the specific activities of human society, the most essential features of education are the training of human and serve the community through this training. This feature is throughout the ancient and modern, as well as all the future education. However, the statement that education is an activity of people cultivation is too general so that only contact with the surface of problem.

From the nature that education is social activity as the direct target of that conscious affect the physical and mental development of human, we believe that the nature is unable to spread around technology while the information technology introduced into the education, but it should spread around the education activity of physical and mental development of human in the information technology conditions. That is another perspective of education information nature which is pedagogy perspective.

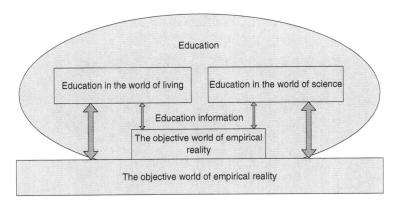

Fig. 111.1 Education information: culture in the digital virtual world

Therefore, the definition of the education information nature should be based on the cognition of education nature (generality) and highlight the nature of information (individuality) so that the education information could separate from other education activities. From this cognition and base on the nature of education and information, the question that what is education information is defined: education information is social activity that conscious affects physical and mental of human in the digital virtual world which is as the direct target (Fig. 111.1).

111.3 Education in the Virtual Life World

The living world theory was first proposed by Husserl. He set up three roads that lead to transcendental phenomenology; they are the road of psychology, the road of Descartes and the road through the living world.

111.3.1 The Connotation of the Life World

From the description of Husserl on living world, living world includes three meanings: the first meaning: The world that we could feel and live every day. The second meaning: The specific and special living environment and life circle of each person which is formed by the practice of people in daily life.

The third meaning: An overall world of life activities by various temporal understandings.

It should be said that the living world concept of Husserl that put forward relative to the science world and try to analyze and solve the crisis of European science based on the theory of living world.

111.3.2 The Significant of Living World to Education

Education aims to make people useful. Therefore, the significance of living world to education is that rediscover the basic significance of science world.

The educational activities in living world are the activities of communication between human. These communication activities are not equal to the daily communication and it could be called educational communication. The educational virtual community is a virtual living world in the network world.

111.4 The Education in Virtual Science World

111.4.1 The Birth of the Science World

Science is developed from the former living world of science; the scientific process is an abstract process of the living world. Husserl believed that the human subject of human life is abstracted and all the spirits and all the cultural characteristics which are attached to material in the human practice are abstracted so that the object becomes pure object.

Science originally from the living world, and ultimately achieve a scientific world picture. A series of meaningful changes are happened in this process. These changes are grouped into three categories:

The first is that the intuition and nature of living world turn to the mathematical nature.

Secondly is that the inaccuracy of living world turn to the accuracy of scientific world.

Thirdly, the living world that is perceived and near the subject is turning to the scientific world which is not perceived and far away from the subject.

The experience real life world has the subjective relativity; only through the rule of univocity could percept the emotional around world and the relativity of subjective interpretation could be overcome, which could realize the objectivity in the principal practical significance. Objectify the living world is a process that far away from the subject of the life world and is a process that non-humane treat to living world.

Science world provides a world picture that the real world is nature of mathematics and concept, and it is a comfortable objects world which is governed by causal law strictly. It could be formulated and explained through the math formula and physical formula. Therefore, the scientific world is constructed by scientific activities, scientific theory and the world picture that is descripted by science.

111.4.2 Education of Virtual Science World

The scientific world provides a mathematical and theoretical nature world picture. The objective scientific world is expressed by binary numbers and presents in front of us. That is a virtual scientific world (Fig. 111.2).

The education of virtual scientific world includes two aspects. One is that the abstract and gray scientific world is presented by digital virtual world intuitively. Another is that utilizes the digital technology and according to the objective knowledge of scientific world to rebuilds a virtual world which fits the scientific theory. The virtual and real world that is virtual and it contains scientific knowledge so that students could immerse themselves in scientific investigation and master the scientific knowledge.

The sentence that is all-encompassing tech methods to cultivate comprehensive talents contains two pairs of contradictions.

(1) From the inner of education, contradictions between students and scientific world which is objectively and abstractly;
(2) From the relations of internal and external education, the contradictions between the limited space–time school and unlimited natural world that is the origin of scientific world. The education of virtual scientific world would break these two conflicts in a certain extent.

From a new perspective, the research of education information could bring some new changes to the nature, research purposes, research value-orientation, research object and research methods of education information which could form a new research paradigm of education information. The education information theory is a huge theory system in the new paradigm. The paper just discussed the nature of education information from the view of pedagogy because of the limitation of personal power and energy, as well as the pages of paper. The other problems remain to be researched. If the paper arouses the concern of researchers and the purpose is achieved; if it could attract researchers to grant instruction, then I will be very happy.

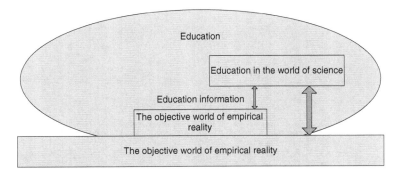

Fig. 111.2 Education of education information and virtual scientific world

References

1. Liu S, Ren H (2006) The comparison between total quality management (TQM) and traditional management (TM). Commer Res 337:122–124
2. He Z, Zhou S (2005) Process management for continuous quality improvement. Ind Eng J 5(8):38–41
3. He Z, Lu J, Liu X, He S (2007) Design and development of the integrated quality management system IQMS2.0. Ind Eng J 10(6):54–58
4. Yuan Y, Liu H (2007) Service outsourcing and promotion of technical innovative efficiency in manufacturing industry. J Dalian Univ Technolo 28(4):1–6 (Social Sciences)
5. Chen G, Meng MA (2000) Studies on the process model of organizational learning. J Manag Sci China 3(3):15–23
6. Edmondson, Mo I (1997) Organizational learning and competitive advantage. Mc Graw-Hill, New York, pp 1–10
7. Dai W, Zhao S, Steve FF (2006) Study on a dynamic model of organizational learning processes under complex system. Stud Sci 24:217–224

Chapter 112
Study on the Construction of General Framework of Educational Cost Management Mode in Colleges and Universities

Xiu Hongbo

Abstract As the core content of the educational cost management in colleges and universities, the educational cost measurement issues have not reached a consensus in theory circle; the cost measurement and cost control have not been formed until they fit the management science law in colleges. In order to research the educational cost management pattern in colleges and universities, the paper is based on the analysis that cost managements in colleges and enterprises are homogeneity and used the cost management pattern of enterprises for reference, and combines with the characteristics of colleges and then constructs the educational cost management pattern of colleges, and describes the characteristics of educational cost management pattern in colleges and universities.

Keywords Continuous improvement · Organization · Organization action model · Comprehensive evaluation system

112.1 Introduction

Pattern is also called paradigm that refers to styles which are able to use as template, model or changed model. As a terminology, pattern has various meanings in different subjects. Based on the understanding of pattern, the paper considered the cost management pattern could be summarized that: the cost management is the sum of generalization of basic regularity in some cost management system and the basic framework and the main operating principles. Cost management pattern reflects the most fundamental things in certain kind of cost management system and it is the theory abstraction of cost management system.

X. Hongbo (✉)
College of Transportation and Civil Engineering, Beihua University, Jilin, People's Republic of China
e-mail: kingmesh@gmail.com

It is a theoretical system that starts from a realistic cost management practices and gets through a comparative analysis and then abstracts out an ideal type or style which could guide cost management practices. Based on the above analysis, the definition of educational cost management pattern in colleges is defined as that the sum of generalization of basic regularity in some cost management system and the basic framework and the main operating principles.

112.2 The Constructional Thoughts of Educational Cost Management Pattern in Colleges and Universities

112.2.1 Cost Management Pattern in Enterprises

Domestic and foreign enterprises have formed a unique cost management pattern with the development of management theory. The standard, target and responsibility cost system are more applied in our enterprises. The standard cost is established by detailed analysis and investigation and technological measurement. It is a target cost that could evaluate actual cost and measure work efficiency. In addition, it is a cost that rule out the cost of consumption which could not occur. The target cost extracts and highlights the cost objective from enterprise target system. The various cost management and other management activities are carried out around the cost objective which could guide, planning and control the costs and expenses. The responsibility cost collects responsibility centers such as cost center, profit center and investment center as the subjects. It belongs to the responsibility range of center management accompanies with controllable costs of the corresponding economic responsibility.

112.2.2 The Homogeneity of Cost Management Between Enterprises and Universities

The cost management pattern of universities could learn from the enterprises or not depends on that whether similarities are existed in universities and enterprises and their operational management activities.

The education teaching, scientific research and social services are the terminal products of universities from the perspective of products. Universities and consumers all have strict quality requirements on products. Universities require promotional planning of enrollment and have human, financial and material management and operation from the perspective of operation. From the view of sales, schools recommend various types of educational services and scientific researches to educator and society are to sell products. The employment rate of graduates reflects the quality of education and the marketable conditions of the education teaching service products. The only difference is that enterprises focus on economic efficiency and universities both need the social and economic benefits.

Therefore, the similarities of universities and enterprises and their operational management activities are greater than the differences. Eliminate the products of the two organizations and from the view of cost management, the cost management of enterprises and universities is homogeneity.

112.3 The General Framework of Educational Cost Management in Colleges and Universities

From the range of cost management and in modern cost management phase, the cost management includes seven components that are forecast, decision, planning, control, measure, analysis and assessment. We generally regard that the cost measurement and control are the two core contents of cost managements. However, the budget and compensation of educational cost should be emphasized while manage the educational cost because of the particularity of the educational cost.

According to the above establishment, a college educational cost management pattern built in this paper can be summarized as: Adapt to the diverse needs of knowledge economy and society for talents and according to the development strategy of colleges, the right educational cost strategy and budget are established. The operating, strategic and total cost managements are comprehensive applied base on the guidance of modern cost management theory. The operating chain of colleges is optimized continuously and the educational cost of colleges is measured accurately and controlled effectively. According to different needs, the educational cost information is disclosed in different levels; the rational tuition policy is developed and the educational cost of colleges to be full compensation. The educational cost of management organization in colleges and system construction are improved. Ensure the various economic activities advanced the way that help control the cost of education and increase the output efficiency of educational resources continuously. The management pattern of educational cost in colleges and universities is shown in Fig. 112.1.

112.4 Characteristics of Educational Cost Management Pattern in Colleges and Universities

Strategy is a plan made by global development goals and trends.

It is also the guidance of the global plans and strategies. Strategy will play a guidance role in the future development of the overall pattern of evolution for a long period while it has been determined. Strategy is always understood as a

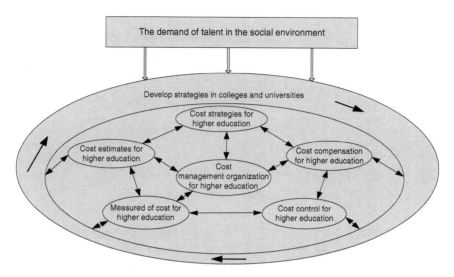

Fig. 112.1 Management mode frame of educational cost in colleges and universities

method of long-term goals achievement in the management area. One strategy applied in the universities is planning which to make the skills and resources to adapt the opportunities in the external environment.

The cost management includes two aspects contents: one is that the university strategy is analyzed, selected and optimized from the view of cost. Another is the strategy to control cost. The former is the cost side of the university strategy; the latter undertakes a planning to educational cost management systems, methods and measures in order to improve the effectiveness of the educational cost management.

Educational cost should be emphasized while universities strategy is formulating, selecting and implementing no matter what strategies are adopted. How to use educational cost strategy to win the cost and competitive advantage in universities is the important content of universities strategy management and educational cost management. The cost advantage protections of cost advantage for universities are provided Based on those foundations and through a series of cost management application.

112.5 DEA Evaluation Model for the Effectiveness of the Cost Management in College Education

112.5.1 Basic Model of Data Envelopment Analysis

Rigorous languages are employed to introduce C^2R model, one of the most basic DEA models, because it is a typical example to regularize and modelize the direct thinking. Assume that there are n $DMU_J(1 \leq j \leq n)$, the input and output of DMU_j are respectively:

$$x_j = (x_{1j}, x_{2j}, \ldots, x_{mj})^T, (j = 1, 2, \ldots, n)$$
$$y_j = (y_{1j}, y_{2j}, \ldots, y_{mj})^T, (j = 1, 2, \ldots, n)$$

Due to the different positions and functions of various input and output in the process of production, it needs to composite the input and output if evaluations are required on the DMU. In other words, they are considered as a production process of total input and output. In this way, each input and output needs to be attached with appropriate weight. For example, the weight of x_j is v_j, and the weight of y_k is $u_k (1 \leq j\ k \leq n)$.

Assume the weight vector of input and output are:

$$v = (v_1, v_1, \ldots, v_m)^T$$
$$u = (u_1, u_1, \ldots, u_s)^T$$

One of the most important thoughts of DEA model is taking the vectors of input and output as variable vectors instead of confirming the value of input and output in advance, and confirming their specific values according to the optimizing principle in the analysis process. Apparently, the weight confirmed through DEA has less artificial interventions and hence is more objective.

C^2R model is:

$$(P) \begin{cases} \max \mu^\tau y_0 = \overline{V_p} \\ s.t\ \omega^T x_j - \mu^T y_j \geq 0, j = 1, 2, \ldots, n \\ \omega^T x_0 = 1 \\ \omega \geq 0, \mu \geq 0 \end{cases}$$

It can be concluded that with the help of DAE analysis, not only the evaluation of past management in the colleges can be conducted, it can also point a direction for future improvements.

References

1. O'Leary DE (2004) On the relationship between REA and SAP. Int J Acc Inf Syst 5(1):65–81
2. Debreceny R, Gray GL (2001) The production and use of semantically rich accounting reports on the internet: XML and XBRL. Int Acc Inf Syst 1:47–74
3. Zhang X, Chai Y(1999)Event driven approach with business rule based modeling. J Tsinghua Univ (Sci Technol), vol 39(7), pp 25–28
4. Jinsong Z, Yifang Z (2006) Research on event-driven based product development process management. Comput Eng Appl 24:94–97
5. Zhi S, Liu J, Yan Z (2005) Relation-based flow control model. Comput Appl 25(11):2693–2697
6. Zhang H(2004)Business process reengineering in the era of information—On updating the accounting business process 19(6):65–69
7. Dao-cai Z (2004) On the audit of accounts and tables in electronic data processing accounting. J Anhui TV Univ 1:35–37

Chapter 113
Study on the Risk Identification and Warning of Tax Administration

Liu Weidong

Abstract It is from a new respective to view the state management activities while the tax administration and risk are associated. The paper analyzed the causes, contents and types of tax administration risk; it raised the basic approach and method of the risk identification and warning of tax administration; it pointed out that the construction of tax administration risk preventions system, the establishment of the risk prevention countermeasures of tax administration and the appropriate risk management organization are the effective measures of tax administration risk warning.

Keywords Tax administration · Mode establishment · Choice of elements

113.1 Introduction

Management activities are the pursuit of effective activities, there are some management risks while pursue the management efficiency. In the tax administration activities, management activities have the potential risks when a new management method or means were adopted, a new management system was formulated, a certain period of work plans were determined in order to improve management efficiency. Therefore, the identification and warning of management risk, the suppression of the negative management are components of the tax administration activities. From vertical angle of the man's general knowledge, management can be defined as an activity of deciding, planning, organizing, coordinating, controlling and supervising the objects of management by managers

L. Weidong (✉)
School of Economics and Management Beihua University, Jilin, China
e-mail: kingmesh@126.com

in a certain organization through powers and some measures in order to attain the set goals efficiently.

Management has dual character, that is, management not only includes the matters related to productivity and scientific technology, from which angle, management objectives in various social forms are different, but also includes the matters related to relations of production and superstructure, from which angle, management in various social shapes is the same on the whole. So we can say that the scientific spirit of management and technology methods of that have characters in common in a variety of management activities whatever is to be managed. Management theory and basic measures are of the same significance to any management activity.

Tax management is a relatively independent subject that touches wider areas. If superstructure and relations of production in different social forms have not been taken into consideration, the scientific spirit of tax management and the advanced spirit of management technology are the focusing problem not only for all the countries in the world, but also facing in the process of tax administration. Given the general analysis of management theory, tax- management is an activity of deciding, planning, organizing, coordinating, controlling and supervising the taxation activities by the state related administrative sectors. Tax management can be divided into three categories, namely, tax management in broad sense, in medium sense and in narrow sense. Tax management in broad sense is referring to all kinds of taxation-oriented management including taxation legislation administration, tax law enforcement administration and taxation judicial administration. The above three together result in tax management in broad sense. The carrier of which contains the state legislation body, tax functionary sectors and the related judicial offices. Tax management in medium sense can be defined as tax law enforcement administration involving tax collection administration for taxpayers and tax administration for workers in the tax authority. The carrier of which is the state tax functionary sectors in theory, but in practice, the state tax authority, financial authority and the Customs at all levels are all the carriers of tax administration in medium sense. Tax management in narrow sense is tax collection administration and whose carrier is the same as that in medium sense. The only difference is the choice and determination of the administration objectives.

113.2 Management Risk and the Risk Management

Management risk and risk management are two different but related things, research and analysis of these two things are very important for improving the identification and warning capability of tax administration. Tax administration for the workers in the tax authority is an important part that cannot be neglected in tax law enforcement administration, which determines the effect of tax collection administration. Tax administration is at present larger in management organization and slow in the process of administration policy decision-making and has the formulation administrative phenomenon brought by the bureaucratic tendency, which has weaken the work efficiency. So requirements and tasks for reforming and improving tax administration are the matters of great urgency. While the research of tax administration have never been studied in the circle of taxation theory and practice in our country. There is a contradiction between the needs of the practical work and the relative weakness of the theoretical research, if which is not solved quickly, tax administration will be in an relatively loose and disorder condition, which will affects taxation efficiency seriously, leading to higher taxation costs which increase not only the financial burden but also the burden on taxpayers and even become a focus of contradiction of the tax collecting part and taxpayers. So strengthening the theoretic and practical work and probing into the mode and methods of practical and operational tax administration is the main way to solve that problem.

113.2.1 Management Risk

Management risk is that due to the adjustment of management method, the changes of management means, system or environment and then the potential risk is formed while the management activities are carried out at the same time. These risks and management activities are presence together and they become potential and direct factors which could impact and restrict the effect of tax administration activities.

113.2.2 Risk Management

Risk management is the identification, adaption and disposal of risk. The purpose of risk management is to avoid risk or makes the loss to the minimum. It is an important complement and extension of organization management strategy and determines the feasibility of its strategy and elasticity, thus it can be seen as a basic management function. It relates to the all levels and departments of organization. The higher the levels of management, the more important of the risk management functions.

113.3 The Prevention Strategies of Tax Administration Risk

In order to avoid losses of tax administration risk to tax administration organizations and society, the tax administration organizations should take initiative to build the risk prevention system and improve the risk prevention measures.

113.3.1 Build the Tax Administration Risk Prevention System

A perfect tax administration risk prevention system includes the following four sections.

(1) Economic and technical measures. Such as monitoring, inspection, legislation and environmental monitoring.
(2) Keep good communication with external. Establish the early warning system and coordinate the relationships between tax departments and government. In the latter case, the aim is to prevent the risks are caused by the system changes such as that government suddenly issued decrees and executive orders.
(3) Improve the internal works. Adjust the organic combination of the management factors, balance the management power, strengthen the coordination and communication of internal departments, ensure the chain integrity of tax administration, and avoid the management risks which are leaded by the internal frictions.
(4) Organize the cultivation of internal psychological prevention mechanism such as internal communications, training and educations of members. On the one hand, the alarm bells should keep ringing, and on the other hand, the risk prevention capacity of members should be trained.

113.3.2 The Risk Prevention Countermeasures of Tax Administration

The premise of solvation of management risk is the recognition of management risk. There should has appropriate preventive measures while solve the management risk.

(1) Avoidance Strategy

The avoidance strategy is the general risk prevention countermeasures which are used by economic organizations, and it refers that achieve the purpose of risk-averse by giving up some interests. In some cases it can play a role of prevention risk while the strategy is used in the tax administration activity. For example, the tax organization plans to use some new management techniques but found that it lacks the ability of management elements adjustment while use new techniques so that the new techniques are stranded, and then resulting in the loss of management efficiency, so organizations decide to give up or put off the new techniques. The essence of avoidance strategy is to avoid the risk source and then avoid the possibility of risk.

(2) Weakened Strategy

The weakened strategy controls the risk losses by decreasing the opportunities of risk occurrence and weakening the seriousness of the losses. The effect of avoidance is always limited and relative because that every management activities accompanies with varying degrees of risks. Therefore, tax administration organization should pursue the expected management efficiency as far as possible the losses are reduced to a minimum.

(3) Separation Strategy

The separation strategy spatial separates the risks that tax administration organization may faces so that the same losses could be avoided. Such as that if the tax administration risk is produced due to the human qualities, organizations could adopt the separation strategy and transfer or stop the works of problem staffs timely in order to avoid a bigger problem.

(4) Decentralization Strategy

Decentralization strategy enhances the resistance risk ability of tax administration organization by increasing the amount of risk carriers or decomposing the management activities links so as to disperse risk.

(5) Transfer Strategy

Transfer strategy controls the risk losses by transferring the risk losses to others. This is a common method that economic organization adopts to avoid the risks. The transferred ways they always adopt are that: transfer the properties or production operating activities which have risks to others; transfer the risk finance and participate in the insurance. In the tax administration activities, the transfer strategy is adopted to avoid risks, which represent that the responsibility of department is detailed to transfer the risks of the whole organization, or transfer the risks that the organization should bear by signing the detailed contract with organization members.

The above risk control strategies with various characteristics and applying conditions and it can be combined utilize and complementary with each other. In practice, the tax administration organization should implement the total combination in order to ensure the preventive effect based on the actual situation.

113.3.3 Establish the Risk Management Organization

In the practice of tax administration, the organizational issues will become unprecedented outstanding when the management risk turned to reality, which is to say that the risk management team should be decided to solve and restrain the risks. Risk management organization includes three aspects contents from a general sense; the provisions of the contents are suitable for the tax administration activities.

113.4 Conclusion

The risk of tax administration has been dealt with. To relate tax administration to the risk is a brand new approach to the state management activities. This thesis analyzes especially the cause of risk and raises identification of that risk and prevention ways. The matters related to performance evaluation of tax administration has been explored such as the multi-criterion and the system of that, which can act as the operational basis for the examination of the performance of tax administration in the practical work. Tax executive administration is a new subject facing our country's tax administration work. This thesis is a tentative and exploratory research, some of whose analyses and adjustments and designs may be found to be inconsistent with the future tax administration practice, but it is held that this beneficial research will bring enlightenment to the future theory research and practice work of tax administration.

References

1. Zhang X, CHAI Y(1999) Event driven approach with business rule based modeling. J Tsinghua Univ(Sci Technol) vol.39(7), pp.25-28
2. Jinsong Z, Yifang Zhong (2006) Research on event-driven based product development process management. Comput Eng Appl 24:94–97
3. Zhi S, LIU J, Yan Z (2005) Relation-based flow control model. Comput Appl 25(11):2693–2697
4. Wei Z, Bao-ping Y (2005) Survey on workflow module. Appl Res Comput 5:11–22
5. Edmondson, Mo ingeon(1997) Organizational learning and competitive advantage. Mc Graw-Hill, New York pp.1-10
6. Wan-wen D, Shu-ming Z, Foster SF (2006) Study on a dynamic model of organizational learning processes under complex system. Stud Sci Sci 24:217–224
7. Zhong-J(2002)On the reasons and countermeasures of the victims in the crimes of seizing the property by computer in economic activities.J Anhui Electr Power Coll Staff vol.7(2), pp.81-83

Chapter 114
Study on the System Design of Sports Public Service Performance Evaluation

Weidong Liu

Abstract Under the guidance of alternative supply mechanism of public service, in order to improve the responsibility and response ability of citizen which are service objects, and inspect the effectiveness of public service supplied and effectively respond to the opportunities and challenges brought by globalization, the paper raises the system design framework of sports public service performance evaluation in order to optimize the operation mechanism of sports administrative power and reflect the public service functions of government in the performance evaluation system. At the same time, it plays as the guidance and oversight roles in the transform of sports administrative functions in order to provide a better institutional environment.

Keywords Continuous improvement · Organization · Organization action model · Comprehensive evaluation system

114.1 Introduction

The performance evaluation of the sports public service mainly aims at the performances, achievements and actual effects that are obtained by government sports public service department in the public management activities. However, these performances, achievements and effects are obtained within the government functions. By dividing the assessment project, the sports public service performance evaluation is conductive to sort out the relationships between the government and market, the government and society, as well as the function differences of various sports administrative departments. Moreover, the results of sports public

W. Liu (✉)
School of Economics and Management, Beihua University, Jilin, China
e-mail: kingmesh@126.com

service performance evaluation also contribute to the optimization of power mechanism of China's sports administration and to the remodeling of the government role so as to promote the reasonable position of the administrative functions of government sports.

114.2 The Process of Sports Public Service Performance Evaluation

Performance evaluation of the sports public service is around the clear goal of performance level of sports public department, and it is a system process that measure and judge the department performance by the index system of system and scientific assessment tools. The performance assessment reflects the management philosophy of "costumer first". The main responsibilities of the sports public departments provide sports public services to social public.

The process of sports public service performance evaluation mainly includes principles and orientation of evaluation, the subject and object of evaluation, examination evaluation model, techniques and methods, index system of evaluation and information systems. The whole process of sports public service performance evaluation is shown in Fig. 114.1.

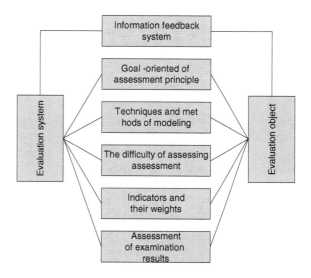

Fig. 114.1 Flow chart of sports public service performance evaluation

114.3 Subject of Sports Public Service Performance Evaluation

114.3.1 Government

Government is one of the evaluation subjects of sports public service. With the deepening of reform of China's sports administration management system, the government should realize the separation of regulatory and supplied functions of sports public service progressively. The institutionalization, professional and scientific evaluations are realized by dependence department to appliers and producers of sports public service and then the diversified subjects of performance evaluation are constructed. Government should establish a scientific evaluation system and detailed examination indicators. It monitors and evaluates the work effect of the supplied department of sports public service, the specification of supplied process and the satisfaction degree of service results. The full range of monitoring could guarantee the smooth running of sports pubic service system and the high quality of sports service enjoyed by citizens.

114.3.2 Citizen

The core functionality of sports public service system supplies the basic sports pubic service to citizens, the participation and satisfaction rate of citizens is a standard which could measure the completion, validation and reasonable of sports public services. For a long time, the absence and the drawbacks of customers in the sports public service are obvious. Customer orientation is one of the main doctrines of the new public management movement. Therefore, the improved performance evaluation mechanism needed to be established that citizens participate in. firstly, the ways that citizens participate in the evaluation should be improved, ensure the objective, fair, transparent and credible of evaluation by means of public exposure, public hearings, opinion polls and interests in consultation with representative. The second is to create evaluation approaches with citizen awareness, participation and evaluation to meet the informed, accountability and supervision of citizen, and reflect the satisfaction of citizen on sports public service and the changes in the sports needs of citizen. The third is to establish fast-track, and combined with advanced network and information technology, the use of a variety of evaluation techniques and methods to facilitate citizen to participate the decision, monitoring and information feedback of sports public service.

114.3.3 The Third Party Subject and Other Social Forces

In the strict sense, the third party evaluation subject refers to that there is no affiliation or fixed interest relationships with the unit which is the object of evaluation and examination. In order to ensure the objectivity and neutrality of the evaluation and examination and prevent the capture of evaluation objects because of the interest reasons, the third-party evaluation subject is introduced. In addition, the evaluation professional standards, levels and human resources of third party can be borrowed while it introduced in. In our country's performance evaluation of sports public service, the third party evaluation subject includes non-profit consulting organization, sports colleges and universities, research institutes and social intermediary. With the development of sports and civil society, the social intermediary organization would develop in the process of maintenance of their own interests, and also can become one of the main evaluations of the sports public service.

114.4 The Index System of Performance Evaluation of Sports Public Service

A effective index system of performance evaluation is the important prerequisite of implement of performance evaluation. In the index design aspect, performance evaluation of sports public service turned to dynamic process evaluation which was static evaluation previously. The goal that improve the execution and social credibility of sports public service organizations can be achieved through evaluate the index of functions, planning, projects, organizational capacity, mass participation and service satisfaction of public departments.

114.5 The Evaluation of the Public Service Performance of PE: the Construction of Index System and Scoring Method

Assume massive communications with related experts, supervising departments and rating agencies on the relative importance of each first-level index {A1, A2, A3} of the public service performance of PE via various forms like questionnaires, interviews, and seminars, etc. Finally, the relative importance of each first-level index {A1, A2, A3} of the public service performance of PE is confirmed based on multiple suggestions and revisions, and the related judgment matrix is formed. The judge eigenvectors of the matrix is $W = [W_1, W_2, W_3]^T = [0.106, 0.634, 0.260]^T$, thus, $AW = \begin{bmatrix} 1 & \frac{1}{5} & \frac{1}{3} \\ 1 & 1 & 3 \\ 1 & \frac{1}{3} & 1 \end{bmatrix} \begin{bmatrix} 0.106 \\ 1.944 \\ 0.789 \end{bmatrix} = \begin{bmatrix} 0.319 \\ 1.944 \\ 0.789 \end{bmatrix}$,

therefore, $\lambda_{\max} = \sum_{i=1}^{3} \frac{(AW)_i}{3w_i} = \frac{(AW)_1}{3w_1} + \frac{(AW)_2}{3w_2} + \frac{(AW)_3}{3w_3} = 3.04$, $CI = \frac{\lambda_{\max} - n}{n-1} = \frac{3.04 - 3}{3-1} = 0.02$, $CR = \frac{CI}{RI} = \frac{0.02}{0.58} = 0.034 < 0.1$.

When n = 3, r = 0.58, the consistency index proportion is calculated. Therefore, the consistency of the judgment matrix is passed, so $W = [W_1, W_2, W_3]^T = [0.106, 0.634, 0.260]^T$ could be considered as the weight vector of the first-level index {B1, B2, B3} of the public service performance of PE.

Assume again that through massive investigation and consultation with related experts, certain public service institution of PE and supervising departments, together with looking up the information about the annual report and interim statements in the recent 3 years of the public service performance of PE of certain area, the mark sheet of the public service performance of PE in the certain area is calculated with the help of the index system of the public service performance of PE.

If 75 out of 100 is set as the standard for fine performance of the public service of PE, the public service performance of PE in that area is below the fine standard, so the public service performance of PE in that area should be improved. Meanwhile, it should also attach great importance to improve the public satisfaction as well as the investment in public service of PE.

114.6 Conclusion

The service-oriented system of sports administration replaces the traditional all-round control of government administration mode which is a profound reform that on the basis of basic framework of sports public service. Its process not only relate to the deepening of all parties recognize, the renewed ideas and the adjustment of interests, but also closely relate to the actual situation of China's society and sports development. Therefore, the transformation from Chinese sports administration system to the service sports administration system will be a gradual process.

References

1. Zhang X, ChaI Y (1999) Event driven approach with business rule based modeling. J Tsinghua Univ (Sci Technol) 39(7):25–28
2. Song Z, Liu J, Zhang Y (2005) Relation-based flow control model. Comput Appl 25(11):2693–2697

3. Zhang J, Zhong Y (2006) Research on event-driven based product development process management. Comput Eng Appl 24:94–97
4. Zhu WD, Jiang Y F, Zhao H F (2003) On the accountancy business process reengineering in the network environment. J Hefei Univ Technol (Nat Sci) 26(1):761–765
5. Debreceny R, Gray GL (2001) The production and use of semantically rich accounting reports on the internet: XML and XBRL. Int Account Inform Syst 1:47–74
6. Zhang H (2004) Business process reengineering in the Era of information-on updating the accounting business process, 19(6) pp 65–69
7. Zeng W, Yan B-P (2005) Survey on workflow module. Appl Res Comput 5:11–22
8. Zhu D-C (2004) On the audit of accounts and tables in electronic data processing accounting. J Anhui TV Univ 1:35–37
9. Edmondson, Mo I (1997) Organizational learning and competitive advantage, Mc Graw-Hill, New York, pp 1–10

Chapter 115
Research on the Construction of Teaching Resources Platform in Universities

Qian Meng

Abstract With the increasing application of network technology, the construction of teaching resources platform is in the ascendant. According to the common problems in the teaching resources platform construction process, such as lack of resources independent, lack of interactivity, lack of personal knowledge management, lack of learning path and process evaluation, put forward corresponding improvement strategy. The teaching recourse platform has been designed for supporting learning process, independent studying, collaborative learning and learning assessment. Through the building of platform, students not only can make full use of teaching resources, but also can improve the efficiency of learning. The platform makes the various works more scientific and standardized and play an enormous role in the development of university's teaching quality.

Keywords Teaching resources platform · Universities · Collaborative learning

115.1 Introduction

As the basic elements of education informationization, teaching resource refers to various resources which support the whole process of teaching to achieve a certain educational purposes, and to achieve a certain function. Those are mainly refer to

---

The paper was supported by education and teaching research project of Jiangsu Normal University (NO. XJG201243).

Q. Meng (✉)
Computer Science and Technology College, Jiangsu Normal University, Xuzhou, China
e-mail: mqzzy2000@126.com

Q. Meng
Information and Electrical Engineering School, China University of Mining and Technology, Xuzhou, China

the network environment which consists of by supporting platform, application software, hardware system, and the software teaching resources that launch on multimedia computer and network environment. With the network teaching platform, teachers can provide students with more learning resources than the classroom, collect students' homework in real-time, timely informed of the students learning. Students are free from the restriction of time and space, according to their actual situation, choose to suit their needs in a variety of learning materials (such as Courseware, video lectures, test questions, etc.) for personalized learning.

Construction of teaching resources platform in Chinese universities has made remarkable achievements. But the numerous present network teaching resources platform is only provided the simple technical support for the network teaching, transplanted directly the traditional classroom instruction to the network teaching. There are lots of the common problems, such as lacked design of platform modules in view of the network teaching characteristic, lack of teaching effect monitoring, lack of learner's personal knowledge management, lack of the study behaviour support, lack of resources, platform independent, lack of interactivity, lack of learning path and process evaluation, lack of an effective organization, the existence of blindness and so on [1–3].

It is necessary to take effective measures to integrate and promote effective teaching resource network construction. This research based on collaborative learning, takes the learning process as the core, carries on the overall construction and function design.

115.2 Architecture of Teaching Resources Platform

The lightweight J2EE software structure is selected. The MVC (Model-View-Controller) exploration model is used in the presentation layer. The distributed application model allows different individual application tiers to focus on different functional elements, thereby improving performance. Teaching resources platform has the following architecture as showed in Fig. 115.1: The whole system can be divided into the client tier and the presentation tie, the business logic tier and the persistence tier.

Client tier: The client tier makes use of the advantage of widely installed browser in every operating system to alleviate the trouble meet in deployment of the client components.

The client side which is simply a browser is where the user accesses the application.

Presentation Tier: The presentation tier is composed of JSPs, servlets, or portlets that get the program data from the business logic layer and create the layout HTML (or another markup language). This tier is responsible for managing the interaction with the end users.

115 Research on the Construction of Teaching Resources Platform

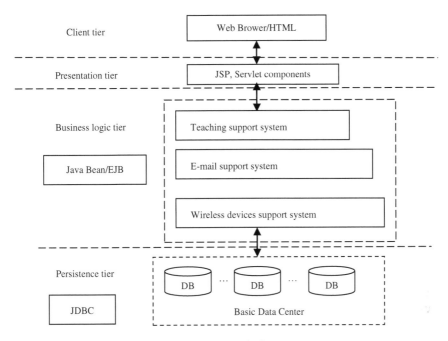

Fig. 115.1 The architecture of teaching resources platform

Business logic tier: The business logic tier acts as a server to serve requests made by the users in the presentation tier. The business logic tier deploys EJB (Enterprise Java Bean) components that encapsulate business rules and other business functions in Session beans.

Persistence Tier: The persistence tier includes the database and any components that are responsible for managing the access to it. In the persistence tier, JDBC (Java database connectivity) is used to connect to databases, make queries, and return query results, and custom connectors [4].

115.3 Function of Teaching Resources Platform

The function of the teaching resources platform showed in Fig. 115.2. University faculty, staff, and students can use their computing account ID and password or a personal digital certificate to log into the teaching resources platform. The teaching resources platform has three kinds of users: student, instructor and system manager.

The key modules are elaborated as follows:

Courses worksite module: A course worksite which set up by instructors is the official worksite for a particular course and can be linked to students' database to

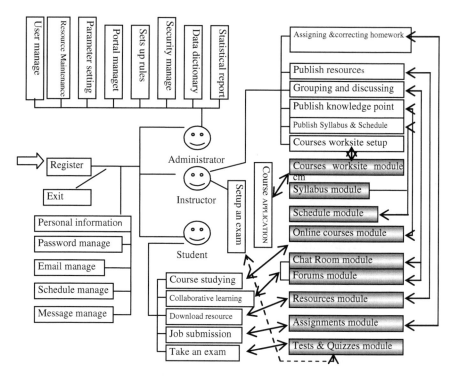

Fig. 115.2 Function of the teching resources platform

automatically populate its roster. When a student log into the system, he'll see a list of all the Courses worksites to which he belong, including courses worksite he have joined and courses worksite to which he have been added as a participant by the creator of the site. Instructor can make changes to information about the site. Usually, after a student takes a course as an elective course, he applies for joining the course worksite, too. He'll become a member of the course after confirmed by the instructor who owns the courses worksite.

Syllabus and Schedule module: The syllabus is the official outline for a course. If instructor or department has prepared an online syllabus already, he can direct the Syllabus tool to link to it. Otherwise, he can enter material to post directly to syllabus.

Online courses module: Online courses, which often wanted to structure material by unit or week. It is easy to link to quizzes and assignments, and to handle common types of content. Online training which needs to define sequences of material. Instructor can import publisher content or content from other systems that support Common Cartridge.

Chat room and forums module: Users can use the Chat Room for real-time, unstructured conversations among site participants who are logged into the site at the same time. Instructors can easily create an "Online Office Hours" chat room for student questions and answers. Dispersed collaboration groups can use Chat as a space to have conversations across distances or catch up with conversations that they may have missed. Forums module allows instructors or site leaders to create an unlimited number of discussion forums, and integrated closely with other tools such as Resources and report book.

Assignments module: For courses, the Assignments module allows instructors to create, distribute, collect, and grade online assignments. Assignments are private; student submissions are not visible to other users of the site.

Resources module: Using the Resources module, instructor can share many kinds of material securely with members of his site, or make them available to the public. Instructor also has his own private resources area in his workspace.

Tests and quizzes module: This module allows instructor to create online assessments for delivery via a web interface to his students or other groups. It was designed primarily to administer tests, but instructor may also create assessments to gather survey information or informal course feedback. Instructor can include multiple question types in an assessment, including ones that require your students to upload files.

115.4 Conclusions

A teaching recourse platform has been designed and variety of teaching resources has been integrated into the unified teaching platform. The platform of each module can be assembled freely. Instructors can be more in-depth understanding of students' learning and thinking, students can have more opportunities to express their ideas and show their talent. The platform can achieve unified management of network teaching resources, expanding the scale of the school teaching. And there is great practical significance in improving teaching quality. Network teaching resources platform has become the important symbol of educational modernization and informatization.

References

1. Xu L, He W (2011) The present situation and improve strategy of network teaching platform in universities, In: International conference on e-education, entertainment and e-management, pp 304–3063
2. Xu ZM, Xia HW (2010) Study on digital instructional resources sharing platform for e-learning, In: International conference on networking and digital society, pp 224–227

3. Liu H, Meng X (2010) Research on network teaching platform based on knowledge Construction teaching model. In: 2nd International Conference on Education Technology and Computer (ICETC), pp 528–532
4. Ren Y, Xing T (2011) Research on structure and functionality of network teaching integrated platform based on MVC. In: International conference on information management, innovation management and industrial engineering, pp 177–180
5. Guo C, Guo K, Lin W, Lin Z (2005) The research on the software architecture of negotiatory synthetical forecasting GDSS based on J2EE. In: 9th international conference on computer supported cooperative work in design, pp 27–32
6. Quick start for collaboration,Available via https://collab.itc.virginia.edu/portal

Chapter 116
Applications of Virtualization Technology to Digital Library

Yu Xiaoyi, Wang Zhengjun, Yu Zhenguo, Jin Yuling, Wang Hong, Liang Yufang, Wang Quanhong, Gao Jian and Wang Haiyin

Abstract This paper takes the construction of a virtual digital library in DUT library for example, emphatically analyzes the system design ideas, structural basis and building measures of virtualization architecture by VMware vSphere four, and gives a detailed proposal of the hardware configuration and the business cluster deployment. Then, this paper describes in detail the significant effect acquired by the specific applications of virtualization in the digital library. Virtualization provides effective approaches to building the digital libraries with high efficiency and stability, sustainable development and green environmental protection. Finally, this paper also introduces the problems which would occur and should be taken into account in the process of virtualization construction and operations.

Keywords Virtualization · VMware · Digital library · HA · DRS

116.1 Introduction

Virtualization is a key building block of dynamic infrastructure. Multiple virtual machines can be operated on a single physical machine by using virtualization; therefore, resources of this computer can be shared among multiple environments.

At present, technology realizations of typical virtual machines on the market are: VMware ESX Server, Microsoft Hyper-V and Critrix XenServer etc., Because Vmware software is better fit for the needs of the digital library's transaction and

---

Y. Xiaoyi (✉) · W. Zhengjun · J. Yuling · W. Hong · L. Yufang · W. Quanhong · G. Jian · W. Haiyin
Dalian University of Technology Library, Dalian 116023, China
e-mail: yuxiaoyi@dhut.edu.cn

Y. Zhenguo
Liaoning Normal University Academy of Mathematics, Dalian 116029, China

S. Li et al. (eds.), *Frontier and Future Development of Information Technology in Medicine and Education*, Lecture Notes in Electrical Engineering 269,
DOI: 10.1007/978-94-007-7618-0_116, © Springer Science+Business Media Dordrecht 2014

services, Dalian University of Technology (DUT)'s librarians have used it to build the virtualization environment. Based on the report "The 2009 investigation report of current situation of virtualization in China" which was released in August 2009 by 51CTO.com, the survey results of more than 10 fields, such as finance, telecommunications, energy and chemical engineering, education and scientific research etc., show that these fields which "have been using virtualization technology, and obtained good results" only possess 12 % of the total number. According to incomplete statistics, during domestic university libraries, only a few libraries, such as Guangdong Provincial Zhongshan Library, University of International Business and Economics Library, Southwest Jiaotong University Library and Tsinghua University Library have completed or are establishing virtualization libraries. At present, viewing from the results which we have achieved, DUT Library has undoubtedly stood in front of the virtual digital libraries' phalanx. Our long-term development goals are to make full use of virtualization technology, gradually transit to private cloud environments, and construct an efficient, automatic, on-demand and convenient infrastructure platform.

116.2 Implementation of the Virtual Program of Digital Libraries

The digitalization of DUT Library has developed rapidly. Its data center has a large number of application software and digital resources, and considerable scale of hardware devices which support the normal operation of these applications. Before the absence of virtualization program, the mode is basically a "one server, an operating system, an application" mode. For overcoming the shortcomings of this mode described previously in this paper, we have already investigated and researched into the virtualization solution programs on the market, and finally decided to use VMware vSphere which is an industry-leading virtualization program to optimize the digital library's services.

116.2.1 Virtualization Hardware Configuration

After the use of virtualization solutions, IT hardware mainly concentrated on several equipment which were installed virtualization ESX. During the last two years, DUT Library's hardware acquisitions took fully into account of the needs of virtualization solutions. We purchased hardware equipment with outstanding configuration and good quality, mainly including three parts of servers, storage and network.

In the first phase, ESX server used the two HP580, configured with four-way CPU and 64G memory. Through the library's application virtualization

Table 116.1 Server configuration

Host computer	Hardware server	CPU	Memory	Hard disk
ESX01	HP580	Intel Xeon E7450 × 4	64G	SAS 136G × 2
ESX02	HP580	Intel Xeon E7450 × 4	64G	SAS 136G × 2
ESX03	DELL PowerEdge R710	Intel Xeon X5660 × 2	128G	SAS 136G × 2
ESX04	DELL PowerEdge R710	Intel Xeon X5660 × 2	128G	SAS 136G × 2
ESX05	DELL PowerEdge R710	Intel Xeon X5660 × 2	128G	SAS 136G × 2
ESX06	DELL PowerEdge R710	Intel Xeon X5660 × 2	128G	SAS 136G × 2
vCenter	DELL PE 2950	Intel Xeon X5355 × 2	8G	SAS 136G × 2

integration, we found that during the running process of the entire virtualization solutions, the memory consumption was relatively large, the occupancy rate of the CPU was not high. Therefore, when we expanded the virtualization solutions in the second phase, 4 DELL R710 servers which we replenished were configured with two-way CPU and 128G memory. A DELL2950 server was used as vCenter server. The server configuration is shown in Table 116.1.

DUT library's storage system consists of the EMC NS960 advanced storage system and EMC CX320 entry-level storage system; of which EMC CX320 has been running for five years and has passed maintenance's warranty period, so it can only operate non-critical businesses and can realize simple data backup at present. The library's virtual infrastructure use NS960 as the main storage medium, which possesses 45T SATA disk space and 13.5T FC optical fiber disc space, whose front and back buses of 8G fibre channel, to provide a strong storage throughput.

At present, gigabit network switching is already completely mature. The library uses Brocade RX-16 gigabit core switches to provide gigabit connection for virtualization servers.

In the library's virtualization solutions, all the physical ESX hosts are connected with NS960 memory via dual 8G fiber link and also connected with the core switch RX-16 by dual Gigabit LAN connection to ensure that the storage and network links are the redundant backup links. ESX are directly installed on the physical server's local hard disk, and two local hard disks work as Raid1. Virtual machines and digital resources are deployed in the store. Hardware diagram is shown in Fig. 116.1.

116.2.2 Programme Planning

According to the number of physical servers, we purchased the software and license of VMware vCenter and VMware vSphere four. The license is 16 CPU license of vSphere four Enterprise Plus. We will not describe the installation and deployment process in detail here. The following highlights the lightspots where

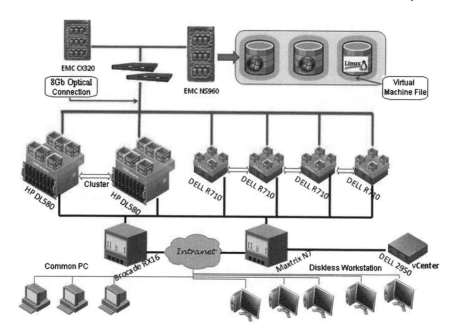

Fig. 116.1 Hardware's schematic diagram

VMware features are fully played during our library's virtualization implementation.

Storage applications are related to the overall system's performances' display, and the different storage media are given according to different applications. The entire library's storage mediums are divided into three cases: 1. High-speed optical disks are mainly provided for the virtual server itself, diskless services, database systems and other key businesses; 2. High-capacity SATA disks are provided for the large number of electronic resources, which mainly offer files storage services; 3. The old CX320 storage space is available to non-critical operations and simple backup.

In order to display VMware virtualization centralized management features, we use cluster management mode. According to the actual application situation of DUT Library's data center, mainly based on the consumption of hardware resources and real-time requirements which business applications need, the virtualization program will be divided into two clusters:

Cluster 1: data services cluster, including the following services:

a. Software services of library business management system, including library automation management systems, OPAC server, ORACLE database etc.;
b. Local mirror electronic resources services, such as e-books, electronic journals, dissertations etc.;
c. Multimedia resources services, such as audio, video and CD-ROM behind books and other non-paper resources;

d. Network management services, such as WEB, DNS, DHCP, FTP, network management, network authentication, remote access etc.;

Library automation system in the cluster is one of the most critical business services. We need to ensure the continued normal operation of library automation system, and provide uninterrupted OPAC service and timing mail sending and other basic services. It is critical to ensure off-screen Oracle database robust, stable and efficient. Through management functions of vSphere Client, we set Oracle's virtual server as the highest prior service level, and through VMware VMotion HA's function we set the hot spare function of virtual server to ensure high availability of database servers.

Resources consumption of services, such as electronic resources, multimedia resources, and network is not very great, and maybe there is a big peak for individual service, so it dynamically allocates resources to virtual service for use by using virtualization after the integration of server resources. VMware DRS can monitor the actual usage of the service, and according to the actual needs of the application, it can allocate the appropriate resources from the resources pool for use. All services are independent from the hardware. High availability of services is ensured through VMware VMotion HA in the cluster.

Electronic resources need to occupy large storage space. In order to allocate storage space flexibly, by using VMware's tidy storage mode, the actual storage space is allocated according to actual requirements of space occupied by resources.

Cluster 2: diskless service cluster. After using the virtualization program, it uses three DELL 2,950 servers as the cluster. Per 60 diskless terminals correspond to a diskless server in the cluster, building five virtual diskless servers. Through resources monitoring and allocation mechanism of VMware DRS, the cluster ensures that each virtual diskless server acquires enough hardware resources as needed, and relying on VMware VMotion HA hardware failure switch application services automatically to ensure the uninterrupted operation of diskless services.

Once a bottleneck takes place in hardware resources of diskless terminals, we need to add the expansion of hardware resources only by adding VMware ESX hosts dynamically in diskless services clusters. Diskless virtual servers can realize rapid deployment by copying the files of virtual machines. DUT Library's virtualization services and business cluster deployment topology map and the virtual machine console's screenshot are shown in Fig. 116.2.

116.3 Virtualization Architecture's Application Results

After we used VMware virtualization to integrate the library's network information services, we have achieved the following results.

116.3.1 We have improved the management efficiency.
116.3.2 We have realized the classification management strategy.
116.3.3 We have enhanced the system's reliability.

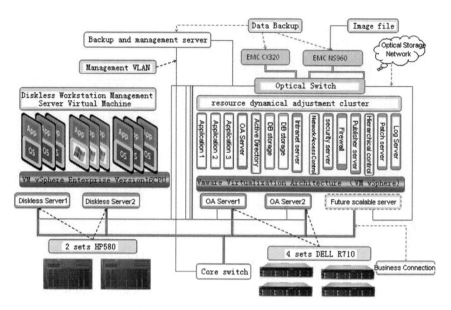

Fig. 116.2 Virtualization services and business cluster deployment topology map

116.3.4 We have efficiently make use of storage space.
116.3.5 We have cut down the application deployment time.
116.3.6 We have enhanced the disaster tolerance capabilities.
116.3.7 All of our work has conformed to the library's low-carbon development strategies.

116.4 Conclusion

It is very significant that digital library integrates the library business by using VMware virtualization. Not only the utilization rate of hardware resources in the digital library is improved, but also the reliability and efficiency of business applications can be raised. The inputs of the library's data center servers and related sets are reduced. And energy consumption is also cut down which is in line with the government's development policy of energy conservation and environmental protection.

In the process of virtualization building, there exist some problems. Firstly, the virtualization software is not free of charge, some manufacturers' products' authorizations are even more expensive than physical servers. So we need to consider our library's economic bearing capacity when we make our plan; Secondly, the maintenance of virtualization platform is more complex and requires some technicians with high level of maintenance; In addition, in the initial construction phase of virtualization platform, the requirements of the hardware configuration are higher than the traditional physical servers. All these factors should be taken into account synthetically.

There are also some problems during the running process of the virtual architecture. Firstly, hardware-level virtualization and software virtualization need to be combined with each other to maximize the system utilization; Secondly, virtualization also has some risks. Putting multiple applications on one server is similar to putting many eggs into one basket. If the major hardware fails, all applications will be affected. It's difficult to eliminate this threat. Thirdly, virtualization may bring about security risks. System-level virtualization technology may cause hackers attack the system when the users are totally unconscious of it. Finally, if the server virtualization should become popular, the application of load balancing is an important problem from a technical perspective. Whether this problem can be solved well or not has a direct impact on the system performances.

References

1. Zhao HM (2009) High availability information service platform based on the virtual machine (in Chinese). Mod Libr Inf Technol 12:18–24
2. Lu S (2008) Computer virtualization technology and application (in Chinese). Mechanical Industry Press, Beijing
3. Zhou CY (2008) Feasibility analysis of the virtualization technology for the server in library (in Chinese). Library Tribune 3:65–68
4. Chen W (2010) Tsinghua University Library: server virtualization to improve service quality (in Chinese). China Educ Netw 10:19–21
5. Jin YL (2010) The application of virtualization technology in the digital library (in Chinese). University Library Forum, China
6. Mache C (2008) CTO virtualization roundtable part II. Commun ACM 12:43–49

Chapter 117
The Health Status Among College Teachers: Taking Jiangxi Local Colleges as Example

Kaiqiang Guo, Weisong Bu and Fangping Li

Abstract This paper examined the health status of college teachers particularly of those in Jiangxi province. With charts comparing, it points to the health status became an important issue among the lecturers that showed obesity problems, cardiopulmonary disease and sub-health etc. The paper suggests the college teachers take part in periodically sports activity; get involved to more body building related study to keep healthy as well as the enhancement of life enjoyment. And there're proper physical methods that help in changing this situation.

Keywords Health status · Teachers · Status · Analysis

117.1 Preface

Good health plays a critical important role in guarantee teachers' teaching and researching work. The teacher position is sacred but his work is hard. In the twenty-first century, however, the technology developed rapidly in modern life, the pace of work to accelerate sharply, brought big pressure to the teachers either on mental or physically. The health status of teachers has become a public topic of the whole society. It's time to concern about teachers' spiritual and physical health, try to protect the candle like persons to be in good condition while light others, no consume itself any more. It's the expectations of the whole society.

K. Guo (✉) · W. Bu · F. Li
Jiangxi Normal University, NanChang, 330022 Jiangxi, China
e-mail: kaiqiang2008@yeah.net

117.2 Research Object with Research Methods

117.2.1 The Research Object

One hundred and sixty-one randomly selected group of teachers in Jiangxi Province "excellent teachers" title, which male 74, female 87.

117.2.2 Research Methods

The State National Physique determination standard test method. Include that physical fitness test, height, standard weight, vital capacity, stepped index; body composition testing; bone mineral density testing and detection of sub-health conditions. Detect objects of men and women groups including; of adult Group A 20–39 years, adult Group B 40–59 years old age group over 60 years. The number of all ages in Table 117.1.

117.3 Results and Analysis

117.3.1 "National Physical Fitness Evaluation Standards" physical fitness assessment a basic briefing: divided into the following four categories based on the completion of the detection and assessment of the crowd:

Class A crowd: complete all indicators detected and assessed for indicators of 0, the composite score more qualified for that type of crowd comprehensive rating based on "National Physical Fitness Evaluation Standards";

Class B crowd: complete detection of all indicators, but at least one indicator assessed as 0 points, more composite score qualified for that type of crowd can not be based on "National Physical Fitness Evaluation Standards" comprehensive rating only on specific indicators-score, therefore, despite the final score of the population is likely to reach excellent, good or qualified, but the level does not reflect the true physical condition of the population.

Class AB crowd: rated as unqualified.

Table 117.1 The number of detected object distribution table n = 161

Gender	Male			Female		
Groups	Group A	Group B	Group C	Group A	Group B	Group C
Age	20–39 years	40–59 years	Aged above 60 years	20–39 years	40–59 years	Aged above 60 years
The number of people	20	50	4	35	49	3
Subtotal	74			87		

Special populations: physical weakness, illness, injury, discomfort or other reasons not to complete the detection of all indicators, the assessment of the type of crowd the crowd with the Class B.

117.3.2 The outstanding teachers constitution test results; comprehensive assessment of the situation on the above classification statistics are shown in Table 117.2.

117.3.3 Can be seen from Table 117.2 **composite score; teachers physique level pass rate of 71.4 %, excellent rate of 42.3 %, it seems that you can also, but the entire ratings system and other rights system, and therefore it can not be completely comprehensive. The scores are used to evaluate the fitness level of the teachers. Can be seen from Tables** 117.3 **and** 117.4, **the specific problems of the physical aspects of the teachers**.

117.3.4 Detection analysis of body composition; Tables 117.5 **and** 117.6 **analysis can be seen; unsatisfactory teachers physique component test results, a total of 56.6 % fat is higher than the standard value, the ratio of male to 77.1 %, the proportion of the female 39.1 and 25.5 % of the people entering obesity. The main features**;

① More serious men of all ages, the ratio at 50 % or more, and are more than 70 % over 30 years old, has entered obesity ratio reached 36.5 %, and the entry of all ages obesity proportion except 30–39 group was 27.3 %, more than 30 %;

② More serious adult women mainly Group B (40–59 years old), the proportion of fat than standard value in more than 50, 25.5 % overall on the entry of women into the proportion of obese and the proportion gradually increased with age-growth trend.

③ Poor women relative to men is 3.4 % edema index abnormal, no case of men. Edema index is associated with the symptoms of kidney disease, high blood pressure, circulatory system diseases, heart disease, systemic or local edema and malnutrition.

④ From Table 117.6 abdominal obesity situation in more serious problems, the teachers into visceral obesity in the general proportion of 42.2 %. Male is more serious, the proportion of 68.9 %, and of all ages in addition to adult Group A (20–39 years old) and slightly lower, the proportion of other ages were above 75 %, and if one adds into the alert from more than 30 years of age, the proportion in more than 80 %, and excessive excessive visceral fat area and visceral fat mass ratio.

⑤ In this respect, Female relatively the male is slightly better, but the overall 19.5 % visceral obesity and the proportion of more than 40 years old are more than 20 %, but the female fat area exceeded Fortunately, the ratio is not high. In visceral obesity hazards relative to the subcutaneous fat super scalar greater, so it should cause attaches great importance to teachers.

117.3.5 Analysis of bone mineral density testing can be seen from Table 117.7;

Table 117.2 Excellent teachers in physical testing overall situation table n = 161

Unit	Complete all indexes detection number and percentage						Do not complete all indexes detection number and percentage	Detection of total number
	A group			B group (%)		Unqualified (%)		
	Very good (%)	Good (%)	Qualified (%)	Sub total (%)				
Total	27 people 16.8	41 people 25.5	47 people 29.2	115 people 71.4	22 people 13.7	10 people 6.2	14 people 8.7	161 people

Note (%) = The classification number/The total number of detection. The B class to achieve excellent have 7 people
① A group and comprehensive score in the above pass, have a total of 115 people, accounting for 71.4 % of the total number
② B group; have a total of 22 people, accounting for 13.7 % of the total number
③ The comprehensive score of unqualified (including AB), total 10 people, accounting for 6.2 % of the total number
④ For weak constitution, disease, injury, physical discomfort or for other reasons not to finish all the indexes, a total of 14 people, accounting for 8.7 % of the total number

Table 117.3 Different gender, category indicators score ≤2 (weak or bad) situation statistical table n = 161

Detection index	Male			Female			Total
	20–39 years (%)	20–39 years (%)	Subtotal (%)	20–39 years (%)	20–39 years (%)	Subtotal (%)	
Standard weight and height	30.0	22.0	24.3	11.4	4.1	7.1	15.0
Vital capacity	55.0	24.0	32.9	24.7	32.7	29.8	30.6
Step index	70.0	49.0	55.1	44.1	31.9	37.0	47.8
Close your eyes standing on one foot	25.0	22.0	22.9	20.0	8.2	13.1	18.0
Sit and reach	70.0	62.0	64.3	29.4	38.8	34.9	48.4
Choice reaction time	45.0	20.0	27.1	25.7	12.2	17.9	21.9
Grip strength	65.0	62.0	62.9	51.4	61.2	57.1	59.4
Vertical jump	30.0	–	30.0	14.7	–	14.7	20.4
Push-ups	30.0	–	30.0	–	–	–	30.0
Sit-ups	–	–	–	9.1	–	9.1	9.1

Note (%) = The classification number finish the gold markers in the total numbers. A man not to do sit-ups, over 40 years old also do not jump and push-ups; female do not do push-ups, over 40 years old of age do not jump and sit-ups

① Teachers bone condition overall better access to reduced bone mass ratio of 14.9, 3.7 % into osteoporosis, and the ages of the men and women into osteoporosis occur at ages above 50 years of age, in line with bone development in the law.

② To be concern; proportion of the 20–29 age segment of the male and female teachers reduced bone mass in more than 20 %, this part of the crowd should cause a certain amount of attention. Should be done early prevention of osteoporosis, early detection of people with osteopenia or osteoporosis, early treatment of science.

117.3.6 Sub-health detection analysis; can be seen from Table 117.8;

Poor teachers sub-health detection, a total of 70.3 % of sub-health state, and the men and women of all ages in addition to female's elderly group, the proportion of 55 %, and the respective proportions of the men and women in general are more than 65 %. From the proportion of the various parts of the energy imbalance, the ratio of more than 50 % of the area are mostly sedentary the lower extremities adverse symptoms caused by adverse symptoms and lack of sleep or poor quality of sleep, fatigue, neck, decreased immunity and lead to adverse symptoms related to inflammation in the body, or infection, gastrointestinal function and urinary system.

Table 117.4 The comprehensive score of excellent population indicators score ≤2 (weak or bad) situation statistical table n = 161

Detection index	The number of excellent	Evaluation of 0 points as the number of	Evaluation of 1 points as the number of	Evaluation of 2 points as the number of	Total
Detection index	75	–	2 2.7 %	–	2 2.7 %
Vital capacity	75	1 1.3 %	–	10 13.3 %	11 14.7 %
Step index	75	3 4.0 %	–	28 37.3 %	31 41.3 %
Close your eyes standing on one foot	75	–	1 1.3 %	2 2.7 %	3 4.0 %
Sit and reach	75	1 1.3 %	3 4.0 %	17 22.7 %	21 20.0 %
Choice reaction time	75	1 1.3 %	–	4 5.3 %	5 6.7 %
Grip strength	75	–	3 4.0 %	28 37.3 %	31 41.3 %
Vertical jump	21	–	–	–	–
Push-up	5	–	–	–	–
Sit-up	20	–	–	–	–

Note (%) = Classification number/The number of excellent. In which have 68 people is class A excellent and have 7 people is class B excellent

① From a general point of view, more than 30 % of the teachers on cardiac pulmonary function, body flexibility, upper limb and hand strength is weak or poor; teachers' physical condition and is not optimistic

② 20–39 year-old male from the ages of view is the most prominent, in addition to balancing capability, more than 30 % of teachers in other indicators for weak or poor, especially heart and lung function, body flexibility and hand strength. This proportion is at least 55 %

③ Overall physical fitness level of the male gender is lower than women, but the common characteristics of men and women is heart function, body flexibility and hand strength is weak or poor

④ Can be seen from Table 117.4 in the composite score of excellent teachers in cardiac function, hand strength and body flexibility still showed weak or poor, the first two terms of the proportion of 41.3 %

117 The Health Status Among College Teachers

Table 117.5 Different gender groups body composition inspection of table

Type		Male						Female						Total
		The adult group A		The adult group B		The old age group	Sub total	The adult group A		The adult group B		The old age group	Sub total	
		20–29 years (%)	30–39 years (%)	40–49 years (%)	50–59 years (%)	60 years (%)		20–29 years (%)	30–39 years (%)	40–49 years (%)	50–59 years (%)	60 years (%)		
Lower than Standard	Very thin	–	–	–	–	–	2.7	–	3.7	–	–	–	1.1	1.9
	Slim	22.2	9.1	–	9.1	25.0	12.2	25.0	33.3	3.8	–	–	13.0	12.0
	Sub total	22.2	9.1	10.7	9.1	25.0	14.9	25.0	37.0	3.8	–	–	14.9	14.9
	Low in fat and muscle	–	–	18.2	–	–	–	–	–	–	–	–	–	–
	Normal	11.1	–	7.1	9.1	–	6.8	50.0	37.0	42.3	30.4	67.7	39.1	24.2
	Muscular over weight	–	–	–	–	–	–	12.5	–	–	–	–	–	–
	Over weight	–	–	–	–	–	–	62.5	37.0	42.3	30.4	–	1.1	0.6
	Subtotal	11.1	–	7.1	9.1	–	6.8	–	–	30.8	48.5	–	40.2	24.0
Higher than Standard	Little weight	22.2	63.6	46.4	31.8	–	39.2	–	–	3.8	4.8	–	20.7	29.2
	Alert obesity	–	–	–	–	25.0	1.4	12.5	14.8	15.4	21.7	–	2.3	1.9
	Obesity	22.2	18.2	32.1	36.4	50.0	31.1	–	–	–	–	–	16.1	22.0
	Extreme obesity	11.1	9.1	3.6	4.5	–	5.4	12.5	14.8	50.0	69.5	67.7	–	2.5
	Subtotal	55.5	90.9	82.1	72.7	75.0	77.1	–	–	–	–	–	99.1	56.6
Abnormal swelling of index		–	–	–	–	–	–	3.7	3.8	–	3.33	3.4	1.9	

Note (%) = The classification number/The number of age group. Male 20–29 1 female 30–39 group 1 metal objects or other reasons because the body can not do body composition testing

Table 117.6 Different gender groups for composition detection abdominal obesity status table

Type		Male						Female						Total
		The adult group A		The adult group A		The old age group	Sub total	The adult group A		The adult group B		The old age group	Sub total	
		20–29 years (%)	30–39 years (%)	40–49 years (%)	50–59 years (%)	60 years (%)		20–29 years (%)	30–39 years (%)	40–49 years (%)	50–59 years (%)	60 years (%)		
Fat mass	Subcutaneous type	22.2	–	–	–	–	2.7	37.5	37.0	–	4.3	–	4.3	9.9
	Balanced type	33.3	9.1	–	13.6	–	9.5	50.0	40.7	46.2	26.1	33.3	39.1	25.5
	Warning admonish	11.1	45.5	17.9	9.1	–	17.6	–	3.7	30.8	43.5	33.3	23.0	20.5
	Visceral adiposity	22.2	45.5	82.1	72.7	75.0	66.2	12.5	11.1	23.1	26.1	33.3	19.5	41.0
	Severe visceral obesity	–	–	–	4.5	25.0	2.7	–	–	–	–	–	–	1.2
	Visceral adiposity and severe visceral obesity	22.2	45.5	82.1	77.3	100.0	68.9	12.5	11.1	23.1	26.1	33.3	19.5	42.2
Fat area	Under	22.2	–	–	4.5	–	5.4	37.5	37.0	–	4.3	–	47.1	28.0
	Standard	44.4	54.5	17.9	18.2	–	25.7	50.0	44.4	77.0	69.6	66.6	49.4	38.5
	Exceed	22.2	45.5	82.1	77.3	100.0	68.9	12.5	11.1	23.0	26.1	33.3	3.4	33.5

Note (%) = Classification number/The number of age group. The group of 20–29 years of male have one people. The group of 30–39 years of female have one people. Because the body has no metal or other reasons to do body composition detection

117 The Health Status Among College Teachers

Table 117.7 Different gender groups of bone density testing table

Type	Male						Female						Total
	The adult group A		The adult group B		The old age group 60 years (%)	Sub total	The adult group A		The adult group B		The old age group 60 years (%)	Sub total	
	20–29 years (%)	30–39 years %	40–49 years (%)	50–59 years (%)			20–29 years (%)	30–39 years (%)	40–49 years (%)	50–59 years (%)			
Normal	55.6	81.8	96.4	63.6	50.0	77.0	37.5	77.8	100.0	82.6	66.7	81.6	79.5
Reduce bone mass	22.2	18.2	3.6	27.3	25.0	16.2	37.5	22.2	–	8.7	33.3	13.8	14.9
Osteoporosis	–	–	–	9.1	25.0	4.1	12.5	–	–	8.7	–	3.4	3.7
Severe osteoporosis	–	–	–	–	–	–	–	–	–	–	–	–	–

Note (%) = Classification number/The number of age group. Have two male of among adult students aged 20–29 years old not to do the physical testing due to special circumstances in the adult male 20–29 age group. Also, there is one female not to do the experiment

Table 117.8 Different gender group sub-healthy testing table

Type		Male						Female						Total
		The adult group A		The adult group B		The old age group 60 years (%)	Sub total	The adult group A		The adult group B		The old age group 60 years (%)	Sub total	
		20–29 years (%)	30–39 years (%)	40–49 years (%)	50–59 years (%)			20–29 years (%)	30–39 years (%)	40–49 years (%)	50–59 years (%)			
Healthy		44.4	36.4	33.3	38.1		34.7	25.0	22.2	20.0	30.4	66.7	25.6	29.7
Sub-healthy	70–79 points	44.4	54.5	55.6	57.1	100.0	56.9	50.0	55.6	56.0	47.8	33.3	52.3	54.4
	60–69 points	11.1		11.1	4.8		6.9	25.0	22.2	20.0	21.7		20.9	14.6
	Under 60 points		9.1				1.4			4.0			1.2	1.3
Sub total		55.6	63.6	66.7	61.9	100.0	65.3	75.0	77.8	80.0	69.6	33.3	74.4	70.3

117.4 Conclusions

117.4.1 The long-term lack of exercise caused by the whole body function decline. Jiangxi elite teachers in physical status as the outstanding performance of cardiopulmonary function are weak, obesity in severe cases.

117.4.2 Owing to the large working load is large, irregular life, low sleeping quality, causing physical and mental fatigue and physiological function, decreased immunity and sub health seriously.

117.4.3 Due to the sedentary, long standing shoulder, neck, in occupation characteristics causing lumbar and lower extremity adverse reactions or symptoms and visceral obesity.

117.5 Suggestions

117.5.1 Perceived importance of health care, improving the quality of life, teachers must form good habits of life, keep the regularity of life, special attention should be paid to the scientific diet structure, according to its own characteristics, physical condition, reasonable arrangements for meals.

117.5.2 Do exercise every day for 1 h. According to one self's body condition to participate in strengthening exercise, Tai Chi, Yi Jingjing, Five-animal boxing etc. Regulation of health psychological health consciousness, maintain a dull quiet state of mind, pay attention to physical and mental health, learning self regulation and relaxation.

117.5.3 Set up actively the new concept of healthy living, the teachers should actively conduct regular health checks, to learn more about the leisure fitness knowledge, through scientific physical exercise to improve their physique, pay attention to timely eliminate fatigue, health hazards in a timely manner to early treatment, nip in the bud.

References

1. Jiangxi physical fitness testing and evaluation database
2. Cao Limin (2006) Analysis to the health status and health of university professors cognitive. J Beijing Sport Univ 5:651–653
3. Yang X, Sheng Y (2006) The study of relationship between obesity index and physical health specification of college students. Hubei Sports Sci Technol 1:44–46
4. Xiong D (1998) Prospects of the national fitness program in China from the trend of the development of mass sports development prospects. Sports Sci 2:3–8

Chapter 118
Research on Students' Perception and Expectations of Printed Materials in Online Education

Jin Yiqiang

Abstract Printed materials are an important part of the curriculum resources for online education. However, the printed materials currently used for online education are with few characteristics and the quality needs to be improved. The paper conducts a survey to find out students' perceptions about the printed materials in use and expectations for ideal printed materials. Based on the data analysis from the survey as well as an examination of the status of printed materials in online education, its integration with the online education technology and the compilation of such printed materials, the paper proposes a new way to design printed materials so as to change the current situation.

Keywords Online education · Printed materials · Perception · Expectations

In online education learning resources, printed materials occupy a special status. "Printed materials in radio and television education are the basis of a variety of instructional media. Both the main carrier of the teaching contents and contacting other instructional media as ties" [1]. Printed materials still have an important position in the online education which taking Internet as the main teaching medium. Various network education colleges still take printed materials as necessary learning resources. The results of surveys in the network education college of South China Normal University also proved this point: in the teaching media, such as "printed materials, online courseware, network broadcast video, BBS discussion, e-mail answering ", students using the most are printed materials, to 43.2 %.

However, in the practice of online education, the quality of printed materials doesn't match their important status. Network education colleges of Renmin University of China and China Petroleum University have expressed their thoughts "the design of printed materials in online education is not satisfactory and does not

---

J. Yiqiang (✉)
Department of Information Technology, Guangdong Teacher College of Foreign Language and Arts, Guangzhou 510640 Guangdong, People's Republic of China
e-mail: hellojinyiqiang@qq.com

reflect the remote features, we should strengthen the research" [2]. Even in CRTVU which has many years of online education experiences, there also had a similar situation.

"We still lack research and exploration of the design and development of a variety of media integration in CRTVU. In recent years, despite a number of multimedia courseware were developed, but the theoretical study and practice of integrated instructional design of printed materials, audio-visual materials, and other media also less, and remained mostly on the initial ideas which didn't put into practice" [3]. "Realistically speaking, we are unable to develop the textbooks which really have the open education characteristics and suit for individualized learning. The excitement was easy to put in the audio-visual teaching materials, now added multimedia courseware" [4]. China Online Education Academic Roundtable also discussed online education printed materials, "Lots of Network Education College have very short experiences in correspondence education stage, or have not gone through correspondence education stage, then directly across to online education, so there are no deep design basis of the printed materials" [1]. So the paper plans to carry out the study of online education participants' perception and expectations of printed materials, investigation of first-line users of printed materials attitude, preferences, habits, seeking their views on the printed materials design.

118.1 The Design of the Questionnaire and Issuance

118.1.1 The Design of the Questionnaire

Before the official release of the questionnaire, the paper selected the 20 students of the network education colleges of South China Normal University to test and individual interview. Then according to test measurements and interviews, the paper fixed the text representation and parts of the questionnaire in order to achieve a unified understanding. At the same time, the master's and doctoral students of the Institute of Online education of SCNU were invited to review the questionnaire; then according to comments to modify the content of printed materials desired part of the investigation. Through test measurement and appraisal to ensure the validity of the questionnaire.

118.1.2 The Questionnaire Issuance

The students who filled out the questionnaire, at least had half a year online learning experiences in the network education colleges of South China Normal University. They could make own choices about the using of printed materials.

The issuance of questionnaires locations scattered throughout Guangdong Province and Guangxi Province and Hainan Province including Guangzhou, Jieyang, Maoming, Shaoguan, Zhuhai, Jingxi, Haikou, Kunming. Though sample control to ensure the reliability of the questionnaire. Finally 240 questionnaires were issued, including recycling 222 valid questionnaires; the recovery rate was 92.5 %. The paper used the SPSS16.0 version to data analysis.

118.2 The Questionnaire Data Analysis

118.2.1 Basic Information

This part contains the age and gender distribution, the enrollment time of the Respondents. In respondents, men account 51.9 %, women account 45.5 %; and missing six. On the age distribution, only three under the age of 20, accounted for 1.4 %, 20–24-year-old accounted for 30.2 %, 25–29 years old accounted for 34.7 %, 30–34 years old accounted for 18.5 %, over the age of 35 accounted for 15.4 %, no missing data. The data indicates that mainly students of online education were working adult, although having begun to appear younger age trend. On enrollment time, the subjects of investigation who had 6 months distance learning experiences accounted for 15.3 %, in a year accounted for 44.1 %, in a year and a half accounted for 12.5 %, 2 years accounted for 4.1 %, and 14.4 % in two-and-a-half years, missing 21 (9.5 %). This indicates that 75.2 % of the students have a year or more online education experiences; they could make their own choices about the use of printed materials.

118.2.2 Perception and Cognitive about Existing Printed Materials

This part aimed to know the students' understanding of the status and role of printed materials, the perception of existing printed materials and textbooks organizations.

118.2.2.1 Students' Understanding of the Status and Role of the Printed Materials for the Internet Age

As previously mentioned, "printed materials, online courseware, network broadcast video, BBS discussion, e-mail answering ", students using the most are printed materials, to 43.2 %, far more than the second online courseware which accounted for 31.5 %.

The students feel online courseware having the largest effect, accounting for 31.5 %. However, there are a total of 66 students feeling printed materials having the largest effect, accounting for 29.7 %; along with 24.3 % students feel printed materials to help the Second.

The survey data show that the printed material in the network education plays an important role: in a variety of learning resources, students applied printed materials most. In the era of online education, the role of the printed materials have been weakened, but still plays an important role; together with network courses, they constitute the main body of teaching content, play the role of connecting other instructional media. At the same time, it maintain long-lasting, easy to use.

118.2.2.2 The Perception of Existing Printed Materials and Textbooks Organizations

About existing textbooks attitude, 43 % of the students thought "printed materials issued by the network education college affected me learn the course confidence", 31.7 % of participants agreed or strongly agreed that "if my own choice, I would not choose printed materials issued by the network education college", up to 71.5 % of the students were tired of using printed materials. This indicated that there were certain problems about the existing teaching materials to attract and maintain student learning; data also revealed that the bad materials would affect the confidence of students.

About textbook organization, 42.8 % of the participants found "the printed materials and online learning content does not close, very loose". This indicates that the existing textbooks need to strengthen relation with online learning content. Meanwhile, 41.1 % of the participants believed that "the language of printed materials obscure and not easy to read", 35.5 % of the participants felt the textbook lack of illustration design, 37.9 % of participants did not agree with "the exercises of existing printed materials, reasonable, the difficulty of properly". These suggested that online education printed materials in the written language expression, illustration, design and exercise arrangements need to specially design to fit the students' learning Table 118.1.

118.2.3 Expectations of the Ideal Printed Materials

118.2.3.1 The Expectations Associated with the Learning Content

This section is intended to understand the expectations of selecting the learning content, learning content associating with the actual life, the practical activities arrangements, the subject learning methods, learning assessment, learning guidance. As can be seen from Table 118.2, the vast majority of students wants to textbook knowledge and real-life close contact, and be able to apply what they

Table 118.1 The perception of existing printed materials and textbooks organizations

Frequency(percentage) cognition textbooks	Strongly agree	Agree	Neutral	Disagree	Strongly disagree
Printed materials issued by the network education college affect the confidence to learn course	8.9	24.1	18.8	43.5	4.7
Printed materials make me feel bored	12.8	58.7	19.9	7.7	1
On my own choice, I would not choose the printed materials issued of network education college	5.7	26	26.8	37.9	3.6
Relationship between printed materials and online content loose	16.2	26.6	28.7	26.9	2.6
Language of printed materials obscure and not easy to read	16.6	24.5	28.1	28.3	2.6
Exercises of textbook have reasonable the difficulty	12.6	24.5	25.1	32.3	5.6

Table 118.2 The expectations associated with the learning content

Frequency(percentage) expectation	Strong desired	Desired	Neutral	Undesired	Strong undesired
Textbook knowledge and real-life close contact	49.2	39.8	10.5	0.5	0
Printed materials provide online extended learning resources	46.6	44.5	7.9	1.0	0
Practice in the textbooks which can contact actual work	42.7	45.8	11.5	0	0
Arrange forms activities in printed materials	26.3	51.5	19.1	2.6	0.5
The reasonable arrangements exercises and knowledge	37	53.6	7.8	1.0	0.5
Each unit has a summary to help seize the key knowledge	44.0	49.2	4.7	2.1	0
Join online learning methods in printed materials	33.0	52.6	12.4	2.1	0

have learned. 90.6 % of students in favor of reasonable arrangements for the exercises in order to deepen the understanding of the knowledge, this indicates that the arrangement of the exercises in the textbook success plays an important role. At the same time 91.1 % of the students want printed materials provide online extended learning resources. Moreover, students support each unit has a unit summary.

118.2.3.2 Expectations of Performance form of Learning Content

Expectations of learning content manifestation contain contacting style between printed materials and online learning materials, compilation of teaching materials,

Table 118.3 Expectations of performance form of learning content

Frequency(percentage) expectations	Strong desired	Desired	Neutral	Undesired	Strong undesired
Hope printed materials close contact with online materials	46.9	45.8	6.8	0.5	0
Textbooks to be written in equality dialogue	28.8	52.1	17.0	2.1	0
Language of printed materials should be easy to understand	29.4	47.9	20.1	2.6	0
Arrangements illustrations to help better understand knowledge	29.4	47.9	20.1	2.6	0
Arrange learning content in a structured way	34	56.2	9.8	0	0

textbooks language features, illustrations arrangements, layout design. As can be seen from Table 118.3, 90.9 % of the students want textbooks to be written in equality, dialogue; similar to this, 77.3 % students think the language of the printed materials should be vivid, easy to understand.

In layout design, 79.4 % students hope to facilitate the reading of the font, the font, the title of printed materials; while students hope more illustrations in textbooks. On the organization of the teaching materials, 90.2 % students would like to arrange the learning content in a structured way, which has a clear knowledge structure diagram. Similarly, most students want printed materials and online learning materials are closely linked. On the style of text explanation, 85.6 % students felt that the teacher should follow terms of printed materials.

118.3 Discussion and Conclusion

According to the above data analysis, this paper discusses the students' cognition and expectations of printed materials, and suggests how to better design and develop printed materials.

118.3.1 Further Understanding of the Status and Role of Network Environments Printed Materials

As previously described, in radio and television education printed materials are the basis of a variety of instructional media. Both the main carrier of the teaching content, and contact other instructional media as ties. However, the survey can be found in the online education environment, printed materials function takes the new changes, and its role has been weakened to some extent. The survey results show that 31.5 % of students believe that the largest help taken to them is the online courseware, more than a printed textbook. Meanwhile, in the internet age, printed materials "low cost, large capacity information and maintain long-lasting, easy-to-use" [5] advantages, in addition to the "easy to use" are still irreplaceable, its large capacity and maintain long-term, "low cost" advantage compared to networks or completely lost, or partially lost. Therefore, in the online education environment, this paper believes we need to re-understand the status and role of the printed materials. The one hand, printed materials are still an important learning resource for online education, its ease of use, the habits of the people that irreplaceable printed materials, it still plays a link to contact a variety of instructional media. The other hand, with the in-depth development of online education, the core position of the printed materials will gradually give way to online courses. Online courses are bound to be the core of the network education instructional media. As to provide more choices to the learner, printed materials and network courses can take together to play a central role in the media mix. No matter what, in the network education, printed materials must be in depth network learning integration, collaborative development, in order to be successful

118.3.2 Integration of Printed Materials and Online Media

As can be seen from the survey results, successful printed materials must be effectively converged network learning methods. One of the main reasons that students do not like the printed materials is "online learning content does not close, very loose". On the way of integration, before developing course learning resources Network Education College should combine printed materials with the network curriculum first, rather than separating printed materials from the network curriculum development, which result in both incompatible phenomenon. In the integration process, we should accord to the characteristics of teaching media to arrange, exert online media advantage to make up for the disadvantage of printed materials [6].

Specific methods can take in media integration: summary presents the main teaching content text and pictures in printed materials; and on the network, through the Teacher Classroom Record course knowledge to provide comprehensive learning content and expansion of resources, such as Knowledge Base, test database. Through printed materials to achieve a one-way exchange of independent learning, through chat rooms, instant messaging, voice answering system to provide network synchronization, asynchronous two-way interactive teaching and collaborative learning.

118.3.3 Printed Materials Design Methods and Precautions

Through Analysis of survey results, we get many specific printed materials design methods and precautions which concluded the organizations selected for the printed textbook content and expression, learning activities, learning guidance design. On the learning content selection, students advocated appropriate to reduce the difficulty of teaching materials, textbooks should be combined with real life, close to the trend of the times. These require that the online education institutions should accord to training objectives to choose learning content.

One of the critical success factors of the printed materials is learning content expression [7]. The survey shows that user-friendly, humorous and vivid language can stimulate learners' interest in learning printed materials. Generally speaking, online education textbooks should be written dialogue, so that learners feel like talk with teachers; language should be a lively, pleasant tone, shorten the distance of the teachers and students [8]. The writers try to read out the written content, avoid heavy incomprehensible tone. Using of graphics, images to express complex things is a good way of expression [9]. The survey shows that the learning activities and the design of the study guide are also very important. Through learning activities deeper meaning can induce the learner's interest in learning, and guide them to positive thinking, mastery learning content [10]. On the study guides, providing more prompt or unit Summary can help students seizing the key content of the textbooks [11].

References

1. CRTVU (1988) Textbooks written specification of the CRTVU Printing (text). CRTVU Education, pp 13 16
2. Li L, Zhang A (2012) To strengthen remote features, promoting the construction of teaching materials. http://www1.open.edu.cn/ycjy/fengmian.php?id=192
3. Ding X (2001) The development and application of educational technology and IT in online education. Hebei Radio and Television University, Zhangjiakou, pp 7–2
4. Bing Y (2001) Basic principles and tasks of teaching resource. Modern Online Educ Res 10–16
5. Yu M (1988) Preparation of principles and basic requirements of the radio and television university textbooks. China Radio and Television University Education, Beijing, pp 13–16
6. Zhang F (2001) Online education printed materials design. E-education, pp 51–54
7. Jia X, Mi Z (2007) "Scaffolding" model design of printed materials in online education. E-education, pp 74–77
8. Desmond K (1993) Theoretical principles of distance education. Routledge, New York, pp 80–84
9. Teli DL (1998) How prepared in open and distance learning materials—teachers' guide to action and action officers. China Radio and Television University Education, Beijing, pp 38–42
10. Chen R (1992) Adult self-learning materials development model. National Open University Press, New York, pp 58–59
11. Li C (2005) Online education learning guide book writing. Distance Education in China, pp 24–26

Chapter 119
Task Driven is an Effective Teaching Model of Discrete Mathematics in High Education

Liu Shuai, Fu Weina, Li Qiang, Zhao Yulan and Duan Chanlun

Abstract With rapid improvement in all domains of computer, discrete mathematics becomes a main professional required course in college of computer science and technology. But this course is full of theoretical knowledge and becomes little interest of students. In this paper, we discuss negative of the classic teaching model in discrete mathematics in high education firstly. Then, we study how to use task driven into teaching method by combined teaching practice in this course for years. Finally, we discuss and study the improvement of teaching model by use task driven.

Keywords Discrete mathematics · Task driven · High education · Teaching model · Teaching process

119.1 Background

Discrete mathematics course is a mathematics course which studies structure and correlation of discrete quantity. Nowadays, it is not only an important part of modern mathematics, but also used widely in many subjects, especially in computer science and technology. Meanwhile, discrete mathematics is a prerequisite course of many professional courses of computer subject. Artificial Intelligence (AI), Theoretical Computer Science (TCS), e.g. Students improved their ability of abstract thinking and logical reasoning [1].

L. Shuai (✉) · F. Weina · L. Qiang · Z. Yulan · D. Chanlun
College of Computer, Inner Mongolia University, Hohhot 010012, China
e-mail: cs_liushuai@imu.edu.cn

F. Weina
Department of Computer Science and Technology, Hohhot University of Nationalities, Hohhot, China

But in modern society, more students show more interests in practice courses. In this case, a new teaching method is analysed to improve students' practical capacity. It is called task driven.

The task driven is a teaching method based on teaching theory of constructivism. It uses a corporate task active centre in teaching process. Under help of teacher and application of resource aggressively, students can study knowledge and synergetic interaction themselves autonomously because they are driven by strong motivation in solution finding of problem. In that way, students study a kind of practical activity when they finish the given task. So a positive cycle is formation from achievement feeling of finished task to thirst of knowledge and exploration [2].

In fact, similar to discrete mathematics, many courses teaching are underlining their theory and ignoring practices. It makes students disgust courses [3]. Contrarily, practical process cannot be easy to lead into teaching because complexity and discreteness of courses. So in this paper, we put forward a teaching model based on task driven. We use the model in teaching and find teaching result is better than before.

119.2 Disadvantage of Classic Teaching Model in Discrete Mathematics

(1) **The classic teaching model**

Since classic class-teaching is constructed by Herbart [4] and improved by Kaiipob [5], it becomes a set of teaching thinking and model. Generalized, it is usually called teaching-in-five-steps. Though there are different versions, teaching-in-five-steps divides a course to five steps.

The classic teaching requires its standard to knowledge achievement. So classic teaching puts knowledge to a sovereign place and trusts others are subsidiary, which contains emotion, attitude, intelligence and ability, and so on. This is the fundamental defect of classic teaching.

(2) **Embodiment of teaching defects in classic model**

The first defect is it requires standard to teaching material. Format of knowledge from book is indirect experience and it accords with rule and feature of teaching process in essence. Meanwhile, students cannot form them to theory model when they have no direct experience. So it breaks balance of experience derivation and lead to that the mountains have brought forth a mouse.

The second defect is it requires standard to teacher/teaching. Through, teaching (teacher) and studying (student) are essential relationship in teaching process. They are both interactivity and retroaction. In classic teaching, it lopsidedly emphasizes teacher and teaching which makes relations between teacher-student and teaching-studying by teacher and teaching standardly.

Table 119.1 Percent of student's reasons for their little interested in discrete mathematics

Reason	Useless	Hard to study (%)	Disgusted (%)	Others (%)
Scale	78	10	7	5

Table 119.2 Percent of student's attitude in discrete mathematics

	Need to study well		Study but NOT need well		No need to study	
	Reason	Scale (%)	Reason	Scale (%)	Reason	Scale (%)
Reson and Scale	Postgraduate	16	Not interesting	27	Useless	18
	Helpful		Knowledge	5	Spend more time	12
	Hard to study	10				
	Other reason	4	Other reason	3	Other reason	5

(3) **Instance of students' attitude in discrete mathematics**

Some researchers investigated 100 students from college of computer if they were interested in discrete mathematics and arrange the result to Table 119.1 [6]. Not long ago, we also conduct an investigation in it with 100 students and arrange the result to Table 119.2.

From these two tables, we find the main reason of students' attitude is invisible value of this course. Generally, it is common in all basis theoretical courses. How to change this case? We trust task driven is the right method.

119.3 Task Driven Model and Application

(1) **Objective and classification of task driven**

In task driven, objective is driven but not task. Driven is achievement motivation of student. So task neither static nor isolated but must promote formation of the motivation [7].

In our opinion, there are two classes in task driven. One is driven by cognition, another is by external cause.

A. **Cognition driven**.

Cognition driven uses cognition driven as kernel. In this teaching process, teaching action is mainly for guide but not interference. There must be a conclusion duly after tasks to make cognition clear and deep.

B. **External cause driven**.

There are environment driven and attachment driven in external cause driven [8]. Environment driven uses inner driven of environment as kernel which is need of gained position (environment) by studying. In high teaching, material award is always used to motivate student. Usually

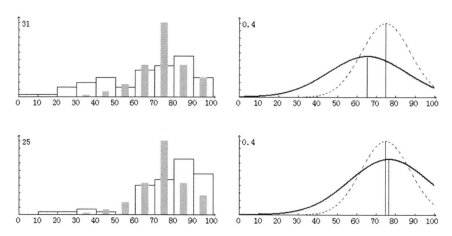

Fig. 119.1 Score analysis for 2010–2011/2011–2012 autumn term

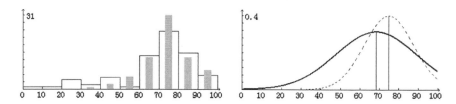

Fig. 119.2 Score analysis for 2012–2013 autumn season

additional score of course is given to encourage great performance of students. Attachment driven is less use in high education because it needs an irresistible relation.

(2) **Application of task driven**

We divide application to two levels, one is macroscopic and another is microcosmic. In macroscopic level, we divide course teaching program and lead a case in teaching process through with difficulty and complexity degree mezzo. In discrete mathematics, there will be 3–4 cases because it needs one case in each part of course. Each case is selected to cover most knowledge of each part of course. Then, at beginning of course, we use each case as task to drive after basis teaching. In this process, students finish work actively and teaching is for work solution. Meanwhile, competition is lead to course to motivate students. In this way, inner-driven replaces outer-driven and better to motivate subjective studying.

In microcosmic level, we study teaching method and inspection in stages for concrete application. It also contains conclusion and analysis of each knowledge point after case teaching and achievement of stage. Students are willing to study and their receptive ability is strengthened based on cases.

119.4 Application

We use task driven model in discrete mathematics by analysed negative of classic teaching model here.

We use the new method in our class and find it motivate interest and excavate capacity of students. Figures 119.1 and 119.2 are shown different scores between two grades. In these figures, we can easily to find the bring benefit by task driven. We find the newer data is (25, 11, 4, 28, 14, 7, 2, 3 and 6 %). Then to compare data (16, 27, 18, 5, 12, 10, 4, 3 and 5 %) in Table 119.2, we can also find the change of students' studying attitude.

Acknowledgments This work is supported by grants programs of higher-level talents of Inner Mongolia University [No. 125126, 115117], National Natural Science Foundation of China (No: 61261019, 61103090, 61170005), Higher Scholastic Science Foundation of Inner Mongolia (No. NJZY13004).

References

1. Kolman RJ (2004) Discrete mathematics (6th ed). Prentice Hall, New York
2. Ausubel DP (1960) The use of advance organizers in the learning and retention of meaningful verbal material. J Educ Psychol 51(5):267–272
3. Prokop P, Tunnicliffe SD, Kubiatko M et al (2011) The role of teacher in students attitudes to and achievement in palaeontology. Energy Educ Sci Technol Part B 3(1):29–45
4. Herbart, J. F (1804) Über die Aesthetische Darstellung der Welt als Hauptgeschäft der Erziehung. In Aus Herbarts Jugendschriften Mit einer Einleitung von H. Döpp-Vorwald. Weinheim/Berlin: Verlag Julius Beltz, without year (1962). (trans: Henry M, and Felkin E (1902) The Science of education, its general principles deduced from its aim and the aesthetic revelation of the world.) Heath & Co, Boston
5. Kaiipob NA (1957) Education. People's education press, Beijing
6. Li F, Sun L (2006) Task-driven of teaching in discrete mathematics. Comp Edu 3:27–29 (in Chinese)
7. Lin W (2006) Revisit the view of Kernberg's integration about object relationships, affects and drives. J Nanjing Nor Univ (Social Science) 5:87–91 (in Chinese with English abstract)
8. Lü J, Ma X, Tao X et al (2008) On environment-driven software model for internetware. Sci China (Ser F-Inf Sci) 51(6):683–721

Chapter 120
Evaluation on Application of Scene-Simulation Teaching Method in Oral Medicine Teaching

Xiaoli An, Qianqian Lin, Wu Fanbieke, YuLin Zhang, Bin Liu and Wang Jizeng

Abstract In order to evaluate the application effect of scene-simulation teaching method in oral medicine teaching. During the teaching process, 75 students participated in traditional teaching methods and 73 students participated in scene-simulation teaching methods, respectively. The performance of the experimental group are better than the control group in the course satisfaction the rate of disease awareness and the reorganization of the extent of teaching methods and etc. The simulation teaching method stimulates students' enthusiasm and improves students' interests and grades as well.

Keywords Scene-simulation teaching method · Oral medicine · Effectiveness of teaching

The simulation teaching method is a kind of important and modern practical teaching method, which combines teaching case, situational- scene with practical method to improve the quality of teaching. Case method originated from Harvard University, the aim of which is to combine theory with practice case act and then to be a type of basical teaching materials, which is widely used for basical and clinical medicine and so on, practically-stronger subject. (1) Scene simulation teaching creates vivid and specific scene consistent with the teaching content in the teaching process, transforms theoretical knowledge into the intuitive cognition. Apart from helping teachers stimulate goal-directed learners' interests, guiding

---

X. An (✉) · Q. Lin · W. Fanbieke · Y. Zhang · B. Liu
Department of Stomatology, College of Stomatology, Lanzhou University,
Lanzhou 730000, China
e-mail: anxl@lzu.edu.cn

B. Liu
e-mail: Liubkq@lzu.edu.cn

W. Jizeng
Institute of Solid Mechanics, School of Civil Engineering and Mechanics, Lanzhou University, Lanzhou 730000, China
e-mail: jzwang@lzu.edu.cn

learners to explore and seek knowledge, the method also helps students understand the theoretical knowledge what they have studied deeply. (2) The teaching method comes from platonic teaching model of ancient Europe. What is called platonic teaching method is a pattern of teaching approach to teach objectives completely by the case and discussion. It changes the teaching of "injection" into "heuristic" method and avoids falling into the simply teach and inject knowledge, it also guides students to ponder independently and actively so that improve students' comprehensive ability. The scene simulation teaching method has many characteristics, such as the highly realistic, targeted clearly, students' initiative, procedure's dynamic and so on. The method can solve the common problem that separates theory and reality in the class teaching.

Oral medicine is kind of clinical disciplines with strong sense of practice in clinical stomatology, which requests students not only grasp the theoretical knowledge solidly but also analyze patients' condition and then cure disease. Traditional teaching method is difficult to expound and manifest the disease and its characteristics completely and multi- perspectively in the limited teaching time, which isolates oral medical students from the study of medical theory. So introduce the teaching method of scene simulation into the class of "Non-Carious Dental Hard Tissue Disease" (the following in short called "NCDHTD") by using the way of scenario simulation, students act as a patient or doctor, reappearing the scene of seeing doctor and treatment process etc. In the classroom, setting up realistic, open, harmony learning and performing situation, providing students with an abundance of opportunities of observing, thinking and practicing. It's helpful to learn and grasp the cause of "NCDHTD" clinical manifestations, diagnosis, treatment more systematically, so help students grasp all kinds of disease of "NCDHTD" overall. This method not only strengths students' ability of analytical thinking and debating skills and problem solving,which then improves the students' comprehensive ability, but also achieves the teaching aim that teach the students how to combine theoretical knowledge with practice. The mentioned above not only contributes to making the class of "NCDHTD" smooth in high quality but also increases effectiveness of teaching the "NCDHTD" class.

120.1 Data and Method

120.1.1 Student Materiels

Choose 75 students (male 39 female 36) in total, who are from 5 year university graduated in 2007 and 2008, majoring in oral medicine, as experimental group, 73 graduated (male 33 female 40) in 2009 as control group. The student in two groups have no difference in the grade and the sex when they came to university ($p > 0.05$). Teachers, teaching time and schedules of two groups are exactly the same

120.1.2 Teaching Methods

The experimental group is taught with the method of simulation. The basic process as follows. First, teachers prepare for scene simulation 2 months before the oral medicine subject begins, disease grouping for "NCDHTD". Students can choose freely which group to stay, then refer to the related information of the disease, design the scene simulation and the role-playing according to the role, purpose and contents of the theme elaborated in detail. Second, carry on either grouping or the whole class discussion. Four students are divided into one group. After discussion, selected a representative as a main speaker, other students adding. Third, on the basis of little group, they discuss again in the whole class. They can debate about it once meeting the focus. By this way, students can express their own points so that they become the real hosts in the class. When students are discussing, teachers do well in organization, inspiration and introduction during the brainstorming process so as to make students speak positively around the central topic. Also, teachers should encourage students dare to tap some sensitive issues at the same time, allow them to express their different ideas freely. When students talked about their different ideas in the whole class, others will know more than before, gain more inspiration to understand and solve problem flexible.

The control group used traditional teaching method. During the whole teaching process a teacher plays a main role in the teaching process according to students' learning needs to explain emphasizes and difficulties, students take notes in the class and finish homework after class.

120.1.3 Evaluation Method

At the end of the semester two group students take a theory test in order to investigate the satisfaction and acceptance of students' about teaching method. The theory examination is closed book, including single choice and multiple-choice, all about the disease of "NCDHTD", 100 points in total. The time is limited in 50 min. Compare scores in two groups; evaluate the effect of the two teaching methods. 148 questionnaires of satisfaction of teaching method coupled with the same number of acceptance of teaching method are sent and then collect all the papers.

120.1.4 Dealing with Statistics

Using SPSS 16.0 statistical software tested it by $x2$ then doing date process. Statistical significance is based on $p < 0.05$.

120.2 Result

120.2.1 The Satisfaction Survey of Students in Experimental Group About Simulation Teaching Method

(See Table 120.1).

120.2.2 Comparing Correct Rate About Disease Between Two Group (%)

(See Table 120.2).

120.2.3 The Survey About Teaching Method's Level of Acceptance Between Two Groups

(See Table 120.3).

Table 120.1 The satisfaction survey of students in experimental group about simulation teaching method

Simulation teaching method	Strongly endorsed		Approved		General		Apposition		Strongly apposed	
	n	%	n	%	n	%	n	%	n	%
Necessary or not	70	93.3	3	4.0	2	2.7	0	0.0	0	0.0
Achieve the desired effect or not	68	90.7	4	5.3	2	2.7	1	1.3	0	0.0
Good for adapting clinical quickly or not	60	80.0	8	10.6	4	5.3	2	2.7	1	1.3
Good for improve the interesting of learning medical department or not	69	92.0	1	1.3	3	4.0	1	1.3	1	1.3

Table 120.2 Comparing correct rate about disease between two group (%)

Class	Number	Clinical manifestation of disease	Disease diagnosis	The method of disease treatment	The diagnosis of disease
Experimental group (grade 07, 08)	75	90.67	93.33	97.33	86.67
Control group (grade 09)	73	82.19	83.56	89.04	80.82

Table 120.3 The survey about teaching method's level of acceptance between two groups

Group	Approve	Interesting	Easy to remember	Inattention
Experimental group	69	57	43	2
Control group	48	30	22	9
X^2	15.39	18.61	11.66	5.02
P value	<0.05	< 0.05	< 0.05	< 0.05

120.3 Discussion

In our country, medical education has used traditional cramming teaching method for many years. Teachers only provide information and knowledge to students, require them remember something important to achieve the goal of learning. Teachers only pay attention to instill transfer knowledge to practice. Because of isolating theoretical knowledge from clinical practice, students can't apply theoretical knowledge to clinical practice, as a result, when they work in the future, they will feel difficult to face complex diseases, so they don't know how to deal with the contradiction produced by the traditional teaching method between teaching reality in class of "NCDHTD" and students 'needs, due to lacking of enthusiasm, initiative and creativity generally, students' leaning interests decrease, effectiveness of teaching also lacks reality. Renee [3] showing active proactively, which as a kind of awareness of vocational education. So we applied the simulation teaching method to oral medicine teaching activities. As can be seen from Table 120.2, the score of experimental group is higher than the control group. From Table 120.1, we know that students in experimental group have greater interests in teaching activities of simulation teaching method, the intention in teaching activities is to arouse students what to learn and create which is premise of innovative education. Simulation teaching method plays an important role in the effectiveness of teaching the class of "NCDHTD". It is good for increasing students' attention and participation in "NCDHTD", which in turn is good for students' interests, learning and emotional sense of identity, making the process of teaching becomes process of teaching and educating. From Table 120.3. We know, if we use simulation teaching method in teaching activities. We can guide students to learn effectively, adding some details to traditional teaching method in order to achieve the purpose what we want. Students' thinking ability will be better and better, which include agile, flexible and critical, students' interests of learning can be improved obviously. Moreover students will sustain to explore a variety of unique or best solution when they take part in the collection, preparation and analysis of case. All is good for increase interesting of learning "NCDHTD" and improve ability of grasp theoretical knowledge, train students' spirit and ability of innovation, help them apply theoretical knowledge to practice at the same time.

Overall, scene simulation teaching is a method that reform education by using this method; we can make teaching of "NCDHTD" achieve more unity between theory and practice, thereby reach the education well. Teaching method is a kind of flexible educational activity. Effect about characteristics of the course, stock knowledge of teachers and psychological and cognitive of students must be reflected in its open, dynamic and effective teaching activity. Then make students have strong enthusiasm to learn theoretical knowledge, put abstract theoretical knowledge into specific case situation. It stimulates students' interests in learning. Scenario simulation teaching method makes teaching atmosphere more relax, in addition,it helps students change the situation of "let me learn" in traditional teaching mode into the situation of "I want to learn".

References

1. Crittenden WF (2005) A social learning theory of cross-function-al case education. J Bus Res 58(7):960–966
2. Lu T, Zhang H (2012).Application of scene simulation teaching method in the clinical teaching of surgical nutrition among associate nursing students.Chin J Nurs Educ 9(6):251–253
3. Renee TR (2009). Assuring ethical treatment of students as research participants. J Nurs Educ 10(48):537–541
4. Duan X, Gao G (2009) Exploratory development of virtual technique in multimedia education domain. IEEE DEC 05–06:25–28

Chapter 121
Research on Three Convolutions Related Issues in Signal Processing

Wei Song

Abstract Convolution computing is an important section in signal processing and it has many applications in the real life, such as medical signal analysis, image and video processing, linear system simulation, communication analysis, electronics, automation and so on. There are there types of convolution algorithms and they are linear convolution, periodic convolution and circular convolution, which are the key points and difficult points in signal processing, because these three concepts are abstract for students to understand and master. In this paper, we will explain the definition of these three convolutions; analyze the relationship between them, especially study deeply on the equalization conditions of these convolutions' transformation.

Keywords Signal processing · Linear convolution · Periodic convolution · Circular convolution

121.1 Introduction

Three convolutions named linear convolution [1, 2], periodic convolution [3] and circular convolution (also known as the cyclic convolution) [4] analyzes the relationship between input and output of linear system in time domain in signal processing. They're not only the key, but also the difficulty. The concepts of three convolutions are too abstract that many students cannot understand them [5, 6].

W. Song (✉)
School of Information Engineering in Minzu University of China, Beijing 100081, China
e-mail: sw_muc@126.com

W. Song
Research Institute of Information Technology in Tsinghua University, Beijing 100084, China

Meanwhile, how to compute these convolutions and how to find the condition, under which these convolutions can transform to each other, is the big problems to students. From the basic definition of the three convolutions, this chapter will explores the teaching method by studying the generation reason of convolutions, the calculation methods and so on. All of these will strengthen mastering and understanding on the related content.

121.2 Linear Convolution: Describe the Relationship Between Input and Output in LTI System

Linear convolution [1, 2, 4] is used to describe the relationship between input and output in linear time invariant system and it is one of the main methods of getting discrete system response. Many important applications are built on the basis of this theory, such as the convolution filtering. First, we study the reason of linear convolution: Known by the property of unit impulse sequence, arbitrary sequence $x(n)$ can be expressed as shift weight sum of unit impulse sequence $\delta(n)$, that is:

$$x(n) = \sum_{m=-\infty}^{\infty} x(m)\, \delta(n-m) \qquad (121.1)$$

Then the sequence $x(n)$ acts as the input of system T that is LTI system. Known by the property of LTI system, the system only affects the sequence $\delta(n-m)$ which is shifted from impulse sequence $\delta(n)$ related to time n, while the input sequence $x(m)$ is preserved after operation as the coefficient of $\delta(n-m)$ that is:

$$y(n) = T[\sum_{m=-\infty}^{\infty} x(m)\, \delta(n-m)] = \sum_{m=-\infty}^{\infty} x(m)\, T[\delta(n-m)] \qquad (121.2)$$

Let $T[\delta(n-m)] = h(n-m)$, named unit response sequence, it becomes:

$$y(n) = \sum_{m=-\infty}^{\infty} x(m)\, T[\delta(n-m)] = \sum_{m=-\infty}^{\infty} x(m)\, h(n-m) \qquad (121.3)$$

The equality describes the relationship between input and output of the LTI system and usually called the equality for the linear convolution. And is expressed as

$$y(n) = \sum_{m=-\infty}^{\infty} x(m)\, h(n-m) = x(n) * h(n) = h(n) * x(n) \qquad (121.4)$$

We can see that, what the linear convolution described is an operation or a relationship. The computation process can be divided into four steps and they are reversal, shift, multiplication, addition. In the solving process, one sequence remains motionless, another sequence flips and move from $-\infty$ to $+\infty$, then multiply the overlapped part and sum. There are two main methods of linear convolution and they are graphing method and analytical method. The first one is intuitive relatively and simple for the solution of finite sequences and the other method is more convenient for sequence whose analysis formula has been gave. However, graphing method is troublesome to make pictures and constrained to the convolution calculation for discrete sequence with a large amounts of data.

The key of the analytic method is confirming the sum space, which is discussing the different overlap of two sequences. For the infinite sequence, the procedure generally can be divided into: non-overlapping, partially overlapping. The calculation process is cumbersome, but can obtain analytic solution.

In addition, there is another method named Multiplication Vertically for two finite length sequences. It needs to be emphasized that multiplication can't carry. Finally, the computing result can be verified by the length. If the lengths of two sequences are N and M, the length of convolution is $N + M - 1$.

121.3 Periodic Convolution

In order to describe the time domain sequence corresponding to the product of the spectral sequence of two periodic sequences, periodic convolution [3,4] is defined:

$$\text{if } \tilde{Y}(k) = \tilde{X}_1(k) \times \tilde{X}_2(k) \text{ then } \tilde{y}(n) = \text{IDFS}(\tilde{Y}(k)) = \sum_{m=0}^{N-1} \tilde{x}_1(m)\tilde{x}_2(n-m)$$

(121.5)

This formula satisfies that multiplication in a domain corresponds to convolution in another domain. There are three steps in periodic convolution and they are multiplication, addition and sum. The two sequences must be with the same period and the convolution result is also a period sequence with the same period as the two input sequences. In the calculation process, when a value in a cycle is shifted out of the one period, the value at the same location of adjacent cycle shifted in this section, so the values of sequence can be always calculated in the section [0, $N-1$] and the total convolution result is a period sequence which make the value in the [0, $N-1$] as one period.

From the analysis, we can get the conclusion that, the meaning values in the periodic sequence are finite. So using circular convolution to describe the convolution of the finite length sequence is effective.

121.4 Circular Convolution

Circular convolution, also called cyclic convolution [4], is the special form of cycle convolution and the convolution is calculated only in one period. So there is no intrinsic difference between the periodic convolution and the circular convolution. Therefore, $x(n)$, $h(n)$ and $y(n)$ are assumed as the input sequence, impulse response sequence and output sequence, respectively.

The detail of the convolution is as Eq. 121.6: the first line is the loop inverse sequence of the sequence $x(n)$. Note that the first value is $x(0)$ and in this row from last to the second is the value with positive order in the sequence. Mobile the sequence in the first line one step towards the right progressively and circularly, we can get the following $L-1$ rows. Therefore, writing the first row correctly is the most important step in the procedure. Correctness of the result can be verified by judging the position of $x(0)$ and it is at the diagonal in the matrix.

$$\begin{bmatrix} y(0) \\ y(1) \\ y(2) \\ \vdots \\ y(L-1) \end{bmatrix} = \begin{bmatrix} x(0) & x(L-1) & x(L-2) & \cdots & x(1) \\ x(1) & x(0) & x(L-1) & \cdots & x(2) \\ x(2) & x(1) & x(0) & \cdots & x(3) \\ \vdots & \vdots & \vdots & \ddots & \vdots \\ x(L-1) & x(L-2) & x(L-3) & \cdots & x(0) \end{bmatrix} \begin{bmatrix} h(0) \\ h(1) \\ h(2) \\ \vdots \\ h(L-1) \end{bmatrix}$$

(121.6)

121.5 The Relationship Between these Three Convolutions

Linear convolution is the foundation of the engineering application. Periodic sequence leads to discretization of spectrum. From the analysis in Sect. 121.4, we know that, the circular convolution is the value in principal value interval of the cycle convolution. And circular convolution can be calculated by fast Fourier algorithm (FFT), which can resolve the real-time processing in real application. Therefore, it is necessary to find out the relationship between circular convolution and linear convolution.

Equation 121.7 shows that: extend the value of linear convolution with period L and get the value in principal value interval; we will get the circular convolution. So if the value of circular convolution with L points can equal to the value of linear convolution with the length $N+M-1$, we must make sure that $L \geq N+M-1$. And it is the condition, under which, convolution can represent the linear convolution.

$$y(n) = x_1(n) \circledN x_2(n) = \left[\sum_{m=0}^{L-1} x_1(m)x_2((n-m))_L\right]R_L(n) = \left[\sum_{m=0}^{L-1} x_1(m) \sum_{r=-\infty}^{\infty} x_2(nrL-m)\right]R_L(n)$$

$$= \left[\sum_{r=-\infty}^{\infty}\sum_{m=0}^{L-1} x_1(m)x_2(n+rL-m)\right]R_L(n) = \left[\sum_{r=-\infty}^{\infty} y_1(n+rL)\right]R_L(n)$$

(121.7)

So, we always add zero of the input sequence to match this condition. For example, assume the lengths of two sequences are M and N, respectively, if you want to use circular convolution take place of linear convolution, you need to add $(N-1)$ zeros to the first sequence and $(M-1)$ zeros to the second sequence. And all of these are to make the length of the circular convolution equals to the length of linear convolution. If you want to use based-2 FFT algorithm, you need to add zeros to make the length is integer power of 2. However, there is also a problem. When the difference between the lengths is big, for example, the long one is 513 and the short one is 10, the length of their linear convolution is $513 + 10 - 1 = 522$. So the number of added zero of the first one is 511 and the second is 1014. The based-2 FFT algorithm is ineffective. So, we should cut the long sequence into small one and two methods named overlap method and overlap add method are proposed [4].

121.6 Conclusions

Three convolutions are the key and difficult sections in signal processing. However, the basic concepts, basic principles and basic methods of these convolutions are hard to understand and master for students. In this chapter, we analyze the generation reason of the linear convolution, which describes the relationship between the input and the output in linear time invariant system. The relationships between three convolutions are also studied. And these are as replenishment the content of textbook to help students understanding and mastering the knowledge of signal processing.

Acknowledgments This work is supported by a grant from the Fundamental Research Funds for the Central Universities (No. 1112KYQN40, No. 1112KYZY49, No. 0910KYZY55) and Cultural heritage protection science and technology project of Cultural relics bureau (No.20110135). Our gratitude is extended to the anonymous reviewers for their valuable comments and professional contributions to the improvement of this paper.

References

1. Hazra J, Kayal D, Dandapat A, Sarkar CK (2011) Design of a high speed low power linear convolution circuit using McCMOS technique. IMPACT'2011. 276–279
2. Martinez J, Heusdens R, Hendriks RC (2011) A generalized poisson summation formula and its application to fast linear convolution. IEEE Sign Process Lett 18(9):501–504
3. Bu HW, Hon TH (2011) Investigation on the FFT-based antenna selection for compact uniform circular arrays incorrelated MIMO channels. IEEE Trans Sign Proc. 59(2):739–746
4. Chen PQ (2008) Digital signal processing, 3rd edn. Tsinghua University Press, Beijing
5. Martinez-Torres MR, BarreroGarcia FJ, ToralMarin SL, GallardoVazquez S (2005) A digital signal processing teaching methodology using concept-mapping techniques. IEEE Trans Educ 48(3):422–429
6. Hu XY, Wang Y, Hu YL (2007) Reform and practice of teaching of digital signal processing. High Educ Forum. 3:67–69

Chapter 122
Evaluation of College Students' Self-Regulated Learning Based on the IT Technology

X. Wang, B. Qu and Ch. Y. Jia

Abstract Information technology (IT) is a dominant factor influencing the development of the 21st century, which has been referred to as the era of information. Computers play an essential role in modern information technology and it demonstrates the development of multimedia, artificial intelligence and global network, which is convenient to facilitate a new self-learning environment. We can introduce the concept of sustainable development into the educational field. The reform of education system aims at training sustainable development talents who are communicative and innovative. How can universities and educating constitutions cultivate students to achieve this goal? In modern society, self-regulated learning ability can influence individual's development. Therefore, analyzing the problem of how to teach college students to use IT technology in self-regulated learning is crucial.

Keywords Information technology (IT) · Self-regulated learning · Sustainable development talents · College students

In the educational field, the reform of education system has brought great challenges to the present teaching mode. Now with the impact of IT technology, modern teaching method is transforming from classical information-transfer method to a method that focuses more on ability training. Furthermore, self-regulated learning is replacing ways of traditional learning, making teaching

---

X. Wang (✉)
Department of the Humanities and Social Sciences, China Medical University,
Shenyang 110001, China
e-mail: 2361522539@qq.com

B. Qu
The Research Center for Medical Education, China Medical University, Shenyang, China

Ch. Y. Jia
7-year Bachelor's and Master's Combined Program, China Medical University,
Shenyang, China

pattern to gradually shift from "knowledge" to "intelligence" and finally to "personal development". In a word, IT offers fundamental guarantee for the reform of educational system.

122.1 Promoting Self-Regulated Learning is a Critical Step for Reform of Higher Education

122.1.1 Self-Regulated Learning Adapts More to the Demand of Educational Reform

In spite of the many versions of the concept of self-regulated learning, the generally accepted one comes from 1986 American educational research association (AERA) annual meeting:

> Students are metacognitively, motivationally, or behaviorally active promoters of their academic achievement [5].

To put it in a simple way, self-regulated learning refers to autonomy of individual learners for learning goals and studying techniques, self monitoring of studying process and self assessment of studying results. As we all know, the goal of educational reform is to provide students with more space and flexibility to organize their own study, so issues in educational reform must be decided on the basis of students. Self-regulated learning is exactly the research aimed to find out how to make students capable of monitoring their own studying process. Research on correlation between self-regulated learning and college students' grades demonstrate that those with higher grades are usually better self-regulated learners, there are also results that suggest after series of curriculum aimed at promoting students' self-regulated learning techniques, their grades are improved [1]. The same results can be drawn from research where most students who excel in their schoolwork master autonomous learning ability, including the whole process of specific learning goal, particular studying method and self evaluating. As the famous Chinese contemporary educator Hushi says:

> Poured-in knowledge serves no great use, real knowledge are those acquired by oneself, self learning ability is the essential condition for seeking knowledge [2].

122.1.2 Psychological Theoretical Basis for Self-Regulated Learning

Self-regulated learning has been a popular topic in educational research since 1960s, it's also well-discussed in the psychology field. Using psychological theory to explain self-regulated learning is a good approach. Constructivism being the leading concept of contemporary Western educational reform, is an important branch of cognitive learning in psychology. Constructivists suggest the best way to enhance students' logical and conceptual growth is to make them experience it in the real world, not merely listening to teachers give lectures [4]. In other words, in order to constitute individual's new knowledge, students' critical role in the learning process should be enhanced, it's also crucial to convert students from passive knowledge accepters to active learners who acquire primary information and process on their own, only through this way can students' creativity and enthusiasm be stimulated. Correspondingly, teachers' role in the teaching process should also be switched, from lecturer to facilitators whose job is to aid students construct concepts actively. Furthermore, teachers should participate in students' learning process by providing inspiration, promoting cooperation and discussion, giving emotional support and as information consultant. In a word, the constructivism theory in psychology accord with learners' cognition pattern, and is put into practice of higher education with the help of information technology.

122.2 Brief Introduction on the Application of IT Technology in China and Abroad

Multi-media has become the fundamental basis of information technology. The modern information technology currently used in schools refers to the digital, networked, multi-media and intelligent IT technology. IT discussed in this article are those that aid students in their self-regulated learning process, such as network, all kinds of media, etc.

First of all, development of IT technology in education in China should be discussed. It is mainly divided into four stages. IT education first started during the 1970s and 1980s, focusing on the teaching of using computers, which goes on to the second stage in the mid and late 80s, applying computer to development of teaching resources and management software. Third stage is reached in mid and late 90s, centering on computer network, and finally, the fourth stage and current IT in education so far has been combined with teaching process. In summary, information technology in our country has been making huge progress but there are still severe gaps in comparison with developed countries and needs to be improved.

Britain as a developed country, attaches great importance to the impact of IT technology on society and on education system. Its IT education started in the 1960s, from primary try-out in elementary and middle schools to wide-spread teaching among citizens. It has experienced three stages to reach the mature growth it is today: first attempt during 60s-gradual spread during 80s-rapid development in 90s. IT education in Britain establishes great significance to national education, it sets as an example for developing countries to learn from.

As for the United States, it has been promoting IT education across the country since 1996, and by 2000 educational IT infrastructure construction has been completed. Apart from setting up specific IT curriculum, there has been successful combination of subject teaching and IT educating, which means the US has formed mature educational IT system. We can see that since IT technology construction in developed countries is gradually reaching perfection, they have many experiences for developing countries like us to refer to.

Japan is the pioneer of Information Communication Technology (ICT). The Japanese government announced the 'IT new reform strategy' in 2006, aiming to make Japan a front runner in global IT. Japan's three goals for IT in education include improving teaching process, information teaching and administrative informationization [3], which is similar to others countries around the world. What is worth noting is the effort Japan made in order to realize these goals, such as establishment of ''Teachers' guide for using ICT in teaching', coming up with development strategies for different stages and launching investigation and research programs, all of these measures are what we can learn from.

122.3 Things Worth Paying Attention to When Applying IT Technology to Self-Regulated Learning

What must be pointed out is that since self-regulating ability, cognitive capacity and ability to use computers all come down to varying levels from student to student, it may result in different learning results in different individuals. Hence teachers' guidance is required in self-regulated learning process to help students build integral knowledge hierarchy and master knowledge in a comprehensive way.

122.3.1 Cultivation of Students' Self-Regulating Ability Should be Emphasized

Research shows many college students lack self monitoring ability in their self-regulated learning process, some of them just simply don't study long enough. As a result of lack of supervision, many students only study when they have free time and we find that one-third of the students do not even have plans for their study. As we all know, self monitoring and regulating abilities have huge impact on students' grades, thus it is required that teachers and teaching administrators pay direct attention to monitoring students' progress and help students make adjustment to studying plans according to feedback information in self-regulated learning.

122.3.2 Provide Students with Timely Studying Guidance

In the self-regulated learning's teaching mode, the major position of students is highly stressed. The current networked environment often leads to deficiency in student–teacher communication. Thus for some students, they can't reach out to teachers' timely help and become afraid of difficulties, in severe cases students may even become hostile towards learning process. That's why we encourage that self-regulated learning should take place under teachers' guidance and encouragement. Teachers offer instructions and students carry on self-regulated learning process. While studying methods and strategies are being carefully studied, significant role of teachers should also be emphasized. Teachers' instructions should be offered based on difference between students' learning ability, cognitive capacity, learning style and self-regulating ability. The instructions should be aimed at helping students make studying plans, choose studying methods and boost studying efficiency. In a word, essence in self-regulated learning lies in students and teachers sharing the right of learning and making decisions together.

122.3.3 Establish Effective Feedback Mechanism

Educational informationization has made IT technology one of the leading factors in educational field, meanwhile also highlighting the teaching of many subjects and curriculum in cultivation of self-regulated learning ability. Self-regulated learning based on IT technology has become the teaching method that lives up more to the demands of modern era, but it's not as easy as it seems as if only to be stacking information on the internet. On the other hand, a lot of other factors remain to be taken under consideration such as arranging reasonable teaching programs, evaluating self-regulated learning methods and results and balancing between intellectual and nonintellectual factors.

References

1. Biemiller A, Shany M et al (1993) Factors influencing children's acquisition and demonstration of self–regulation on academic tasks. In: Schunk DH, Zimmerman BJ (eds) Self-regulated learning: from teaching to self-reflective practice. Guilford Press, New York, pp 203–224
2. Hu SH, Jiang YH (1998) Hushi academic collection. BJ Zhonghua Book Co, Beijing
3. Li KD (2007) Revelation of Japanese IT reform. China Audio-visual Edu 2007(11):38–41
4. Shi LF (2000) Learning strategy-theories of learning psychology. BJ People's education Pub, Beijing
5. Zimmerman BJ (1986) Special issue on self-regulated learning. Contemp Educ Psychol 11:305–427

Chapter 123
The Association Analysis of P16 in Transitional Cell

Yu Hui

Abstract Present study is ready to detect the expression of tumor gene PTEN and the cell cycle depended on kinase inhibitor P16 in bladder carcinoma through immunohistochemical method, and analyze the relation between them and the tumor grade or phase, and exame the correlation of the expression of these two proteinsin bladder carcinoma. It is found that the positive rates of PTEN and P16 protein expression in normal bladder mucosa tissue were higher than in bladder transitional cell carcinoma, and are correlated with pathological grade, the clinical stage and lymph nodes metastasis of BTCC. The expressions of PTEN are positively related to that of P16. They play synergistic action in the occurrence and development of BTCC.

Keywords BTCC · PTEN protein · P16 protein

123.1 Introduction

It is clear that bladder transitional cell carcinoma is one of the most common malignant tumor, the rate of BTCC is around 80–90 %. The mechanism of carcinoma occurrence is not very clear yet, it has been demonstrated that the development of malignant tumors is due to the activation of oncogene and inactivation of tumor suppressor genes, which leading to the loss of control on cell proliferation and apoptosis. With the development of molecular biology, the study in this field is focused on the tumor suppressor genes nowadays. PTEN gene (tensin homology and phosphatase deleted on chromosome ten, namely tensin and auxilin isogenesis, No. 10 chromosome lose phosphatase gene) is the firstly found

---

Y. Hui (✉)
Department of Obstetrics and Gynecology, General Hospital of Wuhan Iron and Steel Corporation, Wuhan 430081, China
e-mail: jinyan203558@126.com

phosphatase oncongene suppressor which regulating cell proliferation, transformation and adhesion etc. On the other hand, P16 is also very important tumor suppressor genes, which inhibit cyclin-dependent kinase 4, CDK4, and regulate cell cycle. When there is mutation or loss of P16 genes, the proliferation of cell is out of control, and for many types of tumors, there is high frequency occurrence of abnormal P16 genes. Present study is ready to detect the expression of tumor gene PTEN and the cell cycle depended on kinase inhibitor P16 in bladder carcinoma through immunohistochemical method, and analyze the relation between them and the tumor grade or phase, and exame the correlation of the expression of these two proteinsin bladder carcinoma. The result may be presumed upon to provide experimental evidence on mechanism of occurrence and development of the bladder cancer, and the treatment on molecular level.

123.2 Materials and Methods

Subjects: 62 cases of bladder cancer tissues were collected from patients in urinary surgery department of Zhongnan Hospital, Wuhan University, and WISCO General Hospital from January 2006 to December 2007. Among them male were 48 cases, female 14 cases. Ages range from 38 to 78 years (mean age 63.2 years). 20 cases of normal tissues were collected as the control group. Pathologic grade by WHO: G1, 22 cases; G2, 24 cases; G3, 16cases. Clinical grade by UICC-TNM: superficial bladder tumor (Ta–T1) period 37 cases, invasive bladder tumor (T2–T3) period 25 cases.

Methods: All the tissues were fixed in 10 % neutral formalin and embedded in paraffin. Immunohistochemistry test (S–P method) was performed to detect the expression of PTEN and P16. The prostate cancer immunostaining act as positive comparison. PBS replace the antibody one make the negative comparison.

Results judgment: Under optical microscope, for PTEN, cell nucleus is stained to brown, and for P16, cytoplasm or cell membrane is stained to brown in bladder cancer tumor. Random sample ten high fields were selected: color absent was 0; light yellow1; brown yellow 2; brown 3; less than 10 %, 1 score; 11–33 %, 2 score; 34–66 % 3 score; >67 % 4 score. Add scores of the two groups: 0–2 score, negative (−); 2–3 score weak positive (+); 4–5 score weak moderate positive (++) and 6–7 score strong positive (+++).

Statistical analysis: SPSS 13.0 software package was used in statistical treatment. Chi square test was used to compare the difference of PTEN and P16. The level of significance was set at a = 0.05. The relation between PTEN and P16 was studied by Spearman analysis.

123.3 Results

123.3.1 Expression of PTEN

Positive immunostaining with the antibody was observed in the cytoplasm of the cells.

The positive rates of PTEN protein expression was 46.77 % in BTCC tissues and 100 % in normal bladder mucosa tissues. The difference between them exists statistical significance ($P < 0.05$) Tables 123.1 and 123.2.

The positive rates of PTEN protein expression in Gl, G2 and G3 were 72.73, 37.50, 25.00 % respectively; and the difference was statistically significant between Gl and G2 or G3 ($P < 0.05$). The positive rate of PTEN protein expression in Ta–Tl was 64.86, and 20.00 % in T2–T4 ($P < 0.05$). The difference between them has statistical significance.

123.3.2 Expression of P16 Protein

Positive immunostaining with the antibody was located to the cytoplasm of the cells.

The positive rates of P16 protein expression was 43.55 % in BTCC tissues and 95.65 % in normal bladder mucosa tissues. There was statistical difference between them ($P < 0.05$) (Tables 123.3, 123.4).

The positive rates of P16 protein expression in Gl, G2 and G3 were 72.73, 33.33, 18.75 % respectively; and the difference exists statistical signifier between Gl and G2 or G3 ($P < 0.05$). The positive rate of P16 protein expression in Ta–Tl

Table 123.1 Expression of PTEN protein in normal mucosa and BTCC

Tissue types	Samples	Expression of PTEN protein		Positive rate (%)	Comments
		Positive	Negative		
Normal Mucosa	23	23	0	100	X^2
BTCC	62	29	33	46.77	$P < 0.05$
Total	85	52	33		

Table 123.2 Relation between expression of PTEN protein and differentiation of BTCC

Differentiation	PTEN		Total	Positive rate (%)
	Positive	Negative		
G1	16	6	22	72.73
G2	9	15	24	37.5
G3	4	12	16	25

Table 123.3 Expression of P16 protein in normal mucosa and BTCC

Tissue types	Samples	Expression of P16 protein		Positive rate (%)	Comments
		Positive	Negative		
Normal Mucosa	23	22	1	95.65	$X^2 = 18.65$
BTCC	62	27	35	43.55	$P < 0.05$
Total	85	49	36		

Table 123.4 Relation between expression of P16 protein and differentiation of BTCC

Differentiation	P16		Total	Positive rate (%)
	Positive	Negative		
G1	16	6	22	72.73
G2	8	16	24	33.33
G3	3	13	16	18.75

Table 123.5 Relation between expression of P16 and PTEN

P16	PTEN		Total	Comments
	+	−		
+	20	7	27	$r = 0.48$
−	9	26	35	$P < 0.05$
Total	29	33	62	

was 62.16 and 16.00 % in T2–T4 ($P < 0.05$). The difference between them has statistical significance. With the increase of pathological grade clinical stage, the expression of P16 decreased significantly (Table 123.5).

The relationship between PTEN and P16 is positively correlation ($P < 0.05$).

123.4 Conclusions

The positive rates of PTEN and P16 protein expression in normal bladder mucosa tissue were higher than in bladder transitional cell carcinoma, and are correlated with pathological grade, the clinical stage and lymph nodes metastasis of BTCC.

The expressions of PTEN are positively related to that of P16. They play synergistic action in the occurrence and development of BTCC.

References

1. Fults D, Pedone CA, Thomas GA (1990) Allelotype of human malignant astrocytoma. Cancer Res 50:5784–5789
2. Rahseed BK, Fuller GN, Friendman AH (1992) Loss of heterozygosity for 10q loci in human glioma. Genes Chromo Cancer 5:75–78
3. Gray IC, Phillips SM, Lee SJ (1995) Loss of chromosomal region 10q23–25 in prostate cancer. Cancer Res 55:4800–4848
4. Li J, Yen C, Liaw D (1997) PTEN, a putive protein tyrosine phosphatase gene mutated in human brain, breast and prostate cancer. Science 275:1943–1947
5. Nevins JR (1992) E2F: a link between the Rb tumor suppressor protein and vival oncoproteins. Science 258:424–429

Chapter 124
Problem-Based Learning (PBL) in Eight-Year Program of Clinical Medicine in Xiangya School of Medicine: New Mode Needs Exploration

Jieyu He, Qingnan He, Xiaoqun Qin, Yongquan Tian, Donna Ambrozy and Aihua Pan

Abstract *Introduction* Problem-based learning (PBL) is an educational method characterized by the use of patient problems as a context for students to learn problem-solving skills and to acquire knowledge on basic and clinical sciences. PBL was introduced to Eight-year program in Xiangya School of Medicine since 2006. Since traditional curricula hardly reach an excellent agreement on the integration of clinical learning and practice, application of PBL into teaching of systematic anatomy can avoid some of the problems existing in traditional curricula. *Methods* A total of 100 students from Eight-year program of clinical medicine participated PBL program. Groups (4–5 students per group) were presented with a certain case a week in advance. Each group worked together to gather information, discuss possible mechanisms and causes, develop hypotheses and strategies to test the hypotheses, and then prepare for presentation and discussion in lectures. In each lecture, the assigned tutor guided students to refine their hypotheses, commented on their presentation and discussion, and introduced updated clinical progresses. *Results* We applied questionnaires with 24 close-set and 2 open-set questions, among a total of 75 students from above after accomplishment of PBL lectures. We demonstrated that greater satisfactions on acquirement of knowledge and roles of tutors were achieved via PBL lectures.

J. He
Eight-year Program of Clinical Medicine of Xiangya School of Medicine, Central South University, Changsha 410013, China

Q. He · X. Qin · Y. Tian · A. Pan
South China Center for Medical Education Research and Development, China Medical University Bookstore, Shenyang, China

D. Ambrozy
Department of Medical Education and Biomedical Informatics, University of Washington, Seattle, China

A. Pan (✉)
Department of Anatomy and Neurobiology of Xiangya School of Medicine, Central South University, Changsha, China
e-mail: panaihua@csu.edu.cn

The survey also suggested more productive approaches to study. *Discussion* PBL motivates students to learn systematic anatomy and improves comprehensive ability. Existed Problems were reflected in the progression of PBL teaching and feedbacks from survey: (1) students can not rapidly adapt themselves to PBL in transforming their thinking pattern, (2) many students are confused about the objectives of PBL and how to concentrate on lectures, (3) resources provided by school are limited. Furthermore, traditional evaluation of students' performance is not favorable in conditions of PBL. Agreement is reached on some details. *Future perspective* Application of PBL in our education system means modification of PBL education based on feasibility of current education and students' abilities. Since PBL is not fixed worldwide, we are required to explore a better mode to fit our education system. To further carry out PBL lectures, some suggestions are given.

Keywords PBL · Medical education

124.1 Introduction

For a long time, China's higher medical education has been adopting three-step pattern—basic learning, clinical education and practice. However, the didactic teacher-centered pattern has been criticized as a serious obstacle in the development of higher medical education and in the cultivation of innovative talents. Reform on teaching methods is called for in medical education of Eight-year program of clinical medicine.

Xiangya School of Medicine opened Eight-year program of Clinical Medicine in 2004. Innovative approaches have been explored for our undergraduates since then. Problem-based learning (PBL) is an educational method characterized by the use of clinical cases as a context for students to learn problem-solving skills and to acquire knowledge on the basic and clinical sciences [1]. It has become increasingly popular in medical education for the benefits of fostering deep learning and motivation of self-learning [2–4]. It meets the challenge of Eight-year Program of Clinical Medicine. In 2006, PBL education was introduced and put into implementation.

In this article, we present the implementation of PBL in eight-year program in Xiangya School of Medicine. We surveyed students who received PBL lectures. Feedbacks of the problems and suggestions in PBL lectures from the questionnaires can be beneficial to improve PBL implementation.

124.1.1 Eight-Year Program: Cultivation of High-Quality Medical Talents

A couple of years ago, Eight-year Program of clinical medicine was established as an ideal educational pattern, in Peking Union Medical College, which is one of the most distinguished medical college in China. Its trial implementation drew a clear perspective blueprint for higher medical education. Xiangya School of Medicine set up this program in 2004. Systematical training scheme was also worked out. The goal of abilities cultivation includes:

- Strong professional ethics
- Wide knowledge of the humanity and social sciences as well as natural sciences
- A firm foundation for scientific medical knowledge
- Systematic knowledge of population health
- Skills of communication and information management
- Abilities of scientific thinking and life-long self-learning
- Capabilities of clinical practice and preliminary clinical research
- Innovation
- Competence in medical practice and international competition.

Briefly speaking, the priority requirement is that students obtain abilities of initiative learning in the process of training. Reform of educational methods is required to fit the scheme of Eight-year Program cultivation.

124.1.2 Traditional Curricula Versus PBL Tutorials

Traditional curricula create division between clinical learning and practice [1]. Acquired knowledge is subsequently forgotten or found to be irrelevant as in the condition of surface learning [5]. Thus application of the acquired knowledge can be difficult. On the contrary, PBL has its own characteristics as student-centered. Its possible advantages over traditional approaches in medical education include promotion of acquiring and application of knowledge into clinical analysis, and encouragement of self-directed life-long learning.

In theory, applying PBL into systematic anatomy can avoid some of the problems existing in traditional curricula. Students may learn more effectively if knowledge and skills acquired are contextualized [1]. As students attempt to understand and solve the case, they apply the acquired knowledge to seeking for a solution. Meanwhile, this process can aid deep learning [6], add interest and increase motivation to learn.

124.2 Methods

Since 2005, educators from our school were designated to University of Washington School of Medicine. They attended PBL curriculum and attained comprehensive knowledge of it. Back at school, they exchanged with other teachers and discussed about the trials of PBL.

Teaching plan was worked out that curriculum of systematic anatomy should be divided into three parts according to its practical situation: 30 % for theory, 60 % for practice, and 10 % for PBL. Cases were selected for analysis and diagnosis. Each one-hour PBL lecture focused on one certain case in alternative two or three weeks.

124.2.1 PBL Implementation

A total of 100 students after two-year study of science courses (humanity and social sciences & natural sciences) participated in the PBL program. Groups (4-5 students per group) were presented with a case a week in advance. Each group worked together to gather information, discuss possible mechanisms and causes, develop hypotheses and strategies to test the hypotheses, and then prepare for presentation and discussion in class. In each lecture, the assigned tutor guided students to refine their hypotheses, commented on their presentation and discussion, and introduced updated clinical progresses.

124.3 Results

To evaluate the achievements and problem of the program, we applied questionnaires with 24 close-set and 2 open-set questions, among a total of 75 students after receiving PBL lectures, who were from eight-year program of Xiangya School of Medicine. Response rate was 100 %. All were available. Results of closed-set questions are showed in percentages (Tables 124.1, 124.2).

Two open-set questions:

25. What are tutors supposed to do in PBL?

Most students thought tutors should delicately select practical cases and prepare lectures well. Also, tutors were supposed to act as facilitators.

26. Give your suggestions for PBL improvement.

Valuable suggestions were concluded as follows: Firstly, cases should be of practical use and be targeted on learned knowledge. Secondly, tutors should provide more sources for PBL. Thirdly, time for PBL should be extended, whereas size of groups should be reduced. Finally, both students and tutors need to summarize the topic case in each lecture actively.

Table 124.1 Results of yes(Y)/no(N) questions

	Questions	Y	N	Y in total (%)
1.	Do you think PBL is superior to traditional teaching methods?	62	13	82.7
2.	Will discussion increase your interest in this course?	62	13	82.7
3.	Will PBL intensify and strengthen your knowledge learned?	66	9	88.0
4.	Will you review related knowledge before PBL lectures?	65	10	86.7
5.	Will you take an active role in preparation for discussion?	51	24	68.0
6.	Do you have many accesses to obtain information?	12	63	16.0
7.	Is teaching resources provided by school sufficient?	18	57	24.0
8.	Are you clear about the goals of the discussion?	54	21	72.0
9.	Are you satisfied with teacher's guidance?	56	19	74.7
10.	Is the atmosphere promotive in study &discussion created in PBL?	64	11	85.3
11.	Do you feel forced to present your opinion in group discussion?	23	52	30.7
12.	Will you listen to your peer's view actively?	57	18	76.0
13.	Is group cooperation helpful to solve problems?	66	9	88.0
14.	Will each discussion meet expectation?	38	37	50.7
15.	Will you review after PBL?	33	42	44.0
16.	Is it worthwhile to take time in PBL lectures?	69	6	92.0
17.	Will PBL increase your ability of self-directed learning?	74	1	98.7
18.	Will PBL provide a platform for practicing presentation?	48	27	64.0
19.	Does PBL make you a listener to other opinions?	69	6	92.0
20.	Is it necessary to start PBL in initial stage of medical study at present?	68	7	90.7
21.	Is PBL teaching method systematic?	43	32	57.3

Table 124.2 Results of multiple-choice questions

	Questions	Results (%)		
22.	Methods to gather information	Via internet 93.3	Library 14.7	Other methods 5.3
23.	Optimal number of group members	3–5 29.3	5–10 54.7	More than 10 16.0
24.	Optimal Academic hour for PBL	Less than 5 26.7	5–0 41.3	More than 10 32

Most Students (82.7 %) considered that PBL was superior to traditional teaching methods. PBL could motivate self-directed learning, intensify and strengthen their knowledge and improve their comprehensive ability. Adequate preparation (68 %) would be made for discussion indicating positive attitudes toward PBL. PBL was widely regarded (92 %) worth time-consuming though it took abundant hours to prepare for PBL. PBL was welcome (91 %) in the initial stage of basic learning. We demonstrated that greater satisfactions on acquirement of knowledge and roles of tutors were achieved via PBL lectures. The survey also suggested more productive approaches to study [7].

124.4 Discussion

PBL emphasizes cultivation of comprehensive abilities, including reasoning, communication and cooperation, self-directed learning and acquisition and integration of basic and clinical knowledge.

PBL motivates students to learn systematic anatomy. Memorizing is crucial in systematic anatomy learning. However, it is a low efficiency for students to acquire knowledge passively in traditional methods. On the contrary, PBL enables students to find the lacking points in their knowledge, and encourages independent learning outside the PBL lectures. Meanwhile, students may try to make use of all available sources to sort out problems without confinement of textbook. Moreover, statements and debates in discussion require flexible application of integrated knowledge. Acquisition from PBL lectures, in turn, motivates further learning, which make for active learning. Summarization after each lecture consolidates the obtained knowledge. Collectively, study on systematic anatomy is transformed from dull memorization to an interesting interacting one, which raises efficiency and interest.

PBL improves comprehensive ability. During PBL discussion, quite many students (72 %) were clear about the focus and objectives. It showed gradual elevation in analytical ability. To solve problems, students have to garner useful information via various media other than textbooks. Almost all students (98.7 %) found improvement in their self-directed learning and information collection & selection. Moreover, over 90 % would listen to and think about peers' views. More than half would present their views and debate actively in PBL lectures. Participation promotes emergence and enhancement of critical thinking. Additionally, work in groups highlights teamwork and cooperation.

Existed Problems were reflected in the progression of PBL teaching and feedbacks from survey.

Students can not rapidly adapt themselves to PBL in transforming their thinking pattern. Instead of the traditional methods' center on class, PBL demands preparation before class. However, lack of abilities, such as independent thinking, self-directed learning, analyzing, and collecting valid information is common among students influenced by traditional education. It implies that tutors need to guide students in a gradual way so as to help them adapt to PBL. It will take time to adjust to PBL both for tutors and students [8].

Resources provided by school are limited. Insufficient information obtained would hamper participation, which may diminish effects of PBL. Meanwhile, students should be introduced to gaining and managing information efficiently.

Many students are confused about the objectives of PBL and how to concentrate on lectures. 49 % thought they failed to meet expectation in discussion. Reasons are that discussion is impaired by unfamiliar information collected and monotonic instruction. Therefore, tutors should act as facilitators to guide the direction of lectures. Besides, problems existed as some cases in PBL lectures are related to other medical courses other than systematic anatomy, which may require integration of multiple disciplinary efforts.

Traditional evaluation of students' performance is not favorable to PBL. First, it can not assess student's performance correctly. Second, it hinders participation in PBL. Some students would muddle through just to complete a task. Assessment in PBL should be incorporated into the evaluation system. Apart from scores and credits, students' comprehensive abilities should be evaluated.

Agreement is reached on some details. The relatively appropriate proportion of PBL lectures in systematic anatomy curriculum is 10 %, as students agree, whereas time of each PBL tutorial needs extension from 1 h to 90 min. Group size of 5–10 is favored considering cooperation and personal ability displaying.

124.4.1 Future Perspective

PBL is considered to be further developed with exploration and reform. Application of PBL in our education system means modification of PBL education based on feasibility of current education and students' abilities. Combination of PBL and traditional methods is our prospective direction, yet now both of them are rather incompatible. Since PBL is not fixed worldwide, we are required to explore a better mode to fit our education system. To further carry out PBL lectures, some suggestions are given as follows.

- Training on document retrieval and other basic skills is necessary. Thus, students can focus on the main parts of PBL.
- Make use of the educational-assisted technology (e.g., computer-assisted learning). Setting up website to promote and exchange PBL lectures. Provision of relevant information online can ameliorate resources limitation. Individual's opinion can be voiced and valued through this democratic platform.
- Tutors need better adjustment. Tutors are no longer instructors or teachers. Instead, they are required to act as facilitators, or education coaches, though it's not easy to change their teaching style. Training of facilitators for PBL lectures should be highlighted.

Acknowledgments This study is supported by China Medical Board of New York (No. 05–820) and the seventh batch of Teaching Reform and Curriculum System Reform Project of Central South University (2012–30).

References

1. Finucane PM, Johnson SM, Prideaux DJ (1998) Problem-based learning: its rationale and efficacy. Med J Aust 168(9):445–448
2. Mansur DI, Kayastha SR, Makaju R et al (2012) Problem based learning in medical education. Kathandu Univ Med J 10(4):78–82
3. Morrison J (2004) Where now for problem-based learning? Lancet 363:174
4. Sulaiman N, Hamdy H (2013) Problem-based learning: where are we now? Guide supplement 36.3- practical application. Med Teach 35(2):160–162
5. Kember D, Biggs J, Leung DY (2004) Examining the multidimensionality of approached to learning through the development of a revised version of the Learning Process Questionnaire. Br J Educ Psychol 74(Pt 2):261–279
6. Azer SA, Guerrero AP, Wals A (2013) Enhancing learning approaches: practical tips for students and teachers. Med Teach 35(6):433–443. doi:10.3109/0142159X.2013.775413
7. Sanson-Fisher RW, Lynagh MC (2005) Problem-based learning: a dissemination success story? Med J Aust 183:258–260
8. Das M, Mpofu DJ, Hasan MY et al (2002) Student perceptions of tutor skills in problem-based learning tutorials. Med Educ 36:272–278

Chapter 125
Design of Virtual Reality Guide Training Room Based on the Modern Education Technology

Zhang Pengshun

Abstract Virtual reality is required to practice the knowledge and skills of tour guides. Considering the current training situation and on the basis of the modern educational technology, the construction of the virtual training room is imperative. It is necessary for us to give full consideration to the design and layout of the virtual training room. Meanwhile, the hardware should be combined with the modern educational ideas so that we can improve the quality and efficiency of the tour guide training.

Keywords Virtual reality · The tour guide training room · The modern education technology · Design

125.1 The Structure of Knowledge and Skills of the Tour Guide

125.1.1 Tour Guide Knowledge Structure

Tour is a occupation, that is guiding tour, letting visitors experience the beauty of the landscape, helping the visitors food, lodging, travel in the process and solving the problems that may occur during the tour. Rich knowledge is the precondition to improve the guide service. The tour guide knowledge includes language knowledge, the history of cultural knowledge, knowledge of policies and regulations and psychology and aesthetics knowledge. The language knowledge is the guide of the most basic skills and the tour guide service tool. If a tour guide has not a solid language skills, he could not be carried out smoothly cultural exchanging with

Z. Pengshun (✉)
Anqing Vocational Institute of Technology, Anqing 246003 Anhui, China
e-mail: zps102388@126.com

tourist and could not finish the tour guide service with high quality. The history of cultural knowledge consists of history, geographical, ethnic, religious, custom, specialty helena hat, literature and art, ancient architecture and gardens etc. Tour guide should be comprehensive understanding ShiDe cultural knowledge and agile using it. Tour guide must master the relevant laws and regulations knowledge, in order to properly address the problem and do it right, favorable, nodulation. Tour guide oneself also can prevent errors from happening. Tour guide should understand tourists to use psychology knowledge and have a definite object to guide and service life in travelling. Tour guide also should provide psychological services so that tourists get psychological satisfaction and get enjoy in spirit. In the same time, Tour guide should use psychology knowledge to do well with all kinds of relations of the tourist reception department. Tour guide will use psychology knowledge adjust their psychological state in order to make oneself always spirit, enthusiasm thoughtful service for tourists.

125.1.2 The Tour Guide Skills

The tour guide personnel should not only have strong strength knowledge but also master the essential service skills. The tour guide skills include ability to work independently, organization and coordination ability, ability to deal with all sorts of people and capability to deal with emergencies and special problems. The tour guide should independently in organizing tourist activities, and independent to deal with all kinds of problems, so strong ability to work independently to tour guide successful completion of the tour guide has special significance. After having a tourist group, tour guide need reasonable arrangement of tourism activities in order to have a satisfaction with life and tourism activities. This requires the tour guide has strong organization and coordination ability. Tour guide need to organize and coordinate all kinds of relationship between team member, travel agency, the travel agency and the scenic area, the travel agency and Hotel, tour guides and tourist etc. In the same time, tour guide need to pay attention to way, method and timely grasp the change of objective condition, nimbly to take the corresponding effective measures to organise and bargain. Tour guide work object surface wide, complex, so it is the tour guide the most important one of the skills good at to deal relationship with all sorts of people. Face danger fearlessly, calm despite the chaos, keep a cool head, resolute, efficient and adjust to changing circumstances is the qualities of tour guides to deal with problems and accidents because of having many problems and accidents in the course of tourism activities.

125.2 Existing Problems in Tour Guide Training

It require the knowledge and skills teaching organically in the tour guide knowledge and skills training. At present, it has four aspects of the problem in our tour guide teaching process. First, it is the students passive learning and the practice teaching effect difference. Second, it is the strongly training by the influence of safety and cost factors. Third, it is teaching experience can not effectively accumulate and facing the difficulty of construction of excellent courses. Fourth, it is less academic exchange of experiences among teachers and slowly raise the level of teaching. From the student's point of view, it has five the main problem in the training of course tourist guide. First, it is the single and boring teaching methods. Second, it is the teaching content based on the point of many local and narrow covering area. Third, it is seldom training opportunity and the weak ability of social practice. Fourth, it is the lack of a comprehensive travel agency business training. Fifth, it is less timely communication and the teacher guidance opportunities with the teacher.

According to the problems in the tour guide knowledge structure and skills training in practice, Tourist guide training can achieve the training goals of qualified tour guides only combination the ideological modern education technology with the means of technique. In recent years, Due to the lack of modern education technology theory, the simulation training room although has been rapid developed at heavy investment, but the training effect is not ideal. Construction simulation guide training room only combining technological innovation and education concept update, it can satisfy the need of the students' class and autonomous learning, accord with the modern education concept of "the teachers guide, the student main body", satisfy the need of Immersive creative teaching of the interaction between teachers and students, strengthen the teaching of vitality and the learning interest of the students.

125.3 Modern Education Technology Concept and Teaching Model

Modern education technology is the theory and practice to the design, development, management, and evaluation of the process of teaching and learning resources. Modern education technical think the student as the center of learning and teaching and emphasize the student will play a main role in the course of teaching. But in the guide in the process of practice teaching, in order to strengthen the contact with knowledge and skills, forms the reliable connection, enhance the learning effect, we emphasize on strengthening to consolidate, the educational thought of the education practice is the coupling theory of learning. Constructing learning psychology think that learning relies mainly on the students' own construction, the teacher is just learning external conditions in the learning process.

Therefore, teachers should mobilize students' learning initiative and enthusiasm, make students practice, learning and thinking. We can achieve the object of reflecting the student-centered through building teaching mode. Student-centered teaching mode mainly has activity teaching, cooperative research learning, independent exploration learning and teaching problems.

125.4 The Construction of Virtual Tour Guide Training Room

The aim of tourism Management Professional which is much application and practical professional is culture talented person with the theory application talents skills and practical ability. Virtual reality technology can help student professional skill training at the same time get hold of the system understanding and overall tourism management professional knowledge, build a reasonable knowledge structure required in tourism management activities, acquire knowledge into ability of knowledge integration.

125.4.1 The Goal of Building a Virtual Tour Guide Training Room

First, situational teaching can help students to improve the overall quality of tour guide. The tour guide training room simulation teaching environment make the students like in real landscape and interpret with the transfer of scenic spots. At the same time, student can correct bad posture at any time, eliminate the students' sense of tension if the student often face the camera lens training, practice courage of speaking in a public occasion which help student play the best state in the future work. Second, controllability of the teaching process to facilitate the teaching goal. Recording whole of teaching activities in the tour guide training room can be played to be commented by teacher. By watching the video, students can also be designed to guide image and have an intuitive understanding of their own guides ability which help student gradually improve the guide ability and shorten the adaptation time of post. Some of the best training material also can be stored for a long time in order for the future teaching demonstration.

125.4.2 The Advantage of Virtual Reality Technology

Virtual reality technology is the combination of computer image technology, sensor technology, computer technology, network technology and man–machine interface technology. Based on computer technology, by creating a three-dimensional visual, auditory and tactile environment, the virtual reality technology can provide interactive tools and help student stay in the real environment and interact with the virtual environment objects. Virtual reality technology can make the participants remain within doors to the outside world or enter the place, such as the distant space, the dangerous environment and the microscopic world, which you can not reach in real life. Virtual reality technology has three basic characteristics in the teaching application, such as immersion, interaction and imagination. Immersion is a feeling of student has a kind of be personally on the scene surrounded by virtual environment, as if it is projected to a simulation in the real world. Student convert from passive observer to active participants and put themselves heart into the virtual world. Interaction is referring student random operation of virtual objects in virtual space and the simulation of space will be the student operation results instant feedback to the student to obtain the human–computer interaction. Imagination is a broad imagination space and advanced consciousness created by the computer virtual world. Imagination not only reproduce once existed or existing scenery, but also construct of things and the environment which is not exist in the real world.

125.4.3 Virtual Tour Guide Training Room Structure

Based on the advantages of virtual reality technology, the modern education technology requirements and the knowledge characteristics of tour guide, the construction of virtual tour guide training room can design from the following aspects. First, virtual tour guide training room process. The core technology of tour guide training room is the virtual studio technology. The virtual studio which is perfect union product virtual reality technology and the traditional matting technology in recent years and a developed new technology based on computer graphics technology and traditional video color key technology compose new picture with camera images and computer generated 3D map image. A virtual environment by computer simulation with some reuse of human–computer interaction and real image can often eliminates the trouble of layout background and save manpower, material and financial resources. The virtual studio is one of tour guide training room which is compose of light group, blue box and camera. When training, students stand in front of the camera, then the camera shoot students training in the blue box in the picture and input to the virtual studio host for chroma-key processing, after, blue box replace the virtual scene made by computer or shoot good landscape, then compose the foreground mask and output new picture. Figure 125.1 is the tour guide training room of the system flow chart.

Second, virtual tour guide training room space structure. In the process of teaching,the synthesis of the tour guide training activities of the image not only can be projected onto the big screen so be observed by the class, but also be played after recording so be commented by teacher. The image can be transferred to the 6

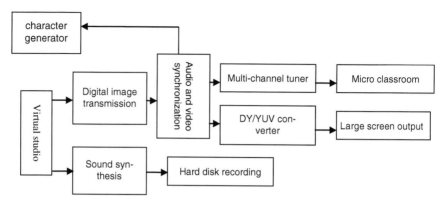

Fig. 125.1 Flow chart of system guide virtual reality training room

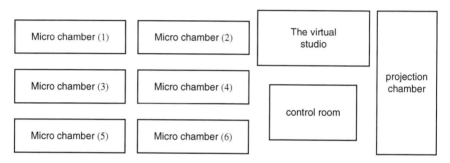

Fig. 125.2 Virtual training room layout

micro teaching classroom so to be watched by grouping the students. In the room, student rehearse as a group according to hierarchical and content. Figure 125.2 is a virtual training room layout.

The virtual training room is divided into three zones. First, it is digital interactive teaching area. In this area, teacher fuse all kinds of information, text, voice, video and other teaching resources into visual guide and play high fidelity through the screen so fully realize the digital interactive teaching function by using the 120 channel stereo screen system and 3D modeling. Second, it is micro teaching training area. Six independent micro teaching training room and 14 micro teaching training flight is placed in the training room. It can train 20 groups of students at the same time. Third, it is teacher control area. Three are one Taiwan and 14 networked computer in it. Teacher or judger observe and record the team training by switching picture.

Three large area is clear division and powerful. Divide three large area not only exerts the hardware function, but also embodies the modern education thought, at the same time, it gives full play to the subjectivity of student learning and mobilizes the enthusiasm of the students.

125.5 Conclusion

Application of Virtual Studio Technology enhance the modernization level of tour guide professional practice teaching, greatly improve the teaching conditions and provide a strong guarantee for the new era of higher vocational training of tour guide personnel.

References

1. Bao Q (2010) The application of VR technology and the digital teaching management system in a simulated tour guide training room. Res Chin Foreign Educ (8):60–62
2. Anfeng F, Yanhua W (2009) Application of three channel stereo projection screen technology in tourism education. Technol Square (7):149–152
3. Rongfang Luo, Huan Liu (2012) The construction of virtual tourism teaching system. Innovation Sci Technol Educ 11:184
4. Danhong C (2007) The use of virtual reality technology in the practical teaching system of tourism management. Cult Educ Mater (4):31–33
5. Wanyin H (2010) Design and research of virtual tour system. J Hubei Univ Econ (Philosophy and Social Sciences Edition) (3):180–181

Chapter 126
Exploration and Practice of Teaching Mode of Mechanical Engineering Control Foundation Based on Project Driving

Tao Wu and Xiao-Bin Duan

Abstract Project driving is one of the methods that implement investigation type teaching mode. Mechanical engineering control foundation is one of the required core specialty courses in the specialty of mechanical engineering and automation. This paper introduces how to use project driving teaching method in this course. Combined with the content and characteristic of mechanical engineering control foundation, a series of experiments or design are developed in the teaching and learning process. The evaluation pattern is discussed as well. Practice makes clear that project teaching method contributes to enhance the students' ability of analysis and solving problem independently, improve the learning enthusiasm and team awareness.

Keywords Project driving · Mechanical engineering and automation · Simulation · Experiment · Education quality

126.1 Introduction

The project teaching method is that students and teachers carry out and fulfill projects together. The teachers organize students to join the whole process of project design, implementation and management.

Mechanical engineering control foundation is based on control theory, which is closely related to practical engineer. It is a required course of mechanical engineering and automation, mechano-electronic and other relative specialties. To achieve good education effect, the student's ability of control system analysis, design and application should be trained. Some examples of relevant establishment

T. Wu (✉) · X.-B. Duan
Faculty of Mechanical and Electrical Engineering, Kunming University of Science and Technology, Kunming 650093, China
e-mail: kmwutao13@126.com

of mathematical model, time domain analysis, frequency domain analysis based on project teaching are discussed in this paper. Through completing concrete project, learners will be familiar with the control system function and property intuitively. So the learning interest is stimulated. It plays positive role to improve the teaching quality.

Depended on the development platform of the mechanic engineering national distinguished specialty of Kunming University of Science and Technology, the project teaching method of the course of mechanical engineering control foundation is probed. The college students of mechanical engineering and automation are the teaching objects. Some creative means have been proposed and some successful experiences have been summarized.

Some practical cases of this teaching mode will be presented as follows.

126.2 Features of Project Teaching Method

There are 3 features in project teaching method.

- Students are the learning core and learn independently.
- Students take part in the whole teaching and learning process: information gathering, plan design, decision making, feedback control, achievement evaluation. The students' comprehensive ability is the focal cultivation point.
- Teachers are organizer, consultant and companion.

126.3 Implementing Process of Project Teaching Method

The concrete implementing process of project teaching method could be classified as the 4 steps: aim definition, project design, project implementation and project evaluation.

126.3.1 Aim Definition

The course of mechanical engineering control foundation is a fundamental specialty course in mechanic engineering and automation specialty. The traditional teaching target emphasizes on "what you have learned". But the target of project teaching method clearly states "what you could do". This will stimulate study enthusiasm and achievement sense.

126.3.2 Project Design

The key link in project teaching is the design and selection of the project. The following two factors should be considered carefully. One is that the project task is related to the students' job. This will make the students feel this course has practical value. So the learning initiative is mobilized. The other is that the project should cover the course knowledge to form a complete knowledge system.

126.3.3 Project Implementation

After the project task has been arranged, the students should discuss and analyze problems to find the key problem and technology, difficulty point and feasibility. Then, according to registrations and individual knowledge difference, the students will be grouped. Usually one group is composed of 6–8 students. In groups, each student is assigned concrete task. Students are encouraged to explore and solve problems through various channels and methods. During this process, the students should be encouraged to cooperate with each other to accomplish knowledge understand and application. Students are asked to master not only knowledge, but also relevant software such as MATLAB and LabVIEW. According to different teaching stage, some projects such as establishment of mathematical model, time domain analysis, frequency domain analysis and comprehensive correction are set.

126.3.3.1 Control System Modeling

To analyze a control system, mathematical model must be established. The DC motor is used as the example to illustrate how to use MATLAB/SIMULINK to establish the mathematical model. The DC motor mathematical model based on SIMULINK is shown in Fig. 126.1.

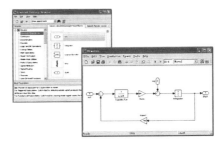

Fig. 126.1 Modeling of separately excited DC motor

Fig. 126.2 Time-domain analysis by LTI Viewer

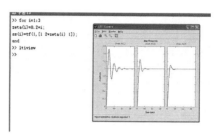

126.3.3.2 Analysis of System Property

In classical control theory, the general system analysis methods have time-domain, root-locus, frequency-domain. Various methods have various features and scope.

Time-domain analysis method has such advantages as audio-visual and accuracy, which could offer total information of time response. The typical 2-order system is shown as Eq. 126.1. When ξ takes 0.2, 0.4, 0.6, its step response curve could be observed by LTI Viewer tool of MATLAB as shown in Fig. 126.2.

$$G(s) = \frac{1}{s^2 + 2\xi s + 1} \tag{126.1}$$

126.3.3.3 Experiment Example Made by LabVIEW

The above example could be realized by LabVIEW software. LabVIEW could not only realize simulation, but also measure and control practical system. National Instruments Corporation provides data gathering card PCI-6024E and SC-2075 breadboard. The electronic component and other hardware circuit could be connected on the SC-2075 breadboard. The data gathering card PCI-6024E could not only gather experiment data, but also output signal. The program of drawing up Nyquist graph is shown in Fig. 126.3a. The signal is output by LabVIEW through

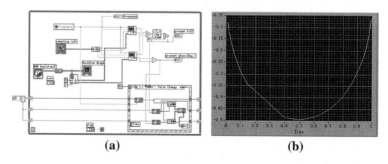

Fig. 126.3 Frequency analysis graph (**a**) Block diagram (**b**) Nyquist diagram of the practical inertia link

PCI-6024E card. The program will measure and record real-time data automatically. According to different magnitude and phase function under different frequency, the Nyquist graph could be drawn automatically as shown in Fig. 126.3b.

126.3.4 Project Evaluation and Examination

During the project complementing process, each group works according to definite procedures and program. They must report regularly, fill in project progress form, and reply periodically. After the project has been completed, every group should estimate the work process and result by himself and write summary report. Then various groups give a mark with each other. Finally, the teachers inspect, reply and evaluate comprehensively.

126.4 Summary

This paper discusses project teaching method and tries to probe teaching contents, project design, and evaluation pattern. Different from traditional teaching mode, the teaching mode based on project drive examines the grasp and application ability of key knowledge and technology depended on focal point, not the test. Through completing concrete project, the students' practical ability, creative ability, team awareness and sense of exploration are enhanced. The above teaching reform has been experimented in the graduates of 2009–2013 of mechanic engineering and automation and achieved excellent effect.

Acknowledgments This work was supported by development of the third distinguished specialty of national education department (Grant No. TS11137).

References

1. Lee Yong (2010) Practice and consideration of project teaching method in computer specialty in medium vocational education. Profession 4:71–72 (In Chinese)
2. Sun Hongmei, Jia Ruisheng (2012) Research on case teaching of software development comprehensive practice based on project driven. Procedia Eng 29:484–488
3. Zhang Guoxiang, Zhang Hao (2010) Application of project teaching method used in mechanic design foundation of mechanical and electrical specialty. Profession 4:49–50 (In Chinese)
4. Deng Xingzhong (2011) Mechanical and electrical drive control. Huazhong University of Science and Technology Press (In Chinese), Wuhan
5. Chang LC, Lee GC (2010) A team-teaching model for practicing project-based learning in high school: collaboration between computer and subject teachers. Comput Educ 55:961–969
6. Divjak Blazenka, Kukec Sandra Katarina (2008) Teaching methods for international R&D project management. Int J Project Manage 26:251–257
7. Sha Shujing, Liu Yamei (2012) Probe and practice of teaching mode of mechanical and electrical specialty based on project driven. J Changchun Univ Sci Technol 7:207–208

Chapter 127
Wireless Sensor Network Distributed Data Collection Strategy Based on the Regional Correlated Variability of Perceptive Area

Yongjun Zhang and Enxiu Chen

Abstract On account of the energy saving problem in wireless sensor network (WSN), this paper proposes the method that classifies sensing area according to the similarity of variability of sensing in terms of fuzzy clustering. Through the head of a cluster in a similar area to sample data to represent approximately collection of the regional sensing data. We through a test manifests data collection of partitioned similar sensing area will implement well in data monitoring and it will reduce the total energy consumption, reduce the computing task for data fusion and lengthen the WSN life circle.

Keywords Fuzzy clustering · Similar sensing area · Energy saving

127.1 Introduction

It is the hot research direction in wireless sensor network (WSN) that is how to utilize the energy of every sensor point effectively to prolong the life cycle of WSN as well as equilibrium of all energy in WSN. LEACH [1] is a typical hierarchical routing protocol. Later the scholarship of MIT Hein Zelman proposes the algorithm of LEACH-C [2] that is based on LEACH algorithm. It solves the problem that hasn't considered the reminder energy in a cluster head election to improve the quality of generated clusters. HEED [3] algorithm through a calculation to broadcast AMRP and to become temporary cluster head with the

Y. Zhang (✉)
Shandong Institute of Commerce and Technology, China National Engineering Research Center for Agricultural Products Logistics, Jinan, China
e-mail: zyj420177@163.com

E. Chen
National Engineering Research Center for Agricultural Products Logistics, Jinan, China

probability of initialization $CH_p = \max(C_p \times \frac{Er}{Em}, p_{\min})$, which select the head of a cluster in terms of reminder energy as first factor and communication in the network as a second factor. The algorithm of HEED is different to the algorithm of LEACH in criteria of cluster head selection and the mechanism of competition, it had improved in speed of clustering and pick more reasonable cluster head to transmit data by considering of inner cluster communication and reminder energy in order to make whole WSN more equilibrium. On the base of above mentioned viewpoints, there are someone propose a method to guarantee the optimized strategy of minimum energy cluster head selection [4, 5], which is based on twice the selection of cluster head and this method makes full consideration of energy parameter and hot zone of WSN. What's more, there are someone use K-MEANS [6, 7] to select a cluster head. These methods, however, are only considered the problem of energy and cost of routing without considering the similarity of sensing in some areas. This paper uses fuzzy cluster method to partition similar area of sensing and use HEED algorithm to select a cluster head to transmit sampling data to SINK point. Therefore, under the condition of request of accuracy and real-time is not high, we can partition similar area to reduce transmission quantity effectively, to reduce the computation of data fusion [8, 9], to cut down the total energy consumption and finally to prolong the life cycle of the whole network.

127.2 Concerned Question Description and Definition

For the area of sensing, the sensing data may have similar change regulation. We can use the similarity of change regulation of sampling data to utilize fuzzy clustering to partition the whole area into several similar areas. In every similar area, we can use HEED algorithm to select a cluster head and utilize it as representation to monitor neighbourhood variation. When inner similar area's real sensing data deviate from the data sampled by cluster head, which exceed threshold *MaxError*. The system should reparation and select the head of clusters to collect the district sensing data. In there, sensing vector is $X = \{p^{(1)}, \ldots, p^{(i)}, \ldots, p^{(n)}\}$ which denote the n sensing data with m sensing results from time t_x to t_y. For example, vector with order number is $p_i = \{p_1^{(i)}, \ldots, p_m^{(i)}\}$, the raw sensing data can be expressed by matrix $\underset{T \in [t_x, t_y]}{SensoringMatrix[n][m]}$.

Definition 1 sensing similarity is $\underset{p_i, p_j \in X}{SimSensoring(p_i, p_j)}$: suppose there are two sensor points p_i and p_j in some area *SimArea* and for the given sensor point set $X = \{p^{(1)}, \ldots, p^{(n)}\}$ has no objects with m dimensions, we define similarity of sensing as follows:

$$SimSensoring(p_i, p_j) = \sigma d_s(p_i, p_j) + (1-\sigma)|\cos(p_i, p_j)| \quad (127.1)$$

Definition 2 max error of sensing *MaxError*: as a classified similar area *SimArea*, we can find two sensor points p_i and p_j they have max dissimilarity, so the *MaxError* in this area satisfy that it $\underset{p_i,p_j \in SimArea}{Min} \{SimSensoring(p_i, p_j)\}$ is true it implicates value $\frac{\sqrt{\frac{1}{m}\sum_{k=1}^{m}(p_i-p_j)^2}}{Max\{p\}-Min\{p\}}$ is close to α, α is max tolerance of real measurement error and range of *MaxError* is (0,1).

Definition 3 similar sensing area (SSA): SSA is a set of sensing points that satisfy the condition $A_j(P_i) = \{P_i | Min\{SimSensoring(P_i, C_j)\} > \delta\}$, C_j is a regional centre of $A_j(P_i)$, so the whole sensing area can be expressed by $sensorArea = \bigcup_{j=1}^{N} A_j(P)$ and for $\forall A_i(P), \forall A_j(P) \in sensorArea$ there is the expression $A_i(P) \cap A_j(P) = \phi$ is correct.

127.3 Distributed Data Collection Strategy

Data collection in the similar sensing area in this paper we can concisely define as SSADC. Firstly, WSN becomes ad hoc network use hierarchical method to collect data from sensing area. Next, using fuzzy clustering to partition data area by using the changing of value of points. Finally, we can use HEED algorithm to select the head of cluster in certain partitioned area. It can represent changing of data by sampling the monitoring areas' data. The criteria for electing of cluster head is to take reminder energy as main factor and to take the density of sensing points as the second factor. With the passage of time, similar area may be changed more or less. Therefore when the sensing error exceeds a certain value, which should do a new fuzzy clustering and reselecting the head of cluster to finish the job of data collection. The algorithm of data collection by using fuzzy clustering as follows:
Method:

Step 1 During the period $[t_x, t_y]$, through statistic we record the sensing data by X, $p_i \in SSA$ (similar sensing area);

Step 2 As for vectors $X = \{p_i^{(j)}\}|_{1 \le i \le m, 1 \le j \le n}$ that with n elements and each has m dimensions, for standardized $p_i^{(k)}$ that can be standardized by
$$p_i^{(k)} = \frac{p_i^{(k)} - \underset{1 \le i \le m}{Min}\{p_i^{(k)}\}}{\underset{1 \le i \le m}{Max}\{p_i^{(k)}\} - \underset{1 \le i \le m}{Min}\{p_i^{(k)}\}}, 1 \le k \le n,$$ to compact data into (0,1) and store the result in $M_{n \times m}$;

Step 3 According to the sensing similarity $SimSensoring(p_i, p_j)$, compute the fuzzy similar Matrix $SimMatrix[n][n]$;

Step 4 For the given level of similarity λ, through the maximum tree algorithm of fuzzy clustering to get clustering result $C = \{c^{(1)}, \ldots, c^{(k)}\}$;

Step 5 If for every clustering result there exist two max dissimilar points that satisfy $\frac{\sqrt{\frac{1}{m}\sum_{k=1}^{m}(p_i - p_j)^2}}{Max\{p\} - Min\{p\}} < \alpha$, then set $\lambda = \lambda + h$ (h is step length) and go to step (4) to redo cluster analysis;

Step 6 For every $c_i \in C$ in clusters result C, we use HEED method to elect the head of cluster in every c_i to sample data and transmit it;

Step 7 At an interval of time β, the system will check periodically if there exist two max dissimilar points $\underset{p_i, p_j \in SimArea}{Min} \{SimSensoring(p_i, p_j)\}$ it satisfies $\frac{\sqrt{\frac{1}{m}\sum_{k=1}^{m}(p_i - p_j)^2}}{Max\{p\} - Min\{p\}} > \alpha$, then go to Step 1 to recompute similar area;

Step 8 The end of this algorithm.

For the convenience of data querying, we build a hash table $I(C)$ to index the final clustering result. In the similar sensing area to take HEED algorithm to select the head of clustering for balance the energy and represent a similar areas' sensing data.

127.4 Experimental Results and its Analysis

We use MATLAB7.0 to analyse 1100×100 m agriculture plant area sensing data. In the monitoring area we randomly and uniformly laid out 300 soil humidity sensors, the collecting point SINK locates in coordination (0,100). We deploy the WSN to compare the performance of our method for collecting data to LEACH, LEACH-C and HEED. Suppose the sensor's initial energy is 0.5 J, $E_{elec} = 50$ nJ/bit, $\varepsilon_s = 0.0013$ pJ/(bit.m4), $E_{com} = 5$ nJ/bit, the length of the message is 500 Bytes, the delay of sending and receiving is 25 μs. The test length is 1200 s and the intervals to repartition the similar area is 120 s.

Through the experiment in Fig. 127.1 we can see HEED method forming speed of the cluster has certainly improved compared to LEACH and LEACH-C, which thought the cost of the inner cluster communication after forming a cluster and select a cluster head that is more suitable to do the task of data transmit. Because this paper also uses HEED to choose the head of cluster in similar area it will be optimized in each partitioned field. What's more, we utilize cluster head to transmit sensing data to represent regional data it will save a lot of cost of energy in data transmission.

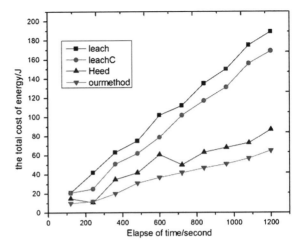

Fig. 127.1 The comparison of 4 cluster head selection methods in total energy cost

127.5 Conclusion

Through the fuzzy clustering method to split the whole monitoring area into many similar sensing areas. As for each similar sensing region we elect the head of cluster by using HEED algorithm to sampling data to represent the areas' sensing data. By using a distributed data collection method to collect monitoring data with less quantity of communication, to decrease the cost of energy in the whole network, to decrease data fusion calculation to improve the reliability of data, finally we can prolong the life cycle of WSN.

References

1. Heinzelman WR, Chandrakasan A, Balakrishnan H (2000) Energy-efficient communication protocol for wireless microsensor networks. In: Proceedings of the 33rd Hawaii international conference on system sciences
2. Heinzelman W, Chandrakasan A, Balarkrishnan H (2002) An application-specific protocol architecture for wireless microsensor networks. IEEE Trans Wireless Commun 1(4):660–670
3. Younis O, Fahmy S (2004) Distributed clustering in ad-hoc sensor networks:a hybrid. Energy-efficient approach, Ieee transactions on mobile computing 3:366–379
4. Peng W, Edwards DJ (2010) K-means like minimum mean distance algorithm for wireless sensor networks [C] 2010. In: 2nd international conference on computer engineering and technology IEEE pp120–124.
5. Zheng J, Wang P, Li C (2010) Distributed data aggregation using Slepian-wolf coding in cluster-based wireless sensor network. IEEE Trans Veh Technol 59(5):2564–2574
6. Chen HF, Mineno H, Mizuno T (2008) Adaptive data aggregation scheme in clustered wireless sensor networks. Comput Commun 31(15):3579–3585
7. Nurdin HI, Mazumdar RR, Bagchi A (2009) Reduced-dimension linear transform coding of distributed correlated signals with implete observations. IEEE Trans Inf Theory 55(6):2848–2858

8. Jiang HB, Jin SD, Wang CG (2011) Prediction or not? An energy-efficient framework for clustering-based data collection in wireless sensor network. IEEE Trans Parallel Distrib Syst 22(6):1064–1071
9. Biswas P, Qi H, Xu Y (2008) Mobile agent-based collaborative sensor fusion. Inf Fusion 9(3):399–411

Chapter 128
The System Design of the Network Teaching Platform of Learning Based on the Concept of Development Evaluation

Liu Yong

Abstract Application of network teaching platform in universities has been more common, organization, network teaching platform common to the curriculum resources learning activities have good support, but in learning evaluation, function is still relatively simple, failed to reflect the current developmental evaluation ideas. This paper analysis of the developmental evaluation based on the concept of network teaching platform, the design elements of evaluation systems and the overall design principle, and on this basis for the design of the system, to support the current study to carry out evaluation standards of evaluation activities.

Keywords Development evaluation · Learning evaluation · Evaluation system

128.1 Introduction

Use of network teaching platform has made college teaching has had the huge change, teachers in classroom teaching, the more the sharing of teaching resources and students on the platform, and the use of the teaching platform to carry out an investigation, discussion, homework, answering, test and other activities, to facilitate the students to learn, to facilitate the teaching management, to strengthen the course interaction, and enhance the teaching effect. Online learning through the network teaching platform has become an indispensable way of learning. The network teaching platform commonly used are Blackboard, Moodle, Sakai and so on, they all can help teachers facilitate the management of teaching resources, organize discussions, chat, Wiki wait for a variety of interactive activities. In the evaluation of learning, they have a strong operation, test function, and can be all

L. Yong (✉)
Shandong College of Electronic Technology, Jinan 250200, China
e-mail: 1125246445@qq.com

the students work for weighted calculation and test results, generating course grade. In addition to the traditional evaluation methods, this platform has some features, Sakai provides bag function of electronic archives, students can design their own layout and style, add content, and can be shared with others, to allow others to comment. Moodle access logs of students have a very detailed records, activities can according to user, time, activities, actions and other conditions in the course of the user:

1. Evaluation of design is not taken seriously.
2. Research on evaluation tools are lack of system. Research on evaluation tool has been focused on the new evaluation tool of the individual, such as electronic files, gauge.
3. N Insufficient attention to the feedback. Feedback is an important part of the evaluation, the present study usually only focuses on the implementation process tracking evaluation part, for how to conduct effective feedback but is often a belt.
4. The evaluation model's operability is not strong. The model is a developing teacher evaluation, two is designed to guide the development of the system.

128.2 The Development of the Concept of Evolution

Nineteen thirties American professor Taylor "eight years on" since, education evaluation has measurement, description, judgment of several stages, continuous development, in recent years, by the constructivist learning theory, multiple intelligence theory and the humanism education thought, education evaluation, especially for student learning assessment is happening tremendous change, a new culture is the rise of educational evaluation. Tendency [1] this new culture of evaluation according to the reality of the existence of the managerialism, utilitarianism and rely on scientific paradigm, the core position of the value returned to the evaluation, the all-round development and personality to promote people's development as the main function of evaluation, to achieve the unification of subject and object of value subject.

128.3 Elements of Design Evaluation System of Network Teaching Platform for Learning

The network teaching platform learning evaluation system [2–5] is a developmental evaluation system. The network teaching platform of learning design evaluation system must be based on the current development of the evaluation of the idea as the instruction, according to the characteristics of the development of evaluation, system should have the following elements: (a) Design of support scheme evaluation; (b) A comprehensive collection of information to support the process; (c) Support for multiple evaluation items and tools; (d) To support the evaluation and self-evaluation; (e) Support for multiple feedback form.

128.4 Learning Design Model of Evaluation System of Network Teaching Platform

One can reflect the current concept of evaluation evaluation system needs to have the above elements, but these elements are far from enough, evaluation system also need to be effective, reasonable organization, formed a complete system. The overall design of evaluation system should adhere to the following principles:

128.4.1 Systematicness

System science thought, composed of several elements, elements connect with organizational structure, elements complement each other to achieve a function of several important features of the system.

128.4.2 Combining with Teaching Evaluations

A small part of learning evaluation is not only the teaching process, not only in learning is complete, it is with every link of teaching integration, during the whole teaching process. The development of the concept of evaluation and its evaluation system, the design of network teaching platform is shown in Fig. 128.1 of the learning architecture evaluation system.

The system will be closely integrated with the network teaching platform of original, acquisition of students in the network course learning, resource utilization and contribution, to discuss and exchange, answer questions and participate in learning activities and other aspects of the process of information, at the same time, the system will also be on the platform in the original evaluation activities and tools for the expansion and improvement of the formation, function more comprehensive evaluation activities and tool libraries. With the system operation and use of the process, the following will be combined with specific stages of preparation, implementation, evaluation, feedback to, as shown in Fig. 128.2.

The interaction degree students and platform can reflect whether the student's learning attitude is positive, teachers in the design of the table "interaction", the

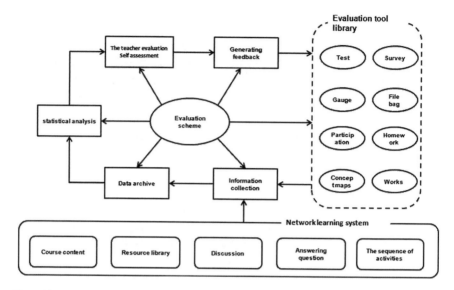

Fig. 128.1 The network teaching platform is shown to study architecture evaluation system

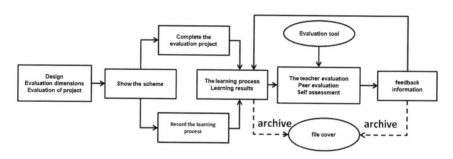

Fig. 128.2 The learning process of evaluation system

first choice to examine the specific project, including task, login times, resource downloads, resource contribution, post a few times, the number of participating in the evaluation study notes, the number, the next also required for each request and weight, students meet the corresponding requirements, can obtain the score. Teaching at the beginning, the system will teachers design scheme evaluation well is presented to students, make students clear direction. Next, the students began to browse learning resources, participation in learning activities, and complete the evaluation scheme within the test, submit the study task. The students participate in the learning process, the system will automatically record their activities in the platform. To overcome the disadvantages, the teacher and students can find the causes together, make improvements.

128.5 Summary and Outlook

The network teaching platform development evaluation concept learning evaluation system can guide, support teachers from multiple dimensions for comprehensive evaluation of students based on the realization of a comprehensive, collecting information, using a variety of evaluation methods and involved in many subjects, embody the concept of the current learning evaluation. However, the platform is only providing the tools, support for the environment to carry out evaluation, to really play the role of evaluation to promote the development of students, but also need the teacher to careful design of the evaluation program, need to pay close attention to teachers in the learning process of students, teachers need guidance on the learning process and all the teachers and students work together to actively participate in the.

References

1. Brown B, Aaron M (2001) The politics of nature. In: Smith J (ed) The rise of modern genomics, 3rd edn. Wiley, New York
2. Dod J (1999) Effective substances. In: The dictionary of substances and their effects. Royal Society of Chemistry. Available via DIALOG. http://www.rsc.org/dose/title of subordinate document. Cited 15 Jan 1999
3. Slifka MK, Whitton JL (2000) Clinical implications of dysregulated cytokine production. J Mol Med 78:74–80. doi:10.1007/s001090000086
4. Smith J, Jones M Jr, Houghton L et al (1999) Future of health insurance. N Engl J Med 965:325–329
5. South J, Blass B (2001) The future of modern genomics. Blackwell, London

Chapter 129
3-Dimensional Finite Element Analysis on Periodontal Stress Distribution of Impacted Teeth During Orthodontic Treatment

Xu-xia Wang, Na Li, Jian-guang Xu, Xu-sheng Ren, Shi-liang Ma and Jun Zhang

Abstract To analyze stress around the impacted tooth by constituting a 3-dimensional finite element model of impacted tooth. The 3-dimensional finite element model of the right upper canine palatally impacted tooth was constituted by CT scan, append periodontal ligament and alveolar bone model was used to constitute impacted model. Three forces were loaded to 3-dimensional finite element model and the periodontal stress of impacted tooth was calculated. When the direction of the force has angle with the central axis of the impacted tooth, if the angle is larger, the maximum stress is larger and the stress distribution is more concentrate, and this goes against the eruption of the impacted tooth. If the angle between the orientation of the traction and central axis of the impacted tooth is smaller, there are more advantages to the eruption of the impacted tooth. When the direction of the force is in line with the central axis, the maximum stress is smaller, and the stress distribution is more even, and this has advantage to the eruption of the impacted tooth. Therefore the angle should be properly selected in order to make sure of the eruption of the impacted tooth. When the angle is quite large, more anchorage is needed to withstand the large force.

X. Wang · J. Zhang (✉)
School of Stomatology, Shandong University, Jinan 250012, China
e-mail: zhangj@sdu.edu.cn

X. Wang · J. Zhang
Shandong Provincial Key Laboratory of Oral Biomedicine, Jinan 250012, China

N. Li
Deptartment of Orthodontics, Shandong Provincial Qianfoshan Hospital,
Jinan 250014, China

J. Xu
School of Stomatology, Anhui Medical University, Hefei 230032, China

X. Ren
Deptartment of Orthodontics, Stomatology Hospital of Jinan, Jinan 250014, China

S. Ma
Deptartment of Orthodontics, School of Stomatology, Binzhou 256603, China

Keywords 3-Dimensional finite element · Impacted tooth · Periodontal stress analysis · Orthodontic treatment

129.1 Introduction

Tooth impaction is one of the most common malocclusions in permanent teeth; it will affect facial aesthetics, cause oral dysfunction, and delay growth and development of children. Without medical intervention, the impacted teeth will lead to many side effects, like root absorption of adjacent teeth, dentigerous cyst, trigeminal neuralgia, and mouth opening difficulties [1–3]. Orthodontic traction is most commonly used by clinicians; it includes three steps: surgical exposure of the crown, bonding of an attachment to the crown, and exertion of a force between the attachment and the fixed orthodontic appliance; as bone remodels the tooth will erupt [4]. Nowadays the treatment of impacted teeth is empirical, because it's difficult to estimate the mode and amount of the tooth displacement and the change of periodontal tissues which largely decreases the controllability and increases the difficulty of the treatment. As the development of computer technology, orthodontists expect to figure out the mechanism of tooth movement through 3-dimensional finite element method. In this study, we constituted a 3-dimensional finite element model of an impacted tooth, different forces were loaded to the model, and the periodontal stress was calculated, aiming to provide fundamental experiment basis for clinical diagnosis, treatment planning and consequence evaluation of tooth traction.

129.2 Materials and Methods

A subject was chosen from the orthodontic department of Stomatology Hospital afflicted to Shandong University, male, 17 years old, with the right upper canine palatally impacted, as is shown in the panoramic radiograph below (Fig. 129.1).

Fig. 129.1 Panorama of patient

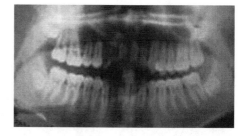

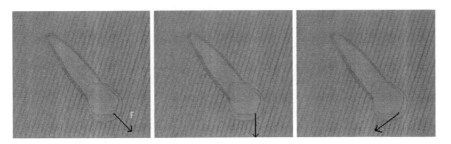

Fig. 129.2 Directions of three loading forces

We carried out a continuous transaction scan on his head by double helix CT whose layer thickness and layer space both were 0.75 mm and acquired the original data of the anatomy shape of the cross-section of the impacted canine. Then the 3-dimensional finite element model containing tooth, periodontal ligament (average thickness was 0.25 mm) and alveolar bone was built. On this basis we picked three conditions to load the canine. In condition 1, the force direction was parallel to the tooth long axis; in condition 2, the force direction formed a 45 ° angle with the long axis of the tooth; In condition 3, the force direction was vertical to the tooth long axis Fig. 129.2.

We set the load to be constant point loading and the loaded part to be the cusp node of the canine. The loaded force was 1.5 N. The software Ansys was used to analyze the loaded model. The distribution of the maximum and minimum equivalent stress and the maximum and minimum first principal stress of the periodontal ligament were evaluated under three conditions.

The mechanical parameters [5] involved in this study are showed below. Elastic modulus of dentin, periodontal ligament, cortical bone, spongy bone is respectively 18,600, 69, 13700, and 1370 MPa; Poisson's ratio is respectively 0.31, 0.45, 0.30, and 0.30. The boundary constraint of this experiment is complete fixation of the surroundings of the alveolar bone. In addition, we assumed that all the components of the model were continuous, homogeneous, and isotropic linear elastic materials and complying with small deformation requirement.

129.3 Results

The distribution of the equivalent stress on the periodontal ligament under three conditions is showed in Table 129.1

The minimum equivalent stress had little difference under three conditions while the maximum equivalent stress sequentially increased. The distribution cloud of the equivalent stress under three conditions is showed in Fig. 129.3.

We can see that in condition 1, the distribution of the equivalent stress was relatively even, while in condition 3, the stress concentrated more on the load

Table 129.1 Stress distribution of periodontal on different force (102 Pa)

Conditions	The minimum	The maximum
Condition 1	0.055662	19.346
Condition 2	0.043085	60.22
Condition 3	0.055348	96.744

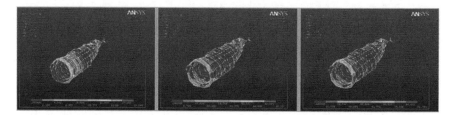

Fig. 129.3 Equivalent stress distribution cloud of periodontal on three different forces

Table 129.2 The maximum stress distribution of periodontal on different force (102 Pa)

Conditions	The minimum	The maximum
Condition 1	−0.003901	19.258
Condition 2	−0.521672	60.214
Condition 3	−0.9521	82.325

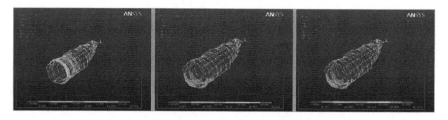

Fig. 129.4 The maximum stress distribution cloud of periodontal on three different forces

pointing side, yet in condition 2, the equivalent stress distributed between the former two.

The distribution of the first principal stress on the periodontal ligament under different three conditions is showed in Table 129.2.

The minimum first principal stress sequentially reduced by condition while the maximum first principal stress sequentially increased. The distribution cloud of the first principal stress under three conditions is showed in Fig. 129.4.

We can see that in condition 1, the distribution of the first principal stress was relatively even, while in condition 3, the stress concentrated more on the load pointing side, yet in condition 2, the first principal stress distributed between the former two.

129.4 Discussion

Tooth impaction is a common disease in stomatology department, causing great damage to patients' oral function and facial aesthetics. It's important to diagnose and cure the disease timely. Finite element research makes it possible to study the biomechanics of impacted tooth's movement which could provide fundamental experiment basis for clinic orthodontic treatment. As we all know, the key to finite element study is to constitute a 3-dimensional finite element model. We compared several kinds of model constitution methods and chose CT image method.

The reverse modeling way was followed [6], which means after getting the information of the tooth impaction patient by CT, we took the coordinates of contour line of the CT images using the software analysis, thus obtained the 3-d entity model of the impacted tooth. Then the periodontal ligament was established through construction method, and we conducted Boolean operations on the ligament and the tooth, thus obtained the highly simulated integral tooth model. This 3-d model we conducted had similar feature with tooth materials, analogous structure and anatomy shape to the real tooth. The model had finely divided units and could be observed, cut, and adjusted through arbitrary rotation. The model also had good measurement accuracy and could be reused easily.

Periodontal reaction is the key to orthodontic treatment. The same force volume and different force direction makes different stress distribution on periodontal ligament, thus different periodontal reaction to the force. It would be best if the orthodontic force is evenly distributed in the periodontal ligament [7]. And this theory also suits the impacted teeth. It's much easier to drag the impacted tooth if the periodontal stress is even.

In this study we found that when the orthodontic traction direction is parallel to the long axis of the impacted tooth, the maximum periodontal stress would distribute evenly and volume moderately which is conductive to the eruption of the tooth. The smaller the angle between the traction direction and the long axis of the tooth is, the easier the orthodontic traction would be, and vise versa. Therefore in the treatment of impacted teeth, clinicians should adjust the force direction as parallel to the tooth long axis as possible.

In summary, in this experiment, we successfully constructed a 3-d finite element model of an impacted tooth, analyzed the periodontal stress under different load conditions, and provided fundamental basis for clinical orthodontic treatment of impacted teeth.

Acknowledgments This study was funded by Shandong Provincial Science and Technology Development Project (2006GG2202031) and Dongying city Science and Technology Development Project (2006-24).

References

1. Xiong XZ, Li XH (2005) Pain with complete denture caused by impacted mandible premolar: Case report. J Dent Prevent Treat 13(1):67
2. Duan SY (2002) Pain with removable partial denture caused by impacted tooth: Case report. Chin J Prosthodont 3(3):179
3. Jiang AN, Xu JK, Qu SY et al (2005) Nasal septum abscess caused by impacted tooth in nasal septum: Case report. Chin J Otorhinolaryngol Head Neck Surg 40(6):457
4. Zhou WG (2002) Correction of impacted maxillary teeth by using both of surgical exposure and orthodontics. Hainan Med J 13(4):29–31
5. Wagner A, Krach W, Schicho K et al (2002) A 3-dimensional finite element analysis investigating the biomechanical behavior of the mandible and plate osteosynthesis in cases of fractures of the condylar process. Oral Surg Oral Med Oral Pathol Oral Radiol Endod 94(6):678–686
6. Liu ZG, Zhao HL, Zhou HF (2002) Tissue modeling and analyzing with finite element method. J Tongji Univ 30(3):356–358
7. Ni L, Wu Y, Dai H (2012) The stress and strain distribution of periodontal ligament of maxillary canine under the orthodontic force. Chin J Tissue Eng Res 16(13):2318–2323

Chapter 130
A Score-Analysis Method Based on ID3 of NCRE

Zeng Xu

Abstract Each paper discussed the data mining technology used in the scoring system for computer rank examination. By applying decision tree rules to analyze the different test types and the scores of the examinee, got the conclusion that the key of passing computer rank examination is "Excel". The conclusion can help the teachers pay more attention to explain that knowledge to the examinee for better teaching effect.

Keywords Data mining · Decision tree rule · Analysis of questions · Computer rank examination · ID3

130.1 Introduction

National computer rank examination is a computer examination system that approved by the ministry of education examination centre and used to investigate the computer application knowledge of examinees. The examination is based on the application of computer in different social departments of different levels and needs. It provides a proof of computer application knowledge and ability level for professional careers.

Traditional paper archive mode has become one of the important factors that hinder the development of health care system. To train a group of staffs who have the ability of using the soft of Office Automation has become an important education target in undergraduate. Zunyi medical college has emphasized the teaching and assessment of national computer rank examination in curriculum specially. In order to make medical examinees target to take part in learning and

---

Z. Xu (✉)
Department of Medical Information Engineering, Zunyi Medical College,
563003 Zunyi, China
e-mail: zengxu27@163.com

being accessed, the department of medical information engineering of Zunyi medical college collects relate data and make an analysis by using data mining technology. The analysis results can help teacher to develop teaching ways.

130.2 Data Ming

Data mining [1] is a technology that could found interesting model from a large number of data. Those data can be stored in a database, data warehouse, or other information databases. The types of data mining technology include classification rule mining, association rule mining, forecast analysis, the summary rule mining, clustering rules mining and trend analysis, etc. The classification rule mining plays an important role in getting knowledge. The decision tree algorithm that in classification rule mining has been paid more attention by its higher efficiency in data analysis.

130.2.1 Decision Tree

Decision tree consists of leaf node, internal node and branch. The branch represents test results, and the internal nodes represent some inspection properties, and leaf nodes represent classification [2].

The process of the construction of the decision tree is from top to down, using the strategy of "divide and conquer". Then test the given data samples starting from the root node, and divide the data samples into a lot of subsamples according to the test results, each component of the subsamples will consist of a new child node. Iterating the building process, until meet the given termination conditions. A constructed decision tree, each branch corresponds to a rule from the root node to the leaf node.

130.2.2 Decision Tree Algorithm

In the 1970s, machine learning researchers J. Ross Quinlan developed decision tree algorithm, called the ID3 [3]. Quinlan developed C4.5 and then it became the new benchmark of supervision and learning performance of the algorithm. In 1984, several statisticians published classification and regression tree. Above two kinds of basic algorithms inspired the cyclone of studying decision tree induction.

This paper using ID3 as the decision tree algorithm which described as the following:

```
Input: samples; attribute_list
Output: decision tree
decision_tree(samples,attribute_list)
{create node N;
if samples in the same class under the C then
return N and mark as C;
if attribute_list ==NULL then
return N as leaf node and mark as the most common class in sample;
select attribute with the highest information gain as test_attribute;
mark node N as test_attribute;
for each ai of given value in test_attribute
grow a new node Ni which meet test_attribute = ai from N;
set si as a set in samples which meet test_attribute = ai;
if si == NULL then
mark Ni as the most common class in sample;
else Ni = decision_tree(si,attribute_list—test_attribute);
return N;}
```

130.3 ID3 for Score Analysis

We can obtain decision tree rules according to the scores by applying the ID3 algorithm in Zunyi medical college computer rank examination scoring system. Taking tested scores that come from grade 2010 clinical professional for example, analyzing related test about "Type", "Word", "Windows", "Choice", "Excel" and "Internet" by using decision tree rule mining technology. There include about 40 pieces of score record, and the basic structure of the original data is shown in Table 130.1.

130.3.1 Data Preprocessing

In order to get better data mining result, we should preprocess the given scores [4, 5], preprocessing process is: mark the examination questions as "Y" while scoring rate is under 60 %, otherwise "N". The preprocessing results are shown in Table 130.2. The preprocessing processes are shown as the following:

Table 130.1 Original data

Student ID	Choice	Windows	Type	Word	Excel	Internet	Score	Result
1020150601	15	8	12	20	0	4	59	Fail
1020150602	12	8	14	20	13	10	77	Pass
......	......	......	......	......	......	......	......	......

Table 130.2 Preprocessed data

Student ID	Choice	Windows	Type	Word	Excel	Internet	Score	Result
1020150601	Y	Y	Y	Y	N	N	59	Fail
1020150602	Y	Y	Y	Y	Y	Y	77	Pass
……	……	……	……	……	……	……	……	……

Choice preprocessing rule: "N" (< 12), "Y" (12-20).
Windows preprocessing rule: "N" (< 6), "Y" (6-10).
Type preprocessing rule: "N" (< 9), "Y" (9-15).
Word preprocessing rule: "N" (< 15), "Y" (15-25).
Excel preprocessing rule: "N" (< 12), "Y" (12-20).
Internet preprocessing rule: "N" (< 6), "Y" (6-10).

130.3.2 Construct Decision Tree

According to the principle of ID3 algorithm, we construct the decision tree model by using the result of whether the students of grade 2010 major in clinical pass the examination or not. The steps shown as the following.

Step 1: Calculate the expected information that the scores sample classification needs coming from grade 2010 clinical professional performance

Divided the sample into two classes: Set C1 as the class whose students pass the examination, Set C2 as the class whose students fail to pass the examination. $S1 = 22$, $S2 = 18$, and total $S = 40$.

Calculate the expected information that the given sample classification needs :
Info(S1,S2) = Info(22,18)
=-22/40*log2(22/40)-18/40*log2(18/40) = 0.992774454

Step 2: Calculate the information gain of each type of the examination questions Calculate the information gain of "Choice"

Case 1:"Choice" = "Y"
S11 = 19(Pass),S21 = 11(Fail)
Info(S11,S21) = Info(19,11)
=-19/30*log2(19/30)-11/30*log2(11/30) = 0.948078244
Case 2:"Choice" = "N"
S12 = 3(Pass),S22 = 7(Fail)
Info(S12,S22) = Info(3,7)
=-3/10*log2(3/10)-7/10*log2(7/10) = 0.881290899
The expected information of given samples classified by "Choice" is:
E("Choice") = 30/40*Info(S11,S21) + 10/40*Info(S21,S22)
=30/40*0.948078244 + 10/40*0.881290899 = 0.931381408
The information gain of this kind of classification is:
Gain("Choice") = Info(S1,S2)-E("Choice")
=0.992774454-0.931381408 = 0.061393046

By using the same way we could get the information gain of other examination questions.

Gain("Windows") = 0.319192829
Gain("Type") = 0.109061966
Gain("Word") = 0.141629148
Gain("Excel") = 0.413954888
Gain("Internet") = 0.009331011
Step 3: make sure the test attribute

"Excel" was selected as the types of test questions and it was used to establish the first node because of its highest information gain. The node divides the sample into two parts, and then work out each part in recursive calculation according to the above methods, the final decision tree we got is shown in Fig. 130.1:

130.3.3 Extracted Decision Tree Classification Rule

We can extract classification rules in this example, and the rules are shown as the following:

1. If "Excel" = "Y" then "Pass"
2. If "Excel" = "N" and "Windows" = "N" then "Fail"
3. If "Excel" = "N" and "Windows" = "N" and "Type" = "N" then "Fail"
4. If "Excel" = "N" and "Windows" = "N" and "Type" = "N" and "Choice" = "N" then "Fail"
5. If "Excel" = "N" and "Windows" = "N" and "Type" = "N" and "Choice" = "N" and "Word" = "N" then "Fail"
6. If "Excel" = "N" and "Windows" = "N" and "Type" = "N" and "Choice" = "N" and "Word" = "N" and "Internet" = "N" then "Fail"
7. If "Excel" = "N" and "Windows" = "N" and "Type" = "N" and "Choice" = "N" and "Word" = "N" and "Internet" = "Y" then "Pass"

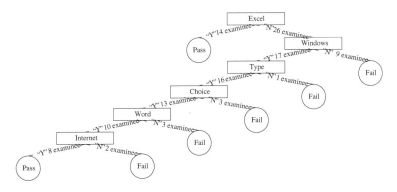

Fig. 130.1 The decision tree

130.4 Conclusion

We can get the following conclusions with the extracted decision tree rules:

1. Those examinees who get "Y" in "Excel" test have already mastered related operations of whole examination. They can get high scores and pass the examination successfully.
2. Those examinees that get "N" in "Excel" test must get high scores in other five tests in order to pass the examination successfully.

We have found out that the "Excel" is the key test after analyzing the six tests by using decision tree mining. The conclusions will guide examinees to master the key of the examination. Meanwhile, Teachers can also emphasize the study of "Excel" in the subsequent teaching process and help the examinees to master the key knowledge and promote the passing rate. The conclusions will give strong guidance to both teachers and examinees.

References

1. Soman KP, Divadar S, Ajay V (2003) Data mining tutorial. Tsinghua University Press, Beijing
2. Xiang W (2011) The application of ID3 algorithm in the analysis of English achievements. J Liuzhou Vocat Tech Coll 11(2):31–34
3. Han J, Kamber M (2007) Data mining concepts and technology. Machinery Industry Press, Beijing
4. Wang Y, Hu X (2011) Research of ID3 algorithm in decision tree. J Anhui Univ 35(3):71–75
5. Tao K (2011) Research based on decision tree technique in the application of university achievement analysis. J Xinxiang Univ 28(1):49–51

Chapter 131
Education Cloud: New Development of Informationization Education in China

Liangtao Yang

Abstract With the development of cloud computing, its application in the field of education has become a hot spot, and people's expectations and demands of the education cloud have been also increasing. This paper analyzes cloud computing and its values in education, points out potential advantages and current applications situation of education cloud. Finally, the author puts forward some proposals on how to construct education cloud.

Keywords Cloud computing · Education cloud · Informationization education

131.1 Introduction

'The Education Informationization 10-year Development Plan (2011–2020)' has just released and established the grand goals 'The overall education informationization will approach the international advanced level in 2020, which will fully show its supporting and leading role in education reform and development'. Because of the location, network transmission speed, the server's data processing capabilities and many other factors, in our process of education informationization, education information platform can not meet the needs of teachers and students, information and resources can not be effectively shared, which has become the bottleneck in the development of education informationization [1]. So it is urgent for us to seek a new technology to solve these problems. Therefore, the Ministry of Education established the implementation of 'The basic capacity-building initiatives of education informationization', arranged the education information network in ahead, built national education satellite broadband transmission network,

L. Yang (✉)
Shanghai Second Polytechnic University, Shanghai, China
e-mail: ltyang@sspu.cn

fully integrated and utilized the information infrastructure of all levels of education institutions to construct the basic cloud environments of nationwide, reasonable distribution, open source and support the formation of the hierarchical structure of the cloud-based platform, the platform of cloud resources and cloud education management service platform.

Currently, education cloud has become the divergent views on the topic. The Ministry of Education and the education authority of every province have clearly regarded the construction of education cloud as one of the priorities of the current work. This paper will analyze cloud technology and the applications of education cloud. The author hopes that education cloud is a solutions which is able to bring real change for the education, also hopes that education authorities, suppliers, schools, academic research team, as well as teachers and learners can maintain rational and positive attitudes to promote the benign development of education cloud applications under the background of education cloud hot [2].

131.2 Cloud Computing and its Application in Education

131.2.1 Cloud Computing

Cloud Computing is the development of distributed computing, parallel computing and Grid Computing. Along with the continuous development of the cloud computing, related technologies such as data storage, data management, programming models, equipment erection, services technology, resource management, task management and many other technologies are constantly developing [3]. Cloud service is the service which cloud can provide. We usually understand that the IT-related capacity is provided to the user as a service which allows the user get the services they need through the Internet when the user do not know technology, relevant knowledge and equipment operating capacity.

While the academia has given a lot of definitions on cloud computing, people have their own understanding. But because of different contexts, it is very difficult for us to give a clear accepted definition. For example, the definition from Wikipedia: it is an internet-based computing mode by which shared hardware & software resources and information can be provided to computers and other devices when user do not know the details of cloud infrastructure and do not have appropriate expertise and direct control; cloud computing provide a new IT services based on the Internet. The definition from The U.S. National Institute of Standards and Technology: Cloud computing is a model [4]. This mode allows the user access easily a shared computing resource library (including networks, servers, storage, applications and services) anywhere through the network. In fact, cloud computing is neither computing nor a pure technical concept. It is how to combine all the hardware and software on the basis of the existing Internet, and fully utilize and mobilize all available information resources, through building a new service mode or a new system structure which can provide service to provide people with the low-cost of different levels, high efficiency intelligent service and information service.

131.2.2 The Application of Cloud Computing in Education

After massive hardware investment, education informationization has gone into the plateau phase. Therefore, we have to reflect how to build new information environment? How to eliminate information silos to realize system interconnection, sharing of resources, application interoperability? How to train professional teacher team to ensure the effective operation of information systems? How to reduce consumption to achieve sustainable development? Cloud computing brings hope. It is an important opportunity for Chinese education informationization to advance education cloud services. In the past, many schools have their own computing cluster, web sites and storage arrays. The inadequate uses cause hardware and software investment to be wasted, these abuses continued to plague education informationization constantly. Education cloud platform adopts virtualization technology, integrates hardware & software resources, weakens the physical dependencies between hardware, software, data, network, storage and other IT systems at different levels of resources, improves the flexibility of computing resources and solves the effectiveness, flexibility, and ease of resource sharing [5].

Future information-based learning environment will be becoming very complex and learning resources will be increasing rapidly. Cloud computing can help solve these new confusion such as the information silos, system interconnection, resources sharing and interoperable application. As a new IT service model, cloud computing is closely integrating with teaching and education. At the same time, the integration of high quality resources and the construction of education cloud are also changing the re-accreditation of education resources [6]. Based on cloud computing, the concept and scope of education resources are expanding continuously, and education resources have much richer epitaxy such as computing resources, platform resources, knowledge and skills, data resources, experience and sharing. Today, education resources are no longer purely digital information resources, but computing, performance, environment and even human resources.

131.3 Superiority of Education Cloud

The application of cloud computing in the field of education can restructure and optimize a variety of information resources, and ultimately achieve extensive and efficient sharing of resources. Based on the following major potential superiority of education cloud, education authorities at all levels promote the construction of educational cloud vigorously.

131.3.1 Rich Resources and Equitable Sharing

One of the characteristics of education cloud is to have a wealth of educational resources and show these resources to the students through the most appropriate ways. Education cloud stores education resources in clouds. We can not only access educational resources from others easily, but also share their own resources with others. Education cloud can realize the openness and the sharing of education resources between schools and schools, between classes and classes. The learners in remote areas can obtain quality education resources from the cloud, which solves effectively the phenomenon of "educational inequality".

Through the construction of large-scale, shared educational resource database, building a digital library, virtual laboratory, we can achieve the sharing of high-quality education and teaching resources, and realize teaching and research inter-regional collaboration to reduce the gap between the different regions and schools to promote the balanced development of education. On Education cloud, the use of resources can be open. At the same time, the resources construction process can also be collaborative and open. It is unnecessary to clear the providers and users of resources [7]. Users sometimes can become providers. Through collaboration platform, both teachers and learners can take part in the construction of educational resources, learn from each other, constantly to provide and update the good resource and maintain its sustainable development.

131.3.2 Easy to Use and Easy to Maintain

Because software stores in clouds, without having to download, install, maintain and upgrade, no matter where, we can learn as long as the Internet and intelligent terminal equipment. Because data of education cloud store in clouds, users do not have to worry about the security of data. The server of education cloud has a professional team to manage information, has advanced data center to save the data, and has strict access strategy to help the user to specify the shared data. At the same time, we do not have to construct the engine room and purchase a large number of software. Therefore, cloud platform is a real convenience, secure, cheap network platform.

Through education cloud platform, we can integrate the hardware and software resources from all types of educational institutions and schools, centralize computing resources, achieve the dynamic sharing of hardware resources, improve the utilization of IT hardware and reduce hardware costs. Cloud platform generally has better stability and security by the construction and maintenance of professional institutions and professionals and users do not need to install software or simply install small client software. In china, educational institutions, especially basic education institutions, are generally short of professional IT technical team. In additional, learners' application of information technology is also limited.

Therefore, the construction of education cloud can make schools and learners spend a lot of energy to buy the service without the need for hardware and software environment. Thus, we may pay more attention to the teaching and learning.

131.4 Analysis of the Construction of Education Cloud in China

According to the case of education cloud in many places, we think that the current construction status of Chinese education cloud can be summarized as follows. Of course, because of the complexity of the construction of education cloud, the following also just list some of them.

131.4.1 Superficial Applications

As the concept of cloud computing has been hyped in the worldwide, the concept of education cloud has been universally accepted, and given the high expectations of education cloud. But all applications have an asymptotic process and the starting point of the application is easy to use. During the construction of education cloud, so-called IaaS just use a part of the cloud computing and the scale of cloud is very smaller. Education cloud is short of the value-added services of cloud computing, especially for teachers and students. Most cloud computing applications is actually a traditional network-based remote application. Currently, the constructions of all types of education cloud are fragmented and are lack of uniform standards and overall plan. If we are not concerned about these issues in a timely manner, the applications of education cloud will become new lonely clouds. Therefore, it should be as soon as possible to construct standard education cloud based on the international standards of cloud computing.

131.4.2 Indeterminate Governance Structure

Education cloud model will make our country gradually form a new pattern managed by education cloud which is led by the education authorities and includes the other participations of the businesses, research institutions, schools. The education authorities should undertake the costs of public education cloud, and at the same time various social organizations can provide a variety of alternative education cloud services to the society under the effective supervision of the education authorities. The service model of education cloud has also brought changes in the management mode of construction funds and education cloud makes education services can be purchased on demand. Pre-fund of education informationization is used mainly for purchasing hardware and software. Purchase services share of funding for information technology in education and cloud environments, the proportion of the fund used for purchasing services will gradually increase under the background of education cloud. Education authority must clearly define the relationship between assets and services in order to guide school actively buy cloud services and benefit from the cloud services.

131.4.3 Repetitive Construction

Cloud computing is not a new round of informationization construction and it should be upgrades of informationization. But now, a lot solutions of cloud computing are based on a completely new system, that is, we must purchase new hardware and software to implement cloud computing. If we do so, it should be out of the question to make full use of IT infrastructure of cloud computing. How to make full use of existing resources rationally, how to transform existing software and hardware to reduce the expense of education cloud and how to continue to add value in education cloud service, all of these are not embodied in all types of construction programs. In addition, our construction of education informationization has been mainly in the form of engineering and project and the management mode of engineering and project makes the information construction project be detained funding cycle. In short, our construction of education informationization has not yet formed a sustainable development strategy.

131.5 Suggestions of the Construction of Education Cloud

131.5.1 Government-Led and Multi-Stakeholder Involvement

In china, the governments play an important role in the process of constructing education cloud. The industry chain of cloud computing is made up of many providers such as cloud computing service providers, network infrastructure providers, cloud computing integrated service providers and terminal equipment manufacturers, which provide services to users. The governments should focus on investing IaaS construction, foster strong PaaS vendors to develop good Paas system according to the demand of resource services and online teaching, develop SaaS software system for educational institutions and gradually build SaaS software distribution channels by which users can easily get cloud services and cloud software according Chinese education system. The governments should supervise the PaaS vendor and SaaS vendors and be responsible to security mechanisms and service quality. For basic SaaS services, the governments may consider collective procurement and free use. The above measures can promote the benign development of education cloud.

131.5.2 To Attach Importance to the Scalability and Security

To build a good education cloud, the key is the on-demand construction and it must solve the problems such as dynamical reconfigurable resources, real-time monitoring and automated deployment, which need to virtualization, high-performance storage, parallel computing technologies and high-speed Internet. It is the key for the development of education cloud to improve some related technologies such as the establishment of the resource library, resource management and scheduling, education cloud services software platform (PaaS) and middleware platform. How to build education cloud? We must effectively integrate the latest achievements of the knowledge engineering, artificial intelligence technology into education cloud services, so as to promote the benign development of education cloud applications.

131.5.3 Close Coordination

The researchers of education technology should conduct in-depth research on education cloud, such as various programs, projects and engineering, implement the test and track of key projects, use the research methods of combination between quantitative and qualitative, carry out cost/benefit study about the education cloud applications as soon as possible and formulate a comprehensive and wide-ranging development path. Standard setters should develop the technology standard of education cloud services to ensure that the data exchange, system interoperability and information security are evidence-based. In addition, education administrators should focus on issues such as the operating model of education cloud, management mechanism and funds management; this is also an important guarantee to ensure that education cloud can really be implemented.

131.6 Conclusion

The construction of education cloud is not a new round of information construction and it should be upgrades of informationization, be a great system of education informationization. Education cloud can promote education reform, improve the overall quality of education, achieve leaps and bounds of education and advance education informationization and the balanced development of education. Of course, it is still a daunting project to make quality educational resources shared through education cloud all over the country and it requires education sectors, schools and social parties attach great importance.

References

1. Feng J (2009) Prospect on modern distance education based on cloud computing. China Educ Technol 10:39–42
2. Lu B, Youqun R (2012) Walk in the clouds: cloud computing in education of china. J Distance Educ 1:62–67
3. Li H (2011) Discussion on education cloud based on concept of cloud computing. J Tianjin Radio TV Univ (3):47–50
4. Ministry of Education of P R C Ten-year development plan for ICT in education in China (2011–2020) [OL]. http://www.moe.edu.cn/ewebeditor/uploadfile/2012/03/29/20120329140800968.doc83c4d329.html
5. Zhang J, Huang R, Zhang L (2012) Smart education cloud: new service model of ict in education. Open Educ Res (3):20–26
6. Xie X, Zhang T (2011) Education cloud is gradually becoming a climate. http://www.edu.cn/ycc_9779/20110621/t20110621_637749.shtml
7. Lei Y, Mei C, Liu D, Li Z (2011) The current situation and development tendency of educational application of cloud computing in China. Mod Distance Educ Res (6):42–46

Chapter 132
CRH5 EMU Fault Diagnosis Simulation Training System Development

Jian Wang, Zhiming Liu, Fengchuan Jiao and Xinhua Zhang

Abstract Today EMU is equipped with a more comprehensive, complex fault diagnosis system, the diagnostic system can report information such as the nature and the location of a fault in the form of fault code the time after the EMU failure occurs, the diagnostic system provides support for maintenance work. But the diagnostic system can't work alone, and only when the train is running the diagnostic system can be used for fault diagnosis and alarm, so this situation makes the motor train-set base can't system comprehensive train drivers and maintenance personnel. According to signal transmission logical relations of CRH5 EMU fault diagnosis system, based on LabVIEW software system hardware modules, we develop a CRH5 EMU fault diagnosis simulation training system. This system mainly includes host teacher machine, simulation of bridge, the main display screen (TS), the driver diagnostic monitor screen (TD), and network systems. Simulation of bridge and TS screen which simulation is according to the composition of CRH5 EMU dynamic system, traction system, the running resistance characteristic, the braking system characteristics, line conditions etc., based on traction calculation theory, under the condition of the LabVIEW software we can build CRH5 EMU driver simulation environment. TD screen is according to the signal transmission CRH5 EMU fault diagnosis system logical relations, based on the LabVIEW software system we can build highly simulation system of fault diagnosis system. Network system adopts the LAN technology by NI Company which provides the DataSocket real-time data transmission technology to transmit data.

Keywords EMU · Fault diagnosis · LabVIEW virtual technology · Simulation training

---

J. Wang (✉) · Z. Liu · F. Jiao · X. Zhang
School of Mechanical, Electronic and Control Engineering, Beijing Jiaotong University, Beijing 100044, China
e-mail: 12125806@bjtu.edu.cn

Z. Liu
e-mail: zhmliu1@bjtu.edu.cn

132.1 Background of EMU Fault Diagnosis Simulation Training System

EMU fault diagnosis system is a set of installations run diagnosis system in real-time on the train. In essence, it is a distributed computer control system, which is responsible for the collection and delivery of information for all parts of the whole train control, detection, diagnosis and recording of the entire train. The control commands of the whole train made by drivers are send to every car of the train, while the work status and fault information of every car can also be transferred to the train communication network driver's display. EMU fault diagnosis system is divided into three levels: the train diagnosis centers, vehicle diagnosis devices, and equipment diagnosis unit. Communication network constitutes the entire diagnostic system.

The purposes of EMU fault diagnosis are to improve the security and availability of the running system and optimize the operational management. What's more, it also makes it easier to use and maintenance. Summary, the fault diagnosis system has the following main features:

1. Fault detection;
2. Fault identification;
3. Fault location;
4. Fault display;
5. Fault recording, storage and transmission;
6. Preparedness operations and regular maintenance inspection.

EMU fault diagnosis system is generally cannot work alone apart from train. It only can diagnoses gives a fault alarm in the case of the operating state of the various components within the system. Therefore, the use of the diagnostic system has brought a certain degree of inconvenience to drivers and maintenance personnel:

1. A wide range of training cannot be on the ground throughout the day;
2. Failure phenomenon can only be decided by the system state of the current car. Staff cannot grasp the nature and location of the various types of failure phenomena systematically and comprehensively.

This article according to the logic relation of signal transmission of CRH5 EMU fault diagnosis system, based on LabVIEW software, is used to develop CRH5 EMU fault diagnosis simulation training system.

132.2 The Composition of CRH5 EMU Fault Diagnosis Simulation System

Fault diagnosis simulation of CRH5 overall framework is shown in Fig. 132.1, including host Teachers machine to simulate the bridge, the driver main monitor (TS-screen), the driver of the diagnosis display (TD screen), and network systems.

132.2.1 EMU Simulation of the Bridge and the Main Display

Based on the composition of CRH5 EMU power system, traction system characteristics, the running resistance characteristics, characteristics of the braking system, line conditions and other factors, CRH5 EMU simulation driving environment is built by using LabVIEW software, as shown in Figs. 132.2, 132.3.

Include:

1. The driver driving simulation platform simulation interface, including traction and braking handle, Pantograph switch, Simulation speed dashboard, The distance from the front of the speed limit point and so on;
2. According to CRH5 EMU traction characteristics, resistance characteristics, line conditions to establish the equations of motion and solving for mileage-time division curve, mileage-speed curve of the EMU;
3. TS screen, TD screen to provide train running status information.

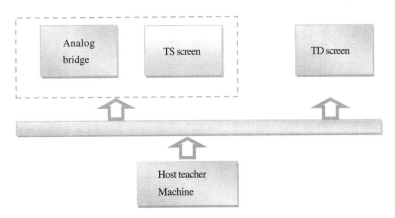

Fig. 132.1 CRH5 fault diagnosis simulation of the overall framework

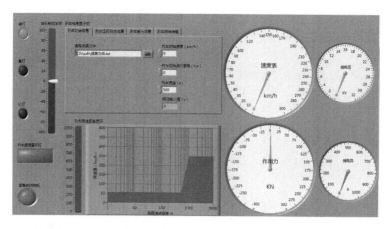

Fig. 132.2 EMU simulation of the bridge and the main display

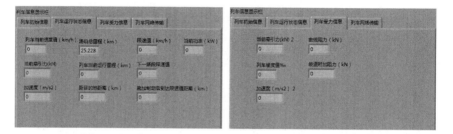

Fig. 132.3 Train information interface

132.2.2 EMU Simulation of Host Teacher Machine and TD Screen

According to the logic relation of signal transmission of CRH5 EMU fault diagnosis system, highly imitative CRH5 EMU system fault diagnosis system is built based on LabVIEW software system, the function of the system:

1. According to the logic relation of signal transmission of CRH5 EMU fault diagnosis system, generation process of failure simulation is prepared on the host teacher's machine, as shown in Fig. 132.4;
2. By getting driving system operation state the from the EMU simulation, the train traction system, braking system, auxiliary system parameters are calculated and set, simulation TD screen control procedures are also prepared;
3. The collection of fault state of the system from the EMU fault simulation is transmitted to the simulation TD screen, as shown in Fig. 132.5.

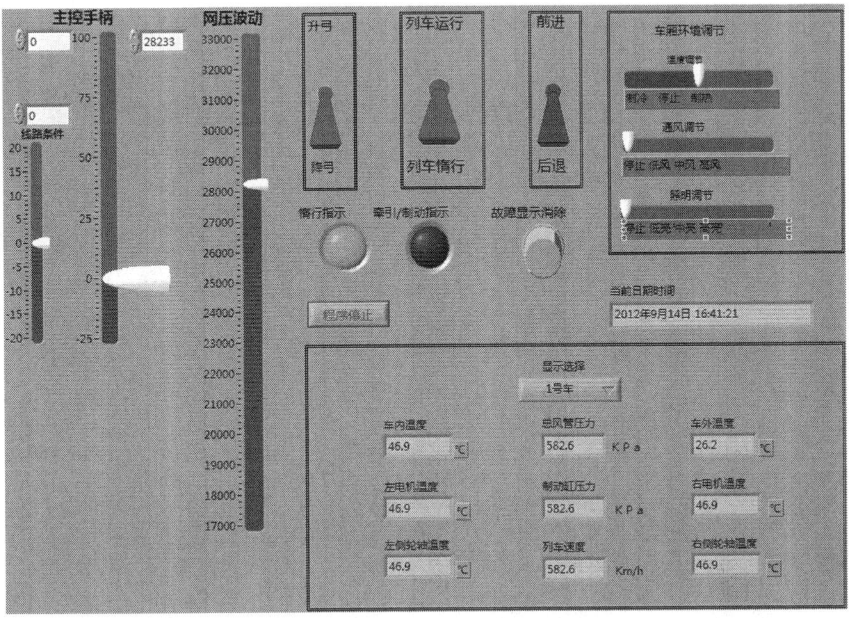

Fig. 132.4 Host teacher machine

132.3 EMU Fault Diagnosis Simulation System Development Program

First, set up a simulation platform of CRH5 EMU which including the power supply system, traction systems, braking systems, ventilation systems, lighting systems and air conditioning systems to simulate CRH5 EMU. During the actual running, the influenced traction by the net pressure change, and the changed Motor torque, braking curve, braking force, motor temperature, axle temperature, ventilation control, conditioning control, lighting control and the inside temperature control through this realistic simulation allow the trainees to be familiar with CRH5 EMU system in the operational status of a variety of conditions and to be able to deal with emergency situations in driving the process and ensure the normal running of the train. In order to provide travelers a comfortable travel environment, trainees need to master systems such as ventilation, lighting, and temperature regulation.

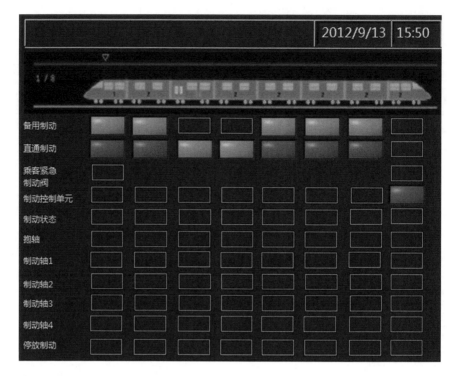

Fig. 132.5 TD screen

132.3.1 EMU Fault Diagnosis Simulation System Hardware Components

The hardware of EMU simulation fault diagnosis system mainly gathers real-time data through a variety of sensors, and then the data is sent to the signal processing circuit. The analog signal is converted into digital signal, which can be recognized by computer by the data acquisition cards, and then is sent to the computer. According to the logic relation between fault EMU equations of motion and the main system through, the LabVIEW software for data processing and analysis obtains the necessary data.

Before using LabVIEW to control the hardware, the first step is to install the hardware and connect it to a computer. Next, install hardware drivers on your computer and make the necessary configuration.

132.3.2 EMU Fault Diagnosis Simulation System Software Configuration

CRH5 EMU fault diagnosis system software has the main function: train operation status signal display, data storage and analysis.

In the fault diagnosis the function of LabVIEW software is mainly: Arrange the sensors in the parts of the train where need to be monitored. Analog signal is converted into digital signal by the data acquisition cards and then is sent to the LabVIEW software platform. On one hand we can do the signal display, signal analysis and so on through LabVIEW software, on the other hand we can do fault analysis and diagnosis with the expert system, neural network, and fault tree analysis.

132.3.3 Data Transfer

CRH5 EMU fault diagnosis simulation system which including teacher machine and trainee builds a LAN through the router between the teacher machine and the trainee machine. Then, the DataSocket real-time data transmission technology is applied between teacher machine and trainee machine which can realize the data exchange and also achieve the goal of real-time controlling and setting up various faults by teachers through the teacher machine. Trainees in the trainee machine determine the conditions of the train and make an emergency handling by observing various display operation status signals and data so that trainees enable to skill to grasp and handle a variety of failures.

132.4 The Realization of EMU Fault Diagnosis Simulation

The fact that the failure of the braking system is more difficult to judge in the main system of EMUD leads to a longer stopping time is the main factor affecting subsequent cross the road and late. Therefore, how to quickly deal with brake failure is an important issue in the use of the EMU. In this paper, the braking system will be used as an example and the technology of fault diagnosis simulation module will be introduced.

In the CRH5 EMU, traction and brake lever is at neutral position. If the trains pipe air pressure is 6.0 bars, safety loop is established, dynamic axial pressure is about 4.4 bar, and drag axial pressure is about 3.2 bar. The malfunction brake does not alleviate is the greatest common brake does not alleviate the fault.

The most commonly used brake failure does not alleviate:

Table 132.1 Maximum braking fault code, fault phenomenon and the processing method does not alleviate

Fault code	Failure phenomenon	Troubleshooting
frdia606f11b4all	1-axis and 4-axis air brake does not alleviate	View fault car 1-axis and 4-axis brake cylinder pressure, if any, isolated 1-axis and 4-axis air brake
frdia606f11b4all	2-axis and 3-axis air brake does not alleviate	View fault car 2-axis and 3-axis brake cylinder pressure, if any, isolated of 2-axis and 3-axis air brake
frbrakedaxleall	When the the traction brake lever traction detected individually axis brake does not alleviate	View the brake cylinder pressure, if any, the parking and isolation brake axis running speed limit regulations by the ministry of railways
frbcudemmiall	Failure of the brake control unit (BCU), the festival train direct braking unavailable	Information BCU1/BCU detected brake and brake cylinder pressure may not be correct, you need to do to the car to close the car handling
cdcavariagwall	WTB Line cut or gateway failure	Train in a degraded mode. Can continue to run in the case of performance degradation

1. Brake WTB network cable is not working;
2. One car or eight car brake control unit fault;
3. ATP exerts maximum service braking without remission;
4. Keep the brake is applied;
5. Network failure.

CRH5 EMU maximum brake does not alleviate fault code, fault phenomenon and the processing method are shown in Table 132.1.

Storing the five fault in the host teacher machine, teachers in the training process can be set to any one or more of the above-mentioned failure, the TD screen of the trainee machine will display maximum service braking fault does not alleviate fault, t in the process of the five kinds of fault to the fault code in the form of existence, in accordance with the CRH5 EMU brake logic diagram (shown in Fig. 132.6) the logic relationship between the information will be transmitted to the TD, and then display the fault occurrence and location.

The above information transfer process is the fault code into binary form can be identified by computer, and then through "or "logic and logic "and" operation, then and fault information comparative analysis, the final result is passed to the TD. If the fault occurs, will display the red; on the contrary, will show the green.

Fig. 132.6 Release brake logic diagram

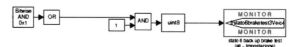

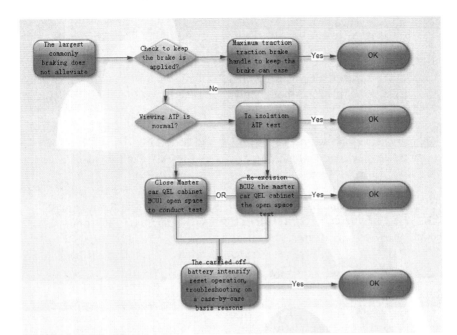

Fig. 132.7 Troubleshooting and processing flow chart

Troubleshooting Manual, the maximum service braking does not ease the troubleshooting process as shown in Fig. 132.7.

When trainee machine appears normal braking does not alleviate the phenomenon, the trainees should be in accordance with the inspection process for troubleshooting:

1. Should first check whether the holding brake applied, the traction and braking handle for maximum traction position can alleviate the holding brake.
2. If you still cannot be restored, the next step view the ATP is normal, trainees can isolate the ATP test, if you still cannot be restored, turn off the master car the QEL cabinet BCU1 open space test, or re-excision master car the QEL cabinet BCU2 empty open test.
3. Finally, still cannot be restored when you need off the battery to increase the reset operation.

In the process teachers can give some instructions and prompts.

Make full use of the EMU simulation system of fault diagnosis for the fault diagnosis of mechanic pre-job simulation, treatment methods and corresponding can tell the mechanic master fault of the EMU.

132.5 Conclusion

The diagnosis system cannot work alone, and only to the operating status of the various components of the train system for fault diagnosis and alarm, which cannot be for drivers and repair personnel how to use the diagnostic system for training problem, this paper proposed the EMU fault diagnosis system of signal transmission logic relations, development dynamic EMU fault diagnosis simulation training system of programs, based on LabVIEW software system and NI hardware module, developed a highly imitative CRH5 EMU fault diagnostic training system.

Make full use of the EMU fault diagnosis simulation training system to allow trainees to the repeated, common treatment methods to make trainees master the EMU emergency fault, the system for drivers and repair personnel comprehensive training provides conditions.

References

1. Xuewen H, Chunming L, Xin FCW, Feng W (2010) CRH3 high-speed EMU fault diagnosis system [J]. Comput Integr Manuf Syst 16(10):2312–2313
2. Fan YX, Liu H (2011) Analysis of data transmission of high-speed EMU fault diagnosis [J]. Lanzhou Jiao tong University 30(4):34–35
3. Wang H (2011) EMU CRH5 type brake does not alleviate the failure analysis and processing [J]. Technological Wind (22):100–101
4. Peng Y, Pan XY, Xie L (2011) LabVIEW virtual instrument design and analysis [M]. Tsinghai University (in press)***
5. Guo S (2008) EMU detection and fault diagnosis technology [M]. Southwest Jiaotong University (in press)***

Chapter 133
A Study on Recruitment Requirements of Small and Medium-Sized Enterprises and the Talent Training of Local Colleges

Zhang Weiwei

Abstract Through empirical analysis, this paper summarizes the recruitment requirements of small and medium-sized enterprises as follows: qualification certificate, job expectation, professional ability, practice experience, professional morality, makes a summary of the characteristics of the recruitment requirements of small and medium-sized enterprises, and then provides some suggestions for the reform of local colleges' talent training.

Keywords SMEs · Recruitment requirements · Talent training

133.1 Questionnaire Design and Data Collection

Along with the popularization of higher education, SMEs have become the major employment channel for the college graduates, especially for the students of local colleges. Therefore, it is extremely urgent for the the local college to improve the model of talent training on the basis of empirical research on SMEs recruitment requirements.

The formal testing chose SEMs in Shandong province of China as the samples, and a total of 500 questionnaires were sent out and 427 valid questionnaires were received. The samples comprised manufacturing industry (25.2 %); wholesale and retail industry (13.3 %); real estate (8.4 %); catering industry (13.6 %); transportation, warehousing, post and telecommunication industry (6.0 %); financial industry (8.3 %); information transmission, computer service and software

Z. Weiwei (✉)
Shandong Polytechnic University, Daxue Road, Jinan, Shandong, People's Republic of China
e-mail: anffieok@126.com

industry (17.8 %); agriculture, forestry, animal husbandry and fishery industry (7.4 %). From the above, we can see the samples had significant representativeness owing to the proper distribution of samples.

133.2 The Analysis of the Recruitment Requirements of SMEs

133.2.1 Mean Analysis

Judging from the interpretation capacity, the higher score of the mean is, the stronger interpretation power a certain item has. This paper firstly analyzed the means of the items (Table 133.1), and then remove all the means which are less than 3.0 in consideration of the project explained. So we could move on to the factor analysis.

133.2.2 Factor Analysis

The factor analysis of the data collected was conducted with SPSS 16.0. Before the factor analysis, we firstly performed the KMO and Bartlett's Test (KMO = 0.845, Sig. = 0.000). It can be seen it is suitable for the factor analysis. After the first factor analysis, it can be found that the loadings of appearance and academic record are below 0.5. Then we make the second factor analysis after deleting the appearance and academic record. It conveyed that all of items were above 0.5, and then we can extract 5 factors (Table 133.2) which accounted for 73.56 % of the overall variables. The 5 factors were defined as qualification certificate, job expectations, professional ability, practice experience and professional ethics.

Table 133.1 The means of the recruitment requirements of SMEs

Item	Mean	Item	Mean	Item	Mean	Item	Mean
Specialty	3.70	Age	2.93	Gender	2.76	Appearance	3.31
Basic abilities	4.07	Job expectations	3.85	Salary expectations	3.56	Professional knowledge	3.85
Association experience	3.46	English certificate	3.07	Working environment expectations	3.62	Employment area preferences	3.14
Driving license	2.51	Professional qualifications	3.28	Experience in social practice	3.91	University reputation	2.93
Academic record	3.58	Computer certificate	3.03	Professional ethics	4.42		

Table 133.2 Rotated Component Matrix(a) of the recruitment requirements of SMEs

Item	Component				
	1	2	3	4	5
English certificate	0.773	0.050	0.267	0.035	0.119
Professional qualifications	0.823	0.096	0.046	0.211	−0.030
Computer certificate	0.850	0.211	0.134	0.119	0.060
Employment area preferences	0.174	0.782	0.063	−0.061	0.025
Job expectations	0.174	0.586	0.004	0.035	0.302
Salary expectations	0.233	0.775	−0.107	0.052	0.041
Working environment expectations	−0.179	0.759	0.081	0.202	−0.135
Specialty	0.246	0.008	0.801	−0.032	−0.204
Professional knowledge	0.240	−0.087	0.775	0.059	0.038
Basic abilities	−0.139	0.212	0.667	0.193	0.425
Experience in social practice	0.138	0.159	−0.028	0.843	0.122
Association experience	0.159	−0.006	0.152	0.787	−0.221
Professional ethics	0.096	0.000	−0.005	−0.108	0.907

133.3 Suggestions for the Talent Training of Local Colleges

133.3.1 Pay More Attention to the Non-major Education

As can be seen from recruitment requirements of SMEs, the mean of basic abilities is 4.07, which implies colleges should strengthen the cultivating of the basic abilities of their students. As we know, enhancing the professional competence of college Students is one of the most important missions of the college. However, non-professional education will also greatly contribute to the improvement of their professional competence. Therefore, local colleges should get rid of the specialization in the undergraduate education, while they should recognize the significance of non-professional education through the requirements in reality, and implement it in the education [1].

133.3.2 Innovate the Mode of Practice Teaching

The mean of social practice experience is 3.91, and the mean of association experience is 3.46, which means that SMEs pay much attention to practice experience in the recruitment. However, classroom teaching has been the major way of the college education since the classroom teaching was born, while extracurricular activities, extracurricular education and second class are in the status of auxiliary supplement. Having life and work experiences has became the college student's expectation. This requires local colleges to keep up with the trend of the times to reform the mode of talent training.

133.3.3 Strengthen the Employment Guidance

At present, college career guidance centers in Chinese colleges often lay more emphasis on offering students employment information. So they should establish a powerful employment service center referring to the Birmingham City University in order to help college students achieve employment [2]. As soon as the students enter the college, local colleges should help them have a good understanding of their own personality and professional interests, then help them establish career goals, give them comprehensive training and guidance to make full preparation for the successful employment.

133.3.4 Strengthen Academic Guidance

Many qualifications are easy to obtain and seem to be useless in the employment. However, college students tend to waste a quantity of time and energy in obtaining them due to the innocence of enterprises' requirements. Instead of guide the students correctly, many colleges promote this tendency by taking CET or other professional qualifications as the prerequisites for graduation. Therefore, local colleges should help college students recognize the effectiveness of the various qualifications, guide them to concentrate on learning and practicing to cultivate college graduates really needed.

133.4 Conclusion

This paper proposed the requirements of SMEs for colleges students, which can be defined as qualification certificate, job expectations, professional ability, practice experience and professional ethics. Based on this, it analyzed the characteristics of the recruitment requirements of SMEs. This paper also offered four pieces of advice for the talent training reform according to the recruitment requirements of SMEs. At last, since this study only focuses on SMEs, the conclusions may be one-sided, so it needs more study at a broader level.

References

1. Ling T (2006) Requirements of the Labor Market for Undergraduate Education. Peking Univ Educ Rev:126
2. Ye X (2011) Developing graduate employability: the experiences of UK and its implications. Educ Sci, pp 94–95
3. Cranmer S (2006) Enhancing graduate employability:best intentions and mixed outcomes. Stud High Educ, pp 169–184

4. Rothwell A, Arnold J (2007) Self-perceived employability: development and validation of a scale. Pers Rev 36:23–41
5. Liu Y (2011) The construction of the training system of the core competitiveness of the undergraduate Employment. J iangsu High Educ:107
6. Li L (2011) Study on the talents requirements of SMEs from recruitment pamphlets. New Educ:34

Chapter 134
Simultaneous Determination of Atractylenolide II and III in *Rhizoma Atractylodes Macrocephalae* and Chinese Medicinal Preparation by Reverse-Phase High-Performance Liquid Chromatography

Xiao-hong Sun and Jian Ge

Abstract This present paper describes the development of a reverse-phase high-performance liquid chromatography (RP-HPLC) coupled with UV spectrometry for simultaneous determination of atractylenolide II and III in traditional Chinese medicines and Chinese medicinal preparation. The standard of atractylenolide II and III was isolated from *Rhizoma Atractylodes Macrocephalae*. From a variety of solvents tested, methanol was found to be the best solvent for simultaneously extracting atractylenolide II and III from *Rhizoma Atractylodes Macrocephalae* and Chinese medicinal preparation samples. RP-HPLC analysis of the extracts was performed on an analytical column (SHIMADZU ODS, 150 × 4.6 mm; i.d., 5 μm) equipped with a security guard pre-column system. The results showed that there was a good linearity over the range 0.5–50.0 μg/ml (r > 0.99). The recoveries were more than 95.0 % in *Rhizoma Atractylodes Macrocephalae*, and the intra- and inter-day coefficients of variation were less than 5.0 % in all cases. The lower limit of quantification (LLOQ) was 0.5 μg/ml. The RP-HPLC method was readily applied to simultaneously quantitate atractylenolide II and III in *Rhizoma Atractylodes Macrocephalae* and Chinese medicinal preparation (Shenlingbaizhu granule).

Keywords Atractylenolide II · Atractylenolide III · RP-HPLC · Rhizoma atractylodes macrocephalae

---

X. Sun
Shaoxing University Yuanpei College, Shaoxing 312000, China

J. Ge (✉)
College of Life Science, China Jiliang University, #258 XueYuan Street, XiaSha Higher Education Zone, Hangzhou 310018, Zhejiang Province, People's Republic of China
e-mail: gejian16888@163.com

134.1 Introduction

Atractylenolide II and atractylenolide III, as marker substances in *Rhizoma Atractylodes Macrocephalae*, possess well-documented gastrointestinal inhibitory effects, anti-inflammatory and anticancer activity [1–3]. *Rhizoma A. macrocephala* is the dried rhizoma of *Atractylodes macrocephala* Koidz, which has been widely used in China as a herbal medicine, and reported as a nutrient for energy and for the treatment of dyspepsia and anorexia [4]. *Rhizoma A. macrocephala* was also contained in many Chinese medicinal prescriptions such as DangguiShaoyao-San (DSS). The essential oil has been isolated and is the major constituent of *Rhizoma A. macrocephala*, which has several pharmacological functions [5, 6]. In the procedures of screening and locating the effective compounds contained in DSS, Gu and his colleagues found that the volatile oil fraction extracted from DSS contributed most to the prevention and treatment of senile dementia [7]. Atractylenolide II and III were found to be the main constituents present in the effective volatile oil fraction [8] which indicate that atractylenolide II and III may be also potential effective compounds for treating senile dementia. These different effects imply that qualitative and quantitative control of the herb to ensure its maximal therapeutic value is very necessary.

Now, lots of interests are focused on describing the determination of active constituents from a lot of herbal medicines by liquid chromatography with UV detection [9, 10], GC-ECD method [11], LC–MS/MS method [12] and by capillary electrophoresis [13, 14]. So far there have been no reports on simultaneous determination of atractylenolide II and III in Chinese herbs and medicinal preparation by RP-HPLC.

Here, we report a simple, sensitive and accurate method of RP-HPLC for the simultaneous determination of atractylenolide II and III concentration in Chinese herb of *Rhizoma Atractylodes Macrocephalae* and medicinal preparation (Shenlingbaizhu granule).

134.2 Material and Method

134.2.1 Material

Atractylenolide II and atractylenolide III were isolated from the rhizome of *A. macrocephala* Koidz. Dried rhizomes of *A. macrocephala* Koidz were purchased from a traditional Chinese medicinal market in Pan'an, Zhejiang Province, China. They were crushed and sifted (i.d. 0.9 mm). Then the powder (3.5 kg) was immersed in petroleum ether (14 L) at room temperature for 5 days. The petroleum ether extract was filtered and concentrated with a rotary evaporator to remove petroleum ether, which produced a dark-brown extract (75 g). Furthermore, the extract was subjected to silica gel column chromatography (9 cm i.d. × 45 cm) with a petroleum-AcOEt gradient (100:0 98:2 95:5 90:10 85:15 80:20). One portion of the petroleum-AcOEt (90:10 85:15) eluate, after being recrystallized with EtOH, gave 0.8 g of atractylenolide II. The petroleum-AcOEt (80:20) eluate was recrystallized with EtOH to give 0.5 g of colorless crystals of atractylenolide III. The two compounds were identified to be atractylenolide II and III, respectively, by UV, IR, LC–MS and ^{1}H and ^{13}C-NMR techniques and also by comparing these data with the authentic compounds [15, 16]. The concentrations of atractylenolide II and atractylenolide III were measured by a RP-HPLC equipped with an ultraviolet (UV) detector and a RP-18C column (4.6 mm i.d. × 150 mm) with acetonitrile–water (60:40, v/v) as the mobile phase. The purity of atractylenolide II and III extracted was determined to be 99.8 and 98.5 %, respectively.

The Shenlingbaizhu granule (Beijing Hantien Pharmaceutical Co., Ltd, Beijing PR China) was purchased from a local herbal store. HPLC grade acetonitrile and methanol were purchased from Hangzhou Jiacheng Chemical Factory (Hangzhou, China).

134.2.2 RP-HPLC Method and Standard Solution

The *RP-HPLC* shimadzu 20 A system consisted of a UV detector and a Zhida N2000 instrument workstation. The analytical column was a SHIMADZU ODS C_{18} column (5 µm, 150 mm × 4.6 mm) which had an ODS C_{18} precolumn (4.6 mm × 12.5 mm). The mobile phase was composed of acetonitrile–water (50:50, v/v). The flow rate was 1.0 ml/min. Column temperature was kept at 30 °C, and the UV detector wavelength was set at 220 nm.

Stock standard solutions of atractylenolide II and III were prepared with methanol. Six concentrations of atractylenolide II and III solution for the calibration curve were prepared by dilution from the stock solution. The calibration range was 0.5 ~ 50.0 µg/ml atractylenolide II and III. Calibration standards were assayed following the method mentioned above. The calibration curve was constructed based on peak-areas of atractylenolide II and III (y) versus concentrations of atractylenolide II and III (x).

134.2.3 Sample Preparation

For the analysis of the atractylenolide II and III, 0.2 g of powdered plant and 2.00 g of powder of Shenlingbaizhu granule were accurately weighed and extracted with 5 and 10 ml methanol separately for 30 min by ultrasonication. After that, it was maintained at room temperature for 30 min. The extracts were filtered through a 0.45 µm membrane before analysis.

The precision and accuracy of the method were assessed for intra-day and inter-day on five different days. The precision was expressed as the percent coefficient of variation. And the recoveries were determined by adding known amounts of the standard of atractylenolide II and III to the samples at beginning of the process.

134.3 Results

134.3.1 Specificity of Chromatograms

The RP-HPLC chromatogram peak of atractylenolide II and III as assayed using the standard solution was at 21.615 and 10.365 min, respectively (Fig. 134.1a). A chromatogram of samples taken from *Rhizoma Atractylodes Macrocephalae* and Chinese medicinal preparation (Shenlingbaizhu granule) showed identifiable atractylenolide II and III peaks (Fig. 134.1b, c).

134.3.2 Method Development

Initially, several mobile phases were selected to separate atractylenolide II and III, including methanol: water (60:40, v/v), acetonitrile: water (50:50, v/v), acetonitrile: water (60:40, v/v). However, only when acetonitrile: water (50:50, v/v) was used as mobile phase, atractylenolide II and III in extracts could be well separated by the RP-HPLC.

134.3.3 Calibration and Validation

Evaluation of the assay was performed with a calibration curve over the concentration range 0.5 ~ 50.0 µg/ml atractylenolide II and III. The slope and

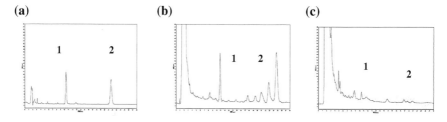

Fig. 134.1 Chromatograms of **a** a standard solution of atractyleolide II and atractyleolide III at 5 µg/mL; **b** *Rhizoma Atractylodes Macrocephalae*; **c** Chinese medicinal preparation, respectively. *Peak 1* atractyleolide III; *Peak 2* atractyleolide II

intercept of the calibration graph were calculated by weighted least squares linear regression. The regression equation of the curve and the correlation coefficients (r) were calculated as followed. Good liner relationship between the peak-area and the concentrations was observed.

$$\text{Atractylenolide II} \quad Y = 47456X + 9489.6 \quad r = 0.9999$$
$$\text{Atractylenolide III} \quad Y = 35397X + 5829.6 \quad r = 0.9999$$

The lower limit of quantification (LLOQ) was defined as the lowest concentration on the calibration curve that can be determined with acceptable precision. The LLOQ was found to be 0.5 μg/ml for atractylenolide II and III. The accuracy and precision of the method were evaluated at concentrations of 0.5, 5, 50 μg/ml. The intra-day precisions and inter-day precisions were less than 5.0 % for all three concentrations (Table 134.1). The data proved good precision and accuracy of the RP-HPLC method developed.

Extraction recovery was determined with the standard addition method for atractylenolide II and III in real sample. The standards of atractylenolide II and III were accurately weighed and mixed with fine powder of *A. macrocephala* Koidz, the mixture was extracted and analyzed using the proposed method. The extraction recoveries were 102.3 % for atractylenolide II (RSD = 1.92 %) and 95.5 % for atractylenolide III (RSD = 2.43 %), which were nearly identical and approaching 100 %, suggesting little atractylenolide II and III were lost in the recovery procedure.

134.3.4 Determination of Atractylenolide II and III in Rhizoma Atractylodes Macrocephalae and Chinese Medicinal Preparations

The extracts of *Rhizoma Atractylodes Macrocephalae* and Chinese medicinal preparation (Shenlingbaizhu granule) were determined under the above method, the calculated contents of atractylenolide II and III were show in Table 134.2. Peaks were identified by the addition of the standard atractylenolide II and III.

Table 134.1 Intra- and interday precision and accuracy of the method (n = 5)

	Accuracy (%)		RSD (%)	
	Intra-day	Inter-day	Intra-day	Inter-day
II	104.82 ± 4.02	96.43 ± 3.09	3.83	3.20
	104.76 ± 1.08	95.82 ± 2.95	1.03	3.08
	103.10 ± 1.73	103.12 ± 2.61	1.58	2.35
III	101.95 ± 3.84	96.37 ± 4.32	3.77	4.48
	104.71 ± 0.89	100.69 ± 0.98	0.85	0.97
	103.62 ± 1.30	101.67 ± 2.05	1.26	2.02

Table 134.2 Percentage content of atractylenolide II and atractylenolide III in real samples (dry plant and Chinese medicinal preparation) (n = 3)

	Rhizoma Atractylodes Macrocephalae		Shenlingbaizhu granule	
	Content (%)	RSD (%)	Content (%)	RSD (%)
II	0.0070	1.46	0.00258	0.56
III	0.021	4.77	0.0008	2.14

134.4 Discussion

A specific, simple, sensitive and accurate RP-HPLC method has been developed and validated for the simultaneously quantitative determination of atractylenolide II and III in *Rhizoma Atractylodes Macrocephalae* and Chinese medicinal preparation (Shenlingbaizhu granule). According to some reported literatures, there were some methods used to determine the atractylenolide chemicals. However, this established RP-HPLC method was also used for determination of atractylenolide compounds in Chinese medicinal preparations including *Rhizoma Atractylodes Macrocephalae*.

Acknowledgments This work was supported financially by the National Natural Science Foundation of China (31100499) and Zhejiang Provincial Analytical Project (2011C37044). Besides, the article was also funded by Shao-xin Sciences and Technology Project (2011A22009).

References

1. Zhang YQ, Xu SB, Lin YC (1999) Gastrointestinal inhibitory effects of sesquiterpene lactones from *Atractylodes macrocephala*. J Chinese Med Mater 12: 636–640
2. Dong HY, Dong YL, He LC et al (2007) Studies on constituents and anti-inflammatory activity of Rhizoma *Atractylodis macrocephalae*. Chinese Pharm J 42:1055–1059
3. Liu Y, Qiu GQ, Zhang M et al (2005) Effects of lactone II from *Atractylodes macrophala Koidz* on cytokines and proteolysis inducing factors in cachectic cancer patients. J First Mil Med Univ 10:1308–1311
4. The Pharmacopoeia Committee of China (2005) The Chinese pharmacopoeia, part I. The Chemical Industry Publishing House, Beijing
5. Endo K, Taguchi T, Taguchi F et al (1979) Antiinflammatory principles of Atractylodes Rhizomes. Chem Pharm Bull 27:2954–2958
6. Matsuda H, Li YH, Taniguchi K et al (1991) Imaging analysis of antiulcer action and the active constituent of *Atractylodis* Rhizoma. Yakugaku Zassh 111:36
7. Gu W, Zhu DN, Yan YQ (2004) Studies on chemical constituents of Danggui Shaoyao and its mechanism in preventing and treatment of senile dementia VI- active chemical components. China J Exp Tradit Med Formulae 10:1–3
8. Li W, Wen HM, Zhang AH (2001) Study on quality of *Atractylodes macrophala* Koidz-determination of 2 atractylenolides by HPLC. Chinese J Pharm Anal 21:170–172

9. Cappra SAP, Koester LS, Mayorga P et al (2007) Development and validation of a LC method for detection of genistein in topical nano emulsions. Pharmazie 62:732–734
10. Kumar V, Mostafa S, Kayo MW et al (2006) Derendorf H. HPLC determination of dexamethasone in human plasma and its application to an in vitro release study from endovascular stents. Pharmazie 61:908–911
11. Sun X, Guo T, He J et al (2006) Simultaneous determination of diallyl trisulfide and diallyl disulfide in rat blood by gas chromatography with electron-capture detection. Pharmazie 61:985–988
12. Xu W, Sun J, Zhang TT et al (2006) A rapid HPLC/ESI-MS method for the quantitative determination of oridonin in rat plasma. Pharmazie 757–759
13. Avula B, Begum S, Ahmed S et al (2008) Quantitative determination of vasicine and vasicinone in *Adhatoda vasica* by high performane capillary electrophoresis. Pharmazie 63:20–22
14. Favier LS, Acosta G, Gomez MR et al (2006) Determination and assay validation of the bioactive sesquiterpene lactone xanthatin isolated from *Xanthium cavanillesii* using capillary electrophoresis. Pharmazie 61:981–984
15. Hikino H, Hikino Y, Yosioka I (1964) Studies on the constituents of atractylodes. IX. Structure and autoxidation of atractylon. Chem Pharm Bull 7: 755–760
16. Pachaly P, Lansing A, Sin KS (1985) Constituents of *Atractylis koreana*. Planta Med 55:59–61

Chapter 135
Research on the Pharmacokinetics and Elimination of Epigallocatechin Gallate (EGCG) in Mice

Yang Liu, Jian Ge, Meng-xin Wang, Lin Cui and Bao-yu Han

Abstract The study was designed to investigate the metabolic kinetics and elimination of Epigallocatechin Gallate (EGCG) in mouse's tissues, basing on establishing a RP-HPLC method for determination of EGCG in mice plasma, liver, heart, spleen, kidney, pancreas, brain, testis, feces and urine. And the results showed that there was a good linearity over the range 0.1–200.0 mg/L (r > 0.999) for plasma and 0.5–200.0 mg/kg (r > 0.999) for other tissues. The recoveries were more than 85.0 % in all samples, and the intra-and inter-day coefficients of variation were less than 15.0 % in all cases. So the RP-HPLC method was readily applied for pharmacokinetics and elimination of EGCG in mice. EGCG was widely distributed in all the tissues of mice. But it was fast metabolized and eliminated from mice, and the main elimination way was metabolized by hydrolysis enzymes and excreted from urine.

Keywords EGCG · Elimination · Metabolism · RP-HPLC

135.1 Introduction

In recent years, with the deep research on pharmacological effects and its biological activity, the biotransformation of green tea extract catechins has also become one of the hot areas of the researchers. The realization of antioxidant and anticancer activity of catechins EGCG depends on its biotransformation in the

---

Y. Liu · J. Ge (✉) · M. Wang · L. Cui
Department of Pharmacy, China Jiliang University, Hangzhou 310018, China

B. Han (✉)
Zhejiang Provincial Key Laboratory of Biometrology and Inspection and Quarantine,
#258 XueYuan Street XiaSha Higher Education Zone, Hangzhou 310018,
Zhejiang Province, China
e-mail: han-insect@263.net

body (absorption, distribution, metabolism, excretion), so it is helpful for understanding the catechins dynamic process in vivo to clarify the relationship of effective ingredients and its health effects [1–4]. Therefore, researching on the pharmacokinetics changes of catechins and evaluating catechin's absorption, distribution and utilization could provide scientific and reasonable evaluation of tea and tea drinks industry development. Scholars at home and abroad for catechin research mainly focuses on the extraction, purification of effective components, concentration analysis and pharmacological activities, while system research on the pharmacokinetics and elimination of catechins in vivo has rarely reported in the literature.

Comparative study on the elimination of catechins in vivo and in vitro is useful to discovery some new substances with high biological activity and it is important for the development of new drugs and new health care products. This paper aimed to investigate the distribution tissues and elimination way of catechins EGCG in mice and explore the clearing rule of catechins in vivo and in vitro. It can provide a reference method and theoretical basis for the study of new catechins drugs or new health production's interaction process in the body. Therefore, it is important for us to further strengthen the clinical application of the catechins health activity and safety, expand catechin compounds usage range and development space [5, 6] and further enhance the technological content and added value of tea.

135.2 Material and Method

135.2.1 Material and Reagents

The EGCG standard (20101012) was purchased from Hang Zhou Hetian Biotechnology Co., Ltd, China. The purity was higher than 98 %. Chromatography methanol and acetonitrile were purchased from Hang Zhou Milk Chemical Instrument Co., Ltd, China. All other agents were analytical grade.

135.2.2 Chromatographic Method of HPLC

The HPLC system used in this research was SHIMADZU-20AT series equipment, with a UV detector and a Zheda N2000 instrument workstation written by Zhejiang University. EGCG separation was achieved on a Hypersil BDS C18 reversed-phase column (5 μm, 250 mm × 4.6 mm). The mobile phase was composed of acetonitrile and 0.1 % citric acid solution (10:90, V/V) at a flow-rate of 1.0 mL/min. The column temperature was kept at 30 °C and the detector wavelength was set at 280 nm. The 20 μL were injected directly into the RP-HPLC system.

135.2.3 Assay of EGCG in Different Tissues

Quantitative homogenates were added into normal saline with a proportion of 1:1. After mixing, 30–150 μL ascorbic acid (20 %) was added to 0.3–1.5 mL homogenates. After vortexing a lot minutes, 3 mL ethyl acetate was added, respectively. The tube was vortex-mixed for 5 min. After centrifugation (6,000 r/min) for 5 min, the organic phase was transferred to a glass test-tube. And this extraction was repeated twice. All the organic phase were blended and evaporated to dryness at 45 °C under a weak stream of nitrogen gas. The residue was reconstituted with 1.0 mL acetonitrile–water (1:4, V/V), vortex-mixed for 1 min and centrifuged (6,000 r/min) for 3 min. And all the supernatant was transferred to a tube and added into 1.0 mL n-hexane. After centrifugation (6,000 r/min) for 3 min, all the n-hexane was discarded. This extraction was repeated twice. After centrifugation (18,000 r/min) for 5 min, 20 μL were injected directly into the RP-HPLC system.

135.2.4 Calibration Curve

EGCG standards were prepared with methanol. Six concentrations of EGCG for the calibration curve were prepared by dilution from the stock solution. The serial solutions were evaporated to dryness at 45 °C under a weak stream of nitrogen gas. Then 1.0 mL of EGCG-free homogenates was added. The calibration range was 0.1–200.0 mg EGCG per liter for plasma tissue (0.5–200.0 mg EGCG per kg for other tissues). Calibration standards were extracted and assayed according to the method mentioned above. The calibration curve was constructed based on peak-area of EGCG (y) versus. concentration of spiked EGCG (x). Then the standard curve equations and correlation coefficient (r) were calculated by the software excel 2003.

135.2.5 Extraction Recovery and Precision

Blank intestine and feces homogenates were spiked with the standards of EGCG at low (1.0 mg/L), medium (10.0 mg/L) and high (50.0 mg/L) concentrations, which were used as quality control samples (QC) later within the calibration curve. Recovery of EGCG with extraction method above was determined by comparing observed peak-area in extracted samples to those of non-processed standard solutions.

Precision of the method were assessed by assaying five replicate QC samples above, respectively. Intra-day precision was evaluated at different times during the same day. Inter-day precision was determined over five different days.

135.2.6 EGCG Concentration Measurement in Mice's Tissue

Male ICR mice (25 ± 2 g) were purchased from the Experimental Animal Center of Zhejiang Academy of Medical Sciences, adaptive feeding for a week in the IVC independent ventilation of the laboratory cage. After fasting 12 h before the experiment, these mice were intraperitoneally injected with catechins EGCG at a dose of 150 mg/kg. Then all the blood and other organs were collected at different time points after injection. And 0–12 and 12–24 h urine and feces were also collected respectively and handled by the method mentioned above. EGCG peak areas measured after sample injection by HPLC method were substituted into the equation of the corresponding standard curve to calculate the concentration in the plasma and tissue samples. Then the EGCG concentration-time curve was drawn according to these EGCG concentrations. EGCG pharmacokinetics parameters were calculated by the formula of pharmacokinetics. And the distribution concentrations of EGCG in other tissues were also determined by the same methods.

135.3 Results

135.3.1 Specificity of Chromatograms

The RP-HPLC chromatogram peak of EGCG assayed by the standard solution was 14.932 min (Fig. 135.1a). No significant interfering peak appeared for normal tissue samples (Fig. 135.1b). Blank tissue samples spiked with EGCG also yielded chromatogram peaks identical to that by the standard solution (Fig. 135.1c). A chromatogram of a liver tissue sample obtained after metabolism in vitro showed that identifiable EGCG peak was clear and strong without any endogenous substances at the corresponding time (Fig. 135.1d).

135.3.2 Calibration Curve

Evaluation of the method was performed with a calibration curve over the concentration range 0.1–200.0 mg • L^{-1} EGCG (0.5–200.0 mg • kg^{-1} EGCG in other tissue). The slope and intercept of the calibration graph were calculated by weighted least squares linear regression. The regression equation of the curve and correlation coefficients (r) were calculated as followed. A liner relationship between peak-area and concentrations was good (Table 135.1).

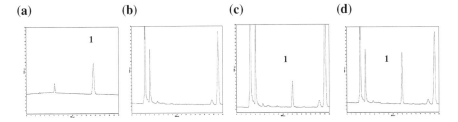

Fig. 135.1 EGCG standard solution chromatogram **a** Blank liver tissue chromatogram; **b** blank liver tissue spiked with EGCG; **c** liver tissue chromatogram after administration; and **d** peak 1: EGCG

Table 135.1 EGCG curve equation and correlation coefficient

Samples	Curve equation	Correlation (r)
Kidney	y = 12101 x−275.53	r = 0.999 9
Spleen	y = 4021.2 x + 1959	r = 0.999 8
Testis	y = 11994 x−1532.9	r = 0.999 8

135.3.3 Recoveries and Precision

The intra-day and inter-day precisions were less than 10.0 % for all three concentrations. Extraction recovery of EGCG at concentrations of 0.5, 5.0 and 50.0 mg • L^{-1} in plasma and tissues were more than 80.0 %, respectively. All the datum of EGCG proved good precision and extraction recovery of the RP-HPLC method developed (Table 135.2).

135.3.4 EGCG Pharmacokinetics and Elimination

Male ICR mice were intraperitoneally injected by the above-described method, and the plasma EGCG peak area was measured at different time points. Then the

Table 135.2 Extraction recovery and precision in different tissues (n = 5)

Samples	Concentration mg/L	Recovery (%)	Precision (%)	
			Intra	Inter
Kidney	1.0	87.41 ± 8.29	6.82	9.49
	10.0	91.86 ± 7.05	5.88	7.67
	50.0	94.36 ± 6.27	6.64	7.86
Spleen	1.0	88.61 ± 8.43	7.38	9.51
	10.0	90.87 ± 8.21	5.26	9.03
	50.0	93.33 ± 6.82	4.52	7.31
Testis	1.0	86.42 ± 7.58	8.71	9.83
	10.0	91.31 ± 9.11	6.28	9.98
	50.0	93.36 ± 7.27	3.28	7.79

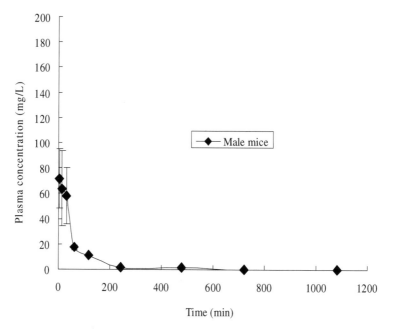

Fig. 135.2 Mean plasma concentration–time curve in male mice. Each point represents the mean EGCG concentration of five mice

concentrations of EGCG in different tissues were calculated by the curve equation established above and concentration–time curve was drawn (Fig. 135.2). Pharmacokinetic parameters were figured out according to the following drug dynamics calculation formula following below (see Table 135.3).

And the distribution and excretion of EGCG in mice was investigated and calculated here (see Figs. 135.3 and 135.4).

$$C = Ae^{-\alpha t} + Be^{-\beta t} \quad AUC = \frac{A}{\alpha} + \frac{B}{\beta} \quad t_{\frac{1}{2}(\beta)} = \frac{0.693}{\beta} \quad t_{\frac{1}{2}(\alpha)} = \frac{0.693}{\alpha}$$

135.4 Discussion

The experimental research clarified the catechin EGCG pharmacokinetics and elimination law, basing on catechin EGCG elimination kinetics and tissue distribution characteristics in plasma, liver, kidney, spleen, pancreas, and testis tissue. The results showed that catechins EGCG was widely distributed and fast eliminated in mice. The distribution half-life and elimination half-life were 25.48 and 182.37 min, respectively. According to the literature, there is significantly difference about catechins bioavailability, pharmacokinetics parameters, plasma concentration–time curve. Besides, there was a markedly difference between the data

Table 135.3 Pharmacokinetics parameters calculated from the EGCG plasma concentration study in male and female mice

Parameters	Unit	Male mice
$t_{1/2\alpha}$	min	25.48
$t_{1/2\beta}$	min	182.37
AUC	mg·min/L	0.81
CL_T	L/min	0.0059
V_d	L/kg	1.55
C_{max}	mg/L	96.48

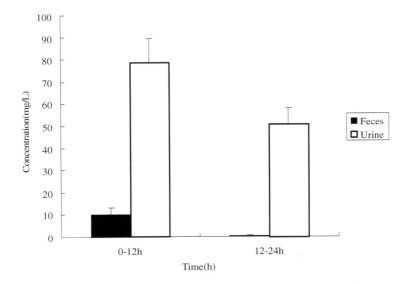

Fig. 135.3 Excretion of EGCG in feces and urine

analyzed from electrochemical detector. EGCG is mainly free form in plasma, which is easy to be metabolism. However, EGC and EC are conjugated with other endogenous compounds, so they are more stable [6]. A few reported showed that the levels of EGCG, EGC, and EC in plasma and tissues were quantified by HPLC with PCNONLIN program. Besides, the plasma concentration–time curves of EGCG, EGC and EC were fitted in a two-compartment model. And only 0.1 % of EGCG was bioavailable by the ratio of AUCi.g./AUCi.v. in plasma. The level of EGCG was found to be the highest in the intestine samples. The levels of EGCG, EGC, and EC in liver and lung were generally lower than those in the intestine and the kidney. The distribution results suggest that EGCG is mainly metabolized by some metabolic enzymes and excreted through bile [7]. A certain experiment show that EGCG was also eliminated in the enterohepatic circulation [8]. Our experiment confirmed that EGCG were widely distributed in mice and it was eliminated fast.

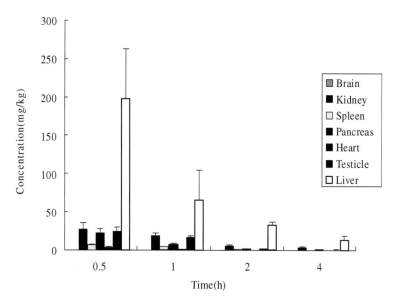

Fig. 135.4 Distribution of EGCG in different tissues

Acknowledgments This work was supported financially by the National Natural Science Foundation of China (31100499 and 31071744) and Natural Science Foundation of Zhejiang Province (Y3080255 and Y3100375). Besides, the article was also funded by Zhejiang Provincial Innovative Research Team Project of University Students (2012R409050).

References

1. Ge J, Lin F, Li MK et al (2011) Research progress on biological activity of epigallocatechin-3-gallate (EGCG). J Anhui Agric Univ 38(2):156–163
2. Ikuo I, Youji I, Eiji S, et al (1992) Tea catechins decrease micellar solubility and intestinal absorption of cholesterol in rats. Biochimica Biophysica Acta (BBA)-lipids and lipid metabolism 1127(2):141–146
3. Lambert Joshua D, Yang Chung S (2003) Cancer chemopreventive activity and bioavalability of tea and tea polypheols. Mutat Res 523–524:201–208
4. Elmets CA, Singh D, Tubesing K et al (2001) Cutaneous photoprotection from ultraviolet injury by green tea polyphenols. J Am Acad Dermatol 44:425–432
5. Williamson MP, McCormick TG, Nance Christina L, et al (2006) Epigallocatechin gallate, the main polyphenoL in green tea, binds to the T-cell receptor, CD4: potential for HIV-therapy. J Allergy Clin Immunol 18(6):1369–1374
6. Lee MJ, Maliakal P, Chen L et al (2002) Pharmacokinetics of tea catechins after ingestion of green tea and (-)-epigallocatechin-3-gallate by humans: formation of different metabolites and individual variability. Cancer Epidemiol Biomark Prev 11:1025–1032
7. Chen L, Lee MJ, Li H et al (1997) Absorption, distribution and elimination of tea polyphenols in rats. Drug Metab Dispos 9:1045–1050
8. Moon YJ, Morris ME (2007) Pharmacokinetics and bioavailability of the bioflavanoid biochanin A: effects of quercetin and EGCG on biochanin A disposition in rats. Mol Pharm 4(6):865–872

Chapter 136
Simultaneous Determination of Five Phthalic Acid Esters (PAEs) in Soil and Air

Tian-yu Hu, Yang Liu, Hua-jun Hu, Meng-xin Wang, Bao-yu Han and Jian Ge

Abstract This present paper describes the development of a gas chromatography(GC) coupled with a Flame Ionization Detector (FID) for simultaneous determination of five Phthalic Acid Esters (PAEs) chemicals in soil and air. Five PAEs chemicals were purchased from J&K Chemicals Ltd, Shanghai, China. From a variety of solvents tested, ethyl acetate was found to be the best solvent for simultaneously extracting five chemicals from soil and air samples. GC (Agilent 6890) analysis of the extracts was performed on an analytical column (HP-5 capillary column, 30 m and 0.25 × 250 μm). The results showed that there was a good linearity over the range 0.625–40.0 μg/mL ($r > 0.99$). The recoveries were more than 85.0 % in soil and air samples, and the intra- and inter-day coefficients of variation were less than 15.0 % in all cases. The lower limit of quantification (LLOQ) was 0.625 μg/mL. The GC-FID method was readily applied to simultaneously quantitate five PAEs chemicals in soil and air extract samples.

Keywords PAEs chemicals · GC-FID · Soil · Air

T. Hu · Y. Liu · H. Hu · M. Wang
College of Life Sciences, China Jiliang University, Hangzhou 310018, China

Bao-yuHan · J. Ge (✉)
Zhejiang Provincial Key Laboratory of Biometrology and Inspection and Quarantine, China Jiliang University, Hangzhou 310018, China
e-mail: gejian16888@163.com

J. Ge
XiaSha Higher Education Zone, Zhejiang Province, #258 XueYuan Street, Hangzhou 310018, China

136.1 Introduction

As important plastic-modifying additives, Phthalic Acid Esters (PAEs) are widely used in the production of plastic plasticizer, agricultural chemicals, coating material, dyeing and finishing, as well as cosmetics and spices. And along with the worldwide consumption of these products by human beings, PAEs have become largely diffused in the environment [1–4]. But as a kind of endocrine-disrupting compounds, PAEs possess estrogenic activities, which can influence the hormone metabolism in animals' reproduction and development process, thus affect the normal behavior of these animals. Further more, the bioaccumulation of PAEs in organisms will bring potential threats to aquatic and human beings through food chain transfer [5–8]. Therefore, the US EPA have classified six kinds of PAEs compounds, including DMP as priority control pollutants [9], and three kinds of PAEs, including DMP are also on China's major pollutants blacklist [10].

In this research, the soil and air concentrations of five PAEs chemicals have been well determined, which included dimethyl phthalate (DMP), diethyl phthalate (DEP), dibutyl phthalate (DBP), butyl benzyl phthalate (BBP) and diethylhexyl phthalate (DEHP). Therefore, the study will provide theory basis for environmental pollution control, food safety, aquatic toxicology, fishing sources protection and aquatic products safety.

136.2 Material and Method

136.2.1 Material and Reagents

The standard DMP, DEP, DBP, BBP and DEHP (purity ≥99 %) were purchased from J&K Chemicals Ltd, Shanghai, China. All chemical agents, including ethyl acetate, methanol and acetonitrile for the analysis of five chemicals were of the HPLC grade, which were all obtained from Hangzhou Milk Chemical Instrument Co., Ltd, China.

136.2.2 Chromatographic Method of GC-FID

The GC system was Agilent 6890 GC series equipment, with a Flame Ionization Detector and Capillary Column (HP-5, 30 m and 0.25 × 250 μm). And the carrier gas was high-purity Helium, with a flow rate of 40 mL/min, while the combustion gases were high-purity Hydrogen and air. In the study, the splitless injection model was used and the volume was 1 μL. And the column temperature was maintained at 80 °C for 1 min at first, then it would be increased to 235 °C at a rate of 30 °C/min. Then the temperature would be maintained at 235 °C for 15 min and increased to

290 °C at a rate of 5 °C/min. The temperatures of injection port and detector were 280 °C and 300 °C, respectively.

136.2.3 Assay of Five PAEs Chemicals in Soil and Air

For the analysis of the five chemicals, 2 g soil was powdered and accurately weighed. Then a 3 ml ethyl acetate was added to the soil sample, which would be vortex-mixed and centrifugated (6,000 rpm) for 5 min separately hereafter. Then the organic phase was transferred to a glass test-tube. And this extraction would be repeated twice. After that, all the organic phase were collected together and evaporated to dryness at 45 °C under a weak stream of nitrogen gas. Then the residue was reconstituted with 0.4 mL n-hexane, vortex-mixed for 1 min and centrifuged (18,000 rpm) for 5 min. The 1 μL were injected directly into the GC system.

PAEs chemicals in air were collected via a custom-made push–pull aeration system that included a glass cylinder (18 cm internal diameter, 10 L volume) with one air-in adapter (7 mm ID) on one end and one air-out adapter (7 mm ID) on the other end. Once started, the air in our lab or outside the lab was pumped into the cylinder at 100 mL/min, and PAEs chemicals from air were trapped onto 80 mg of Super Q absorbent (80/100 mesh; Alltech Associates., Inc., Deerfield, IL, USA) at the outlet end. During the collection, flow-meters were used to calculate the air volume and insure that the air flow was not stead-going (See Fig. 136.1). After 1 h, the absorbent was eluted with 3 mL ethyl acetate. Then these ethyl acetate was evaporated to dryness at 45 °C under a weak stream of nitrogen gas. Then the residue was reconstituted with 0.4 mL n-hexane, vortex-mixed for 1 min and centrifuged (18,000 rpm) for 5 min. The 1 μL were injected directly into the GC system (Fig. 136.2).

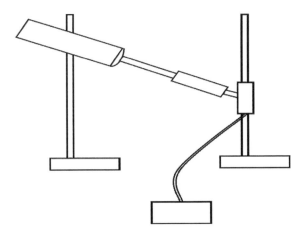

Fig. 136.1 The collector of air

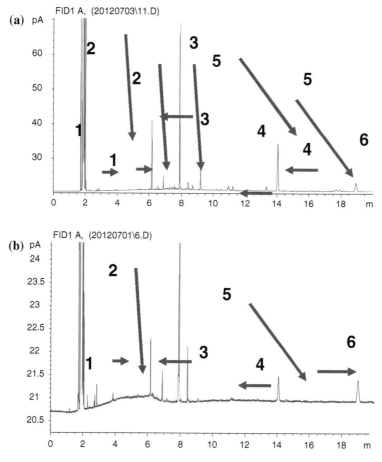

Fig. 136.2 PAEs chromatogram **a** PAEs standard solution chromatogram; **b** Blank soil chromatogram; *Peak 1* DMP; *Peak 2* DEP; *Peak 3* DBP; *Peak 4* BBP; *Peak 5* DEHP

136.2.4 Calibration Curve

PAEs chemical standard solutions were prepared with methanol. Six concentrations of PAEs chemical for the calibration curve were prepared by dilution from the stock solution. The serial solution (0.6 mL each concentration) were evaporated to dryness at 45 °C under a weak stream of nitrogen gas. Then 0.6 mL of PAEs-free soil was added. The calibration range was 0.625–40 μg PAEs chemical per milliliter. Calibration standards were extracted and assayed according to the method mentioned above. The calibration curve was constructed based on peak-area of PAEs chemical (y) versus concentrations of spiked PAEs chemical (x). Then the standard curve equations and correlation coefficient (r) were calculated by the software excel 2003.

PAEs chemical standard solutions (0.625–40 μg PAEs chemical per milliliter) were indirectly injected into GC-FID, and the calibration curves were established and used to calculated PAEs concentrations in air.

136.2.5 Extraction Recovery and Precision

Blank soil samples were spiked with the standards of PAEs chemical standard solutions at low (1.25 μg/mL), medium (5.0 μg/mL) and high (20.0 μg/mL) concentrations, which were used as quality control samples (QC) later within the calibration curve. Recovery of PAEs chemical standard solutions with extraction method above was determined by comparing observed peak-area ratios in extracted soil samples to those of non-processed standard solutions.

Precision of the method were assessed by assaying five replicate QC samples above, respectively. Intra-day precision was evaluated at different times during the same day. Inter-day precision was determined over five different days.

136.2.6 Determination of PAEs Chemicals in Soil and Air

The soil used to determine PAEs chemicals was collected from the farm in our campus, and these soils were assayed and determined by the methods mentioned above. The air was also collected in our campus by the collector mentioned above.

136.3 Results

136.3.1 Determination of PAEs Chemicals in Soil and Air

The soil used to determine PAEs chemicals was collected from the farm in our campus, and these soils were assayed and determined by the methods mentioned above. The air was also collected in our campus by the collector mentioned above.

136.3.2 Calibration and Validation of Method

Evaluation of the method was performed with a calibration curve over the concentration range 0.625–40.0 $\mu g \cdot mL^{-1}$ (g^{-1}) PAEs. The slope and intercept of the calibration graph were calculated by weighted least squares linear regression. The regression equation of the curve and correlation coefficients (r) were calculated as

Table 136.1 Curve equation and correlation coefficient of PAEs chemicals in soil

PAEs	Curve equation	Correlation
DMP	$Y = 0.9371X + 0.1151$	$r = 0.9992$
DEP	$Y = 1.1806X + 0.1922$	$r = 0.9992$
DBP	$Y = 1.1219X + 0.7801$	$r = 0.9993$
BBP	$Y = 1.1291X + 1.8493$	$r = 0.9991$
DEHP	$Y = 1.8189X + 0.9528$	$r = 0.9992$

Table 136.2 Recovery and precision of DMP and DEP in soil (n = 5)

Samples	Recovery (%)	Precision(%)	
		Intra day	Inter day
DMP	84.31 ± 7.09	8.15	9.21
	87.76 ± 6.05	7.24	7.95
	91.26 ± 6.37	6.14	7.66
DEP	85.24 ± 7.05	8.01	9.11
	90.21 ± 7.01	8.58	9.02
	93.14 ± 6.52	6.19	8.05

followed. A liner relationship between peak-area and concentrations was good (Table 136.1).

The lower limit of quantification (LLOQ) was found to be 0.625 µg · mL^{-1} (g^{-1}) for PAEs in soil. The intra-day and inter-day precisions were less than 15.0 % for all three concentrations. Extraction recovery of PAEs at concentrations of 1.25, 5.0 and 20.0 µg · mL^{-1} (g^{-1}) in soil were more than 80.0 %, respectively. All the datum of PAEs proved good precision and extraction recovery of the GC-FID method developed (Table 136.2).

136.3.3 Recoveries and Precision

The intra-day and inter-day precisions were less than 10.0 % for all three concentrations. Extraction recovery of EGCG at concentrations of 0.5, 5.0 and 50.0 mg · L^{-1} in plasma and tissues were more than 80.0 %, respectively. All the datum of EGCG proved good precision and extraction recovery of the RP-HPLC method developed (Table 136.2).

136.3.4 Determination of PAEs Chemicals in Soil and Air

After determination of PAEs chemicals in soil and air, the PAEs contents in soil were calculated in Fig. 136.3. Besides, their concentrations in air was followed in Fig. 136.4.

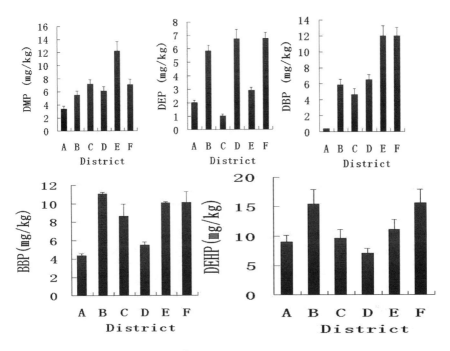

Fig. 136.3 PAEs concentrations in soil

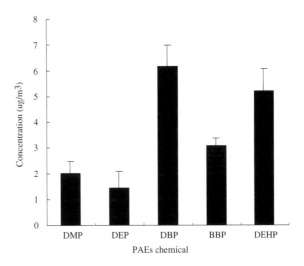

Fig. 136.4 PAEs concentrations in air

136.4 Discussion

As PAEs chemicals are classified as endocrine-disrupting compound, they will disrupt animals' endocrine function through hypothalamus-pituitary–gonadal axis, resulting in endocrine disturbance, and affect the normal reproduction and development of animals finally [5–8]. Besides, the animal's endocrine system is closely connected with immune system, so the DMP will also diminish the immune system because of the endocrine system disturbance, making animals liable to disease [11]. So the distribution of PAEs chemicals in soil do have great impacts on the accumulation and toxicological effects of PAEs.

Here the GC-FID method was specific, simple, sensitive and accurate for determination of PAEs chemicals in soil and air. And this method was successfully applied to PAEs chemicals distribution study in soil and air.

Acknowledgments This work was supported financially by the National Natural Science Foundation of China (31100499) and Natural Science Foundation of Zhejiang Province (Y3080255). Besides, the article was also funded by Zhejiang Provincial Analytical Project (2011C37044).

References

1. Wu PG, Han GG, Wang HH et al (1999) An investigation on phthalates in drinking water. J Environ Health 16(6):338–339
2. Lin XT, Chen M, Wang XY et al (2004) Analysis of phthalate esters of environmental hormone in waste water treatment plant. Environ Sci Technol 27(6):79–83
3. Chen ZL, Huang YK, Wang GM et al (2007) Detection method of phthalates of environment hormone in cosmetics. Environ Sci Technol 30(4):43–47
4. Yang Q, Zhang MS, Chen WS et al (2008) Determination of 6 kinds of phthalate ester in edible oils by Gas Chromatography. J Chin Cereals Oils Assoc 23(5):171–174
5. Van Meeuwen JA, Weterburg AH, Piersma M et al (2007) Mixture effects of estrogenic compounds on proliferation and pS2 expression of MCF-7 human breast cancer cells. Food Chem Toxicol 45(11):2319–2330
6. Salazar V, Castillo C, Ariznavarreta C et al (2004) Effect of oral intake of dibutyl phthalate on reproductive parameters of Long Evans rats and pre-pubertal development of their offspring. Toxicology 205(1):131–137
7. Foster PMD, Cattley RC, Mylchreest E (2000) Effects of di-n-butyl phthalate (DBP) on male reproductive development in the rat: implications for human risk assessment. Food Chem Toxicol 38(Suppl 1):97–99
8. Ema M, Miyawaki E, Kawashima K (2000) Effects of dibutyl phthalate on reproductive function in pregnant and pseudopregnant rats. Reprod Toxicol 14(1):13–19
9. Wang LS (1995) Chemistry of environmental pollution. Press of chemical industry, Beijing, pp 316–318
10. Hu XY, Zhang KR, Sun JH (2003) Environmental contamination by phthalates in china. Chin J Health Lab Technol 13(2):9–14
11. Lin XT, Wang XY, Lv WT et al (2009) Research progress in metabolism of phthalate esters. J Environ Health 26(2):182–184

Chapter 137
The Relationship Between Employability Self-Efficacy and Growth: The Mediator Role of e-Recruiting Perceived

Chun-Mei Chou, Chien-Hua Shen, Hsi-Chi Hsiao, Hui-Tzu Chang, Su-Chang Chen, Chin-Pin Chen, Jen-Chia Chang, Jing-Yi Chen, Kuan-Fu Shen and Hsiang-Li Shen

Abstract This study examines 672 tertiary education students' EG and its influencing factors. The results show that students' e-Recruiting perceived (ERP) has a

---

C.-M. Chou (✉)
Institute of Vocational and Technological Education, National Yunlin University of Science and Technology, Yunlin, Taiwan
e-mail: choucm@yuntech.edu.tw

C.-H. Shen
Department of Business Administration, Transworld Institute of Technology, Yunlin, Taiwan
e-mail: shen17@ms51.hinet.net

H.-C. Hsiao
Department of Business Administration, Cheng Shin University, Kaohsiung, Taiwan

H.-T. Chang
Institute of Education, National Chiao Tung University, Hsinchu, Taiwan

S.-C. Chen
Department of Marketing and Logistics and Management, National Penghu University of Science and Technology, Penghu, Taiwan

C.-P. Chen
Department of Industrial Education and Technology, National Changhua University of Education, Changhua, Taiwan

J.-C. Chang
Institute of Technological and Vocational Education, National Taipei University of Technology, Taipei, Taiwan

J.-Y. Chen
Department of Information Management, National Yunlin University of Science and Technology, Yunlin, Taiwan

K.-F. Shen
Department of Finance, Chien Hsin University of Science and Technology, Taoyuan, Taiwan

H.-L. Shen
Chien Hsin University of Science and Technology Secretariat Office, Taoyuan, Taiwan

significant direct effect on employability growth (EG), and employability self-efficacy (ESE) has a significant effect on EG through ERP. The influence pattern and empirical data of ESE and ERP on EG has a good fit.

Keywords e-Recruiting · Employability growth · Employability self-efficacy

137.1 Introduction

There are 55 % of university graduates who uncertain future career direction, and more than 50 % of university students are unsure whether the election of professional study in Taiwan [1]. Employability is becoming an important topic to promote economic growth and development in the economies of Taiwanese high education [1, 2]. As the domestic unemployment rate climbs, employment-oriented tertiary education programs urgently need to find the teaching resources for employability education in Taiwan. Development employability education plays the role of helping to reduce the unemployment rate in a country [1]. The National Youth Commission study college students' career needs, the results found career counseling services of college students most looking forward to provide employment information [3]. It is important that university education content and employment force is an urgent need to effectively link issues that enhance college students' employability and employment force [1, 3].

Employability self-efficacy was define that individuals' cognition of employment force and understand the current situation of the job market, including the social environment, employment opportunities, economic development, market conditions, work ability assessment, and awareness of the work [4, 5]. Some research found students' employability self-efficacy, e-Recruiting perceived and employability growth have provided them with chances to learn new employment skills and career making-decision, which may be helpful for their future employability and career development [6–8].

From a theory of planned behavior theory point of view, the e-Recruiting perceived (ERP) to become employability growth (EG) has been depicted as actively intention of employability [9, 10]. The availability of a validated instrument to measure skill development, employment choice, and creating job towards EG could help students' employability growth [11, 12]. e-Recruiting perceived was define the attitude towards include employment information, workplace analyses, manpower demands analyses, employment market analyses for media reports, salary level surveys, and labor market conditions [11, 12]. Therefore, high ERP of students has actually indicates towards high work capacity, social environment, and employment opportunity [13, 14].

Employability growth and given feedback from the employability self-efficacy results in which employment information processing is raised. Research suggests that employability self-efficacy (ESE) is important to affect workplace analyses and manpower demand [9, 14]. It is positively related to students' skills development, employment choice, and creating job. It is suggested that the concept of e-Recruiting, derived from planned behavior theory plays an important role in the development of ESE and EG [15, 16].

The paper, Analysis of factors in tertiary students' perceived ESE and EG, using ERP as a mediator variable, discussed the variables which may influence tertiary education student's EG and found the relationships among the variables.

137.2 Methodology

137.2.1 Subjects

This study 326 tertiary students were collected as the population, and adopts random sampling and cluster sampling for survey.

137.2.2 Research Tools

The research tool is a 'Questionnaire of Factors Which Influence Tertiary Education Students' Employability Self-Efficacy and Growth'. The questionnaire includes e-Recruiting perceived scale, employability self-efficacy scale and employability growth scale [14–16]. The "Questionnaire of Factors Which Influence Tertiary Education Students' ESE and EG" was reviewed by five experts for subject contents' suitability to ensure the scale's expert validation. Five tertiary education students were invited to answer the questionnaire to enhance the validity of the scale's contents. In addition, five tertiary education schools were selected for a pre-test, and 126 students were selected as the pre-test objects in total. The scales used in this study are in self-assessment form, and a Likert 5-point scale is used as the scoring method. The scales' factors, number of questions reliability and validity are shown in Table 137.1.

137.2.3 Data Analysis

In processing the survey data used in this study, the collected questionnaires were coded, and Statistical Package for Social Science (SPSS version 12.0) and linear structural analysis (LISREL version 8.5) were used to verify model.

Table 137.1 An overview of factors, number of questions, reliability and validity for tertiary students' ESE, ERP and EG scale

Employability self-efficacy scale				e-Recruiting perceived scale				Employability growth scale			
Factor name	No.	Cronbach α	Factor loading (%)	Factor name	No.	Cronbach α	Factor loading (%)	Factor name	No.	Cronbach α	Factor loading (%)
Work capacity	4	0.89	24.13	Employment information	4	0.89	25.20	Skills development	4	0.88	25.77
Social environment	4	0.88	22.91	Workplace analyses	4	0.87	20.93	Employment choice	4	0.87	22.23
Employment opportunity	4	0.86	18.11	Manpower demands	4	0.85	18.91	Creating job	4	0.86	18.65
Total reliability cronbach α		0.90		Total reliability cronbach α		0.91		Total reliability cronbach α		0.92	
Accumulated explained variance			65.15	Accumulated explained variance			65.04	Accumulated explained variance			66.65

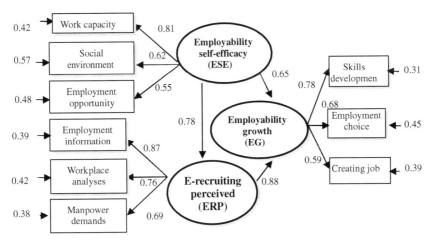

Fig. 137.1 Path of technical and vocation school students' EG

137.3 Results

The empirical results of tertiary education students' EG are shown in Fig. 137.1, and are analyzed as follows:

1. The estimated value of the direct affecting parameter between ERP and ESE is 0.78 (t = 6.19, p < 0.05). This means that ERP has a significant effect on ESE.
2. The estimated value of the direct affecting parameter between ERP and EG is 0.65 (t = 5.81, p > 0.05). This means that ERP does not necessarily have a significant effect on EG.
3. The estimated value of the direct affecting parameter between ESE and EG is 0.88 (t = 4.91, p < 0.05). This means that ESE has a significant effect on EG.

In summary, in this study of tertiary education students' EG and its influence pattern, ERP has a significant effect on ESE, but does not have a significant effect on EG, and ESE has a significant effect on EG.

137.4 Conclusion

Students' ERP has a significant direct effect on EG, and ESE has a significant effect on EG through ERP. The influence pattern and empirical data of ESE and ERP on EG has a good fit. The influence effects of ERP, ESE and EG shows that for tertiary students, the influence of ESE on EG comes mainly through their awareness of ERP. In addition, ERP has a direct and significant effect on EG. From the influence of ERP, ESE and EG, we can clearly see that compared with ESE, ERP has a greater influence on EG [11, 12].

Regarding the test results, according to the goodness of fit test standard by Hair et al., the model in this study has a good overall fit. In the absolute fitness and incremental fitness tests, all indices meet the standard, and have the best fit. Most of the parsimonious fitness indices meet the test standard, and have a good fit. Overall, in the EG and its influence model established in the study based on theories, both the model and the data have a good fit, and in the parameter estimation most of the estimated values are significant. This shows that all the indices of latent variables have their importance, and only the parameter value of ESE on EG is low. Overall, the empirical data have a good explanatory power. Students' ESE influences ERP and 'Work capacity' is an important factor which influences ESE. Students' ESE influences EG, 'skills development' and 'employment choice' are important factors which influence EG [12, 13].

The results show that among all latent variables in the model, the direct influence of ESE on EG is not significant, indicating that the assumed influence of ESE on students' EG needs further testing; this is something worthy of a more in-depth study and validation in the future. Based on test results, although the overall result is acceptable, the model consistency level is not entirely satisfactory, and its e-Recruiting perceived has a relatively low explanatory power for EG.

Acknowledgments This paper was written while the authors were supported by a grant from the National Science Council, Republic of China (NSC 101-2511-S-224 -002; **NSC** 99-2511-S-224-001-MY3).

References

1. Wu CC (2011) High graduate unemployment rate and Taiwanese undergraduate education. J Edu Deve 31:303–310
2. Shafie LA, Nayan S (2010) Employability awareness among Malaysian undergraduates. J Bus Manag 5(8):119–123
3. The National Youth Commission (2009) 98 years of the current situation of the the college youth employment force survey. Youth Commission, Taipei
4. Gracia L (2009) Employability and higher education: contextualising female students' workplace experiences to enhance understanding of employability development. J Edu Work 22(4):301–318
5. Jones B, Iredale N (2006) Developing an entrepreneurial life skills summer school. Inno Edu Tea 43(3):233–244
6. Braddy PW, Meade AW, Michael JJ, Fleenor JW (2009) Internet recruiting: effects of website content features on viewers' perceptions of organizational culture. Journal Sele Asse. doi:10.1111/j.1468-2389.2009.00448.x
7. Bohnert D, Ross WH (2010) The influence of social networking web sites on the evaluation of job candidates. Cybe Beha Soci. doi:10.1089/cyber.2009.0193
8. Walker JJ, Field HS, Giles WF, Armenakis AA, Bernerth JB (2009) Displaying employee testimonials on recruitment web sites: Effects of communication media, employee race, and job seeker race on organizational attraction and information credibility. J App Psy. doi:10.1037/a0014964

9. Van der Heijden BIJM, Boon J, Van der Klink M, Meijs E (2009) Employability enhancement through formal and informal learning: an empirical study among Dutch non-academic university staff members. J Trai Deve 13(1):19–37
10. Juhdi N, Pa'Wan F, Othman NA, Moksin H (2010) Factors influencing internal and external employability of employees. J Bus Eco 11:1–10
11. Maurer SD, Cook DP (2011) Using company web sites to e-recruit qualified applicants: a job marketing based review of theory-based research. Com in Hum Beha. doi:10.1016/j.chb.2010.07.013
12. Braddy PW, Meade AW, Michael JJ, Fleenor JW (2009) Internet recruiting: effects of website content features on viewers' perceptions of organizational culture. Int J Sele Asse. doi:10.1111/j.1468-2389.2009.00448.x
13. Guerrero M, Rialp J, Urbano D (2008) The impact of desirability and feasibility on entrepreneurial intentions: a structural equation model. J Ent Mana 4:35–50

Chapter 138
A Study to Analyze the Effectiveness of Video-Feedback for Teaching Nursing Etiquette

Xiaoling Zhu, Mulan Wei, Ruoyan Chen, Daolin Jian and Xiaofei Chen

Abstract Objection: To investigate the effects of a video-feedback method in nursing etiquette class of undergraduate nursing students. Method: The video-feedback method was applied among 36 female nursing undergraduates of Grade 2009 to a grooming etiquette class of nursing etiquette. Then the participants were given a questionnaire. Result: The survey show that the initiative enthusiasm and self-confidence of students were greatly improved after the video-feedback method being applied to the grooming etiquette class. Conclusion: The video-feedback method can greatly strengthen the self-learning and learning efficiency of students as well as reinforce the teachers' teaching ability and quality, especially in operational course.

Keywords Video-feedback method · Nursing etiquette · Grooming etiquette · Applicational effect

138.1 Introduction

Nursing etiquette is one of an important part of nursing curriculum of university, including not only some general etiquette knowledge, but also some behavior criterions and norms of nursing [1]. The appropriate choice of teaching method of nursing etiquette which is the key to completing the task of teaching and achieving teaching goals. Which is related to the level of efficiency in education and quality of

X. Zhu (✉) · M. Wei · R. Chen · D. Jian · X. Chen
China Three Gorges University Second Clinical Medical College, Yichang 443002, Hubei Province, China
e-mail: zhuxl@ctgu.edu.cn

teaching. Recently, many vocational college are still using traditional method teaching nursing classes, and the imparting of nursing etiquette knowledge has been confined to the mode that the teacher teach and the students just learn passively [1]. Taking one's self-consciousness and self-evaluation as the core, video-feedback method is a flexible teaching method with video equipment reflexing information [2]. It has been mainly applied to the field physical education [3], while less in nursing education. Now, we do a survey to investigate the effectiveness of video-feedback for teaching nursing etiquette, reporting as follows.

138.2 Sample

The study was conducted in SanXia university whose population selected probability was composed of 36 female nursing students of Grade 2009. All the participants have computer and mobile phone.

138.3 Method

Before class All the students were given clear clarification about the process of video-feedback method for grooming etiquette.

In class First, the teacher taught theoretical knowledge of make-up skills by traditional teaching method. Second, The teacher selected a students as model to demonstrate makeup process, recording the process as a standard video. Third, The students practiced in their own or others' face according to what the teacher had explained and demonstrated, recording every students'process as their individual student video. Last, the teacher selected several student videos, commenting on the process that was easy to be made mistakes to all the students.

After class the individual student video and the standard video were given to every participants to help them practice autonomously. Then, every participant was required to hand in the best demonstrated video and a picture after putting on make-up they had thought in 3 or 5 weeks.

The video and the picture handed in accounted for 40 % of the course examination results (the ending theory test accounted for 60 %).

138.4 Evaluation

The 36 students in the survey were given a homemade bearer survey questionnaire. The questionnaire included 11 items such as the understanding and satisfaction of video-feedback method interest confidence and effectiveness in learning after video-feedback method being applied to the grooming etiquette class and so on. Every item contained 6 levels (fully agree basic agree unclear basic disgree fully disagree abstention). And one open-ended questions that what was the advantage and disadvantage of video-feedback method compared with traditional method in operational class. After explaining the purposes of the research and the fill method, the 36 questionnaires were handed out. Recovery and efficiency rate of them were 100 %.

138.5 Results

Sense of identification

According to all the questionnaires, 83.4 % students had some understanding of the video-feedback method after attending the experiment. And almost 2/3 students agreed with the 11 items among which the students had the highest sense of agreement on the thought that the video-feedback method could help them review and consolidate what the had learnt in class, reaching to 94.4 % (Table 138.1).

Table 138.1 Students' cognitive evaluation of video-feedback method (n = 36)

Statement	Fully agree (%)	Agree (%)	Unknown (%)	Disagree (%)	Fully disagree (%)	Foreit (%)
I enjoy video-feedback method in grooming etiquette class	27.8	55.6	8.3	8.3	0	0
The video-feedback method can improve my interest of learning	58.3	30.6	11.1	0	0	0
The video-feedback method can increase my confidence of learning	33.3	52.8	5.6	5.6	0	2.8
The video-feedback method can raise my learning efficiency	83.3	11.1	5.6	0	0	0
The video-feedback method can fully increase my enthusiasm of learning	55.6	36.1	8.3	0	0	0
The video-feedback method can urge me to learn proactively	50.0	33.3	13.9	0	2.8	0
The video-feedback method can spur me on reviewing and consolidating what I have learnt	55.6	38.9	5.6	0	0	0
The video-feedback method can improve my ability of theory with practice	41.7	44.4	8.3	2.8	0	2.8
The video-feedback method can provide a lively atmosphere	41.7	41.7	8.3	8.3	0	0
I think the video-feedback method can enhance teachers, teaching quality	33.3	50.0	11.1	5.6	0	0
I think the video-feedback method is creative	36.1	41.7	13.9	5.6	2.8	0

In the open-ended question, most students think the video-feedback method is novel and it help them improve their interest of learning, self-confidence in learning and efficiency of learning. However, some students hold the view that the video-feedback method somehow occupies personal spare time.

138.6 Discussion

- The video-feedback method can improve students' initiative and enthusiasm, changing students' learning from passive learning to active learning, and increase their learning efficiency. Recently, the teaching method of nursing etiquette of many Chinese universities are just limited to the traditional teaching method. That is to say, teachers give lesson through PPT discs and demonstration and so on. While the students receive the lesson through chalk and talk and can't have a full understanding of what they have learnt if the teacher doesn't give them a specific requirements. The traditional one is so boring that many students have little interest in class and what they have learnt is easy to forget. What's more, the traditional one have some disadvantages that the students' self-learning as well as self-practice is blind after class and their learning effect isn't obvious, especially in operational knowledge, for the teacher can't give students an objective evaluation and feedback on their technical skills without targeted videos. However, judging from the questionnaires, more than 3/4 students considered that the video-feedback method aroused their interest of learning, and raised their initiative and enthusiasm greatly. Meanwhile, the video-feedback method applied to the operational class was equivalent to a novel teaching mode, which appealed to students with curiosity. Furthermore, the vivid screen concise explanations normative deno video of video-feedback method had made the design of curriculum more interesting, which also improved students' enthusiasim. Students practiced as the teacher's standard video and found out their weaknesses, which is an active learning process with practice feedback repractice, refeedback. At last, the handed in one of the best videos and pictures of theirs to the teacher, which increased students' learning efficiency. In addition, when students were told that the video and picture would become process grade which is one part of the final grade, they were driven to practice actively.
- Video-feedback method give students' learning more flexibility and freedom. As we all known, every student has his or her own schedule, so they always fail to get together to learn the same lecture after class. However, students had access to teacher's standard video and theirs so they could practice according to their respective schedule without waiting others. What's more, the video was available to them wherever and whenever they wanted if it was convenient to them to open their computers. It was also a process to review and consolidate which could not only deepen their understanding of nursing etiquette, but also offered students an opportunity to view the demonstration of skills, by an expect, an unlimited number of time.

- Video-feedback method can improve the evaluation or judgment of the worth of one's performance and the identification of one's strengths and weaknesses to enhance one's reviewing and consolidating of learning. In the study, students become aware of their weaknesses by watching the teacher's standard video others' practicing, then they corrected their mistakes. As they identified others' mistakes, they would be reminded not to commit the same ones. Thus, they would keep error-prone process in mind, which was a process to impel students to review and consolidate. In the survey, about 94.5 % students thought the video-feedback method could spur them on reviewing. Meanwhile, the bystander's friendly smile at one's non-verbal wrong skills such as wrong make-up skill and wrong hair flattening may lead to one's emotional attitude towards study changing, and the changing attitude is closely related to one's brain. Consequently, students' study may reach to a higher level they have expected from a primary level, promoting their self-improvement and consolidation.
- Video-feedback method can help create a relaxed pleasant atmosphere. The study proved that the atmosphere was lively and the students discussed fiercely. In the process of recording video, students assessed and evaluated others' practice, finding shortcomings of each other and giving mutual feedback. In this process, students discussed with each other, asking questions, clearing up doubts exploring innovation and transmitting information, turning mechanical and boring technical skills into vivid activity in which the students can learn from each other and make progress. From the questionnaire, there were 83.4 % students agreed that the video-feedback method could make the atmosphere vivid.
- Video-feedback can help teachers improve self-quality and teaching ability. Etiquette norms is closely related with people's live, especially nurse and etiquette teachers. When teachers instill etiquette knowledge in class, they at the same time become aesthetic and appraisal object of students after class. Therefore, video-feedback method put forward higher requirement for its teachers. The teachers need first to cultivate the conduct and behavior of themselves, to demand strict on themselves, to dig out the most aesthetic and appealing highlight to present to the students, guiding students to sentiment beauty and find beauty, helping students form a positive attitude to learning. Meanwhile, the teachers are supposed to master the theoretical and practical knowledge of the integrated use of a variety of etiquette teaching method. The video enabled teachers to watch the process of teaching, which is beneficial to help teachers find their weaknesses and improve their technical skills, and find find the students' mistakes to make a timely explanation, which help teachers and students build a friendly teaching bilateral relationship, rather than one-way primary and secondary relationship, heightening the flexibility of teaching and improving teachers'teaching ability. According to questionnaire, more than 4/5 students thought the video-feedback method could help increase tearchers' teaching ability and quality.
- Video-feedback method has posed a new challenge to the traditional assessement method, changin "terminal evaluation" to "process evaluation + terminal evaluation". The ultimate purpose of teaching evaluation is testing the

effectiveness of teaching to improve teaching and teaching quality. The traditional assess system of nursing etiquette just test students' master of theory through theoretical examination papers rather than the level of operational skills. That which is easy to be made mistakes by students can't be well known to teachers. When the video-feedback method was applied to nursing etiquette, the assessment evaluation consists of operational video which makes up 40 % and the terminal theoretical examination grade which makes up 60 %. It not only test students' practical ability and theory knowledge, but also find out the dynamic learning process of students, so the teacher can adjust his teaching according to the master of students.

138.7 Conclusions

Though the study video-feedback method in grooming etiquette of nursing etiquette, the study has revealed that the use of video-feedback method in operational class enhance students' active engagement with the feedback they received and their interests in learning as well as efficiency of learning can be improved obviously, and for teachers, the use of video-feedback method can improve their teaching ability and quality.

138.8 Suggestion

As the preparation and implementation of video-feedback method is a little time-consuming and not all part of nursing etiquette is suit the video-feedback method, teachers should choose which part suit this method according to the specific requirement of syllabus. In addition, colleges and universities are appreciated to provide teaching equipment and condition to promote the use of video-feedback method in nursing education.

References

1. Liudan (2012) The investigation of demonatration teaching method in nursing etiquette class. Educ Innov Guid 19
2. Fukkink RG, Trienekens N, Kramer LJC et al (2011) Video feedback in education and training: putting learning in the picture. Educ Psychol Rev (23):45–63
3. Wangqi, Sunxia (2011) The use of video feedback method in fosbury flop of unniversities. Paper of Shanxi Normal Institute of Physical Education, vol 26, No. 3
4. Hongyun Z (2005) The investigation of teaching practice of nursing etiquette of nursing profession. Nurs Educ 24

Chapter 139
A Biomedical Microdevice for Quantal Exocytosis Measurement with Microelectrodes Arrays

Liguo Sun, Zhimeng Zou, Haifei Li, Peizheng Liu, Keping Tan and Jun Li

Abstract A microdevice was developed for cell trapping and exocytosis monitoring. The microdevice was assembled by two-layer poly(dimethyl siloxane) slab and microelectrodes integrated glass slide. The top layer with a depth of 20 μm was manufactured for cell flowing and the bottom layer with a depth of 2.5 μm was manufactured for cell trapping. Chromaffin cells can be trapped on top of indium tin oxide electrodes with this microdevice, and amperometric signals originated from catecholamine oxidation were obtained by flowing high K+ stimulating solution. The time course and areas of spikes recorded show that the manufactured device can provide sufficient sensitivity for quantal exocytosis measurement, and this biomedical device can be used for measuring cell exocytosis as traditional carbon fiber microelectrodes. By coupling with the multi-channel amplifier, high throughput analysis of cell exocytosis can be achieved with this microdevice, which is obviously superior to the carbon fiber microelectrodes based method.

Keywords Microdevice · Exocytosis · Poly(dimethyl siloxane) · Chromaffin cells

139.1 Introduction

Measurement of transmitter release from living cells has always been an area of great interest in biological and medical science as the study of single cell dynamics could help us better understands diverse processes such as exocytotic pathway vesicle fusion dynamics and presynaptic regulation of neurotransmission, etc. To obtain fast, sensitive, spatially resolved analysis of exocytosis, robust and reliable

L. Sun (✉) · Z. Zou · H. Li · P. Liu · K. Tan · J. Li
Department of Radiology, Binzhou Medical College Affiliated Hospital at Yantai,
Takustr. 7, Yantai 264100 Shandong Province, China
e-mail: zisetasong@sina.com

cellular analysis systems are required. Several well-established techniques, including patch-clamp capacitance detection, optical spectroscopy, and electrochemical sensing with ultramicroelectrodes [1], have been employed to investigate these events. Despite of excellent time resolution of vesicle fusion event provided by the state-of-the-art techniques, these techniques are, to a certain extent, labor intensive and low-throughput, because they require highly skilled lab technicians for the manual positioning of the electrode to the cell surface using micromanipulators, and only one cell can be detected at a time. In addition, the glass pipette and carbon fiber electrodes are manually fabricated individually or in small lots.

In our work, a two-layer AZ positive photoresist was patterned based on standard photolithography, and elastomeric poly(dimethyl) siloxane (PDMS) substrates were casted to trap cells. Similar to carbon fiber microelectrodes monitoring the quantal exocytosis adjacent to the cell surface, the surface-patterned indium tin oxide (ITO) microelectrodes can measure the vesicle fusion and transmitter release events when cells in direct contact or approxmity of the electrode surface. By utilizing the cell trapping devices, cells can be automatically trapped at the entrance of the shallow microfluidic channels at mild hydraulic pressure, while the cell debris was allowed to pass through and exit to the waste reservoir.

139.2 Results and Discussion

After successfully assembling the biomedical microdevice by integrating indium tin oxide electrodes with cell trapping structures, experiments for characterization microelectrodes, cell trapping and exocytosis were performed.

139.2.1 Characterization of Microelectrodes

Precise amperometric measurements requires electrode surface areas small enough to minimize non-faradic information such as electrical noise and capacitive currents, because larger electrodes cannot ensure all the quantal release events be detected due to the high background noise, although, electrodes need to remain large enough for allowing a quantitative collection of released molecules from releasing point distributed on the surface of a single cell or from a collection of cells depending on the scope of the measurements. Therefore, we measured the standard deviation of background current of the fabricated electrodes under the same conditions as exocytosis measurement was performed. Table 139.1 showed that the 100 μm^2 yielded lowest current, and the noise performance of planar microelectrodes is superior to that of the carbon fiber microelectrodes of the same area.

Table 139.1 The standard deviation of the background current versus electrode area

Electrode area (μm²)	100	200	1000	2000
Background noise (pA)	0.25	0.52	1.75	2.69

The data was recorded at a bandwidth of 2.9 kHz while holding the electrode at 0.7 V versus Ag/AgCl

139.2.2 Cell Trapping

Hydraulic pressure pumping and vacuuming were usually chosen over electroosmotic pumping to transport cells along the channel, because high voltage may affect the cell state and vitality. The schematic diagram of microfluidic chip with cell trapping design is shown in Fig. 139.1. It shows that cells traveled through the inlet channel, trapped along the entrance of the shallow channel, while solutions and small cell debris can flow freely inside all the channels.

139.2.3 Amperometric Measurement

Arrays of microelectrodes can be used to electrochemically measure the released neurotransmitters from exocytosis, which offer the unique advantages of providing quantitative information about the amount of released molecules and precise kinetic characteristics with high sensitivity and sub-millisecond time resolution 2. By placing microelectrodes at the entrance of the shallow channels, single cell exocytosis measurement can be achieved. Figure 139.2a displays a 120 s amperometric recording of exocytotic events detected at a single bovine adrenal chromaffin cell by ITO microelectrode. Each current transient reflects the release dynamics during exocytosis, most of the spikes started with a sharp increase in the current, as is shown the amperometric spikes on expanded time scale in Fig. 139.2b. (a) while some of the events are, however, preceded by a foot signal, as is in Fig. 139.2b. (b), which is similar to those reported recordings with conventional carbon fiber electrodes.

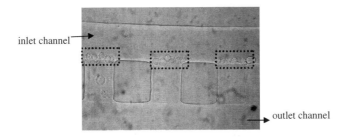

Fig. 139.1 Micrograph of chromaffin cell trapping at a 50 μm wide, 2.5 μm deep channels

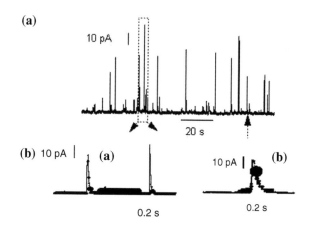

Fig. 139.2 Amperometric detection of quantal exocytosis of catecholamines from chromaffin cells using microfluidic cell trapping devices. (B) a, Expanded scale of the amperometric spikes within the dashed box in Fig. 5(A), b, Expanded view of the foot signal

139.3 Conclusions

We have designed and manufactured an effective cell trapping device suitable for high-throughput amperometric measurement of quantal exocytosis from individual cells. It offered an efficient method to target cells to electrode in a relatively simple manner without the need for precise pressure control and fluidhandling. The obtained data from the microfluidic device was in agreement with those published from measurements using conventional carbon fiber microelectrodes.

References

1. Kennedy RT, Huang L, Atkinson MA, Dush P (1993) Detection of exocytosis at individual pancreatic beta cells by amperometry at a chemically modified microelectrode. Anal Chem 65:1882–1886
2. Dod JT, Schroeder J, Borges R, Finnegan JM, Pihel K, Amatore C, Wightman RM (1996) Biophys J 70:1061–1068

Chapter 140
The Construction of Comprehensive Financial Evaluation System in Higher Vocational Colleges Based on Connotation Construction

Zhongsheng Zhu and Fei Gao

Abstract The connotation construction is indispensable to the development of higher vocational colleges. On the basis of practical experiences, this paper introduces the overall financial strength, the teaching quality performance, the skill training performance and the development potential of higher vocational colleges. The comprehensive financial evaluation system that embodies the connotation construction of Higher Vocational Colleges is thus constructed.

Keywords Higher vocational colleges · Connotative development · Finance · Appraisal system

140.1 Introduction

Several Opinions on Improving the Overall Quality of Higher Education (released by The Ministry of Education) pointed out that colleges and universities should firmly focus on talent training and set up the scientific development concept of higher education. They must stabilize the scale, optimize the structure, strengthen the characteristics, pay attention to innovation and take the quality as the core. That's what we call connotative development. Only by strengthening the connotation construction, and improving the quality of talent training can higher vocational education meet the requirements of China's social and economic development. Because there are differences in location advantages, history of running schools and the capital investments, there are some differences in the quality of education between colleges. How to objectively evaluate the differences so as to analyze the development potential of higher vocational colleges is an

Z. Zhu (✉) · F. Gao
Anqing Vocational and Technical College, Anqing 246003 Anhui, People's Republic of China

important subject. It is necessary to establish the financial appraisal of higher vocational colleges so that we can have a comprehensive understanding of the situation. At the same time, we need to find out the gap between the colleges, the characteristics and the strength of each college by comparing the related indexes of different types of higher vocational colleges in different regions. Financial appraisal can not only reflect the comprehensive strength and the level of single indexes of a higher vocational college, but also can provide more detailed first-hand information for the education department to make decisions.

140.2 Establishment of Financial Appraisal System of Higher Vocational Colleges

We can generalize the basic principles that higher vocational colleges should follow on the basis of the previous theories on comprehensive financial appraisal system of colleges and universities. The principles include scientificity, generalizability, whole optimization, comparability, feasibility and dynamic improvement.

Financial appraisal system of higher vocational colleges is a multi-objective system. It should correctly reflect the management requirements to the benefit of running a school as the core and the educational goal based on connotative development of vocational education. Connotative construction of vocational education should highlight the characteristics and the law of vocational education. Colleges should focus on monitoring the teaching quality and skill training. In analytic hierarchy process, we regard dynamic management as the target and highlight connotative construction of vocational education to establish the appraisal system of performance, which should focus on the performance of teaching quality and skill training. The comprehensive financial strength needs to be used as a reference. The financial indexes can reveal the comprehensive levels of higher vocational colleges. The appraisal system includes the overall financial strength, performance of teaching quality, performance of skill training and the development potential. There are four first level indexes and 31 s level indexes.

140.2.1 Comprehensive Financial Strength

Comprehensive financial strength of higher vocational colleges refers to the ability to obtain funds from the government and self-financing channels through their own efforts. Such indexes as the total outlay per capita for the students, the proportion of government funds to the total outlay, the proportion of self-finance to the total outlay can reflect the ability of the colleges to obtain funds from various channels. These indexes do not use absolute gross indexes due to the influence of the scale and the area factors. Generally speaking, the larger the scale is and the more developed the region is, the more revenue the college gets. The eight detailed second level indexes are as follows: the total outlay per capita for the students, the proportion of financial allocation to the total outlay, the proportion of donations and sponsorship to the total outlay, the proportion of self-finance to the total outlay, the proportion of expenditure to the total outlay, the annual growth rate of self-finance, total outlay for the staff per capita and the proportion of personal expenses to the total expenditure.

140.2.2 Performance of Teaching Quality

The efforts to improve the teaching quality in higher vocational colleges and the results got are the key points for assessment of the performance of teaching quality. The 10 detailed second level indexes are as follows: the average student's training funds, the staff-student ratio, the proportion of teacher training funds to the total outlay, the proportion of teaching business funds to the total outlay, annual growth rate of teaching business funds, the proportion of the income of teaching activities to the total outlay, the annual growth rate of the income of teaching activities, the proportion of teachers to the staff, the proportion of spending on social services to the total outlay and student enrollment.

140.2.3 Performance of Skill Training

The work for the training of students' and teachers' skills and the effect of acquisition of skills are the key points for assessment of performance of skill training. The detailed second level indexes are as follows: the proportion of teaching equipment investment to the total outlay, funds for the teachers' skill training, the average teacher's research funds, the average student's practical training funds, the proportion of the income for social services and technological activities to the total outlay, the annual growth rate of the income for social services and technological activities, research awards, the number of specialized experiment (training) rooms.

140.2.4 Development Potential

Whether the present situation agrees with the social development trend is the key point for assessment of the development potential of higher vocational colleges. The detailed second level indexes are as follows: the growth rate of the total revenue, the proportion of double-professional teachers to all the staff, the annual growth rate of the income for social services and technological activities, the proportion of high-end teaching equipment, the annual growth rate of college students.

140.3 Determination of the Weights of Various Indexes in Financial Appraisal System of Higher Vocational Colleges

Many scholars have talked about the connotation of each index in different academic papers.

140.3.1 Methods Used to Determine the Weights

Weight or weighted coefficient means a quantitative distribution of importance degrees of something. Comprehensive appraisal conducted by the author is the appraisal of indexes. Each index in the system has its weight. Based on a questionnaire survey, we use the Delphi method to determine the weights and to establish the appraisal index system.

Financial appraisal has the characteristics of fuzziness and comprehensiveness. According to the research of scholars home and abroad, there are different methods to determine the weights. This paper uses the fuzzy statistical method. Detailed calculation process is as follows:

Firstly, some experts and the persons engaged in relevant work are asked to propose the most appropriate weight according to the various elements in $U = \{U1, U2, U3, \ldots, Un\}$. The expression $Aj = (a1j, a2j, a3j, \ldots, aij)$ shows what the first person grades each factor. Then, each factor of $Ui = (1, 2, 3, \ldots, n)$ is analyzed by univariate statistics. In $\sum_{i=1}^{n} a_{ij} = 1, (j = 1, 2, \ldots \ldots m)$, each factor of Ui ($i = 1, 2, 3, \ldots, n$) finds the maximum value Mi and the minimum value mi in its weight $aij = 1$ ($j = 1, 2, 3, \ldots, m$). $Mi = \max\{aij\}, mi = \min\{aij\}(1 \leq i \leq m$, $1 \leq i \leq M)$. Select a positive integer K and group the data, calculate the distances of the weights in K groups and divide the weights into K groups in ascending order. Calculate the weights and the frequency of each group. Determine the weights ai according to the distribution of the weights and the frequency, then the weight vectors $A = (A1, A2, A3, \ldots, An)$ can be got.

140.3.2 Determination of Weights of Financial Indexes

In the course of the study, the weight calculation of financial appraisal index system of higher vocational colleges is shown in Table 140.1. The experts firstly grade the weights of the first level indexes, grade again according to the influence that the second level indexes have on the first level indexes and calculate with normalization method, then we can get the actual weights of the second level indexes (calculated by SPSS13.0).

Table 140.1 The weight calculation of financial appraisal index system of higher vocational colleges

Overall performance	First level index	Weight	Second level index	Weight
Comprehensive financial level of higher vocational colleges	The overall strength of the finance	30	The total outlay for the students per capita	5.12
			The proportion of financial allocation to the total outlay	2.42
			The proportion of donations and sponsorship to the total outlay	4.46
			The proportion of self-finance to the total outlay	1.94
			The proportion of expenditure to the total outlay	4.11
			The annual growth rate of self-finance	1.05
			The total outlay for the staff per capita	8.88
			The proportion of personal expenses to the total expenditure	2.02
	The performance of teaching quality	30	The average student's training funds	4.12
			The staff-student ratio	1.54
			The proportion of teacher training funds to the total outlay	3.16
			The proportion of teaching business funds to the total outlay	3.74
			The annual growth rate of teaching business funds	2.91
			The proportion of the income for teaching activities to the total outlay	1.15
			The annual growth rate of the income for teaching activities	3.34
			The proportion of teachers to the staff	2.32
			The proportion of spending on social services to the total outlay	1.94
			Student enrollment	5.78
	Performance of skill training	25	The proportion of teaching equipment investment to the total outlay	3.44
			Funds for the teachers' skill training	3.32
			The average teacher's research funds	3.65
			The average student's practical training funds	2.91
			The proportion of the income for social services and technological activities to the total outlay	2.45
			The annual growth rate of the income for social services and technological activities	3.54
			Research awards	2.72
	Development potential	15	The number of specialized experiment (training) rooms	2.93
			The growth rate of the total revenue	4.04
			The proportion of double-professional teachers to all the staff	3.21
			The annual growth rate of the income for social services and technological activities	2.38
			The proportion of high-end teaching equipment	2.23
			The annual growth rate of college students	3.14

140.4 Conclusion

Establishment of financial appraisal system of higher vocational colleges should obey the law of vocational education. It should have the characteristics of vocational education and focus on the connotative development of vocational education with emphasis on the examination of teaching quality and skill training. Comprehensive financial appraisal system of higher vocational colleges based on connotative development not only reflects the overall financial strength of a higher vocational college, it reflects more importantly the social service ability, quality of the graduates and the level of coordinated development with local economics. The indexes can reflect the level and characteristics of a college. It is necessary to think about the teaching quality and the skill training of higher vocational colleges from the viewpoint of connotative development, which can be helpful for coming up with better ideas for education and for appraisal of the comprehensive teaching levels and the development potential of higher vocational colleges.

References

1. Qiao Chunhua College Accounting (1998) Financial and Economic Publishing House, Beijing
2. Zhoufu Y, Jianjun S (2002) Comprehensive evaluation of financial research. Renmin University Press of China, Beijing
3. Zhang S (2004) Research on comprehensive financial evaluation system of colleges and universities. Stat Forecast
4. Ma M (2011) Study on connotative development of higher vocational colleges in 10 years of the new century. J East China Normal Univ

Chapter 141
Spatial Covariance Modeling Analysis of Hypertension on Cognitive Aging

Lan Lin, Wei-wei Wu, Shui-cai Wu and Guang-yu Bin

Abstract It's becoming increasingly clear that hypertension (HTN) is at the root of much cognitive decline previously attributed to aging. Long before patients in clinical stroke, HTN has caused a certain degree of damage on brain cognitive function. In this study, magnetic resonance images (MRI) of hypertensive and control group will be first collected, then processed by voxel based morphology (VBM), and further studied with spatial covariance modeling. Testing the effect of HTN on the expression of the age-related gray matter pattern revealed that hypertensive showed higher expression of age-related pattern than normotensives. HTN may have an accelerated effect on normal cognitive aging process.

Keywords Hypertension (HTN) · Spatial covariance modeling · Voxel-based morphometry (VBM)

141.1 Introduction

The population of elder adults is expected to grow rapidly over the next decades, reaching more than 248 million in the china alone by 2020. Associated with the increase of elderly population is the increase of age-related cognitive decline. An article published recently in PNAS [1] revealed that cognitive ability is a more important indicator than age distribution. Preservation of cognitive functions is an

---

Supported by Scientific Research Foundation for Doctors of Beijing University of Technology.

L. Lin (✉) · W. Wu · S. Wu · G. Bin
College of Life Science and Bioengineering, Beijing University of Technology, Beijing 100124, China
e-mail: lanlin@bjut.edu.cn

essential factor for supporting the skills and abilities needed to maintain full and active participation in society [2], as well as for maintaining quality life.

With the increasing of the population base and the acceleration of the aging people, hypertensives continue to increase, and their ages tend to be younger. HTN is a common health risk factor with a high prevalence in the healthy aging population. Because its influence on the cognition is relatively light and easily overlooked, HTN tends to produce long-term, sustained adverse effects on the brain tissues. There is considerable evidence that HTN has a significant impact on age-related cognitive abilities [3]. It is directly related to the brain atrophy which is associated with aging [4]. A recent study [5] had found that the risk of cognitive impairment for elderly hypertensive was 40 percent higher than normotensives.

Most neuroimaging studies [6] for HTN to date have used univariate analyses which identify changes at the voxel level. Multivariate network analysis methods evaluate brain changes as network interactions that reflect the regionally distributed effects of age or disease. In the current study, we employed a multivariate spatial covariance methodology, the Scaled Subprofile Model (SSM) [7, 8] to evaluate the effect of HTN on normal cognitive aging process.

141.2 Method

141.2.1 Experiment

68 right-handed healthy elderly subject were included in this study. This cohort includes 35 normotensives (NT) and 33 hypertensive (HT). Participants underwent an extensive screen to exclude significant medical, neurological or psychiatric disorders or injury that would affect cognitive performance. Subject characteristics are shown in Table 141.1. The NT and HT groups did not differ significantly in age ($p = 0.51$), education ($p = 0.16$), or gender distribution ($p = 0.53$). Structural MRI scans for the NT and HT groups were performed with a 3T GE Signa II scanner with an eight-channel phased array coil (HD Signa Excite, General Electric, Milwaukee, WI) and a T1-weighted, 3D Spoiled Gradient-echo (3DSPGR) sequence (TR = 5.3 ms, TE = 2.0 ms, TI = 500; flip angle = 15°; matrix = 256 × 256; FOV = 256 × 256 mm^2) with 204 contiguous 1.0 mm thick coronal slices.

Table 141.1 Subject characteristics

N	68
Age (years)	68.7 ± 5.2
Age range (years)	57–82
Gender, M/F	29/39
Education (years)	15.4 ± 2.2
MMSE, mean ± SD	29.1 ± 0.8
HTN status (yes/no)	33/35

141.2.2 Image Analysis

141.2.2.1 Voxel Based Morphometry (VBM)

Images were pre-processed using a procedure outlined by Pereira [9]. The images were first skull-stripped by a hybrid watershed algorithm. Next, the extracted brains were bias-corrected using the non-parametric non-uniform intensity normalization (N3) [10]. Finally, images were manually aligned to the SPM8 T1 template. The parameters for N3 correction were selected from a procedure described by Boyes [11] in which accuracy is favored over speed.

After preprocessing, images were processed using voxel-based morphometry (VBM) [12] with Statistical Parametric Mapping (SPM8) and the DARTEL toolbox. DARTEL was used to segment gray matter (GM) and white matter (WM) and simultaneously register and create a customized template in the subject's native space. The individual segmented gray matter images were brought into Montreal Neurological Institute (MNI) space and the smoothed segmented GM images were used for subsequent spatial covariance analyses.

141.2.2.2 Spatial Covariance Analysis

SSM toolbox (http://feinsteinneuroscience.org) was used for spatial covariance analysis. The steps of analysis are as follows: (1). Mean voxel values across regions and subjects for the natural log transformed at each voxel for each subject were subtracted. (2). The processed data were included in a principal components analysis (PCA). Voxels participating in each PC have either a positive or negative

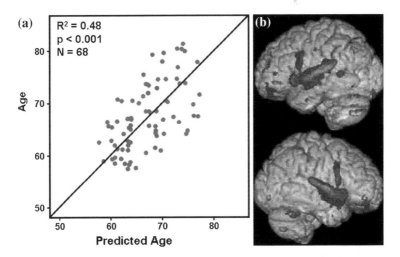

Fig. 141.1 Multiple regression of subject scores from the prospective application of the age-associated pattern, predicting HT group and NT group

loading: Positive loadings represent age related relative GM preservation whereas negative loadings represent brain atrophy. The expression of each PC for each subjects were quantified by a subject score. A higher score indicates greater manifestation of age associated PCs. (3). Patterns which explained at least 2 % of the variance in the overall subject by region and that caused the overall Akaike Information Criterion (AIC) value to decrease were included in analyses to create a linear combination of patterns that maximally predicted condition. (4). A bootstrap re-sampling procedure was performed with 500 iterations to provide reliability estimates for the observed SSM pattern weights in this sample (Fig. 141.1).

141.3 Results

The prospective application of the age-associated pattern into the NT and HT groups produced subject scores representing the degree to which each subject manifested the age-related pattern. In a multiple regression model, expression of age-related pattern was a significant predictor of group membership, with the HT patients expressing the aging pattern to a greater degree than NT (Fig. 141.2), and it was also associated with a poorer performance on a factor score of information processing speed ($p = 0.002$).

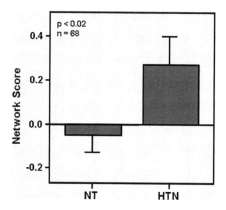

Fig. 141.2 a Subject predicted age from the spatial covariance analysis associated with real age b Projection map of MRI gray matter reflecting the combined SSM component patterns which are associated with aging. The *blue scale* indicates areas of decreased GM with aging, whereas the *orange scale* indicates areas of relative gray matter preservation with aging ($Z > 3$). SSM analysis identified a linear combination of the first two component patterns that was associated with age ($R2 = 0.48$, $p < 0.001$). This effect remained significant after controlling for eTIV, education and gender. The pattern was characterized by brain atrophy mainly in bilateral dorsolateral and medial prefrontal, anterior cingulate, lateral cerebellum, precuneus regions and superior temporal, with relative preservation in bilateral fusiform, lingual and thalamic

141.4 Discussion

Network analysis showed brain atrophy associated with age in bilateral dorsolateral and medial prefrontal, anterior cingulate, lateral cerebellum, precuneus regions and superior temporal. These regional reductions were associated with poorer performance on a cognitive factor score of information processing speed. The HT group showed a higher expression of the age-associated atrophy pattern than NT despite being matched in age. These results suggest that HTN, this common cerebrovascular risk factor may contribute to an accelerated normal brain aging process.

References

1. Vegard S, Elke L, Daniela W (2012) Variation in cognitive functioning as a refined approach to comparing aging across countries. Proc Natl Acad Sci 109(3):770–774
2. Ritchie K, Artero S, Touchon J (2001) Classification criteria for mild cognitive impairment: a population-based validation study. Neurology 56:37–42
3. Elias PK, Elias MF, Agostino RB et al (1997) NIDDM and blood pressure as risk factors for poor cognitive performance. Diabetes Care 20(9):1388–1395
4. Raz N, Rodrigue KM, Acker JD (2003) Hypertension and the brain: vulnerability of the prefrontal regions and executive function. Behav Neurosci 117(6):1169–1180
5. Reitz C, Tang M, Manly J et al (2007) Hypertension and the risk of mild cognitive impairment. Arch Neurol 64(12):1734–1740
6. Glodzik L, Mosconi L, Tsui W et al (2012) Alzheimer's disease markers, hypertension, and gray matter damage in normal elderly. Neurobiol Aging 33(7):1215–1227
7. Moeller J, Strother S, Sidtis J et al (1987) Scaled subprofile model: a statistical approach to the analysis of functional patterns in positron emission tomographic data. J Cereb Blood Flow Metab 7(5):649–658
8. Strother S, Anderson J, Schaper K et al (1995) Principal component analysis and the scaled subprofile model compared to intersubject averaging and statistical parametric mapping: I. "Functional connectivity" of the human motor system studied with [15O]water PET. J Cereb Blood Flow Metab 15(5):738–753
9. Pereira JM, Xiong L, Acosta-Cabronero J et al (2010) Registration accuracy for VBM studies varies according to region and degenerative disease grouping. Neuroimage 49(3):2205–2215
10. Sled JG, Zijdenbos AP, Evans AC (1998) A nonparametric method for automatic correction of intensity nonuniformity in MRI data. IEEE Trans Med Imaging 17(1):87–97
11. Boyes RG, Gunter JL, Frost C et al (2008) Intensity non-uniformity correction using N3 on 3-T scanners with multichannel phased array coils. Neuroimage 39(4):1752–1762
12. Ashburner J, Friston KJ (2001) Why voxel-based morphometry should be used. Neuroimage 14(6):1238–1243

Chapter 142
A New Practice Mode and Platform Based on Network Cooperation for Software Engineering Specialty

Ling He

Abstract College students of software engineering specialty hope to develop a practical software project in practice, but practice resource is inadequate. In order to integrate practice resource of college, enterprises and students, this paper presents a practice mode based on network cooperation. Research of the mode includes: source of software project, organization of practice process, and management of software result. In addition, Practice platform according to this mode is developed. Design method and technology is described in this paper. Effect of this practice mode is analyzed in the paper end. This practice mode more exploits the practice resources of enterprise and college. The platform improves practice quality, and it reduces practice cost.

Keywords Practice mode · Practical project · Software engineering

142.1 Foreword

Software engineering is a specialty which attaches importance to practice. In the 4 years of university education, it is arranged that theoretical teaching in classroom and one or two visit to the enterprise for learning. But those are not enough to exercise ability of resolve practical problems. Because be faced with intense competition for jobs, many students hope to develop an actual software project in school. Students want to accumulate experience to improve the employment confidence. The best way is that the students join a software company for a period

---

This paper is research findings of TJAU education reform project (NO.B-10-11).

L. He (✉)
Tianjin Agriculture University, Tianjin, China
e-mail: heling@tjau.edu.cn

of time. During the internship, students will develop a software project leading by professional engineer. Students can study the process of software development, experience the way of cooperate. Unfortunately, the software company can only accept a few students due to limited conditions. Most students still develop the imaginary software project in laboratory. In addition, in order not to affect the project progress and quality, companies are unwilling to let students really involved in the development work. Then the practice becomes a mere formality.

The mode of "Witkey Network" is that people can release problems on Internet, and people who resolve that problem will receive reward. These problems mainly depend on the intelligence to solve. Software can be developed without any limitations of time and space. As long as there is a fit computer, we can develop software by intelligence. So "Witkey" mode is suitable for software specialty. By using "Witkey" mode, students can acquire lots of actual software requirement. Inspired by "Witkey" mode, this paper proposes a practice mode based on network cooperation. This mode builds a platform on Internet. Then enterprises, teachers and students cooperate to complete a practice process. More specifically, firstly enterprises release real software requirement. Then students organize teams to apply for the software project. And then teachers of software specialty lead students to develop the software. Next engineers of enterprise check software results and give their advice. Finally some satisfactory software results will be accepted and paid by demander. The practice mode is good to motivate the enthusiasm of students. The practice mode can lessen interference to enterprises' normal work. At the same time the practice mode makes teachers out of the ivory tower and to be involved in the practical project. Then teachers get the opportunity to communicate with the enterprise, and teachers understand the student's actual level of specialty, these experiences will guide the reform of theory teaching in the further.

142.2 Research of the Practice Mode

Research of the practice mode based on network cooperation mainly includes the following three problems.

142.2.1 Source of the Software Project

Source of software project is the prerequisite in the practice mode. It determines whether the practice mode can work as expected. The most important is that software must come from the practical demand. In order to ensure a sufficient number of software projects for practice, we have signed contract with some software enterprises. Every semester, they will release software requirement according to the agreed quantity. These software may be being developed, it also probably prepare to be developed. Though, practice students and engineer of the enterprise develop the same projects, they do not interfere with each other, so it does not involve copyright and technical secrets. In addition, teachers of any department in our university are encouraged to release software requirements which come from their teaching or research.

142.2.2 Organization and Management Method

How to organize a practice is the key of the practice mode research. The practice mode mainly applies to students' practice. If students have the ability to complete some projects at spare time, they also can receive reward by this way. The process of practice as follows.

First, some enterprise or teacher can release a software project by submitting a detailed requirements specification. A teacher of software specialty must evaluate difficult grade of the software project, explain the difficulty and give some advice to the development.

Then, students freely organize teams to apply for a software project. The number of a team according to the difficult grade of the project, and a project manager is elected to be responsible for coordinating the overall work. Each team chooses a practice tutor to guide the development process. Team applied for the project, must have a clear division of labor. They should sign a contract with project releaser, mainly making agreement on the development Schedule, software quality, and rewards. If some teams choose the same project, they will compete. Of course, the best software result will be accepted by the project releaser.

Next, Students develop the software in a computer laboratory. The laboratory is rebuilt as enterprise workroom. There are about thirty suitable computers, two servers, and some switches in a laboratory. Every student can use a computer independently. They can install software on the computer, and a group of students can set up a local area network. During software development, discussion between developers and demander is important. This discussion is asked by student, and organized by practice tutor. Students, tutor and project releaser take part in the discussion. The thought of software engineering requires that software development process is divided into stages: requirement analysis, system design, coding and system test. Each stage finished, project manager submits the document of this stage, and every member needs to submit a work report. Practice tutor should respond to the stage document and work report. During the development process, students should develop the ability to think independently and solve problems jointly, while tutor only guides the direction of working.

Finally, development completed, software should be evaluated openly. Software will be tested respectively by requirement releaser, practice tutor and users who are students have nothing to do with this project. Then each of them submits an evaluation report. Evaluation report includes: whether functions of the software are completed as requirements specification, whether interface is friendly, found bugs of the software, advantages and defects, advice to improve the software.

142.2.3 Practice Score and Software Result

In every stage of development, tutor gives a stage score according to student's performance. Practice completed, tutor gives a project score according to evaluation report. Count up these scores in proportion is the student's final practice score.

Practice completed, software result should be backup into database. Software result includes not only the program code, but also the software development documents. If the software demander thinks the software result is satisfied by and large, he will give rewards for the software, and students should continue to improve this software as demander's opinion.

142.3 Design of a Practice Platform

142.3.1 Functions of the Platform

According to the analysis of above practice mode, a practice platform is designed. The platform makes it more efficient to manage the process of practice. Practice platform provide functions for four roles of users: software releasers, project tutors, students of software engineering specialty and administrator. All users need username and password to login platform in a certain role, and then use the certain functions platform provides. Software releasers and software professional teachers can register themselves through the registration interface. There is only one administrator in the platform system, he can clear data, backup data, and check the authenticity of the registered users. Function of this platform system is shown in Fig. 142.1. The platform system includes four modules. Function of each module is shown in Figs. 142.2, 142.3, 142.4 and 142.5.

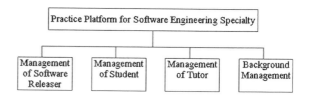

Fig. 142.1 Function of platform system

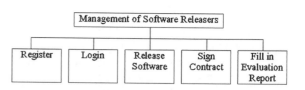

Fig. 142.2 Function of software releaser module

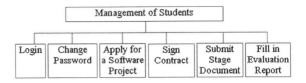

Fig. 142.3 Function of student module

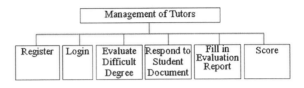

Fig. 142.4 Function of tutor module

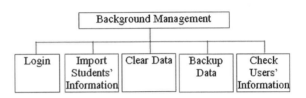

Fig. 142.5 Function of manager module

142.3.2 Technology Used in the Platform

When developing this platform system, technology of ASP.NET is used, C# language is used as programming language, and SQL Server is used as database management system. In addition, security method based on role is used in the system. Software releasers, practice tutors and students are three different roles, system provide different function interface to each role. By this way, data security is stronger, and users are clear to his work.

142.4 Analysis About the Practice Effect

Students have practised on this platform for 1 year long. Through the following numbers, we can see that the new practice mode is effectual.

Previously, software enterprises can only accepted about 30 students to practise every semester, other students need to contact practice companies themselves. In order to the practice task can be finished on time, enterprises reduced the difficulty of task. The 30 students only developed 3 smaller programs, and these programs didn't be used in actual. Students reaped little from this practice.

Platform has been used over the past year, we have obtained 8 projects from the software enterprises, and 5 projects have been obtained from our teachers' research. All 57 students of software specialty have participated in the practice, and another 6 students have applied for projects form the network platform voluntarily. 6 software results have been recognised fully by the software demander and have been used in actual. At the same time 9 graduates have been employed by software companies because of their excellent practice work.

The practice mode breaks the limits of practice space and practice time. This mode integrates practice resources of college and enterprises as far as possible.

References

1. Liu Y, Chen Y (2009) Construction and practice of the training base of software engineering specialty. Comput Educ 20:141–144
2. Tim W (2012) Further and higher education adviser to the department for education and employment. Comput Educ 37:4–8
3. Related rules of Time wealth nets. http://help.680.com/canyu.asp.2009
4. Colin J, Harry M, Alex M (2012) Enterprise education: for all, or just some. Internet High Educ 54:30–35
5. Huang F, Ren S (2010) Discussion on the mode of software engineering practice based on project practice. Hunan Soc Sci 5:175–178

Chapter 143
Post-Newborn: A New Concept of Period in Early Life

Long Chen, Jie Li, Nan Wang and Yuan Shi

Abstract Post-newborn infants refer to infants fromnbsp;>28 days to <100 days after birth. During this period, infants are still completely dependent on breast milk or/and formula milk for feeding. Up to now, the concept of post-newborn has not been mentioned in classic textbooks. With the development of perinatal medicine, mortality rate of diseases in neonates such as premature infants, asphyxia, infectious diseases have decreased significantly, and consequently, issues of the quality of life for these survivors have aroused widespread concerns. The post-newborn infants have some important characteristics differing from both newborn infants and infants after the period: (1) different fatal diseases and mortality rate; (2) the diseases inherited from newborn period requiring early and prompt treatments; (3) some peculiar diseases during this period requiring much attention; (4) either similar or different immune function; (5) rapid growth and uneven development of organ systems. Establishment of the new concept of post-newborn will further reveal the nature of life, reduce the mortality rate of infants, and improve the quality of life.

Keywords Infant · Newborn · Post-newborn

L. Chen and J. Li (Equal contributions to the study).

L. Chen · N. Wang · Y. Shi (✉)
Department of Pediatrics, Daping Hospital, Third Military Medical University,
Chongqing 400042, China
e-mail: neuroclong@126.com

L. Chen
e-mail: 476679422@qq.com

J. Li
Department of Obstetrics, The First Affiliated Hospital, Chongqing Medical University,
Chongqing 400014, China
e-mail: doralijie@hotmail.com

143.1 The Establishment of the Neonatal Intensive Care Unit (NICU) Could Greatly Reduce the Mortality Rate of Newborn Infant, but not Improve the Quality of Life Synchronously

In the early 1960s, the world's first NICU was established at New Haven Hospital of Yale University, which became a milestone in the developmental history of modern neonatal medicine. After that, NICU has been established in the world in succession and developed rapidly, and thus, neonatal medicine has entered a booming era. With the establishment of transfer and treatment network for the critically ill neonatal infant in the developed areas, the constant in-depth development of the relevant basic and clinical research, improvement of the treatment techniques, and especially the use of pulmonary surfactant, the mortality rate for the seriously ill newborn infants such as low birth weight newborns, extreme low birth weight newborns, severe respiratory distress syndrome have been decreased significantly. The mortality rate of the newborn in United States in 2006 has been dropped by nearly half as compared with that in 1980 (from 8.48 to 4.45 ‰) [1], where as the neonatal mortality rate in China in 2008 has been decreased by 70 % as compared with that of 1990 (from 34.0 to 10.2 ‰) [2]. However, a few surviving infants suffered from different kinds complications in the post-newborn, such as recurrent respiratory infections, physical retardation, cerebral palsy, bronchopulmonary dysplasia, retinopathy, and congenital heart disease requiring early surgical treatment [3–7]. Moreover, the complication and sequelae could change the way of life and learning of the children to some extent, affect their formation of good personality and mentality, lead to various kinds of personal and social problems in adults, add a great deal of disease burden to the countries, families and individuals [8, 9]. Although most of these children in the post-newborn have obtained some treatment and their prognosis has been improved, the post-newborn is still a very fragile, important and special stage in early life, which lacks a specific concept to define the short but crucial time.

143.2 The Definition for the Post-newborn

The post-newborn is a continuation of neonatal period. In addition to the above-mentioned sequelae and complications during the neonatal period, there is no clear distinction between the physiological and pathological condition of early infants. Because the symptoms and signs of diseases are more atypical in early infants, pediatricians should hold very cautious attitude. Nevertheless, it's lack of a specific term to cluster the infants during this period. So far most of literatures have described the early infant as "baby", "early baby", or "small baby". A clear and specific concept has not been mentioned in the previous classic textbooks. With the development of perinatal medicine, the neonatal mortality rate has been gradually decreased. Chinese Ministry of Health recently announced the infant mortality rate was run down from 32.3 ‰ in 2000 to 13.1 ‰ in 2010, achieving the UN Millennium Development Goals [10–12] ahead of schedule. Consequently the issues of quality of life for these infants surviving in the neonatal period have caused widespread concerns. The task of pediatrics is not only to focus on reducing morbidity and mortality rate, but also to guarantee children's health, improve the quality of life. The disease sequelae of the post-newborn might affect the health and well-beings of future life. Within this period, the infant have a very strong repair and remodeling capacity. When given appropriate rehabilitation, the infant could obtain unimaginable therapeutic efficacy. At the same time, early prevention of some adult diseases such as hypertension and diabetes should be paid much attention. Studies have suggested that these main diseases in adulthood have a close relationship with early infancy, especially nutritional status of the post-newborn [13]. How to further promote the growth and development and correct the complications and sequelae at the post-neonatal period, make the ill infants reach the level of normal infant development as early as possible, and reduce the incidence of adult-related diseases has become an important issue. It is necessary to carry out professional studies. For this purpose, we give the definition for this period which refers to post-newborn from >28 days to <100 days. In this period, the infant still completely depend on breast milk and/or formula milk for feeding. Up to now, the concept of post-newborn has not been mentioned in classic textbooks. The concept of post-newborn is mainly based on the following reasons:

(1) The supplementary food is usually introduced from the 4th month after birth. After this period, the gastrointestinal function of infant begins to adapt to the supplementary food and has significant changes.
(2) After 100 days, most of the common neonatal diseases and complications have been cured.
(3) For most infant medications at this period, no reference for dosage has been made yet, which is not consistent with evidence-based medicine: whether the application of various drugs has an effect or not? How the level of such drug's effect is produced? Is there any possible side effects or delayed benefits? The emphasis on this period is helpful for promoting the drug research and development in this specific period. After this period, most of the medications have some reference usage, which has greatly enhanced the safety.
(4) In this period, the antibody levels of infants from breast milk are high, while its own immune function is low, and there are few autoimmune diseases. Investigation of the immunity and its tolerance in this period is expected to provide new treatment methods for immunological disease/rheumatic diseases in the future.
(5) People in a lot of countries usually have the historical tradition and habit to invite relatives and friends to congratulate the baby on the 100th day after birth on spending the most vulnerable period of life. The time is easy to remember.

143.3 The Post-newborn Infants Have Some Important Characteristics Differing from the Newborn and Infant After this Period

143.3.1. **Post**-newborn infants have different fatal disease and mortality. An important indicator for reflecting children's health issue is the infant mortality. However, due to different kinds of reasons, there is no infant mortality reported within 3 months alone. It is reported that in some Asian developing countries, neonatal disease is still the first cause of death, and infectious disease is the major killer after the neonatal period. In western developed countries, the first cause of death is the congenital malformation, and the death age of those infants is not at the neonatal period [1, 14]. Because of high infant mortality rate and various kinds of complicated diseases, this indicator can not fully reflect the health level of infants. Clinical practice experience suggests that most of the deaths occurred in younger infants after the neonatal period, especially within 100 days. In the United States, sudden infant death syndrome is one of the main causes of infant mortality [15], the peak age of death appeared in 2–4 months after birth, and the infant mortality rate decreased after 4 months [16, 17].

143.3.2. The disease inherited from neonatal period requires early and prompt treatment. There might be a distinct defect in terms of the time concept for neonatal period. Although during neonatal period, a few of the mother-born diseases have been corrected, such as hemolytic disease of newborns, premature rupture of membranes, gestational diabetes etc. [18], it is impossible for the sequelae and complications of neonatal diseases to be fully corrected in this period. How to better diagnose and treat these diseases in post-neonatal period is the issue which the pediatricians have to pay much attention to. These diseases often require the full co-operation of many specialties including screening and correcting for hearing anomalies, treatment of persistent pathological jaundice, rehabilitation for hypoxic ischemic encephalopathy, screening and treatment for retinopathy, therapy for repeated infection of bronchopulmonary dysplasia, congenital heart disease requiring early surgical treatment due to repeated or fatal respiratory infections affecting infant growth and development.

143.3.3. In this period, some special diseases need attention, such as late-onset vitamin K deficiency, which is frequently present in infant with exclusive breastfeeding, chronic diarrhea, and malnutrition. It is prone to have fatal intracranial hemorrhage, and the survivors often leave behind the neurological sequelae, seriously harming the health of babies. During this period, the nerve myelin development is obvious. Early diagnosis and treatment of cerebral palsy can help reduce neurological sequelae.

143.3.4. The immune function has similarities and differences. The common point of post-neonatal infant and other infancy stages is the low immune function. During this period, the non-specific immunity, humoral and cellular immune function are very immature, and levels of sIgA and IgG are low, with low resistance to infection, prone to have various bacterial and viral infections. Clinical manifestations of pneumonia in the post-newborn is more insidious than those of children's pneumonia, The post-newborn infants suffering from pneumonia have usually very light and a typical symptoms such as refusing milk or milk feeding decreasing, no weight increasing, weak cry, and some even lack any clinical manifestation but with rapid disease progress. The difference between neonatal and post-neonatal infants is that the neonatal babies have significantly increased resistance because of colostrum feeding. As the time going on, the maternal antibodies decrease obviously, leading to a variety of infectious diseases such as respiratory syncytial virus, EB virus and EV71 virus.

143.3.5. There is a conflict between the rapid development and growth and uneven development of organ systems during the post-newborn period. This period is the stage for extremely strong growth. The weight of infant has been more than doubled that at the birth. The nutritional requirements are relatively high. At the same time, the uneven development of organ systems, especially the digestive system is often difficult to adapt to a large number of food digestion and absorption. It has been suggested that both nutritional deficiencies and overnutrition are able to significantly affect adult metabolic diseases [13, 19, 20]. The fine mapping of the human genome indicated that diseases were genetically related. Not only genetic (congenital) disease but also risk of acquired and some so called adulthood-starting diseases (such as diabetes, hypertension) might start to be increased before birth or at the infancy and childhood. Moreover, it has made people realize that gene could not be the only factor to decide the human disease. Through epigenetic modifications of gene, early nutrition and its regulation could alter genetic pathway, and then prevent or inhibit the occurrence of disease in adulthood. Classical genetics indicated that individuals of the same gene should have exactly the same phenotype, but the truth is not the case. One pair of identical twins often has the differences in terms of appearance, personality of many aspects, which might be the result of epigenetic modifications. The epigenetics has made the research that under the situation gene DNA sequence has not changed, the gene expression has the inheritable changes. The epigenetics has three important features: (1) not involving DNA changes; (2) gene functions have changed; (3) the change of gene function has heritability and reversibility. Food, as a source of methyl donor may change the gene expression and thus affect the development of various organ systems, possibly through epigenetic methylation modifications.

143.4 Strengthening Investigation of Post-newborn Could Further Reveal the Nature of Life and Improve Life Quality of Children

Pediatrics is the only vertical division of subject in clinical medicine in accordance with the process of human life (age group). The division of each age group has accordingly promoted the research progress of the stage. Especially the establishment of neonatology and its specialties has made remarkable achievements. The infant stage, especially post-newborn is one of the critical periods for individual physique and neurogenesis, with time and spatial differences. Not only the normal anatomy and physiology have the characteristics, but also diseases in different system in terms of etiology, clinical phenotype, assessment method, diagnosis and treatment are quite different from those newborns, children and adults. The research on the developmental law of post-neonatal infants will help to find new diagnosis, treatment and prevention methods for the diseases of children and adults.

The task of the post-newborn research remains how to better promote physical and neurological growth and development of the infants, which are the most basic features and the most common issues in children's life course. The physical development integrates child nutrition, endocrine and metabolic diseases, genetics and environmental medicine. Nutrition is the material basis for physical growth and development, whereas environmental factors are the important aspect affecting development. Researches have revealed that developmental abnormalities are related to human abuse of the environmental substances such as melamine and phthalate esters, whose mechanism may be through endocrine and epigenetic modification. It's important to maintain the balance of nutrients, trace elements, minerals and vitamins. The neurological development is the essence of life quality, which includes the prevention and treatment of children's neurological diseases and mental illness, and promotion of neural development level. Although neurological rehabilitation medicine has been significantly improved, the number of children with neurological and intellectual disabilities has been not significantly decreased because the mortality for neonatal disease, especially preterm infants, severe asphyxia, severe respiratory distress syndrome has been dropped significantly and many survivors suffer from neurological complications. It is a big challenge for pediatrician to carry out the early identification and intervention for the infants with the intellectual disability and high risk factors, and finally reduce the incidence of children with intellectual disabilities.

Prevention of infectious disease and immunization is important for infants during post-newborn. Infectious diseases once led to the death of large number of infants. Along with development of antibiotics and vaccine work, infectious diseases have been obviously under control. However, a few of infectious diseases such as tuberculosis and measles have flared up in recent years. More seriously, at the same time, new resistant strains such as the production NDM-1 "super bacteria" have been emerged constantly. In addition, a number of newly-emerging viruses including H1N1 avian flu virus, EV71 virus, SARS virus have brought forward new challenges. The strengthening of the development for anti-infective drugs, vaccines and vaccination during this period will help decrease the illness of infant, reduce costs for health care, lower the social and family burden, and thus abate infant mortality.

The strengthening of the post-newborn research, especially the research on translational medicine [21], may help to find new ways and methods for the treatment of diseases in infants, children, and adult caused by nutritional abnormalities. The nutritional abnormalities could cause disease by means of epigenetic modification. DNA methylation depends on the dietary intake of methionine and folate which are subject to individual nutrient levels. Low dietary intake of methionine in rats could lead to the occurrence of DNA demethylation, more prone to liver cancer [22]. It has been suggested that mammals should have a critical developmental period before and after birth, and nutrition as well as other environmental stimuli have an impact on developmental processes and cause permanent change in terms of metabolism and susceptibility to chronic disease [23–26]. A few of population epidemiological and animal model experimental data support this view, but the complex biological mechanism is still unclear. Future research in this area is to select possible target goal to improve the nutritional regulation of intestinal development, namely the detailed understanding of the relationships among nutrients, epithelial cells, intestinal flora, enteric nerves and endocrine. It's of great value to find what nutrients and metabolic pathways get involved in regulation of early life and adult dietary regulation of epigenetic mechanisms. More importantly, epigenetic modifications might occur in the critical window period of early life, especially in the post-newborn.

The premise of research is to enhance the degree of concerns on post-newborn. First of all, it is to strengthen the promotion of concept of post-newborn. In the 1980s, the textbook set the "newborn of diabetic mothers" as the independent chapter for etiological diagnosis, which caused a high degree of perinatal medical attention, hence greatly contributed to the research on this disease. For this reason, it's strongly recommend that post-neonatal should be defined as an independent age group and be regulated. The post-newborn should be write into pediatric articles and textbooks. In addition, the relevant theoretical system should be built in time. At the same time, specialized training courses and academic conferences should be held to study on the basis of post-newborn so that the concept of post-newborn could go deep into the field.

References

1. Melonie H, Donna LH et al (2009) Deaths: final data for 2006. Natl Vital Stat Rep 57:1–134
2. Rudan I, Chan KY, Zhang JS et al (2010) Causes of deaths in children younger than 5 years in China in 2008. Lancet 375:1083–1089
3. Kinsella JP, Greenough A, Abman SH (2006) Bronchopulmonary dysplasia. Lancet 367:1421–1431
4. Lillian RB, Avroy AF, Raju TNK (2004). Research on prevention of bilirubin-induced brain injury and kernicterus: national institute of child health and human development conference executive summary. Pediatrics 114:229–233
5. Davidson S, Quinn GE (2011) The impact of pediatric vision disorders in adulthood. Pediatrics 127:334–339
6. Gergely K, Gerinec A (2010) Retinopathy of prematurity–epidemics, incidence, prevalence, blindness. Bratisl Lek Listy 111:514–517
7. Brown KL, Ridout DA, Hoskote A (2006) Delayed diagnosis of congenital heart disease worsens preoperative condition and outcome of surgery in neonates. Heart 92:1298–1302

8. Uzark K, Jones K, Slusher J (2008) Quality of life in children with heart disease as perceived by children and parents. Pediatrics 121:1060–1067
9. Pramana IA, Latzin P, Schlapbach LJ (2011) Respiratory symptoms in preterm infants: burden of disease in the first year of life. Eur J Med Res 16:223–230
10. UN (2009) The Millennium Development Goals report. United Nations, New York
11. Countdown Coverage Writing Group, on behalf of the Countdown to 2015 Core Group (2008) Countdown to 2015 for maternal, newborn, and child survival: the 2008 report on tracking coverage of interventions. Lancet 371:1247–1258
12. Ministry of Health of the People's Republic of China (2009) China health statistics yearbook 2008. Ministry of Health of the People's Republic of China, Beijing
13. Sallout B, Walker M (2003) The fetal origin of adult diseases. J Obstet Gynaecol 23:555–560
14. Xia L, Zhong D (2010) Evolution of cause of infant and mortality in Some countries and regions in the world [Chin]. Chin J Evid Based Pediatr 5:151–154
15. Moon RY, RSC Horne, Hauck FR (2007) Sudden infant death syndrome. Lancet 370:1578–1587
16. Ponsonby AL, Dwyer T, Michael EJ (1992). Sudden infant death syndrome: seasonality and a biphasic model of pathogenesis. J Epidemiol Community Health 46:33–37
17. Task Force on Sudden Infant Death Syndrome (2005) The changing concept of sudden infant death syndrome: diagnostic coding shifts, controversies regarding the sleeping environment, and new variables to consider in reducing risk. Pediatrics 116:1245–1255
18. Z Feng (2011) Attention to mother-born diseases of newborn[Chin]. Chin J Pediatr 49:405–407
19. Barker DJ, Osmond C (1986) Infant mortality, childhood nutrition, and ischaemic heart disease in England and Wales. Lancet 1:1077–1081
20. Hales CN, Barker DJ, Clark PM et al (1991) Fetal and infant growth and impaired glucose tolerance at age 64. BMJ 303:1019–1022
21. Morrow GR, Bellg AJ (1994) Behavioral science in translational research and cancer control. Cancer 74:1409–1417
22. Wilson MJ, Shivapurkar N, Poirier LA (1984) Hypomethylation of hepatic nuclear DNA in rates fed with a carcinogenic methyldeficient diet. Biochem J 218:987–990
23. Lucas A (1991) Programming by early nutrition in man. Ciba Found Symp 156:38–50
24. Waterland RA, Garza C (1999) Potential mechanisms of metabolic imprinting that lead to chronic disease. Am J Clin Nutr 69:179–197
25. Gluckman PD, Hanson MA (2004) Developmental origins of disease paradigm: a mechanistic and evolutionary perspective. Pediatr Res 56:311–317
26. McMillen IC, Robinson JS (2005) Developmental origins of the metabolic syndrome prediction, plasticity, and programming. Physiol Rev 85:571–633

Chapter 144
Analysis of the Characteristics of Papillary Thyroid Carcinoma and Discussion on the Surgery (Experience of 392 Cases)

Jia Liu, Guimin Wang, Guang Chen, Shuai Xue and Su Dong

Abstract The incidence of papillary thyroid carcinoma is increasing in recent years. In order to investigate the biological characteristic of papillary thyroid carcinoma and to discuss on the surgery, we collected clinical data of 392 patients who were diagnosed thyroid papillary carcinoma and underwent total thyroidectomy and conventional central lymph node dissection from January, 2010 to December 2012 in the First Hospital of Jilin University. The operations of 392 cases were all successful. There was no permanent iatrogenic injury of recurrent laryngeal nerve. Only one patient had a permanent hypoparathyroidism. There was bilateral cancer in 112 cases (28.6 %). Thyroid membrane invasion was found in 249 cases (63.5 %), in which the invasion rate of bilateral cancer rate was 44.6 % (50/112). Central cervical lymph node metastasis was found in 191 cases (48.7 %), in which central cervical lymph node metastasis of bilateral cancer rate was 53.6 % (60/112) and of unilateral cancer rate was 46.8 % (131/280). The central cervical lymph node metastasis of thyroid membrane invasion rate was 48.6 % (121/249). The thyroid membrane invasion or cervical lymph node metastasis rate in all cases were 81.4 % (319/392). 62 cases of 112 cases bilateral thyroid papillary carcinoma were diagnosed suspicious unilateral cancer and the rate was 55.4 % (62/112). According to the results, papillary thyroid carcinomas often occur bilaterally and the ration of central cervical lymph node metastasis is very high. We suggest most patients with thyroid papillary carcinoma should undergo total thyroidectomy and conventional central lymph node dissection and combined with I131 and hormonal treatments.

Keywords Papillary thyroid carcinoma · Thyroidectomy · Neck dissection

---

J. Liu · G. Wang · G. Chen · S. Xue
Department of Thyroid Surgery, The First Hospital of Jilin University, Changchun 130021, China

S. Dong (✉)
Department of Anesthesia, The First Hospital of Jilin University, Changchun 130021, China
e-mail: dongsu327@sina.com

144.1 Introduction

Thyroid cancer is the most common endocrine malignancy, although representing less than 1 % of all human tumors. Papillary carcinoma accounts for 85 % of differentiated thyroid cancers and the bilateral accounts for 60 %. We witness a yearly increased incidence and this is may be, in part, due to the increasing use of neck ultrasonography [6]. Nowadays the most commonly occurring differentiated thyroid cancer in many countries is a microcarcinoma in patients older than 45 years, incidentally found during neck ultrasound [10]. In view of their low morbidity and mortality, the crucial point is how to manage such carcinomas. Recently published European and American guidelines aim to minimize the diagnostic and therapeutic procedures without affecting the diagnostic accuracy and the therapeutic effectiveness, keeping in mind that we are dealing with patients who have a normal life expectancy and to whom we have to guarantee an excellent quality of life. Currently there is considerable controversy about the most appropriate treatment of patients with the papillary thyroid cancer. This report concerned the author's experience with 392 patients who were underwent total thyroidectomy and conventional central lymph node dissection in two years, which aim to investigate the biological characteristics of papillary thyroid carcinoma and to discuss on the surgery.

144.2 Materials and Methods

144.2.1 Clinical Data

We collected clinical data of 392 patients who were diagnosed thyroid papillary carcinoma (all confirmed by pathological diagnosis) and underwent total thyroidectomy and conventional central lymph node dissection from January, 2010 to December 2012 in the First Hospital of Jilin University. There were 289 women and 103 men whose mean age was 38.7 years. 212 cases (54.1 %) were found by thyroid ultrasonography during the physical examination.

144.2.2 Methods

144.2.2.1 Preoperative Preparation

Preoperative evaluation mainly included the thyroid and their lymph node ultrasound examination, chest X-ray, fiberoptic laryngoscopy and thyroid function.

144.2.2.2 Surgical Procedure

These operations were performed by the same surgeon and medical group with routine thyroid operation equipment and Heine 3.5 times operation magnifier. We performed general anesthesia with endotracheal intubation. The patient was supine and appropriately positioned with the neck extended with a pad pillow under the shoulder. A transverse incision about 6–12 cm was made about one fingerbreadths above the cervical anterior sterna notch. If possible, the incision incorporated normal skin lines to aid in optimal cosmetic healing. We use electric knife to dissect skin, subcutaneous tissue and the platysma in turn to the anterior cervical muscles surface. Then we dissect neck line and divide neck anterior muscle group to exposure the thyroid glands. The nodule and the surrounding portion of the gland were excised by electric knife or scalpel and were sent for rapid pathologic frozen section. After we received the report about the rapid pathological diagnosis as papillary carcinoma, total thyroidectomy and conventional central neck lymph node dissection were performed. All 392 patients were underwent total thyroidectomy and conventional central lymph node dissection and of which 18 cases were combined with lateral cervical lymph node dissection.

144.3 Results

The operations of 392 cases were all successful. There was no permanent iatrogenic injury of recurrent laryngeal nerve. Only one patient had a permanent hypoparathyroidism (The postoperative pathology confirmed ectopic parathyroid was in the thyroid gland) who was taking oral calcium 1800 mg/day. There was bilateral cancer in 112 cases (28.6 %). Thyroid membrane invasion was found in 249 cases (63.5 %), in which the invasion rate of bilateral cancer rate was 44.6 % (50/112). Central cervical lymph node metastasis was found in 191 cases (48.7 %), in which central cervical lymph node metastasis of bilateral cancer rate was 53.6 % (60/112) and of unilateral cancer rate was 46.8 % (131/280). The central cervical lymph node metastasis of thyroid membrane invasion rate was 48.6 % (121/249). The thyroid membrane invasion or cervical lymph node metastasis rate in all cases were 81.4 % (319/392) (Table 144.1). 62 cases of 112 cases bilateral thyroid papillary carcinoma were diagnosed suspicious unilateral cancer and the rate was 55.4 % (62/112). It included suspicious unilateral cancer and the other side lobe without nodule or with benign nodules which diagnosed by preoperative ultrasound examination. The majority of these were microcarcinomas which diameter were less than 2 mm.

All postoperative cases were taking oral levothyroxine tablets, calcium 1200 mg and vitamin D 300 u. Radioactive iodine treatment was given to the cases with multifocal carcinoma accompanied by lymph node metastasis or by

Table 144.1 Total thyroidectomy and conventional central lymph node dissection (392 cases)

	Cases	Central lymph node metastasis	Membrane invasion	Central lymph node metastasis with membrane invasion
Unilateral cancer	280	131/280 (46.8 %)	199/280 (71.1 %)	79/280 (28.2 %)
Bilateral cancer	112	60/112 (53.6 %)	50/112 (44.6 %)	42/112 (37.5 %)

membrane invasion which confirmed by postoperative pathology. All cases were followed up after operation. The duration of follow-up evaluation is 2–26 months. No recurrence occurred temporarily.

144.4 Discussion

144.4.1 The Thyroid Papillary Ultrasonography

Thyroid papillary microcarcinoma is being diagnosed with increasing frequency and generally has an excellent prognosis with less than 0.5 % disease-specific mortality. Better prognostic stratification, especially for high-risk patients, helps to optimize surgical care. Older age, extrathyroidal invasion, lymph node involvement, and distant metastases are usually regarded as the most potent risk factors for patients with Thyroid papillary microcarcinoma. Total or near-total thyroidectomy is advocated as the initial therapy for most primary microcarcinomas. But it is easy to miss diagnosis because microcarcinoma was small, asymptomatic and often coexisted with benign nodules. Consequently, most cases were found incidentally in the operation of thyroid gland or by postoperative pathological diagnosis. Ultrasound examination for diagnosis of thyroid microcarcinoma had incomparable superiority than others [9].

Ultrasonic examination could even detect microcarcinoma foci which were 1–2 mm diameter. 212 cases were diagnosed by routine thyroid ultrasound examination during physical examination in 392 cases (54.31 %). From the above data we can conclude that thyroid ultrasonography is indispensable to diagnose thyroid microcarcinoma earlier [11]. Through the thyroid ultrasonography, we can know the presence of tumor and its nature, size, number, lymph node metastasis and other information.

144.4.1.1 The Ultrasound Typical Features of Thyroid Papillary Cancer

We can see hypoechoic nodules, unclear boundary, irregular shape, and the aspect ratio is greater than 1. At the same time, we can find calcification in it and the nodules membranes are not continuous. The infiltrations are around the trachea, esophagus, vascular and the internal rich blood vascular display disorder.

144.4.1.2 The Ultrasound Typical Features of Regional Metastatic Lymph Nodes

The metastatic lymph nodes can mostly be found in neck III, IV, VI zones. The shape of lymph node changes to be rounded and the lymph nodes become calcifications, liquefaction and vacuolar. Lymph node portal structures disappear and there are rich blood flow signal in the lymph node.

144.4.2 Central Cervical Lymph Node and Membrane Metastasis

The report demonstrated that bilateral cancer took a significant large proportion in papillary thyroid carcinoma, which was in 112 cases (28.6 %). In addition, the rate of central cervical lymph node metastasis in thyroid papillary carcinoma was high. Central cervical lymph node metastasis was found in 191 cases (48.7 %), in which central cervical lymph node metastasis of bilateral cancer rate was 53.6 % (60/112) and of unilateral cancer rate was 46.8 % (131/280). There were 62 cases (55.4 %) only found suspicious unilateral cancer before the operation in bilateral thyroid papillary carcinoma by postoperative pathological diagnosis. It included suspicious unilateral cancer and the other side lobe without nodule or with benign nodules which diagnosed by preoperative ultrasound examination.

Clinical studies have found neck lymph node metastasis was relevant with membrane invasion of primary tumor. Bardet reported thyroid papillary carcinoma invasion was an independent risk factor to cervical lymph node metastasis and recurrence [5]. The rate of central cervical lymph node metastasis in 211 cases with thyroid membrane invasion was 48.7 % (191/392), which demonstrated that central cervical lymph metastasis was easier occurred in patients with thyroid membrane invasion.

144.4.3 Discussion on Surgery

At present, some domestic scholars endorsed that they could achieve the radical effect by total lobectomy plus isthmusectomy and conventional central lymph node dissection for the patient with unilateral papillary thyroid carcinoma [1]. Based on the statistical analysis, we found the ratio of bilateral central cervical lymph node metastasis were very high in thyroid papillary carcinoma patients. We would easily missed may existent carcinoma foci in the other side lobe if we only performed total lobectomy plus isthmusectomy and lead to early recurrence [4]. Radioactive iodine may be used for diagnosis and treatment of recurrent thyroid cancer and is useful for treating microscopic disease after the entire thyroid gland has been removed. Thyroglobulin (TG) levels may be used to screen for recurrent or persistent disease. After total thyroiddectomy serum TG levels should be low unless the disease is present. Therefore we suggested that the vast majority of patients with papillary thyroid carcinoma should be treated with total thyroidectomy and central cervical lymph node routine dissection [3], followed by I131 therapy and endocrine therapy. Total lobectomy plus isthmusectomy and conventional central lymph node dissection apply only to the lesions confined to one side lobe, the single suspicious lesions, and lesions of less than 1 cm, limited to the membrane and not associated with lymph node metastasis. Nearly decade increasing reports illustrated that cervical lymph node metastasis was a significant prognostic factors of thyroid carcinoma. Lymph node metastasis of papillary thyroid cancer is regular, which mainly concentrated in the VI, IV, and III zone. We found that lymph node metastasis rate of thyroid papillary carcinoma in central zone was up to 43 %. Some domestic research reported that it could be about 60 %. Therefore the central lymph node dissection is indispensable.

144.4.4 Prevention of Complications

The keys to prevent the operation complications are solid understanding of patients' anatomy and skilled surgical technique. Total thyroidectomy is performed not so much because of the worry about postoperative complications including permanent recurrent laryngeal nerve and parathyroid injury [2]. In recent years, along with the anatomical research, the development of operation devices, the improvement of meticulous capsular dissection technique based on the operative field amplification, an experienced surgeon can reduce the incidence of complications [7]. The operations of 392 cases were all successful. There was no permanent iatrogenic injury of recurrent laryngeal nerve. Only one patient had a permanent hypoparathyroidism (The postoperative pathology confirmed ectopic parathyroid was in the thyroid gland) and its rate was 0.25 % (1/392). On the protection of recurrent laryngeal nerve, routine exposure of the recurrent laryngeal nerve is recommended. We should see the never clearly and protect neurovascular bundle with meticulous and no violent operation. We should not blindly cramp until the operation field is clear when bleeding, especially at the top of the point where recurrent laryngeal nerve enter into the larynx. A great deal of emphasis should be laid on the process of dividing the cross site between inferior artery and recurrent laryngeal nerve [8]. Recurrent laryngeal nerve often have multiple branches, we should pay close attention to the protection of branches. If it is difficult to find the nerve, we can look for it further down along the point where recurrent laryngeal nerve enters into the larynx. The inferior thyroid artery and inferior horn of thyroid cartilage are often good masks for looking for recurrent laryngeal nerve. In addition, the conception of nonrecurrent laryngeal nerve should exist (right, left nonrecurrent laryngeal nerve is not reported). Heat injury is cared during application of high-frequency electric knife and ultrasonic scalpel. We should maintain lower power and a certain distance during dissection in the vicinity of recurrent laryngeal nerve. The distance between the ultrasonic scalpel and the never should be 5 mm above while electric knife working distance is larger. Careful ligation and sharp transection to the small vessels near the nerve are advised. For patients with second operation, we can use the recurrent laryngeal nerve detector to help identify, protect and reduce the damage of the recurrent laryngeal nerve as far as possible.

References

1. Abboud B, Tannoury J (2011) Surgical treatment of papillary thyroid carcinoma. J Med Liban 59(4):206–212
2. Giordano D, Valcavi R, Thompson GB (2012) Complications of central neck dissection in patients with papillary thyroid carcinoma: results of a study on 1087 patients and review of the literature. J Thyroid 22(9):911–917
3. Lanq BH, Nq SH (2013) A systematic review and meta-analysis of prophylactic central neck dissection on short-term locoregional recurrence in papillary thyroid carcinoma after total thyroidectomy. J Thyroid [Epub ahead of print]
4. Mazeh H, Chen H (2011) Advances in surgical therapy for thyroid cancer. Nat Rev Endocrinol 7(10):581–588. doi:10.1038/nrendo.2011.140
5. Moo TA, Umunna B, Kato M (2009) Ipsilateral versus bilateral central neck lymph node dissection in papillary thyroid carcinoma. J Ann Surg 250:403–408
6. Pacini F (2012) Thyroid microcarcinoma. Best Prac Res Clin Endocrinol Metab 26(3):3819
7. Sadowski BM, Snyder SK (2009) Routine bilateral central lymph node clearance for papillary thyroid cancer. J Surg 146:696–703; discussion 703–705
8. Steward DL (2012) Update in utility of secondary node dissection for papillary thyroid cancer. J Clin Endocrinol Metab 97(10):333–3398
9. Wang Y, Li L, Wang YX (2012) Ultrasound findings of papillary thyroid microcarcinoma: a review of 113 consecutive cases with histopathologic correlation. J Ultrasound Med Biol 38(10):1681–1688
10. Wu AW, Nguyen C, Wang MB (2011) What is the best treatment for papillary thyroid microcarcinoma? J Larynqosc 121(9):1828–1829. doi:10.1002/lary.22033
11. Yu XM, Lloyd R, Chen H (2012) Current treatment of papillary thyroid microcarcinoma. J Adv Surg 46:191–203

Chapter 145
Skills of Minimally Invasive Endoscopic Thyroidectomy via Small Incision of Neck (Experience of 1,226 Cases)

Jia Liu, Su Dong, Xianying Meng, Shuai Xue and Guang Chen

Abstract Minimally invasive endoscopic thyroidectomy is being adopted by an increasing number of surgeons around the globe. We analyzed clinical data of 1,226 cases of endoscopic thyroidectomy via small incision of neck in the First Hospital of Jilin University in China from June, 2006 to December, 2012. During Surgical procedure, we recorded operation time, blood loss, incision size, the postoperative drainage, beauty score, whether the use of analgesics, postoperative time to discharge, hospitalization costs, with or without tumor recurrence, wound infection and other complications. Thousand two twenty six patients were all successfully operated. The mean operative time of the first 50 cases was (60 ± 13) min; A mean operative time of later 1,176 cases was (41 ± 6) min. 10–82 mL of intra-operative blood loss and 3–35 mL of postoperative drainage were confirmed. After two days drainage tubes were removed. Postoperative hospital stay was (3 ± 1) d. The incision size was 2.0–3.5 cm. Patients were all satisfied with the scar. No analgesic was acquired after the operation. Four cases occurred postoperative transient hoarseness, one case occurred subcutaneous emphysema, 14 cases transferred to open surgery because of thyroid carcinoma with cervical lymph node metastasis. All cases had no postoperative bleeding or infection. The whole group were followed up for 3–12 months, no recurrences happened. The endoscopic thyroidectomy is a feasible and safe procedure. The short postoperative stay, better cosmetic results and less postoperative stress and pain are obvious. It is believed that endoscopic thyroidectomy would become widely used as a surgical procedure for treating small thyroid nodules.

Keywords Thyroidectomy · Endoscopy

J. Liu · X. Meng · S. Xue · G. Chen (✉)
Department of Thyroid Surgery, The First Hospital of Jilin University, 130021 Changchun, China
e-mail: sosea@sina.com

S. Dong
Department of Anesthesia, The First Hospital of Jilin University, Changchun, China

145.1 Introduction

Minimally invasive is the result of the efforts of several surgeons to extrapolate the proven benefits of minimally invasive techniques in the abdomen, chest, blood vessels, and joints compared with the traditional technique of open thyroidectomy. Although endoscopic and minimally invasive surgery is not a new concept, the past decade has seen an explosion in the number of reports in peer-reviewed journals dedicated to this subject. Minimally invasive techniques are classified into two major categories based on whether a skin incision is made in the neck or away from the neck. The first complete endoscopic thyroidectomy was performed by Huscher et al. [7] which created several complications to the initial patients including massive subcutaneous emphysema. In 1999, Miccoli et al. [9] and Bellantone et al. [2] developed a technique that combines elements from the endoscopic thyroidectomy and the traditional open technique. The main idea of this minimally invasive video assisted thyroidectomy (MIVAT) is based on a small horizontal cervical incision approximately one finger breadth above the sternal notch. The cosmetic implications of neck surgery have motivated surgeons and investigators to develop new approaches to access the neck, skull base, and other tracks using minimally invasive techniques. The goals of these techniques are to reduce postoperative recovery time, reduce postoperative pain, and limit external scarring, and to achieve these ends without compromising treatment efficacy. Furthermore, endoscopic thyroidectomy has gradually become a popular approach for surgical treatment in patients with nodular goiter, Graves' disease, and even thyroid carcinoma. This article summarized 1,226 cases of neck minimally invasive endoscopic-assisted thyroidectomy in our department from June, 2006 to December, 2012, which discussed the skills and relevant experience about the operation at the same time.

145.2 Materials and Methods

145.2.1 Clinical Data

We collected clinical data of 1,226 patients, 812 women and 414 men with a mean age of 36.8 years (range: 14–74), from June, 2006 to December 2012 in the First Hospital of Jilin University. Preoperative diagnoses were: PTC in 154 cases, nodular goiter in 551 cases, thyroid adenoma in 355 cases, nodular goiter with adenoma in 101 cases, Hashimoto's goiter in the remaining 55.

145.2.2 Methods

145.2.1.1 Preoperative preparation Preoperative preparation Preoperative evaluation mainly included the thyroid and their lymph node ultrasound examination, chest X-ray, fiberoptic laryngoscopy and thyroid function.

145.2.1.2 Surgical procedure The operation was performed under general anesthesia and tracheal intubation. The patient is positioned supine with slight neck extension. The open component consists of a 20 mm horizontal cervical incision along the cervical crease usually about a fingerbreadth below the lower edge of the cricoids' cartilage. The incision is carried through the skin and subcutaneous tissue to the superficial layer of the deep cervical fascia. Neck flaps are not raised. This is followed by identification and vertical dissection of the anterior cervical muscles at the median raphe. With blunt dissection, a surgical space is obtained around the thyroid gland. This marks the beginning of the endoscopic portion of the procedure. We should pay much attention to protect the recurrent laryngeal nerve, superior laryngeal nerve and parathyroid during this procedure. The choices of surgical approach were: single adenoma for partial thyroidectomy, unilateral multiple nodules for subtotal thyroidectomy, bilateral multiple nodules for subtotal thyroidectomy, unilateral differentiated thyroid carcinoma for the ipsilateral lobe and isthmus resection and contralateral subtotal resection. Bilateral multiple differentiated thyroid cancer for total thyroidectomy. Resection specimens removed from the incision and sent to the frozen section. The residual gland was sewed up with 5–0 polyglactin. Then we rinsed the surgical field, placed a drainage tube in the cavity and used absorbable suture to close the incision.

145.2.1.3 Observation indexes During surgical procedure, we recorded operation time, blood loss, incision size, the postoperative drainage, beauty score, whether the use of analgesics, postoperative time to discharge, hospitalization costs, with or without tumor recurrence, wound infection and other complications.

145.3 Results

Thousand two twenty six patients were all successfully operated. The mean operative time of the first 50 cases was (60 ± 13) min; A mean operative time of later 1,176 cases was (41 ± 6) min. 10–82 mL of intra-operative blood loss and 3–35 mL of postoperative drainage were confirmed. After two days drainage tubes were removed. Postoperative hospital stay was (3 ± 1) d. The incision size was 2.0–3.5 cm. Patients were all satisfied with the scar. Patient satisfaction with the cosmetic result was expressed by a verbal response scale (VRS) after surgeries. Cosmetic results of all were evaluated one month after the operation. Most of the patients were satisfied with the scar, especially in young female patients. We evaluated the sense of pain with the VAS (Visual analogue score). 83 % of the patients were below 60 in the first day and were below 30 in the second day in my study. No analgesic was acquired after the operation. Four cases occurred postoperative transient hoarseness, one case occurred subcutaneous emphysema, 14 cases transferred to open surgery because of thyroid carcinoma with cervical lymph node metastasis. All cases had no postoperative bleeding or infection. The whole group were followed up for 3–12 months, no recurrences happened.

145.4 Discussion

Minimally invasive video-assisted thyroid surgery (MIVAT) was invented by Miccoli [9, 10]. Plenty of groups contribute new improvements or surgical studies with comparable results [11]. Even in pediatric patients the minimally invasive technique (MIVAT) is described to be a proper surgical procedure for certain patients [13]. Other work groups extend the MIVAT technique to functional lateral neck dissections during surgery for metastatic papillary thyroid carcinoma [8]. Being a novel technique, the aspiring surgeons who want to introduce it in their departments have to be aware of ways to do so successfully without compromising current standard of care. An up-to-date knowledge of literature, training opportunities and audit requirements are essential. Del Rio et al. [5] reported their learning curve for minimally invasive video-assisted thyroidectomy (MIVAT). The mean operating time for the first 50 cases (100 cases in total) was significantly higher than the mean operation time for the remaining 50 cases ($p < 0.004$).

The endoscopic system provides an amplified operating field greatly facilitating tissue identification and leading to a reduction of recurrent laryngeal nerve and parathyroid gland injury frequency. Therefore, nerve monitoring applied during surgery in several institutes worldwide can help to protect the recurrent laryngeal nerve [14]. The magnification by endoscopic equipment simplifies the identification of the exact location of parathyroid gland. However, several publications have reported that complications of endoscopic thyroidectomy occurred more frequently during the early application stage of this technique [12]. Improvements in the surgical instruments and skills significantly reduced post-operative complications of endoscopic thyroidectomy. Intra-operative conversion to open surgery is inevitable in certain patients who undergo endoscopic thyroidectomy. Arterial bleeding and large tumor size are both difficult to deal with under endoscopic procedures in comparison to open surgery, especially in the cervical group, where the visual field is easily disturbed within such a relatively limited operating space. In addition, identification of the RLN would be difficult in a narrow space, especially given the anatomical variations of the RLN. Dangerous operative bleeding in endoscopic thyroidectomy usually results from the superior vessels of the thyroid, which is similar to open surgery. Therefore, handling the superior vessels in thyroid surgery is of critical importance. The application of the ultrasonic scalpel has shortened the duration of operating time for endoscopic thyroidectomy and reduced blood loss [4]. Barczyn'ski et al. [1] found that blood loss was significantly lower in the ultrasonic scalpel group than the group that did not use the ultrasonic scalpel (12.9 ± 5.7 vs. 32.8 ± 13.0 ml, $P < 0.001$). In fact, intraoperative blood loss is more relative to the tumor location, tumor size, disease type, and technical skill of the surgeon. In general, there will be more intraoperative blood loss for patients with thyroiditis or (and) Graves' disease, and with a tumor located at the upper thyroid pole. Bellantone et al. and Hegazy et al. [3] both recorded a low volume total intra-operative blood loss (<40 ml) associated with cervical endoscopic thyroidectomy in their RCT studies.

Surgeon should have some tips during surgical procedures. The author believes that surgeon can retreat the lens to reveal a wider range of vision when exposing and put the lens near to the operative field to get a clearly exposure when operating. The endoscope should keep the proper angle with instruments in order to show the sense of depth of the organ and not obstruct the vision of manipulation. It is very important. The surgeon assistant must be familiar with the specific anatomic landmarks. This is a guarantee of success. Sharp head and fast block to cut can be used to separate general adhesion; Blunt head and slow block to cut can be used for the tissue which is relatively thick or estimated that the vascular adhesion or important parts of the organization. when using the ultrasonic scalpel to stop bleeding, for the smaller vessels less than 2 mm, we suggest to use blunt head and mid-range speed directly to cut the organization without first separation of blood vessels; While thick blood vessels should be repeated freezing and not cut off by the blunt instrument head and slow block until we confirm that the organization solidified in order to prevent blood pressure so high to open solidification end or organization be broken so quickly to cause coagulation is not completely. Techniques to prevent the recurrent laryngeal nerve injury are maintaining a clear operative field. We should discern the relationships and do not blindly stopping bleeding and cutting, do not over- stretching the thyroid tissue. Blunt dissection is wiser when operating in recurrent laryngeal nerve region and prolonged use of ultrasonic scalpel should be avoided [4]. Endoscopic recurrent laryngeal nerve revelation can be operated by the positioning of the inferior thyroid artery or throat room. It is easier to identify the parathyroid glands by the virtual zoom vision of endoscope than direct vision. In accordance with the principles of fine capsule anatomy, we can dissociate parathyroid glands, even if we can not confirm the parathyroid (mainly inferior parathyroid), and can also leave it safely.

In 2007, Terris et al. [15] defined the essential principles for cosmetic thyroid surgery. The biggest advantage of endoscopic thyroidectomy in comparison to conventional open surgery is the cosmetic results. Patient satisfaction with the cosmetic result was expressed by a VRS after surgeries. The VRS had four options: 1, poor; 2, acceptable; 3, good; 4, excellent. According to the only available cost analysis study, there is no difference in the total cost between the video-assisted and conventional thyroidectomy [3, 6]. The harmonic scalpel does however reduce operating times for some additional cost. Therefore, initial costs are more related to increased operating time rather than equipment required.

In summary, endoscopic thyroidectomy for patients with thyroid diseases should be personalized. The surgical approach should meet the patients' requirements. Our study demonstrated that endoscopic thyroidectomy is a feasible and safe procedure. The short postoperative stay, better cosmetic results and less postoperative stress and pain are obvious. It is believed that endoscopic thyroidectomy would become widely used as a surgical procedure for treating small thyroid nodules.

References

1. Barczyński M, Konturek A, Cichoń S (2008) Minimally invasive videoassisted thyreoidectomy (MIVAT) with and without use of harmonic scalpel—a randomized study. Langenbecks Arch Surg 393:647–654
2. Bellantone R, Lombardi CP, Raffaelli M, Rubino F, Boscherini M, Perilli W (1999) Minimally invasive, totally gasless video-assisted thyroid lobectomy. Am J Surg 177:342–343
3. Bellantone R, Lombardi CP, Bossola M, Boscherini M, De Crea C, Alesina PF, Traini E (2002) Video-assisted vs. conventional thyroid lobectomy: a randomized trial. Arch Surg 137:301–305
4. Carlos C, Rafael F, Jaqueline R, Herrera MF (2005) A randomized, prospective, parallel group study comparing the Harmonic Scalpel to electrocautery in thyroidectomy. Surgery 137:337–341
5. Del Rio P, Sommaruga L, Cataldo S, Robuschi G, Arcuri MF, Sianesi M (2008) Minimally invasive video-assisted thyroidectomy: the learning curve. Eur Surg Res 41:33–36
6. Hegazy MA, Khater AA, Setit AE, Amin MA, Kotb SZ, El Shafei MA, Yousef TF, Hussein O, Shabana YK, Dayem OT (2007) Minimally invasive video-assisted thyroidectomy for small follicular thyroid nodules. World J Surg 31:1743–1750
7. Huscher CS, Chiodini S, Napolitano C, Recher A (1997) Endoscopic right thyroid lobectomy. Surg Endosc 11:877
8. Lombardi CP, Raffaelli M, Princi P, De CC, Bellantone R (2007) Minimally invasive video-assisted functional lateral neck dissection for metastatic papillary thyroid carcinoma. Am J Surg 193(1):114–118
9. Miccoli P, Berti P, Conte M, Bendinelli C, Marcocci C (1999) Minimally invasive surgery for thyroid small nodules: preliminary report. J Endocrinol Invest 22:849–851
10. Miccoli P, Berti P, Ambrosini CE (2008) Perspective and lessons learned after a decade of minimally invasive video-assisted thyroidectomy. ORL J Otorhinolaryngol Relat Spec 70(5):282–286
11. Ruggieri M, Straniero A, Mascaro A, Genderini M, D'Armiento M, Gargiulo P, Fumarola A, Trimboli P (2005) The minimally invasive open video-assisted approach in surgical thyroid diseases. BMC Surg 5:9
12. Sasaki A, Nakajima J, Ikeda K, Otsuka K, Koeda K, Wakabayashi G (2008) Endoscopic thyroidectomy by the breast approach: a single institution's 9-year experience. World J Surg 32:381–385
13. Spinelli C, Donatini G, Berti P, Materazzi G, Costanzo S, Miccoli P (2008) Minimally invasive video-assisted thyroidectomy in pediatric patients. J Pediatr Surg 43(7):1259–1261
14. Terris DJ, Anderson SK, Watts TL, Chin E (2007) Laryngeal nerve monitoring and minimally invasive thyroid surgery: complementary technologies. Arch Otolaryngol Head Neck Surg 133:1254–1257
15. Terris DJ, Seybt MW, Elchoufi M, Chin E (2007) Cosmetic thyroid surgery: defining the essential principles. Laryngoscope 117:1168–1172

Chapter 146
Research on the Contemporary College Students' Information Literacy

Zhong Wenjuan, Wang Jing, Wang Mei and Guan Yanwen

Abstract *Objective* In order to learn about the current situation of information literacy of the college students in China. *Methods* we take the random sampling method and carry out questionnaire survey in certain groups of students in Nanyang Normal College. This study will cover College students' information awareness, information knowledge, information skills and information ethics. *Result* The contemporary college students have certain information literacy, but their ability needs to be improved urgently. *Conclusion* It is suggested to take appropriate measures to improve their information literacy according to the characteristics of the colleges students.

Keywords Information literacy · College students · Resolving measures

The twenty first century is a period of rapid technological development and rapid expansion of information. People must learn to acquire and apply the resources needed in the vast ocean of information and get the ability to explore the knowledge and to bring different knowledge into mastery. Therefore, information literacy has become one of the most important contents of the learning ability in digital age, at the same time it is important for today's college students whose information literacy should be paid more attention [1]. Information Literacy Competency is the ability of individuals who can obtain the information they needed, it is the basic ability of individuals to survive and develop in the information society [2, 3]. Therefore, the author makes a survey to partly students of Nanyang Normal College in terms of information awareness, information knowledge, information skills, information ethics, by analyzing the survey, the

---

Z. Wenjuan · W. Jing · W. Mei
Health and Nursing College of Wuhan Polytechnic University, Wuhan 430023, China
e-mail: zhongwenjuan2726@sina.com

G. Yanwen (✉)
Huazhong University of Science and Technology, Wuhan 430073, China
e-mail: yanwenguan@hust.edu.cn

author summarizes the shortcomings of college students' information literacy and then proposes the corresponding countermeasures in order to improve Chinese college students' information literacy competency in obtaining information, analyzing information and evaluating information in science and technology developed today.

146.1 Objects and Methods

146.1.1 Research Objects and Contents

This paper chooses Nanyang Normal College students as research objects. By using the way of survey questionnaire, the author randomly selected some certain students and hand out information literacy questionnaire in different majors, To some degree, it controls samples' proportion in terms of students' sex, household register, major, training direction and grade, which makes samples get a better average in each dimension and makes the sample representative broader in order to make research result broad promotion, handing out 200 copies of questionnaires, getting back 190 copies of questionnaires, three copies of invalid questionnaires. Finally, the number of valid questionnaires are 187, effective recovery rate of 93.5 % (See the Table 146.1).

Table 146.1 The general situation construction of college students being investigation

Research objects		Number	Percentage (%)	Cumulative percentage (%)
Sex	Male	96	51.3	51.3
	Female	91	48.7	100.0
Household register	Country	128	68.4	68.4
	City and town	59	31.6	100.0
Majors	Literature and history	64	34.2	34.2
	Science and engineering	62	33.2	67.4
	Arts	61	32.6	100.0
Grade	Freshman	46	24.6	24.6
	Sophomore	48	25.7	50.3
	Junior	48	25.7	75.9
	Senior	45	24.1	100.0

146.1.2 Research Tools

The questionnaire based on Normal students' information literacy questionnaire adopted by Huang Lilii on the East China Normal University [4]. The author partly modifies the questionnaire and designs Nanyang Normal College students' information literacy questionnaire consists of four parts: Information awareness, information knowledge, information skills, information ethics, there are totally 19 questions.

146.1.3 Data Processing

Using the SPSS 12.0 statistical software to describe statistics and process the data by frequency analysis in the descriptive statistics.

146.2 The Results

146.2.1 The Analysis on The College Students' Information Awareness

9.1 % of the students understand the term information literacy well, 42.2 % of the students have only heard of it, 48.7 % of the students do not know the term information literacy at all Table 146.2.

36.4 % of the students take a casual look at it, 52.4 % of the students sometimes think about it and 11.2 % of them often visit it when browsing online news or reports Table 146.3.

Table 146.2 The college students' attitude toward needing information

Information needs of attitude (take the initiative to find)	Frequency	Percentage (%)	Cumulative percentage (%)
Always look for it actively	41	21.9	21.9
Most of the time	108	57.8	79.7
Sometimes	27	14.4	94.1
Rarely	11	5.9	100.0

Table 146.3 The college students would track their interested information

Attitude to tracking information	Frequency	Percentage (%)	Cumulative percentage (%)
Frequently	74	39.6	39.6
Sometimes	86	46.0	85.6
Occasionally	24	12.8	98.4
Never	3	1.6	100.0

146.2.2 Analysis on the College Students in the Aspects of Information and Knowledge

On the degree of understanding of the basic principle of computer networks, 12.3 % of the students are familiar with it, 24.6 % of the students know most of the principles, 56.1 % of the students just know a little, 7.0 % of the students do not understand it at all. As for the needed information and material, 7.5 % of the students know clearly where to find it, 61.5 % of the students relatively know where to find it, 27.3 % of the students don't know clearly where to find it, 3.7 % of the students know nothing where to find it. The situation of the college students on studying the related document searching and database searching courses (see Table 146.4).

Understanding degree of the information retrieval methods is shown in Table 146.5.

146.2.3 Analysis on the College Students in Information skills

Using Baidu or Google and other related searching engines to solve the problems in daily life or study problems, 59.9 % of the college students often use it, 27.3 % of college students occasionally use it, 12.8 % of the college students have not used it yet.

About the mastery degree of Excel, 15 % of college students are good command of using Excel, 75.9 % of college students know some basic operations, 9.1 % of college students don't know how to use Excel.

Ability to take effectively measures to stop hackers or virus from attacking computers, 40.1 % of the students can take effective measures to prevent, 59.9 % of the students are not able to.

Table 146.4 The college students have learned the related courses of the document searching and database searching

Related courses	Frequency	Percentage (%)	Cumulative percentage (%)
Yes	81	43.3	43.3
No	106	56.7	100.0

Table 146.5 The college students' understanding degree of the information retrieval methods

Degree of understanding	Frequency	Percentage (%)	Cumulative percentage (%)
Know well	18	9.6	9.6
Know some	105	56.1	65.8
Just heard of	47	25.1	90.9
Do not know	17	9.1	100.0

146.2.4 Analysis on the College Students in the Information Ethics

In light of situation of browsing Pornographic and violence web sites, 5.9 % of college students frequently browse, 33.2 % of college students occasionally browse, 61 % of college students have not browsed.

On the situation of using books from the library, 18.2 % of college students have made marks on books borrowed from the library. 16.6 % of college students have damaged the paper of books borrowed from the library. 65.2 % of college students have never damaged books borrowed from the library Table 146.6.

146.3 Discuss

146.3.1 The Information Awareness

The college students have a basic sense of information, but the degree of information awareness is not high, The psychological needs for the information is not strong. Some reasons may be that Nanyang Normal College is lack of popularity and publicity of information literacy, so nearly half of the college students have not heard of the term—information literacy. Other reasons may be due to college students' lazy psychological [5]. Those who think carefully when browsing the news reports online take the initiative to find the information needed and always keep tracking the information interested, which takes up low proportion.

Table 146.6 The college students' situation of making personal attacks online

Personal attacks online	Frequency	Percentage (%)	Cumulative percentage (%)
Frequently	5	2.7	2.7
Sometimes	19	10.2	12.8
Seldom	60	32.1	44.9
Never	103	55.1	100.0

146.3.2 The Information Knowledge

The Information knowledge of college students is not rich, For some basic information knowledge, college students just reach low cognitive level. Some reasons may be that the college does not attach importance to information knowledge and college students do not have more channels to obtain the relevant information knowledge. Other possible reasons may be that college offered fewer relevant courses and the teachers didn't make further explanation, so many college students only stay low cognitive level to computer theory and information retrieval methods.

146.3.3 The Information Skills

The college students with basic information skills can master the Searching engine, Excel and other basic computer skills to operate, but most of college students can not master highly specialized skills to take measures to prevent hackers or virus from attacking computers. The reason is that most college students are able to master the basic computer operation, but they failed to master the operation of specialized computer skills unless they learned or are trained. The Information knowledge survey shows that college did not take the information knowledge seriously, for example, the relevant courses are not opened well and the specialized computer skills training is not enough, either.

146.3.4 The Information Ethics

Generally speaking, most college students have the information ethics and only a minority of college students do not have information ethics or their level of information ethics are relatively low. The reason why a small part of the college students have low level of information ethics is that, on the one hand, the chances of college students, on the other hand, the herd mentality of college students.

146.4 Suggestions

146.4.1 Building a Beautiful Campus Environment and Creating a Healthy Study Environment

Colleges should pay more attention to the popularization and promotion of information literacy, organize college students to introduce information literacy and put information literacy into the daily life of college students [6]. Opening document searching courses and colleges should highly emphasize to foster college students' information awareness and improve their ability to get, process and use information, to foster their ability to retrieval, process and apply the information and foster and improve the college students' information ethics.

Colleges should focus on college students' education of information ethics. First, we must attach importance to the teaching of legal basic courses in information law and regulations. Second, teaching information ethics in document retrieval must be focused on, what we add contents of information ethics into document retrieval courses can directly make college students know which behaviors are illegal. Finally, reforming moral education in universities and emphasizing on college students' construction of information ethics should be done [7].

146.4.2 Developing Good Personal Habits and Practicing Independent Learning Style

Colleges students should develop their awareness and ability of independent learning by overcoming their personally lazy psychology. At the same time, college students should make their learning plans and goals by adopting science learning method in order to read faster, better and more relaxing. Colleges students should constantly put knowledge into practice and sum up experience in practice, only doing that they can master the learned knowledge more solidly.

146.4.3 Building Sound Elementary Infrastructure, Coordinating Material and Spiritual Guidance

In the social aspects, the construction of information elementary infrastructure should be accelerated [8]. Nowadays, although China has possessed a certain material and technical basis, further accelerating the research and development of science and technology and the elementary infrastructure construction to meet the needs of the constantly deepening information technology. China should speed up the information' popularization and application and promote the process of education information in the whole society. Meanwhile, we should purify the information cultural environment by legal and ethical means.

In today's era, information literacy has gradually become an important indicator to evaluate the overall quality of talents. College students are high-tech talents and scientific research talents of country's future, their level of information literacy will affect their lifelong study and work [9], higher levels of information literacy for them will play invaluable role in obtaining the information knowledge actively in the future and improving their business level and innovation ability. In order to improve college students' information literacy, it is necessary to efficiently combine the external influence factors with the internal influence factors, to enhance their information literacy education, which can transit high-tech talents and scientific research talents with high level of information literacy to the society, bringing enormous promotional role for our country's technological, economic and cultural development [10].

Acknowledgments The research is supported by the project of 12th five-year plan of educational science in Hubei Provice (No. 2011B327), Doctor's research project of Wuhan Polytechnic University (09y036).

References

1. Ping S, Xiaomu Z (2005) Oriented information literacy outline. Libr Forum 25(4):12–18
2. Haiqun M (1997) On the information literacy education. Libr Acad J 23(2):84–87
3. Wang M (1997) Analysis on the demanding of modern information society for librarian. Gui Tu Acad periodical (4):67–69
4. Huang L (2009) Research on training strategies of normal students information literacy in modern educational technology environment. The East China Normal University, Shanghai
5. Wang J (1999) Information literacy theory. Shanghai Education Press, Shanghai
6. Sang X (2000) Into the learning theory and practice of the information age. Central Radio and Television University Press, Beijing
7. Taiping L (2001) On the information quality and training. High Educ Res (4):99–105
8. Kekang H, Wenguang L (2002) Educational technology. Beijing Normal University Press, Beijing
9. Zhong Z (2001) Information literacy: develop your eight capacities. China Education Newspaper. 1st Mar 2001
10. Zhang Y, Li Y (2003) Information literacy a new definition. Educ Res (3):47–49

Chapter 147
The CEMS Research Based on Web Service

Wenke Zang and Xiyu Liu

Abstract This paper has studied and applied the technology of web service to design a set of continuing education management system (CEMS). Through the web service technology, this system has solved the complex issues in the course of the education management and network data transmission, and improved the efficiency of education management. In accordance with the characteristics of web service and application requirement, the system has designed a unique architecture. The client called by web service communicates with the remote server, achieves lightweight data access to the local xml database operations and a message broadcast mechanism. With its novel design, advanced technique and stable operation, this system has been adopted in many colleges and universities.

Keywords Web service · Continuing education · Educational management

147.1 Introduction

In recent years, with the continuous reform of education system, the size of continuing education has been growing gradually. However, continuing education has some distinctive characteristics that is different from general education: scattering students, scattering classes, repeated admissions, the students' partition according to teaching points, education, learning hierarchy, learning form, which make its management intricate. All the continuous education colleges in the universities are charged with the overall management and control functions of the

W. Zang (✉) · X. Liu
School of Management Science and Engineering, Shandong Normal University, Jinan, 250014 Shandong, China
e-mail: zwker@163.com

X. Liu
e-mail: zwker@163.com

secondary colleges and teaching points, management and maintenance of teaching information of all the colleges, and the implementation of the relevant academic teaching of every secondary colleges and teaching points. At present, there are many teaching system software for general undergraduates, which are mature as well, while the information management is far below the needs of development. In order to meet the increasingly complex requirements of management, the paper proposes an idea of designing the management software of continuous education based on Web Service, and plans to develop a set of continuous education management system which is multi-level distributed, safe and reliable, easily maintained, and of good scalability and openness (Table 147.1).

This paper analyzes and studies the web service technology with the actual needs of the system, and then elaborates the characteristics and advantages of web service technology. On the basis of deep analysis of architecture of web service and implementation mechanism, web service is applied in the design of the system, and the educational management system that is based on web service is successfully developed and applied in many universities in Shandong province. The paper gives a detailed description of relevant technology, design of architecture and the implementation of the system.

147.2 Web Service Technology

147.2.1 Overview

Web Service is a kind of new technical architecture, as well as new application environment of software. Its architecture and implementation technology fully inherited the original technology, and the Web Service is currently regarded as the better extension of internet for interoperability. Web Service ensures the dynamic link between procedures through a series of standards and protocols. Web service technology is a standard mechanism that application releases and exploits software maintenance through intranet or internet, also a component deployed on the web, providing objected-based interface, its client programs find the web service components deployed on the server-side through UDDI(universal description, discovery and integration) protocol, and get the interface to call the service through reading WSDL (web service description language) files that describe the interface of components, and then use the SOAP messages (XML documents based on simple object access protocol) to change data with the server-sided web service through the common ways of transmission (XML can communicate across the firewall) such as HTTP, FTP and SMTP.

Web service makes the combination of component-based development with web best. The component-based object models have been released for a long time, and those models depend on special object model protocol, while web service makes further expansion for the models in the communications to remove obstacles of special object models. Web service mainly makes the business data

Table 147.1 Case models

No.	Functional requirements	Description	Actor
1	Admission management	Processing of the enrolled students' information, including the distribution of schools, teaching points and classes, as well as the registration, generation of student ID, and notice print for college students	College user
2	Enrollment management	Management of the students' basic information, including registration, modification, and the processing of enrollment changes, the print of the list of student status changes, and the various statistics	Teaching point user
3	Teaching management	The management of teaching tasks, including the information management such as teaching plans, arrangement of classes, and the test etc.	Teaching point user
…	……	……	……

transmit on the web through HTTP and SOAP protocol, and web users can use SOAP and HTTP to call the remote object through the web calling.

147.2.2 Web Service Architecture Model

As a new generation of distributed computing model, web service provides a standard method of profession and achieves a distributed communication by using the web requests and responses based on XML, providing unparalleled support for different distributed computing platform and achieving interoperability between languages. The proposal of web service solved the traditional problem of application of indirect techniques, making the architecture which lies on different platforms and uses different object technology remove the differences of platform and implementation and unite on the technology layer of web service.

The architecture of web service is based on the interaction of three roles (service provider, service registry and service requestor), and the interaction is specifically related to the operation of publishing, seeking and binding, all of which act on the components of web service. In a typical case, service providers provide software modules (a web service implementation) which can be accessed by network; they define the service description of web service and publish it to the center of service requestor or service registry. The service requestors use the seek operation from the local or service registry center to search for the description of service, binding it with the service providers by using the service description, and calling the corresponding implementation of web service to interact with it. The role of service providers and service requesters is logic contracture. Figure 147.1 describes the relationship between the three roles and three operations.

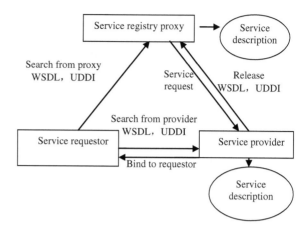

Fig. 147.1 Relationship among three roles and three operations

147.3 Architecture and Design of Educational Management System

147.3.1 Objectives and Requirements of the System

The objective to develop the system is to achieve automation and standardization of continuing education management and to provide integrated management services for layers of educational management by means of computer. The educational management can complete all the daily tasks of educational administration through the system, from the beginning of student enrollment to graduation, all of the education-related data in schools are managed through educational system. Students can query their personal information (curriculum, examination arrangements and results) through the system. Teachers can query their curriculum arrangements and input the results and so on. After the investigation of needs, we determined the basic needs and application details. According to its function, the system mainly include enrollment management, status management, teaching management, examination management, fee management, textbook management, degree management, graduate management. Besides, it also provides file settings for system initialization and the function of online help.

147.3.2 Architecture of the System

The successful experience shows that currently it is right for developing software system especially the large-scale projects to choose the object-oriented. The system builds the system framework and software model by applying unified modeling language UML, combining the rational unified procedure RUP, and using rational software engineering tools Rational Rose etc.

In terms of architecture, the system uses the software engineering theory and tools of Rational Company. In terms of design, the system adopts the specific client + web service + local XML + remote database mode to access the data. The client programs access the data of remote database server by calling web service, including read and write operations; some common data such as parameter settings, learning forms, learning hierarchy and so on are stored in local data sets of XML, whose access does not need network transmission, improving the efficiency finally.

The mechanism of message queue MSMQ in the system can achieve active communication [2] between the different transfer stations through the broadcast.

147.3.3 Functions and Processes of the System

147.3.3.1 Functional Requirements and Case Models

Case, which can be described as an interaction between the actors and the system, is a functional unit in the system. The application of the case models is to list the cases and the actors in the system, and to show which actor involves in the implementation of which case.

147.4 Implementation of the System and Application Results

According to the analyses of the system, we achieve the functions step by step. In the specific implementation processes, we mainly achieve the following two steps:

The first step: to complete basic functions. The proposed development project is a set of complicated rich clients and web applications, which as well can predict various types of data and tables. Therefore, the completion of the basic parts early in the project is in line with the development ideas of "interaction" "progressive" which required by Rational unified process.

The second step: to complete extension. We will complete the rest in the trial run of the beta. The benefit is: if we complete extension on the basis of stable basic functions, the system will have a stable structure, which facilitates future expansion, improvement and perfection.

147.4.1 Development Platform of the System

1. Development Platform: Visual Studio.Net 2010. ASP.NET is one component of Visual Stueio.NET, and the core technology of Visual Stueio.NET, which

represents the latest thinking in a new generation of software development. The applications which adopted the technology have a great improvement in performance, features and system security. Client uses Delphi 7, Web Service server uses C#.NET written.
2. Database: SQL Server 2008.
3. Database access technology: ADO.NET:.NET Framework includes a set of data access technology, which is called ADO.NET, it is easy to connect to data source, and it is one of the most advanced data connectivity technologies.

147.4.2 XML Schema Definition

As the XML document is used between the layers in the system model as the carrier of information interaction, the design of the interface between layers becomes the data modeling for the XML documents to be transmitted [3]. Now, two techniques can be used for data modeling for XML: DTD and XML Schema, among which the XML Schema uses namespace and has rich embedded data types and powerful functions of data structure definition, it is a response to the shortcomings of DTD technology. Compared with DTD, XML Schema has following characteristics which DTD has not in data modeling:

XML Schema is described by XML syntax. Unlike the DTD whose definition complies with their own definition of the syntax, XML Schema definition complies with XML syntax. XML documents determined that the XML Schema has good scalability and flexibility. At the same time, all the tools to parse and process XML documents can be used in XML Schema, which brings a big convenience for XML document processing.

XML Schema owns rich data types. XML Schema provides a wide range of built-in data types, and supports user-defined data types, while DTD only provides a small amount of built-in data types. DTD to data modeling is hard to establish an ideal data model in lack of strong support of data types, but XML Schema seldom has the problem [4].

In this system, the XML document schema that is self-descriptive is established. Among them, the document code of the student information model and professional information model is shown as following:

```xml
<? Xml version="1.0"?>

<xsd: schema xmlns:xsd="http://www.w3.org/2001/XMLSchema">

<xsd: element name="student">

  <xsd: complexType>

    <Xsd: sequence>

      <xsd: element name="studentid" type="xsd: string" minOccurs="0"/>

      <xsd: element name="Student_IDcardNo" type="xsd: string" minOccurs="0"/>

      ......

    </xsd: sequence>

  </xsd: complexType>

</xsd: element>

</xsd:choice>

</xsd: schema>
```

The document models in other modules are similar to student information tables, at this point, we will not go into.

147.4.3 Implementation of Web Service

147.4.3.1 The Establishment of Web Service

At first, we build a web service project, then add the method to achieve system function into the file code in the project, the slight difference between the implementation of the method and the method of other types of projects is to add [Web Method] before the method name, and then to compile and generate DLL files for external client to access.

Take the example of system log to illustrate. Users login server, accept the user name and password, respectively correspond to the parameters of user and pwd. Return code of 1 indicates a successful landing, you can work; return code of 0 indicates failure of landing, you cannot continue to work, and it will provide the reasons for failure.

The format of the return code: 1: successful landing. Data type: string
[Web Method (Description="login service, accept user name and password!")]
Public string Login (string user, string pwd, string hostname)
{
   (...code omitted)
}
[Web Method (Description="......")]// more modular approach to implementation is omitted here.

147.4.3.2 XML Web Service Application

Deploying the web service involves copying all the programs that are used by .asmx files and web service but not part of microsoft.NET framework to the web server.

We designed a web service called DBService. Deploying web service, is then to create a virtual directory and to place the web service.asmx files in this directory. Virtual directory should also be an internet information service web application. A typical deployment has the following directory structure.
\Inetpub
\Wwwroot
\DBService
DBService.asmx
\Bin

Items with the release of web service: web application directory, .asmx file .disco file, web.config file, Bin directory.

Web service discovery is a process to locate the web service description and to inquire, it is also a preliminary step to visit the web service. Through the discovery process, web service clients can understand what functions the existing web service has and how to properly interact with them.

We can find the web service provided by remote server to go into the project and to complete the call through this positioning, when designing clients by using Delphi.

147.5 Conclusion

The system is a set of teaching management software based on web service, designed for continuing education management. Through the communication with many Colleges of Education, the system can now successfully run after more than 6 months' exploitation. However, due to various reasons, there are still some problems to solve and some room to improve.

1. Due to the larger changes in demand, the system cannot make adjustments for all the changes. Since some management changes at any time in practical work, this requires the system to change to adjust. While so far the system has not yet been able to achieve automatic adjustment for the modules, and it can only modify in the background according to the requirements of the users.
2. The need to improve the data backup and data recovery program. The system has provided the function of data backup and data recovery. The system administrators can back up the system at any time to ensure data integrity to certain extent. However, if the data loss is caused by external factors such as virus, disk damage, and natural disasters and so on, this requires a set of rigorous data backup program.

Acknowledgments The research is supported by the College Science and Technology Project of Shandong Province (No: J12LN65), and Jinan Youth Science and Technology Star Project (No: 20120108).

References

1. Wan H, Zhu G (2010) Access control integration of multi-web application system based on web service. Comput Appl Softw 26(7):28–30
2. Liu D, Liu R (2009) Research and implementation of asynchronous web service based on WSE and message queue. Comput Eng 33(08):127–129
3. Jin R, Zhao J-F, Gao Y-B, Shi H-J (2009) Dynamic web services composition based on active XML. Comput Eng 33(18):125–127
4. Wu J, Deng C, Shao X-Y, You B-S (2008) Research on enterprise application integration based on web services. Appl Res Comput (8)
5. Deng S (2010) Using Axis2 asynchronous call to implement large data transportation web services. Comput Appl Softw 25(7):200–201

Chapter 148
Enterprise Development with P Systems

Xiuting Li, Laisheng Xiang and Xiyu Liu

Abstract Enterprises are both an emerging force in national reform and a major force in its future economic development. The professors in China and on abroad have do much research on enterprise development and put forward lots of valuable theories. P systems have been proposed for about 14 years, and its applications refer to numbers of areas. However, to investigate the survival and development of firms in the aspect of P systems is rarely. In this study, it makes analysis on the survival and development of small and medium-sized enterprises in an aspect of bionics, trying to find out the origin which makes the enterprise exuberant and everlasting. Have the enterprises compare to biological cells and construct a membrane framework in order to interpret an enterprise's survival. At the same time it also highlights the irreplaceable role of enterprise DNA in the inheritance of the enterprise entity.

Keywords Enterprise cell · Enterprise DNA · P systems · Bionics

148.1 Introduction

Development of small and medium-sized enterprises is essential to development of national market economy. And they are becoming the most vital growth point in national economy. Researches on how enterprise survive, develop and evolve are

---

X. Li · L. Xiang (✉) · X. Liu
Management Science and Engineering, Shandong Normal University, Shandong, China
e-mail: sunnysddy@gmail.com

X. Li
e-mail: sunnysddy@126.com

X. Liu
e-mail: sdxyliu@163.com

always a main stream of enterprise theory study since the born of enterprise. Management has gone through several stages: Traditional experience management, Classical science management, Behavior science management and Culture management. Why there is more short-lived cooperates than longevous? Various theories give numerous explanations while the problem has not been solved very well. Based or analyzing the basic theory of regarding enterprises as living organism is always been there, because we see them really like an organism with life, living or die, old or young, healthy or sick, and there's life cycle fluctuation. Now, it is the stage of Bionic Management.

148.2 Enterprise Bionics and P Systems

148.2.1 Enterprise Bionics Theory

Until now, there's no certain conclusion on what enterprise bionics is. In the study we consider enterprise bionics as a new management pattern on enterprises' mechanism, which simulates living beings so that to make new design on its structure and function with the purpose of healthy development. It derives from culture management, but has more meanings beyond culture management. It becomes more specific, more maneuverability, and more practical. Properly to handle the relationships between persons, enterprises, society and the environment may be the realization of enterprise's longevity.

There is a great deal of researches concerning the theory of enterprise bionics. The American scholar entrepreneur Ken Baskin [1] holds up the concept of market ecology, organic company, and synergism evolution hypothesis. His book mirrors the origination of organism system over these years, and exposes the basic motivate of business development. Neilson et al. [2] defines the basic factor of enterprise is enterprise DNA, just the same as a person is decided by a series of complicated genes, the enterprise DNA controls the enterprise gene. Professor Li [3] studies the enterprise evolution process from the aspect of enterprise genes and thinks that genes self-organization is the basic mechanism of enterprise evolution. He also points out this mechanism contains the DNA replication, differentiation, recombination and diagnosis—four mechanisms. Liu [4] studies the innovative small and medium-sized enterprises' genes, identifies its structure and analyses its

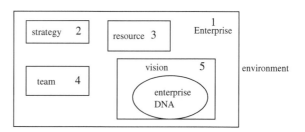

Fig. 148.1 Membrane structure of enterprise cell

activities. He constructs a unity of theoretical framework so that deepens the effect of enterprise genes on its growth of internal mechanism theory research (Fig. 148.1).

148.2.2 P Systems Research

Membrane computing is an emergent branch of natural computing, first introduced by Păun [5]. This unconventional model of computation is a type of distributed parallel system, which is inspired by the structure and function of living cells. The devices of this model are called P systems. For more information, refer to [6, 7].

A P system can be defined as follows: $\Pi = (O, \mu, w_1, \cdots, w_n, (R_1, \rho_1), \cdots (R_n, \rho_n), i_0)$, where,

(i) O is an alphabet of objects, its elements are called objects;
(ii) μ is a membrane structure consisting of n membranes (and hence the regions) injectively labeled with $1, 2, \cdots, n, n \geq 1$;
(iii) w_i are strings that represent multisets over O;
(iv) R_i are finite sets of evolution rules;
(v) ρ_i are a partial order relation on R_i;
(vi) i_0 is the output membrane.

Some basic rules are:
endocytosis rule: $[u]_i[\ ]_j \rightarrow [[v]_i]_j$ exocytosis rule: $[[u]_i]_j \rightarrow [v]_i[\ ]_j$
divide rule: $[u]_i \rightarrow [v]_j[w]_k$ reproduction rule: $[u]_i \rightarrow [\ ]_i[u]_j$
evolution rule: $[u \rightarrow v]_i$ dissolve rule: $[u]_i \rightarrow v$ creation rule: $u \rightarrow [v]_i$
communication rules: sending in: $u[\ ]_i \rightarrow [v]_j$
sending out: $[u]_i \rightarrow [\ ]_j v$.

148.3 Construct the Enterprise Cell Membrane Structure

In the view of enterprise bionics, enterprises also have there life just like any other livings. They have the process of birth, growth, strong, and finally go to die. Considering enterprises as the "cells" of market economy, so enterprises have the structure of P systems. We define a small and medium-sized enterprise as:

$$Enterprise = (O, \mu, w_i, \cdots, w_n, (R_i, \rho_i), \cdots (R_n, \rho_n), i_0)$$

where,

(i) O is an alphabet of objects, its elements are strategy, resource, team, vision and its components respectively;

Fig. 148.2 Inlayer membranes

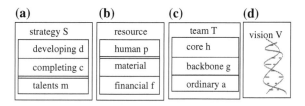

(ii) μ is an enterprise basic structure consisting of n membranes (and hence the regions) injectively labeled with $1, 2, \cdots, n, n \geq 1$;
(iii) w_i are strings that represent multisets over O, as enterprise DNA in vision membrane, we write $w_6 = $ *enterprise DNA*;
(iv) R_i are finite sets of evolution rules, as mentioned upwards, $u \to [v]_i$ can be used to express the creation of an enterprise, company's merger and restructuring is in explanation with $[u]_i [\ ]_j \to [[v]_i]_j$ and so on;
(v) ρ_i is a partial order relation on R_i;
(vi) i_0 is the outside market environment.

There are 6 membranes, and we show it as: $\left[{}_1 [2]_2 [3]_3 [4]_4 [5[6]_6]_5 \right]_1$. Membrane 1 is the skin membrane that separate the enterprise from the market environment; membrane 2 is the strategy membrane, it consists of 3 elementary membranes: developing strategy, competing strategy and talents (Fig. 148.2a); membrane 3 is the resource membrane, it also include-human resources, material resources, financial resources (Fig. 148.2b) three kind of resources; team membrane is labeled with 4, there are: core leadership layer, backbone layer and ordinary employees layer (Fig. 148.2c); membrane 5 is the vision membrane, the enterprise DNA is included(Fig. 148.2d).

The vision of any organization or enterprise decides the enterprise mission, and the enterprise vision membrane contains the enterprise's genetic material—enterprise DNA, and the quality of DNA has a great influence on the enterprise's survival and development, so the vision must be clear, not vague, also cannot change randomly. And the vision's realization needs a series of goals to achieve, and correct strategies to choose. For any goal, needs certain resources, needs to construct and cultivate a team adapting with resources, needs to make corresponding strategies, and then achieve the goal in a proper environment. So when everything is ready, with the rule $SRTV \to [Enterprise]_1$, a new enterprise is born. Strategies need to change with the great change of market environment by $[d_1 c_1 m_1 \to d_2 c_2 m_2]_i$, so that we can adjust ourselves in the increasingly cut-throat competition and to find out effective measures in time. The replication and transfer of enterprise DNA is the enterprise core values' copy and transfer process. The accurate replication of DNA guarantees the core value's correct transformation with $[[enterpriseDNA]_i]_j \to [DNA_1]_i [DNA_2]_j$, just like the model of Mcdonald's. In the time when an enterprise cell actively makes a choice, the choice may turns to some different directions. However, choice itself is an important part in making strategies. The company's core value is actually the core teams' common values to the enterprise operation management. So, when any one conforms to the enterprise value, then the choice will be on behalf of all staffs' will. When the resources are not sufficient, the team's ability is without development, the environment becomes more uncertain, and in a short time finding no corresponding strategy to sharp expansion goal, any of the proposed "strategy" is a dream. With no twist, the company may be die and the resources dissolved by $[SRTV]_i \rightarrow environment$. Therefore, the enterprise's survival and development is the mutual connection of the enterprise vision, strategy, resource, team and external environment.

148.4 Conclusion

From the inorganic machinery without evolution processes to organism with life, we can see that the purpose of enterprises is not simply to maximize profit, but in order to grow or stay longevity. The enterprise strategies should coexist with other components and rely on each other. Considering enterprise as cells, it has its life characteristics, and it can be the foundation and basic basis to use membrane computing theory to carry on the analysis.

By constructing enterprise cell membrane structure, using membrane rules to simulate the growth of enterprises, can be regarded as a major innovation in the point of bionics research on enterprise's development and evolution. However, its live application is not common, and the combination of enterprise development is just a theoretical exploration, the theory and application research remains to be perfect.

Acknowledgments This paper was finally supported by National Natural Science Foundation of China (61170038), Shandong Province Natural Science Foundation (ZR2011FM001), Humanities and Social Sciences Project of Ministry of Education (12YJA630152), Shandong Province Social Science Foundation (11CGLJ22), Project of Shandong Province Higher Educational Science and Technology Program (J12LN22).

References

1. B Ken (2001) Enterprise DNA-Inspired from organism. Citic Press, Beijing
2. Neilson G (2004) Organization DNA. strategic finance. 86(5)
3. Li G (2007) Enterprise evolution mechanism research in the perspective of enterprise gene. Fudan University, Shanghai
4. Liu DS (2011) Study on the gene and Its mechanism of innovative small and medium-sized enterprise. Shandong University, Shandong
5. Păun G (2000) Computing with membranes. J Comput Syst Sci 61(1):108–143
6. Păun G (2002) Membrane computing. An Introduction, Springer, Heidelberg
7. http://ppage.psystems.eu/[C]

8. Zhang YM, Li WW (2009) Constructing the Internal growth mechanism in the small and medium technical enterprise from bionics View. J grad sch of Chin acad of soc sci 4:37–41
9. Păun, Gh (2010) The oxford handbook of membrane computing. Oxford University Press, Oxford
10. Yan, b (2010) The theory of evolution for company reproduction. Hangzhou: Zhejiang People's Publishing House

Chapter 149
Application of Microblog in Educational Technology Practice Teaching

Jiugen Yuan and Ruonan Xing

Abstract Along with the educational reform, the normal students' practice teaching ability of Educational technology is related to its future on their job performance. The emergence of new technology can help us to improve the effect of practice teaching. Microblog's educational potential is proved by a lot of educational practice. Based on the problems existing in the practice teaching of normal students and combined with microblog's characteristic, this study creates the microblog practice teaching process according to three stages: the mobilization preparation, practice teaching and summarize evaluation. We hope it can improve the practice teaching effect.

Keywords Microblog · Educational technology · Practice teaching

149.1 Introduction

Educational Technology is a subject of both theoretical and practical; there are many problems to be solved during its practice teaching. For example, the practice courses ineffective teaching guide normal school students and the instructor in the course of practice due to the characteristics of spatial and temporal dispersion of practical activities, lack of communication, lacking of communication opportunities between students of different practice base. Therefore, normal students need to make some improvements when practice teaching.

J. Yuan (✉)
Education School, Vocational Education Institute, Jiangxi Science and Technology Normal University, Nanchang 330000, China
e-mail: yjgnine@163.com

R. Xing
Communication School, Jiangxi Normal University, Nanchang 330000, China

Social Software (SS) is a application software built on information technology and the internet, its functions can reflect and promote the development of real social relations and the formation of exchanging activities, making the integration of human activities with the software function [1]. Currently, the fastest growing social software is microblog, which is a platform for information's sharing, dissemination and achievement, it is based on users' relationship, users can set up individual communities through WEB, WAP, and a variety of clients, update information in 140 words and share instantly [2]. The perspective of this study is to explore how to use the microblog platform in normal students' practicing teaching, to research the normal students using microblog platform to communicate during the hands-on learning and to explore how to use microblog correctly and effectively to promote normal students' practicing teaching.

149.2 Application Status of Microblog in Teaching

Microblog has already widely played its role on various courses' learning, it used actively by domestic and international teachers in teaching. In our country, the teaching application research about microblog technology is still in its infancy, Haozhaojie, comes from Henan University, introduced microblog to the "C Program" classroom teaching, teacher released the important points of this chapter, a typical example, the job, learning methods, views solicitation and other contents, then students read knowledge points, examples, procedures, learning methods, asked questions, participated in discussions, provided suggestions or recommendations [3]. Researchers confirmed that Twitter can be used as an educational tool to help students to participate in the learning process actively, and mobilize teachers' interest of research [4].

149.3 Practice Teaching Process Based on Microblog

Education practice is designed to make students understand the middle school's teaching situation, its task is to view the classroom teaching and all kinds of research activity through the initial contact with the middle school's teaching practice. To make the students understand each link and operation mechanism in middle school's education teaching, and test their professional basic theory, basic knowledge, basic skills through the education teaching practice, have more definite studying direction in the future. At present normal education practice have many problems, in order to improve students' education practicing effect, strengthen the relationship between students and teacher. The process will be carried out according to Fig. 149.1, and practice teaching process shows as following:

149 Application of Microblog in Educational Technology Practice Teaching

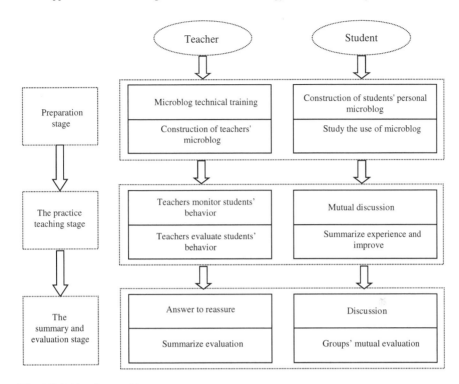

Fig. 149.1 Practice teaching process

149.3.1 Mobilization and Preparation Stage

149.3.1.1 Preparation Before Practice Teaching

Before the teaching practice, teachers should give students an opening meeting, let the students have a preliminary understanding about the purpose and significance of education practice, we can make a preparation for using microblog in advance and qualify basic information literacy in advance.

Although some students have heard or used microblog newly emerged social software, not every student used systematically, especially used it for learning, so it is very necessary to implement microblog technical training before the curriculum. Training includes how to use mobile phones, register web, land microblog account and how to add attention, find someone, release microblog, comments and so on.

149.3.1.2 Teachers and Students Establish Microblog Account and Add Attention

Class participants including teachers are required to use real name to establish microblog account for convenient recognition and supervision. Students practicing in the same school are in a group, members in the same team add attention on each other. In addition, users can add attention on their interested students, teachers focus on each team's leader. All members pay attention to their teachers.

149.3.2 Practice Teaching Stage

149.3.2.1 Arrange Teaching Task and Monitor Students' Behaviour

Through the microblog, teachers issued practice requirement, homework and notice, etc. It requests the normal students' discussions in microblog during practicing, is one of the reference standards of the practicing performance assessment. Student's practicing situation is monitored through the microblog, and for the same practicing group, mainly through browsing apprentice leaders' microblog to understand practice progress. Teachers evaluate students' work through browsing the groups' work released by the leaders, reply and evaluate students' discussions. Students can communicate with their partners and teachers, share their feelings and what they saw and what they heard in practice through the microblog.

149.3.2.2 Students Discuss, Summarize and Improve

Release whatever happened in the practicing school, like your work and things you know in microblog. The other students gathered and comment their interested microblog. The application of microblog in education technology professional practice teaching will show the degree of freedom, live, promptness and structure, which other network interactive tools not have.

149.3.2.3 Teachers Evaluate Students' Behaviour

Students use microblog platform to interact, its using time is not fixed, making the microblog become the main tool for sharing internship experience, solving practice confusion, and testing practice live. Therefore, the teacher needs to regard students' performance in the practice expressed by the microblog as the important basis to evaluate practicing result.

149.3.3 Summary and Evaluation Stage

The concept of microblog is to communicate at anytime and anywhere, it can help students overcome the barriers of time and distance for free communication. Students' evaluation can not only see the team work and their attention, but also the problems' thinking depth, these can improve the accuracy of the practice teaching evaluation.

Through the microblog platform, users can discuss the practicing problems, although users can't participate in others' practice, but can see others' working environment and working characteristics, to broaden normal students' practicing horizon. At the same time, the time of practicing class is limited. It is not enough if only using class time to improve students' practical ability. Normal students can discuss interaction for more information after class through the microblog platform.

149.4 Conclusion

Based on the microblog, practice teaching is positioned at the basis of sharing experience, it transcends the limitations of time and space, share experience, knowledge and tips, and these are the biggest advantage of microblog. Based on microblog, practice teaching should regard microblog as a platform sharing resource and feeling, as an auxiliary practice teaching tool, to help students communicate with their peers, for guidance, self records and reflection. The educational technology professional students can gain more experience from the practical teaching, broaden their thought and vision. Based on its own propagation characteristic, microblog have offered some help to improve the students' practice teaching effect.

References

1. Social Software. http://baike.baidu.com/view/609640.htm. Accessed 28 Feb 2013
2. Microblog. http://baike.baidu.com/view/1567099.htm. Accessed 25 Feb 2013
3. Hao Zhaojie (2011) Application research of microblog in C program design teaching. China Educ Tech 01:101–105, 109
4. Junco R, Heiberger G, Loken E (2011) The effect of Twitter on college student engagement and grades. J Comput Assist Learn 27:ll9–132
5. Ting Luo (2011) Researching into interactive application of microblog in college english teaching for the second classroom. J Hubei Radio Telev Univ 31(02):118–119
6. 10 high files on Twitter. http://chronicle.com/article/10-High-Fliers-on-Twitter/16488

Chapter 150
Ultrasound Image Segmentation Using Graph Cuts with Deformable Prior

Lin Li, Yue Wu and Mao Ye

Abstract Graph cuts for medical image segmentation with graph cuts without prior information is difficult, especial for ultrasound image segmentation. This paper presents a graph cuts algorithm with deformable priors, which can successfully seize clinical ultrasound image features. The experiment shows the success of the proposed approach.

Keywords Ultrasound image · Segmentation · Graph cuts · Deformable prior

150.1 Introduction

The ultrasound imaging is widely used in medical applications for its simplicity, flexibility, cost effectiveness, harmlessness and other advantages. The segmentation for ultrasound image is strongly influenced by the data quality [1]. However, there are factors such as poor signal-to-noise ratio (SNR) and the speckle noise which complicate the segmentation task [2]. So, the segmentation of ultrasound image segmentation is complex.

This paper presents method based on graph cuts with deformable prior to model this kind of situation. In the past decades, Interactive segmentation [3–7] became popular because in different domains, user interaction is available, and it can greatly reduce the ambiguity of segmentation caused by complex object appearance, weak edges, etc. Global optimization [8–15] for graph model, became

---

L. Li (✉) · Y. Wu · M. Ye
University of Electronic Science and Technology of China, No. 2006, Xiyuan Ave,
West Hi-Tech Zone, Chengdu 611731 Sichuan, People's Republic of China
e-mail: lilin200909@gmail.com

L. Li
Sichuan TOP IT Vocational Institute, Chengdu 611743, China

popular because it is more robust compared to the local methods such as thresholding or region-growing.

Our method is mostly inspired by Schoenemann [15], which use the prior knowledge to model the specific scene. We presents the deformable priors information to catch the tumour feature in ultrasound image and graph cuts to seize the global optimization. See Eq. (150.1).

$$Energy = Data + Boundary + Deformable\ Prior \qquad (150.1)$$

Energy is the overall energy. Data represents the point energy. Boundary consists of interaction energy between points. Deformable Prior indicates the objects deformable shapes prior energy.

150.2 Graph Cuts Algorithm with Deformable Prior

Segmenting an object from its background is formulated as a binary labeling problem, i.e. each pixel in the image has to be assigned a label from the label set $L = \{0, 1\}$, where 0 and 1 stand for the background and the object respectively.

Let P be the set of all pixels in the image, and let N be the standard 4 or 8-connected neighborhood system on P, consisting of ordered pixel pairs (p, q) where $p < q$. Let $f_p \in L$ be the label assigned to pixel p, and $f = \{f_p \in P\}$. Our model has the form.

$$E(f) = \sum_{p \in P} D_p(f_p) + \lambda \sum_{(q,q) \in N} V_{pq}(f_p, f_q) + \eta \sum_{(p,q) \in N} DF_{(p,q)} \qquad (150.2)$$

In Eq. (150.2), the first term is called the regional or data term because it incorporates regional constraints. The second sum is called the boundary term because it incorporates the boundary constraints. A segmentation boundary occurs whenever two neighboring pixels are assigned different labels. $V_{(pq)}(f_p, f_q)$ is the penalty for assigning labels f_p and f_q to neighboring pixels. $\eta \sum_{(p,q) \in N} DF_{(p,q)}$ is the deformable shape prior for ultrasound image.

We now show how to implement the deformable shape prior in the graph cuts for ultrasound image segmentation. We assume that the center of the deformable shape C is known (see Fig. 150.1).

Our intrinsic assumption is that the tumor in the ultrasound image is a deformable shape object (see Fig. 150.2 the blue block). Our core task is to model the preassumption. In the third item of Eq. (150.2), η is the weight for its significance in overall energy and $DF_{(p,q)}$ is the deformable prior between pixel p and q. We model it as follow:

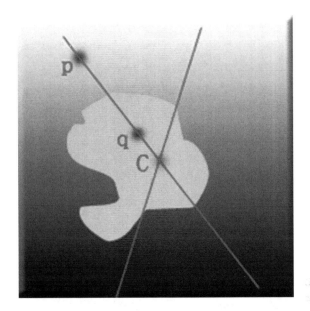

Fig. 150.1 Our deformable shape prior assumption

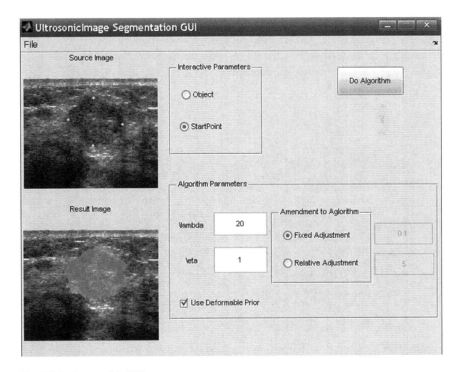

Fig. 150.2 Our matlab GUI

$$DF_{(p,q)} = \begin{cases} 0 \text{ if } f_p = f_q \\ -\|p - C\| + \|q - C\| \text{ if } f_p = 1 \text{ and } f_q = 0 \\ \|p - C\| + \|q - C\| \text{ if } f_p = 0 \text{ and } f_q = 1 \end{cases} \quad (150.3)$$

where C is the start point pixel, $\|.\|$ means the intensity norm between two pixels. $f_q = 1$ means that pixel q belongs to object. $f_q = 0$ means that pixel q belongs to background.

Like Veksler's [16] method, our shape prior also needs revision. We consider two types of revision. One is fixed adjustment which the constance energy is set between pixels. The other one is relative adjustment. We use this formula.

$$D_{relative(p,q)} = \|p.\text{int} - q.\text{int}\| + \|p.x - q.x\| + \|p.y - q.y\| \quad (150.4)$$

where $p.\text{int}$ means that pixel p 's intensity. $p.x$ means that pixel p 's X coordination value in image. $p.y$ means that pixel p 's Y coordination value in image $\|.\|$ means the norm between two values.

150.3 Segmentation Experiment

We used our algorithm to segment a tumor from a ultrasound image. Our implementation consists of two parts: the core algorithm part and the GUI part. The core part was implemented in C++ based on Boykov's [7] code for maxflow computation and CImg for basic image processing. The GUI part was implemented in Matlab for interactive parameters input and segmentation result display (see Fig. 150.2).

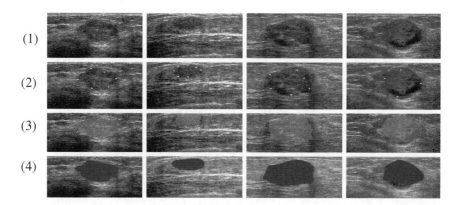

Fig. 150.3 Graph cuts illustration. Row (1) is original ultrasound images. Row (2) shows the start point and object point seed. Row (3) shows the according segmentation results. Row (4) is the Gold standard segmentation

Table 150.1 The comparisons of our method with Schoenemann et al. [15] on four ultrasound images

	B16	B19	C28	C28
Schoenemann et al. [15]	0.854	0.840	0.831	0.879
Our method	0.776	0.791	0.813	0.830

Table 150.2 The running time of our method for four ultrasound images

Image	B16	B19	C28	C28
Running Time (second)	0.673	0.681	0.632	0.709

As shown in Fig. 150.3 row (2), a user initializes the segmentation by clicking on the image to generate seeds for start point (only needing one start point) and object points (see Fig. 150.3 Row (2)). An immediate result is shown in (see Fig. 150.3 Row (3)). The segmentation completes in less than one second on a machine with a Pentium 4 2.0 GHz processor (see Table 150.1).

150.4 Conclusions and Future Works

Although ultrasound segmentation is widely used in medical imaging. It's still a challenge task for ultrasound image segmentation due to the intrinsics characteristics such as speckle noise and poor signal to noise ratio(SNR). Compared with active contours and edge based methods, Graph cuts can escaped from local minima.

Interactive graph-cuts proposed by Boykov is an excellent method for common image boundary segmentation. However, directly using the method for ultrasound image is still challenging. We incorporated the deformable prior in our new energy formula. With the deformable prior, our method can successfully apply to ultrasound image segmentation.

Our segmentation method runs more accuracy than Schoenemann et al. on on four clinical images (see Table 150.1).

Our segmentation method runs fast enough for real time processing, the average time less about 0.7 s per image. However, the actual running time depends on the object seed location and amount of seed. The average range of segmentation running time is about 0.65–0.75 s per image (see Table 150.2).

However our method also have some weakness. The initial start point and object point plays significantly roles in the segmentation results. This will be our future work to find more general energy formula to eliminate the location sensitivity.

References

1. Noble AJ, Boukerroui D (2006) Ultrasound image segmentation: a survey. IEEE Trans Med Imag 25(8):987–1010
2. Pathak SD, Chalana V, Haynor DR, Kim Y (2000) Edge guided boundary delineation in prostate ultrasound images. IEEE Trans Med Imag 19(12):1211–1219
3. Kass M, Witkin, Terzopoulos AD (1998) Snakes: active contour models. IJCV 321–331
4. Mortensen EN, Barrett WA (1998) Interactive segmentation with intelligent scissors. Graph Models Image Proces 60:349–384
5. Boykov Y, Jolly MP (2001) Interactive graph cuts for optimal boundary and region segmentation. ICCV 1:105–112
6. Blake A, Rother C (2004) Interactive image segmentation using an adaptive GMMRF model. In: ECCV
7. Boykov Y, Lea GF (2006) Graph cuts and efficient n-d image segmentation. Int J Comput Vision 69(2):109–131
8. Wu Z, Leahy R (1993) An optimal graph theoretic approach to data clustering: theory and its application to image segmentation. PAMI 15(11):1101–1113
9. Shi J, Malik J (1997), Normalized cuts and image segmentation. In: IEEE Conference on Computer Vision (ICCV), pp 731–737
10. Veksler O (2000) Image segmentation by nested cuts. CVPR I:339–344
11. Jermyn I, Ishikawa H (2001) Globally optimal regions and boundaries as minimum ratio weight cycles. PAMI 23(10):1075–1088
12. Felzenszwalb P, Huttenlocher D (2004) Efficient graph-based image segmentation. IJCV 59(2):167–181
13. Wang S, Kubota T, Siskind J, Wang J (2005) Salient closed boundary extraction with ratio contour. PAMI 27(4):546–561
14. Grady L, Schwartz EL (2006) Isoperimetric graph partitioning for image segmentation. PAMI 28(3):469–475
15. Schoenemann T, Cremers D (2007) Globally optimal image segmentation with an elastic shape prior. In: ICCV, pp 1–6
16. Veksler O (2008) Star shape prior for graph-cut image Segmentation. In:ECCV

Chapter 151
Classifying and Diagnosing 199 Impacted Permanent Using Cone Beam Computed Tomography

Xu-xia Wang, Jian-guang Xu, Yun Chen, Chao Liu, Jun Zheng, Wan-xin Liu, Rui Dong and Jun Zhang

Abstract Grasping the position of embedded teeth in jaw bone and their spatial relationship with neighboring anatomical structures accurately is the foundation of orthodontic and maxillofacial surgical treatments. Cone beam computed tomography (CBCT), a newly developed imaging technique, which produces high definition and high resolution three-dimensional volumetric images, can provide accurate dynamic 3D images and six-surfaces visual angle for locating embedded teeth to get intuitive fault images in comparison with conventional CT. CBCT is being used in the practice of oral and maxillofacial radiology with increasing frequency to make up the shortcomings of traditional plane images. The purpose of this prospective study was to use CBCT to locate 199 impacted teeth of 103 patients, and make a classification.

Keywords Embedded teeth · Cone beam CT · Classification · Diagnosis · Orthodontics

---

X. Wang · Y. Chen · J. Zheng · W. Liu · R. Dong · J. Zhang (✉)
School of Stomatology, Shandong University, Jinan 250012, China
e-mail: zhangj@sdu.edu.cn

X. Wang · J. Zhang
Shandong Provincial Key Laboratory of Oral Biomedicine, Jinan 250012, China

J. Xu
School of Stomatology, Anhui Medical University, Hefei 230032, China

C. Liu
Department of Orthodontics, Shandong Provincial Shengli Hospital, Jinan 250021, China

151.1 Introduction

When tooth eruption has been mechanically impeded by the proximity of adjacent teeth, including supernumerary teeth, one speaks about impaction. Impacted teeth can get infected or damage neighboring teeth, Impacted teeth often or lead to some complications, such as odontoloxia, adjacent root absorption, odontogenic cyst etc., often requiring early intervene. However, the determination of treatment schemes depends on correct diagnosis and localization [1]. The traditional imaging technology plays an important role in the diagnosis of embedded teeth, but it can only show 2D image information, having obvious limitations. Exact three-dimensional localization of impacted teeth is invaluable in orthodontic diagnosis and treatment planning. Cone beam computed tomography (CBCT) is able to provide image scanning and 3D volume data for patients quickly. Also owing to its less irradiation dose and lower cost, CBCT is widely used in oral clinical examination [2–4]. The author of 199 impacted permanent teeth of 103 clinically treated cases retrospectively, now reports as below.

151.2 Materials and Methods

151.2.1 Materials

151.2.1.1 Clinical Material

Cone beam computed tomography (CBCT) images were collected from 103 patients who visited consecutively the orthodontics department of Shandong University Stomatological Hospital (mean age 18.2 ± 6.7, range 8–42 years old).

151.2.1.2 Diagnosis Standard

Diagnosis standard: Impacted permanent teeth except the mandibular third molars still remain embedded in the jaw bone or within the gum and mucous membrane beyond the normal eruption time. X-ray shows: roots are full-grown.

151.2.2 Methods

Making inductive analysis of 199 impacted permanent teeth positions and their types. CBCT enables three-dimensional imaging but has the additional advantages of lower cost, smaller device size, and smaller radiation dose when compared to conventional CT. CBCT has been evaluated for localization of impacted teeth and shows distinct advantages compared to the pantomographic images [1].

Patients were placed in a horizontal position, stabilized with custom-made head bands and chin support, and monitored to ensure that they remained motionless throughout the duration of the scan (36 s).

151.3 Results

151.3.1 Tooth Bit of 199 Impacted Permanent Teeth

(1) Thirty-nine impacted maxillary central incisors come from 33 cases (15 males; mean age 12.2; 18 females; mean age 8.9). Six patients of which have bilateral central incisors impacted, 11 also have maxillary lateral incisor or canine impacted.
(2) Among 94 impacted maxillary canines of 75 patients (34 males, mean age 14.5; 41 females, mean age 13.8); 19 have both maxillary canine impacted; 67 teeth belong to lip-angular impaction; 27 belong to palatal-angular impaction (of which, 10 couple with abnormal lateral incisors).
(3) Among 20 impacted mandibular canines of 11 patients (6 males, mean age 13.7:5 females, mean age 13.2), nine have bilateral mandibular canines impacted simultaneously.
(4) Fourteen impacted maxillary lateral incisors come from nine patients, five of which also have maxillary canines impacted.

151.3.2 Classification

According to the position and their adjacent relationship of embedded teeth, these teeth are divided into the following four basic types:

(1) Horizontal impaction: total 49 teeth, accounting for 24.6 % of all.
(2) Translocation: total 20 teeth, accounting for about 10.1 %.
(3) Lip-angular impaction: total 84 teeth, accounting for 42.2 %.
(4) Palate-angular impaction: total 46 teeth, accounting for 23.1 %.

151.4 Discussion

151.4.1 The Prevalence of Impacted Permanent Teeth Except Mandibular Third Molars

There are many reports about impacted permanent teeth at home and abroad, but the prevalence is different, because of the diversity of race and respondent. As Moyer [5] reported, the rate of impaction is upper canine > upper and lower second premolar > upper central incisor. However this study's result is: upper canine > upper central incisor > lower canine > upper lateral incisor > upper and lower second premolar.

This study demonstrates that the incidence of maxillary central incisors between male and female subjects is 1:1.2. But Witsenburg and Boering [6] reported the rate of that between males and females is 5:3; Geng and Gao [7] publicated the rate is 1.1:1.

The maxillary incisors are the most prominent teeth in an individual's smile, they are crucial to occlusion, facial esthetics and phonetics, in addition, its occurrence rate is high in the population, so it draws much attention. Our researchful results show impaction of maxillary permanent incisors occurs in 3.9 % of outpatients, male to female ratio is 1:1.2. Of these people, about 25 % have bilateral canines impacted. It is different from the occurrence rate reported by some foreign literature [8] (female 1.17 %, male 0.5 % of people with the problem, 8 % have bilateral canines impacted inconformity).

Foreign scholars' study [9] reports, the rate of maxillary canine linguoangular impaction is about $2 \sim 3$ times as high as that of lipoangular impaction, whereas this result is the rate of lipoangular impaction is 1.4 times higher than that of linguoangular impaction. It may result from racial differences or Chinese children' crowded dentition [10]; foreign literature reports the prevalence of impacted mandibular canine is lower, about 0.35 %. The study' results shows that the prevalence is relatively lower, about 1/5 the morbidity of that of maxillary canine, but higher than other teeth sites' occurrence. The ratio of the prevalence of maxillary and mandibular impacted canines is $10 \sim 20:1$ reported by foreign scholars [11], which is very different from our result; Excepting the three tooth bits above, the prevalence of other teeth is quite low.

151.4.2 Impacted Teeth of Typing

According to the position and their adjacent relationship of embedded teeth, divided into the following four basic types: horizontal type, translocational type, lipoangular type and palate-angular type. The horizontal type means that embedded teeth are parallel to the occlusal plane basically, around adjacent root apex or above, visible at lip and palatal side, there are 49 teeth of this kind in this study, accounting for 24.6 % of the total; and the ratio in lip and palate side is no difference. Translocational type means the site of embedded and adjacent teeth switch with each other. We have 20 teeth of this kind, accounting for 10.1 % of the total, often seen in incisive area, seen in premolar area by chance; mostly appear in lip side, rarely in palatal side, and the long axis is upright. Lipoangular type means that embedded teeth locate in the lip side of the dental arch, we have 84 teeth of this kind, accounting for 42.2 % of all, the proportion is the largest of all kinds of embedded teeth; Comparing with lipoangular impaction, palatal type means that embedded teeth are located in the palatal side of the dental arch, we have 46 teeth of this kind, accounting for 23.1 % of all.

Acknowledgments This study was funded by Shandong Provincial Educational, Scientific and Cultural Special Subject (2011107).

References

1. Tymofiyeva O, Rottner K, Jakob PM et al (2010) Three-dimensional localization of impacted teeth using magnetic resonance imaging [J]. Clin Oral Investig 14(2):169–176
2. Tsiklakis K (2010) Cone beam computed tomographic findings in temporomandibular joint disorders [J]. Alpha Omegan 103(2):68–78
3. Cantelmi P, Singer SR, Tamari K (2010) Dental caries in an impacted mandibular second molar: using cone beam computed tomography to explain inconsistent clinical and radiographic findings [J]. Quintessence Int 41(8):627–630
4. Peck S, Peck L, Kataja M (1994) The palatally displaced canine as a dental anomaly of genetic origin [J]. Angle Orthod 64(4):249–256
5. Moyer RE (1988) Handbook of Orthodontics, 4th edn. Year Book Medical, Chicago
6. Witsenburg B, Boering G (1981) Eruption of impacted permanent upper incisors after removal of super numeraryteeth. Int J Oral Surg 10(6):423–431
7. Geng F, Gao X (1995) The diagnosis and treatment of maxillary impacted central incisors. Orthodontics 2(1):25–26
8. Duncan WK, Ashrafi MH, Meister F (1983) Management of the unerupted maxillary anterior tooth. JADA 106(5):640–644
9. Bishara SE (1992) Impacted maxillary canines : a review. Am J Orthod Dentofac Orthop 101(2):159–171
10. Xianglong Z (2000) Modern OrthodonticsDiagnostic Manual. Beijing Medical University Press, Beijing
11. Kerr WJ (1982) A migratory mandibular canine. Br J Orthod 9(2):111–112

Chapter 152
Research Status and Development Tendency of Multi-campus and Two Level Teaching Quality Monitoring and Security System

Mu Lei, Liu Xilin, Wang Keqin and Sun Ye

Abstract In the context of popular education, multiple-campus teaching is a brand-new type of model of teaching with the expansion of enrolment amount. As a kind of immature teaching management mode, multiple-campus teaching faces a serial of obstacles which challenge the effective teaching quality and security system. Therefore, many an institution and scholar at home and abroad conducted all round and multi-level studies on it. Based on the research status of the brief overview of the present multi-campus and two stage teaching quality monitoring and security system, the paper points out some gap and weakness in the present research field and pave the way for future exploration and study.

Keywords Multi-campus · Two level teaching · Teaching quality · Quality assurance · Quality monitoring

152.1 Introduction

Multi-campus universities have a short history in China, which have existed four of six types of international multi-campus universities. (six types: 'self-broadening', 'attached to another university', 'merging and recombination', 'extension mixed with merging', 'public systematic' and 'affiliated colleges' except for public systematic in USA and affiliated colleges in UK and in India). At present, many domestic researches mainly focus on affiliated colleges universities. With a view to some specific features such as regions scattered of multi-campus universities, boosting college and department two level management is an effective means to solve many teaching management problems which caused by enlarging scale of the

---

M. Lei (✉) · L. Xilin · W. Keqin · S. Ye
School of Management, Northwestern Polytechnical University, NPU, Xi'an 710072, China
e-mail: mulei@nwpu.edu.cn

school and complicating organization structure. Under the college and department two level management pattern, teaching quality management and teaching quality security system should make some changes. Therefore, related researches have been conducted at home and abroad. However, some major aspects still don't involve. Thus, purpose of this paper is to come up with further research direction based on research status.

152.2 Research Status at Home and Abroad

152.2.1 Research Status of Teaching Quality Monitoring System

Teaching quality monitoring is a vital sub-system during teaching system, which serves as teaching monitor, evaluations and feedbacks and determines teaching operational direction. All aspects of teaching management, each link is inseparable from the teaching quality monitoring. Teaching quality monitoring including objective monitoring, process monitoring and effect monitoring etc., which is a multi-facet and multi-perspective monitoring and regulating system.

In the perspective of teaching quality monitoring and evaluation, the representatives abroad include International student assessment project hold by Organization for Economic Cooperation and Development, The Third Trends in International Mathematics and Science Study hold by International Association for the Evaluation of Educational Achievement, National Assessment of Educational Progress hold by National Center for Education Statistics and so on. Regarding evaluation method, there are stratification samplings about national students score sample test, matrix way to design test questions, Structure Equation Model to guarantee the structure validity of questionnaires, using multilevel linear model to analysis data with nested relationship.

The domestic researches principally center on classification of teaching quality monitoring, universities and colleges education quality system research, existing questions, graduate design quality control and the role of quality management theory in teaching monitoring. Here, it is necessary to lay emphasis on monitoring taking Hong Kong university education funding council and Hong Kong Council for Accreditation of Academic and Vocational Qualifications as buffer organization, which has an important effect on higher education through Education and Manpower Bureau, Education Commission, Hong Kong university education funding council and Hong Kong Council for Accreditation of Academic and Vocational Qualifications.

With regard to general teaching quality monitoring system, different scholars have different ideas. Some people regard it as an independent environment and constructing teaching quality monitoring closed loop system. Some suggests adopting dynamic school, monitoring group, college, students and teachers five level quality monitoring mode, or college, university two level teaching quality monitoring system. Others construct two level operational and concrete modes.

Other literatures analyze and conclude problems existing in teaching quality monitoring system, and point them out: (1) Unscientific for teaching quality monitoring system. (2) Narrow for the sphere of teaching quality monitoring. (3) Imperfect for evaluation of teaching quality. (4) Insufficient for advocating. (5) Weak for self-monitoring and self-control. (6) Rough for operation. (7) Imperfect for monitoring system. (8) Poor in collecting information. (9) Lack in encouraging and restriction.

Domestic researches partly involved in high school design quality monitoring. And they study the graduate design of general disciplines and mechanical graduate design. Some researches propose application of quality management theory on teaching quality monitoring. For example, some employ all-round quality management of concept and methods, some use all-round quality management and ISO 90000 quality management of concept and methods for reference, forming effective monitoring system. Some refers to ideas of hall three dimensions structure to build the teaching quality monitoring system. And others conduct survey on teaching quality monitoring system based on PDCA circle; other scholars mirror TQM, ISO 9000 to do research on quality management, quality security, quality monitoring, quality feedbacks and control system of college graduate design. And combine practical teaching experience to construct and carry out a set of regular, advanced and practical graduate design quality management and monitoring system.

152.2.2 Research Overview of Teaching Quality Security System

Teaching quality security system of certain education level and education type exert object-orientation, condition guaranteed, restriction, and monitoring and control function in teaching process which makes educational outcomes match certain quality standards to large extent and fits for public demand and expectation.

Research at abroad such as America, Britain and Austria bring in teaching quality security system from Columbia University and Pennsylvania University and introduce unique England teaching style, Cambridge University quality security system and the implications on Chinese high education. Specifically, Cambridge University has a set of teaching quality security system including objectives, structure and organization, plan, internal and external complete teaching quality security system which is scientific, systematic, normative and creative and so on and conforms to international standard and whose modern quality management concept and methods fits for college and university teaching quality management. Open University in Britain pays more attention to teaching quality and establishes strict quality security system: (1) Teacher recruits. (2) Drawing up and publishing high quality textbooks and using multi-media effectively. (3) Establishing strict post responsibility system. (4) Establishing testing system. And also it introduces teaching quality security strategy, Evaluation strategies; Optimization strategies; Heavy release strategies; Role points bear strategies; Information strategies; Internationalization strategies in Australia.

The researches at home mainly focus on the implication and classification of security system and under the level to level system of teaching quality security, graduate teaching quality security system and quality management theory and etc.

Under the classification of teaching quality security system, there are two typical categories. One is external security and internal security; the other is identified teaching quality security and developmental teaching quality system. Therefore, it is about the basic exploration on teaching quality security.

In the context of popular education, many scholars hold different ideas. Some suppose we must establish education teaching quality security system with a core of marketing system, and set up sub-type and sub-level higher education teaching evaluation system. Some study it from perspective of management concept, discipline melting, and teaching quality monitoring and system and culture construction. Others try to construct three dimensional and interactional college internal teaching quality security including teaching condition and teaching reform and teaching management. Besides, some experts do special research on graduate teaching quality system.

As for the application of quality management theory to teaching quality security, a few of literature is involved. They introduce the implication of all-round quality management concept on college education quality management, and elaborate how to mirror all-round management belief to construct education quality. And the literature proposes that we should use Baldrige education quality management to control computer and network communication.

152.3 Further Research in the Future

Based on the above analysis, many scholars and institutions did a large number of researches on multi-campus colleges and universities, colleges of two-level management model under the teaching quality monitoring system, teaching quality security system, etc. But in the context of the popularization of education under the background of multi-campus universities, colleges of two levels of teaching quality monitoring and security system, the following aspects need researching.

(1) Research on multi-campus university management which is composed of 'self-broadening' and 'extension mixed with merging'. (2) In the context of popular education background, multi-campus and two level teaching quality monitoring and security system. (3) How to strengthen the teaching quality monitoring and security of postgraduate design. (4) Research and practice on quality management theory and the standard in the multi-campus schools, two levels of teaching quality monitoring and security system. (5) Research on young

teachers' teaching quality monitoring and security. (6) Research on foreign college teaching quality monitoring and security experience.

152.4 Conclusion

In China, higher education has come into the stage of popular education, and many universities become multi-campus universities and schools. Two levels of teaching quality monitoring and security system gradually become the research hot spot. Therefore, the trend of higher education in china is multi-campus and college and university in the context of popular education, and the eternal theme is teaching quality. Therefore, based on the present research work, we should do the further research, which is an important way to secure and promote teaching quality, and core competitiveness, and is also a band-new tendency to how to promote teaching quality in colleges and universities.

References

1. Gu J (2006) Construction of the dynamic and multilevel supervision system and model of college teaching quality. J Taiyuan Univ Sci Technol 27(5):393–396
2. He G (2005) Foreign teaching quality monitoring and evaluation and its characteristics analysis. J Jiao xue yu guan li 8:75–77
3. Hu C, Tan X, Wu Y (2007) Undergraduate course colleges and universities build and implement the whole process of teaching quality monitoring system.Continue Educ Res 25(8):87–88
4. Jin L (2005) A preliminary study of the problems and strategies in the Multi- Campus University educational administration. J Taizhou Coll 27(5):58–61
5. Lu J (2005) A discussion of diversified Hong Kong higher education quality assurance system. J Technol Coll Educ 24(4):82–84
6. Pan X, Zheng J (2005) Constructing of efficient Undergraduate teaching quality monitoring and security system. China Univ Teach 1:42–44
7. Shi Q, Ning B (2006) Structural and designing ideas of teaching quality monitoring system in American community college. J Higher Educ Res 16(4):92–93
8. Song N, Xiong G, Chen Y (2000) Monitoring system in academic quality based on the model proposed by Baldrige-Winn and C3 techniques. J Taiyuan Univ Sci Technol 18(1):46–53

Chapter 153
Analysis of the Research and Trend for Electronic Whiteboard

Guiying Guo and Baishuang Qiu

Abstract In CNKI, putting "electronic whiteboard" as the title keywords, there are 474 articles retrieved form Periodicals. By the method of content analysis, we analyze the published journal articles on the electronic whiteboard from time distribution, contents of the field, and the change of the concerns in order to research the electronic whiteboard development and application trends. The development proposals are put forward to promote further research and application of the electronic whiteboard.

Keywords Electronic whiteboard · Educational applications · Research

153.1 Research Background

As a new teaching media and technology, electronic whiteboards have a lot of advantages, such as technology integration, resource integration, ease of interaction, and close to the teachers and students and so on. The teaching equipments bring us classroom ecological environment changes, new teaching design and teaching practice. It also supplies a new feature of the classroom culture of teacher-student relationship and interactive classroom atmosphere. From the start of this century, scholars began to focus on the educational applications of the electronic whiteboard, and the deepening research on this teaching equipment. Research results overall

---

G. Guo (✉)
School of Informational Technology, Tianjin University of Technology and Education, Tianjin 300222, China
e-mail: guiyingguo@foxmail.com

B. Qiu
Multimedia Teaching Management Center, College of Light Industry Hebei United University, Tangshan 063000, China
e-mail: qbskeer@126.com

showed an increasing trend. In the context of the electronic whiteboard research concern, combing the state of research, analysis of research trends, and providing references for further study are all the necessary and meaningful works.

153.2 The Course of the Study

In the paper, the research subjects are papers published by the domestic Periodical, in which "Electronic whiteboard" retrieved in the CNKI by "title". Retrieval date is December 2012, and the search result is 474 articles.

The documentary research mainly refers to collecting, identifying, organizing the literature in order to form a scientific understanding of the facts by the study of articles. This paper begins in the collection of the literature, and then collates literature. By the study of literature, we clear the studying situation of electronic whiteboard, then find out its research trends, finally find some problems in the research and then to propose appropriate.

Content analysis is to achieve a scientific understanding of the facts by quantitative analysis of the literature, and with a statistical description of the way. This paper is quantitative analysis of 474 literatures, from distributing of the time, the content changes, and research trends to depict our electronic whiteboard contours and the development in order to raise valuable reference for future research.

153.3 Research Results and Analysis

153.3.1 Articles Time Distribution

The number of papers for electronic whiteboard is rising every year. Began research is seen in 1988, and then the newspapers every year after 1997 studied the electronic whiteboard. The number of articles one year from several to 135 in 2012 has been increasing fast. Before 2007 the quantity was a slowly climbing upward. Annually since 2008, a substantial increased in the number of articles and had been increased to 135 in 2012, which show electronic whiteboard good posture and a wide range of applications trends.

153.3.2 Content Analysis of the Articles

153.3.2.1 Product Development Stage

From 474 papers, the research and development of the electronic whiteboard is divided into two stages by the author, the study and application of the electronic

Table 153.1 Content analysis data in product development stage

Years projects	System implementation and hardware	Function introduction	Applied research	Total of articles
1988		1		1
1997	2		1	3
1998	2			2
1999	3		1	4
2000	6			6
2001	3	4		7
2002	10	4		14
2003	8	1		9
Total	34	10	2	46

whiteboard before 2003 uninvolved education. The papers in 2004 are related to the field of education which developed rapid in the field of education, and the study points were continuously enriched. However the papers in 2003 and before can be referred to as the product development stage, called after the applied research stage. Table 153.1 is the content analysis data in product development stage. Be seen from the table, the system and the number of hardware research articles accounted for 34. Ten articles were about Features, while only two were applied research. This time period electronic whiteboard application in China was still relatively small, there was no scale.

153.3.2.2 Applied Research Stage

Electronic whiteboard field of study began from the 2004 expansion, in addition to mainstream research direction of hardware system. The study applications and prospects of the electronic whiteboard were begun, and finally opened the curtain of applied research, emerging new research results all the time. As shown in Table 153.2, it is the content analysis data in applied research stage.

The articles' content distribution and time distribution in the applied research stage have a detailed analysis in Table 153.2. Combined with the study of the articles contents, the following information can be obtained.

Applied research in the stage is one major research content of the electronic whiteboard. The quantity and quality of the articles have a lot of progress, and the application of research is divided into different directions, disciplinary applications, instructional design, classroom applications, interactive applications, online education applications, the application of academic levels etc. The trend is to constantly refine research directions, making the electronic whiteboard in Education research scene prosperity.

Electronic whiteboard in the various disciplines of mathematics, English, chemistry, physics, geography, art, biological research is the most abundant. The number of the articles is 163, accounting for 34.4 % of the total number of articles. Not only the Number is large, but it also contained more comprehensive learning

Table 153.2 Content analysis data in applied research stage

Project years		2004	2005	2006	2007	2008	2009	2010	2011	2012	Total
Hardware		6	11	12	6	7	8	11	7	9	77
Applied research	Disciplinary applications			2	1	1	8	25	48	78	163
	Instructional design						3			2	5
	Classroom teaching	2	2	4	1	8	5	15	12	19	68
	Application status trend	1		1	1		3	11	9	11	37
	Interactive applications		1			1		2	1	3	8
	Applications of online education			1		1	1	1	1	2	7
	Different academic levels								12	4	16
	Teacher development								3	2	5
Various activities	Spread							1		1	2
	Survey							1		1	2
	Competition						1		2	2	5
	Product introduction		2	1	5	5	2	1	1	1	18
	Conference					2	1	1			4
	Journals						8	1	2		11
Total		9	16	21	14	25	40	70	98	135	428

phase, involving a kindergarten, primary and secondary schools, higher vocational education in colleges and universities, among which the secondary research is most.

Electronic whiteboard disciplinary applications in special education also play a role, such as the deaf school English teaching. Course of the study, the author also found that a feature of the research direction is mostly concentrated in the same unit of researchers. Research papers focused study of a small number of nursery education and vocational education, which researchers are come from the same school.

Product development stage system and hardware accounted for the proportion is high of 74 % and the target is 18 % in applied research stage, ranking second. Therefore, scholars attach great importance to the system development and hardware design. There are more extensive research, such as wireless electronic whiteboard, portable electronic whiteboard Design and Implementation, positioning method, interactive system design.

Acknowledgments This study was part of the research project of "Study on vocational classroom teaching reconfiguration based the interactive electronic whiteboard (KJ10-07)" by the grant from the research and development fund of Tianjin University of Technology and Education.

References

1. Zhan QL (2008) A model for knowledge innovation in online learning community. LNCS 5093:21–31
2. Laurillard D (2002) Rethinking University Teaching. Routledge Falmer, London, pp 81–180
3. Ma N, Chen G, Liu J, Ding J, Yu S (2011) National educational technology guides for teachers in higher education. J Dist Educ 6:3–6

Chapter 154
Study on Multi-faceted Teaching Model of Common Courses in Stomatology: Taking Curriculums of "The Oral Prevention and Health Care" as an Example

Yanyang Xu, Qian Zheng, Yuting Du, XueLi Gou, Guilong Gu, Jianhua Huang and Bin Liu

Abstract In this paper, based on the investigation of the oral prevention and health care, after three years of exploration, we put forward the diversified teaching mode applying on the oral medicine courses open teaching, teaching race, combining intuitive teaching with the comprehensive assessment. During diversified teaching mode, satisfaction of students' listening, interesting of learning, active classroom atmosphere and the students' comprehensive qualities have significantly improved, which is compared with traditional teaching mode.

Keywords Medical general class · Diversified teaching mode · Investigation and research · Satisfaction

In the history of human higher education, it appears successively four training talent modes: free education mode, science education mode, professional education mode and general education mode. With the development of era and the inspection of time, although the professional education is still within the scope of the world widely exist, more and more people heavily rely on general education. General Education is an effective training talent mode, it demonstrates the knowledge and exploration form in these different areas guide students to achieve a variety of different methods of analysis and to understand how to use these

---

Y. Xu · Q. Zheng · Y. Du · X. Gou · J. Huang · B. Liu (✉)
Department of Stomatology, College of Stomatology, Lanzhou University,
Lanzhou 730000, China
e-mail: Liubkq@lzu.edu.cn

Y. Xu
e-mail: xuyanyang@lzu.edu.cn

G. Gu
Science and Technology Agency, Lanzhou University, Lanzhou 730000, China

methods, as well as their value, and it emphasizes the cultivating of ability, method and temperament [1].

To improve the effect of course teaching, it must break through the mode of traditional teaching boldly, and explore a variety of teaching methods actively to enhance the "attraction" of the general education courses [2]. This paper uses the general class named "oral preventive and health care" opened by Lanzhou university of Stomatology school as the research foundation, course teachers and 360 students who selected the course in three semesters of the course as the research object. After exploration and attempt of three years, a combination of open teaching, competition teaching, intuitive teaching and overall evaluation diversified teaching mode have been put forward. The new mode is the innovation of medical general class teaching; meanwhile it achieves the fundamental purpose of stimulating students' interest with students as center.

154.1 The Innovation of Stomatology Medicine General Teaching Model's

(1) Open teaching advocates students to walk out of the classroom and go into the society. The stomatology general education course is a science course, students can understand the clinical characteristics and preventive principle of oral common diseases through learning and master the basic oral health care knowledge, it helps and guides others to conduct oral prevention and health care. In the process of "oral preventive and health care" teaching, it enhances the students' dedication and service awareness, and encourages students to walk out of the classroom and go into the society. By the September 20 "Love Teeth Day", students are mobilized to participate in the theme propaganda of "Love Teeth Day" actively, to temper oneself and to increase their abilities sequentially in practice. In the teaching program it adds the practice step, the questionnaires are to survey about community service, social investigation and so onto develop students' practical and analytical skills, Scientific theory, innovative thinking comes from the practice, and serves to the practice [3]. In the modern teaching environment, open teaching conforms the requirement of teaching reform and respect students' self-behavior, it is the benign teaching mode of "carrying students to knowledge".

(2) Competition teaching cultivates the students' sense of community and problem. How to guide students to find problem actively and solve problems is always focused on by course teachers. Competition teaching is through the form of team competition to teach, pays attention to the cultivation of the spirit of innovation and team spirits, strengthen the students' awareness of problems, the timely feedback of information, and stimulate interest in learning. In the process of the "The oral preventive care" course, students based on study group or study team as the foundation are to participate in various oral competition activities, such as oral preventive and health care non-professional knowledge contest, oral carved

teeth competition, oral skill operation, etc. They are not only strengthening collaboration and cooperation of the team, but also giving full play to the students' competition spirit and competition consciousness, mobilize the study enthusiasm, it is helpful to the cultivation of student consciousness, laying the solid foundation for improving teaching methods and teaching qualities.

(3) The intuitive teaching uses a variety of teaching methods to promote knowledge transferring. From the students' cognitive point of view, the students' vision is broadened through the visit and exchange of classic case, pictures exhibition etc., making the dull knowledge become vivid. Teachers of oral prevention and health care organized the students in beaches to visit the Dental Hospital of Lanzhou University, allowing students to intuitively understand the diagnosis and treatment of common dental diseases, knowing the content of the work of dentists and equipment operation procedures. We utilize the most intuitive ways to help them to realize the importance of oral preventive and health care. With the rapid development of modern information technology, we play videos of classic cases in the classroom and exchange their ideas to make the class more vividly. Apart from that, we collect some classical films, stories and pictures related to oral preventive and health care, introducing and explaining the expertise through the free and easy ways. Intuitive teaching is a common teaching method in medical teaching, especially using in the Medicine General History lesson. Knowledge is more easily accepted by students, it is beneficial to the knowledge dissemination as well.

(4) The intuitive teaching utilizes a variety of assessment methods and comprehensive assessment to promote the enhancement of students' comprehensive qualities. The traditional mode of examination is the one-time examination after the end of the courses, However, they do not pay attention to the usual process of learning. There are many drawbacks about the traditional method, such as the one-sideness of examination function, the contents of examination are similar to teaching materials, and the simplification of examination method [4]. Papers are not the only indicator to assess students' abilities, combining a panel the contents of discussion with research of review, the daily performance of many aspects to assess their comprehensive abilities, which are new methods of assessment of common courses. Oral prevention and health care encourage interdisciplinary, different grades, and different levels of students to discuss the topic. When the courses are end, students should write a review about oral medicine-related problems, according to their interests. The performance of students in study groups or learning teams is focused on by teachers to strengthen the students' teamwork and collaboration capacity-building and make the team promote individual. This class use comprehensive assessments to encourage students to achieve their potentials, enhancing the awareness of innovation. Meanwhile, the students are couraged to explore and think, and cultivate interests and correct learning attitudes, finally, their individual ability can be rapidly promoted.

154.2 Conclusion

General courses are not only focusing on the thought-provoking methods teaching and guiding students to learn forwardly, but also cultivating students' abilities of problems identifying, analyzing and solving, and promoting the development in an all-around way of students. Based on students' psychological, cognitive ability and basic needs, this article summarized, from a new perspective, open, competitive, intuitive and comprehensive assessment, which consist of a diversified curriculum teaching mode. However, the four teaching modes have an influence on each other, and build a complete diversification of common courses teaching mode. Open mode teaching gets rid of the monotonous classroom teaching, which puts emphasis on developing the students' social practical abilities. This method has integrated social organism into the teaching, enhancing students' abilities and strengthening their minds in society. Competitive teaching and intuitive teaching are based on the specific mode of operation to promote the reform of medical general knowledge teaching. They combine the different teaching stages and teaching contents to conduct various forms of group and team competitions. They use the modern multimedia means to improve intuitive teaching, promoting changes with innovation in the pattern of teaching to accomplish teaching programs better. Comprehensive assessment is focused on both of the teaching process and teaching results to fulfill the teaching objectives of enhancing students' comprehensive ability.

In order to understand the diversified teaching mode in the general effect and the role of teaching, a questionnaire survey was conducted in "preventive oral health" of the teacher and the student elective course, a total of 372 questionnaires were handed out, 355 questionnaires were recovered, 321 questionnaires were effective. After investigation and research, we have found that the diversified teaching mode is far superior to the traditional teaching mode, the students' satisfaction about lessons is up to 81.22 %, 89.13 % of the students consider that their interest in learning is enhanced by the diversified teaching mode, 76.34 % of the students think the classroom atmosphere is very active, 81.46 % of the students deem that the new curriculum teaching mode plays an vital role on the promoting the comprehensive quality, 86.37 % of the students hope that the diversified teaching mode is popular in class.

The exploring of the diversified teaching mode is the innovation and experiments of teaching reform, the application of new teaching methods, which is to enhance the teaching quality. The oral prevention and health care lessons let students as a center, the diversified teaching mode is put forward after we research repeatedly, which has a good response in the teaching process. This subject can not only create a free and relaxed atmosphere in the classroom, but also enhance the effective dissemination of knowledge, while is beneficial to improvement of students' comprehensive quality and research ability.

References

1. Li N, Zhou J (2011) Comparison and revelation of university general education course construction in China and USA [J]. Sci Technol Prog Policy 14(28):147–151
2. Li B (2011) How to improve effect of classroom teaching of a curriculum in local colleges [J]. Curriculum Teach Mater (9): 148–149
3. Hu J (2001) Speech in celebrating the anniversary of the Tsinghua University conference. EB/OL, 201(1)
4. Hu J (2008) On the reform of the test system in Chinese higher education [J]. Soc Sci 5(41):25–28

Chapter 155
Teaching Discussion on Pattern Matching Algorithm in the Course of Data Structure

Yang An and Bo Zhao

Abstract Pattern matching algorithm, such as KMP, is one of the most important and difficult problems in the course of data structure. In order that students could better grasp the algorithm, Algorithm KMP is analysed in detail, and relevant examples are illustrated in this article.

Keywords Pattern matching · KMP · Function next · Function nextval

155.1 Introduction

Pattern matching is one of the most important problems in the course of Data Structure, which occurs naturally as parts of data processing, text editing, term rewriting, and natural language processing. However, students usually complain about the pattern matching algorithm that is difficult to understand. In order that students might better grasp the algorithm, Algorithm KMP is analysed in detail, and relevant examples are illustrated in this article.

Assume s is a main string and t is a pattern string, the pattern matching is to find the identical substring in s that is equivalent with the pattern string t and return the beginning location of the t in s. There are a number of string pattern matching algorithms in existence today, such as (BF) and KMP. The simplest matching pattern algorithm is Brute-Force (BF). However a large number of comparisons are occurred without consideration of previous comparisons result in BF algorithm. In fact, this kind of backtracking is not necessary. Therefore the Algorithm we shall discuss in this article is KMP.

Y. An (✉) · B. Zhao
School of Computer, Wuhan University, Wuhan 430072 c, China
e-mail: yangan@whu.edu.cn

155.2 KMP Algorithm

KMP algorithm developed by Knuth, Morris and Pratt is an improvement of the BF algorithm. KMP algorithm is similar to BF algorithm: it considers shifts in order from 1 to n − m, and determines if the pattern matches at that shift. The difference is that the KMP algorithm uses information gleaned from partial matches of the pattern and text to skip over shifts that are guaranteed not to result in a match.

In common cases, assume the main string $s = \text{"}s_0 s_1 \ldots s_{n-1}\text{"}$ and pattern string $t = \text{"}t_0 t_1 \ldots t_{m-1}\text{"}$. Suppose that "$s_{i-j} s_{i-j+1} \ldots s_{i-1}$" is matched with "$t_0 t_1 \ldots t_{j-1}$" and a mismatch then occurs: $s_i \neq t_j$, two situations should be discussed.

(1) If the pattern t contains the proper substring such as "$t_0 t_1 \ldots t_{k-1}$" = "$t_{j-k} t_{j-k+1} \ldots t_{j-1}$" and "$t_0 t_1 \ldots t_{k-2}$" $\neq$ "$t_{j-k+1} t_{j-k+2} \ldots t_{j-1}$", we know that "$t_0 t_1 \ldots t_{k-1}$" has matched with "$s_{i-k} s_{i-k+1} \ldots s_{i-1}$". In this case, the algorithm slides the pattern j−k positions to the right so that s_{i-1} is lined up with t_{k-1}. The next comparison is between s_i and t_k. The procedure can be illustrated in Fig. 155.1.

(2) If the pattern doesn't contain proper substrings, we could deduce that the pattern string "$t_0 t_1 \ldots t_{j-1}$" does not contain any substrings beginning with t_0 that matches a substring ending with s_{i-1} in "$s_{i-j+1} s_{i-j+2} \ldots s_{i-1}$". The next comparison is between s_i and t_0.

Assume next[j] = k, and next[j] is the new position of the pattern that compares with s_i of the main string when the mismatch occurs: $s_i \neq t_j$. The function next[j] is defined as follows:

$$\text{next}[j] = \begin{cases} \max\{k | 0 < k < j \text{ and } \text{"}t_0 t_1 \ldots t_{k-1}\text{"} = \text{"}t_{j-k} t_{j-k+1}\text{"}\} & \text{if this set is not null} \\ -1 & \text{else if } j = 0 \\ 0 & \text{others} \end{cases}$$

The calculation of next[j] and KMP algorithm are described as Algorithm 1 and Algorithm 2 respectively:

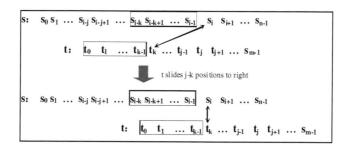

Fig. 155.1 The pattern slide to the right after mismatch in KMP

Algorithm 1: calculating next[j]
```
void GetNext(SqString t,int next[])
{    int j,k;
    j=0; k=-1; next[0]=-1;
    while (j<t.len-1)
    {   if (k==-1 || t.data[j]==t.data[k])
        {    j++;k++;
            next[j]=k;
        }
            else k=next[k];
    }
}
```
Algorithm 2: KMP algorithm
```
int KMPIndex(SqString s,SqString t)
{    int next[MaxSize],i=0,j=0,v;
    GetNext(t,next);
    while (i<s.len && j<t.len)
    {   if (j==-1 || s.data[i]==t.data[j])
        {  i++;j++; }
        else j=next[j];
    }
    if (j>=t.len)  v=i-t.len;
    else  v=-1;
    return v;
}
```

Assume m and n are the length of the main string s and the pattern respectively. The time complexity of calculation of next[j] is O(m). And the time complexity of KMP is O(m + n).

For example, assume s = "aaabaaaab" and t = "aaaab". The corresponding value of next[j] is given in Table 155.1. And the matching process of KMP is shown in Fig. 155.2.

155.3 Improved KMP Algorithm

The KMP algorithm above is more efficient because it doesn't need backtracking of the main string pointer. However, Fig. 155.2 shows that repeated comparisons between the main string and the sequential, identical same characters in the

Table 155.1 Value of next[j] for the example that t = aaaab

j	0	1	1	3	4
t[j]	a	a	a	a	b
next[j]	−1	0	1	2	3

Fig. 155.2 The matching process of KMP

First match	s=aaabaaaab	i=3
	t=aaaab	j=3,j=next[3]=2 failure
Second match	s=aaabaaaab	i=3
	t=aaaab	j=2,j=next[2]=1 failure
Third match	s=aaabaaaab	i=3
	t=aaaab	j=1,j=next[1]=0 failure
Fourth match	s=aaabaaaab	i=3
	t=aaaab	j=0,j=next[0]=-1 failure
Fifth match	s=aaabaaaab	i=9
	t=aaaab	j=5,return9-5=4 success

pattern. For example, when $i = 3$ and $j = 3$, there is $s3 \neq t3$; at this time according to next[j], three comparisons are still required, which are $i = 3$ & $j = 2$, $i = 3$ & $j = 1$ and $i = 3$ & $j = 0$. In fact, the first, second, third and fourth character in the pattern are the same, therefore the pattern string can be slide four characters to right and perform the next comparison ($i = 4, j = 0$).

This indicates another finding. If next[j] = k is derived according to the above definition, and $t_j = t_k$ in the pattern string, then there is no need to compare s_i with t_k if $s_i \neq t_j$. In other words, next[j] equals next[k] at that time. Therefore we revise next[j] to be nextval[j]. Each time nextval[j] is calculated, if $t_j \neq t_k$, then nextval[j] = next[j]; else if $t_j = t_k$, then nextval[j] = nextval[k].

The improved algorithm for calculating nextval[] and the improved KMP are shown respectively in Algorithm 3 and Algorithm 4.

Algorithm 3: The improved algorithm for calculating nextval[].

```
void GetNextval(SqString t,int nextval[])
{   int j=0,k=-1;
    nextval[0]=-1;
    while (j<t.len)
    {   if (k==-1 || t.data[j]==t.data[k])
        {   j++;k++;
            if (t.data[j]!=t.data[k]) nextval[j]=k;
            else nextval[j]=nextval[k];
        }
        else k=nextval[k];
    }
}
```

Table 155.2 Values of next[] and nextval[] of the pattern

j	0	1	1	3	4
t[j]	a	a	a	a	b
next[j]	−1	0	1	2	3
nextval[j]	−1	−1	−1	−1	3

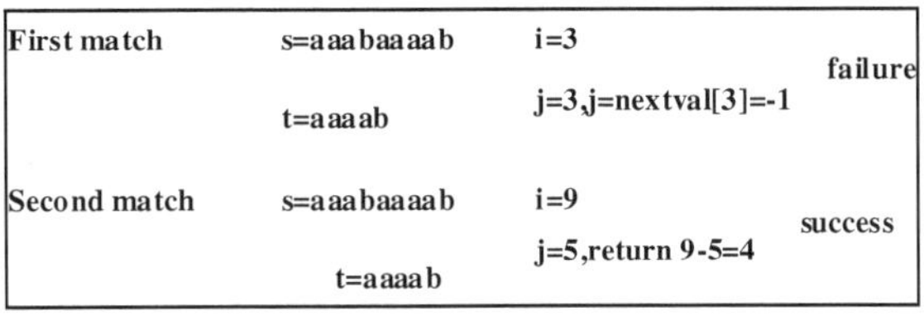

Fig. 155.3 Match process of improved KMP Algorithm

First match	s=aaabaaaab	i=3	failure
	t=aaaab	j=3,j=nextval[3]=−1	
Second match	s=aaabaaaab	i=9	success
	t=aaaab	j=5,return 9-5=4	

Algorithm 4. The improved KMP algorithm.

```
int KMPIndex1(SqString s,SqString t)
{   int nextval[MaxSize],i=0,j=0,v;
    GetNextval(t,nextval);
    while (i<s.len && j<t.len)
    {   if (j==-1 || s.data[i]==t.data[j])
        {  i++;j++; }
        else j=nextval[j];
    }
    if (j>=t.len) v=i-t.len;
    else  v=-1;
    return v;
}
```

The improved KMP algorithm also has a time complexity of $O(n + m)$.

Take the former example, i.e. s = "aaabaaaab" and t = "aaaab". The values of corresponding next[] and nextval[] of the pattern are given in Table 155.2.

According to Table 155.2, the match process is shown in Fig. 155.3.

155.4 Conclusions

String pattern matching is not only one of the most important contents in data structure, but also difficult to understand. It is not easy for students to understand it via simply reading the algorithm or relevant programs. To address this problem, this article proposed a new way to understand the theory of KMP. The article introduced theory of KMP, which eliminates the backtracking of the main string pointer and simply relies on sliding of the pattern pointer. Finally, analyzing two functions of KMP (next and nextval) with relevant examples made students better understand this algorithm comprehensively.

References

1. Weiss M A (2007) Data structures and algorithm analysis in C. Posts & Telecom Press, Beijing
2. Flaming B (1994) Practical data structures in C++. Wiley, New York
3. Sedgewick R (1990) Algorithms in C. Addison-Wesley, Reading

Chapter 156
The Optimal Medical Device Order Strategy: An Improved EOQ Model in Hospital

Wei Yan, Yong Jiang and Huimin Duan

Abstract *Objective* To minimize total stock cost, we make an optimal strategy by which we can submit an appropriate order sheet. *Methods* According to the properties of medical consumables,we list three strategy models: multi-variety in deterministic demand, solo variety in indeterminate demand and multi-variety in indeterminate demand.What's more,we use improved EOQ model to calculate optimal order period and quantities. *Results* We give some formulas which comprise all stock cost parameters.If these costs were confirmed,we can calculate an appropriate order sheet. *Conclusion* A case has been shown to illustrate the method of our order strategy.

Keywords Order form · Stock · Strategy · EOQ (economic order quantity model)

156.1 Introduction

In hospital, medical device storeroom department, which is a key sector connected purchase unit and users, undertakes such works as keeping stock, commodity distribution and order submission. According to 80/20 regulation, stock in hospital always comprises high-cost consumables and common consumables. Purchasing agent often spend only 20 % of their time and energy to transact orders from common consumables. A common way of doing that is that they choose several long-standing suppliers and each takes the responsibility for some varieties. This means that storeroom department should submit economic orders of common

---

W. Yan (✉) · Y. Jiang
Department of Medical Engineering, The Second Artillery General Hospital PLA,
Xinjiekou wai 16# Str, Beijing, China
e-mail: Leucocyte@sina.com

H. Duan
Department of Medical Engineering, The First Affiliated Hospital of the General
Hospital PLA, Beijing, China

consumables for less stock cost and purchasing workload. This order is economic order quantity model (EOQ), which calculates an optimal quantity of minimizing fund occupation but maximizing client's satisfaction.

156.2 Inventory Cost

What we have researched for is to calculated optimal order periods and quantities for a minimum inventory cost. To describe inventory cost precisely, we divide it into acquisition cost, holding cost, shortage cost and prepare cost. All these costs should be estimated in actual cases.

156.2.1 Acquisition Cost

Acquisition cost means costs payed for acquiring goods, include of price, freight and other costs related with order quantity. For example, a one-off injector sells one yuan, its unit acquisition cost is one yuan. Sometimes unit acquisition cost is not a constant, because supplier often gives a discount to encourage a large order sheet. In this article, K is the symbol of unit acquisition cost.

156.2.2 Holding Cost

Holding cost are costs occurred from keeping stock, which include of warehouse rental fees, management fees, employee salary, inventory capital cost, etc. In this article, c_1 is the symbol of unit holding cost in unit time.

156.2.3 Shortage Cost

Shortage cost are direct or indirect losses caused by stock shortage. In this article, c_2 is the symbol of unit shortage cost.

156.2.4 Prepare Cost

Prepare cost are expenses in order submission, include of management fees, commission charge, labor cost and any other costs occured from prepare order and receive goods. In this article, c_3 is the symbol of prepare cost.

If all these costs are confirmed, we can begin our EOQ calculating.

156.3 Methods

In 1915, Ford W. Harris (Westinghouse Corporation) mentioned Economic Order Quantity Model (EOQ) firstly, which is an order strategy to make total inventory costs minimum. There are some postulates in EOQ: ① Never permit shortage. That means shortage cost never can be considered. ② All goods can be delivered instantly. There are not in-transit inventory. ③ Purchasing price and order cost are invariable and not related with quantity.

To adapt demands from medical device stock department, we improved this model. The new model can calculate order quantities of several varieties from one supplier so that various goods can be delivered at same time. This model can reduce expenses of stock department. Many medical consumables in hospital like one-off injectors, infusion devices and etc. can use this model to calculate their order quantities.

156.3.1 Order Periods and Quantities of Multi-variety in Deterministic Demands

In this model, there are n varieties to be ordered. We presume that every variety has a fixed consumption rate (recorded as D_n) and unit acquisition cost. All varieties ordered from one supplier. We complement our stock in t time and never permit shortage. The order quantity is recorded as Q_n. Stock curves are shown as in Fig. 156.1.

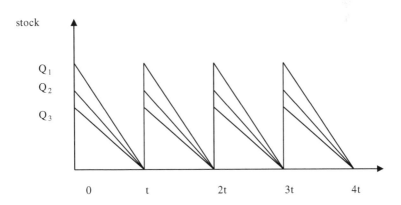

Fig. 156.1 Quantity and time of the order

In this figure, subscript of Q shows its variety. Order quantity Q must satisfy demands in t time. That is to say $Q_n = D_n t$

In t time, average stock is showed as: $\frac{1}{t}\int_0^t D_n t\, dt = \frac{D_n t}{2}$. Average holding cost in t time is $\frac{c_1 D_n t}{2}$. Average prepare cost in t time is $\frac{c_3}{t}$. Because we presumed that c_1 has a unit like box and each box has approximately same bulk, so c_1 is unrelated with its variety. What's more, according to our previous assumption, we needn't to think about unit acquisition cost and shortage cost. We can get average total cost which is recorded as $C(t)$ in t time by adding average unit holding cost and average prepare cost.

$$C(t) = \sum_{n=0}^{n=n} \frac{1}{2} c_1 D_n t + \frac{c_3}{t}$$

$$\frac{dC(t)}{dt} = \frac{1}{2} \sum_{n=0}^{n=n} D_n - \frac{c_3}{t^2}$$

To get minimum of $C(t)$, make $\frac{dC(t)}{dt} = 0$ and then we can calculate optimal order periods which is recorded as t^* $t^* = \sqrt{\frac{2c_3}{c_1 \sum_{n=0}^{n=n} D_n}}$, order quantity

$$Q_n^* = D_n t^* = \sqrt{\frac{2 c_3 D_n^2}{c_1 \sum_{n=0}^{n=n} D_n}} \tag{156.1}$$

156.3.2 Order Period and Quantity of Solo Variety in Indeterminate Demands

Some varieties, like one-off injector or infusion device, can be regarded as fixed consumption rate varieties in hospital, because they have large demands. Some other varieties, like stent or balloon, have such smaller and indeterminate demands that we should use indeterminate demands model to analyze them. In this model, we calculate solo variety firstly. We presume that the variety have a random demand but its distribution is clear. We use a random variable X denote its everyday demand and X obey the law of normal distribution $U(\mu, \sigma^2)$. We use subscript n denote day and every n days is an order period. Q is also quantity, $Q = \sum_{n=0}^{n=n} X_n$. In an order period, the n-th day has a inventory $Q - \sum_{n=0}^{n=n} X_n$. Average stock in n days is

$$\frac{\sum_{n=0}^{n}\left(Q - \sum_{n=0}^{n} X_n\right)}{n} = Q - \frac{\sum\sum X_n}{n} = \frac{1}{n}\sum_{n=2}^{n}(n-1)X_n.$$

Average total cost in n days is the sum of average unit holding cost and average prepare cost. We also record it as C(n).

$C(n) = \frac{c_1}{n}\sum_{n=2}^{n}(n-1)X_n + \frac{c_3}{n} + C(n)$ has a mathematical expectation $E(C) = E\left(\frac{c_1}{n}\sum_{n=2}^{n}(n-1)X_n + \frac{c_3}{n}\right)$. Because variable X obey the law of normal distribution, its linear function has a mathematical expectation as its mathematical expectation of the linear function. In this formula, X_n can be regarded as a constant μ to skip out, $E(C) = \frac{\mu c_1(n-1)}{2} + \frac{c_3}{n}$. To get minimum of E(C), we regarded n as a continuous variable and use derivative method to get a optimal

$$n^*, n^* = \sqrt{\frac{2c_3}{c_1\mu}}, \text{ quantity } Q^* = \mu n^* \quad (156.2)$$

Variable obey the law of normal distribution or uniformly distribution have a characteristic that its linear function still obey its original distribution, but its function has a mathematical expectation as its mathematical expectation of the same function. Because of this characteristic, results of (156.2) are same as (156.1). We only use its mathematical expectation μ instead of D_n

156.3.3 Order Periods and Quantities of Multi-variety in Indeterminate Demands

We can see from (156.1) and (156.2) that order periods and quantities of multi-variety in indeterminate demands are

$$t^* = \sqrt{\frac{2c_3}{c_1\sum_{n=0}^{n=n}\mu_n}}, Q_n^* = \mu_n t^* = \sqrt{\frac{2c_3\mu_n^2}{c_1\sum_{n}= 0^n = n\mu_n}} \quad (156.3)$$

Table 156.1 Consumptions and order quantities in a hospital

Varieties	Everyday consumption (box)		Order quantity after calculate (box)
Injectors of 2 ml	0.3	D_1	6.3
Injectors of 5 ml	0.5	D_2	10.5
Injectors of 10 ml	0.2	D_3	4.2
Injectors of 20 ml	2	D_4	42
Injectors of 50 ml	0.3	D_5	6.3
Infusion devices	1.5	D_6	31.5

In this formula, we can endue time with a unit of day and μ_n means the mathematical expectation of everyday's consumption in the n-th variety.

156.4 Results

A case of EOQ strategy as follows:

In a hospital, one-off infusion devices and injectors of 2, 5, 10, 20, 50 ml are in common use. After statistics, their everyday consumption are listed as follow:

We presumed that 12 boxes could be packed in 1 square meter in the storeroom and each box should expend 0.1 yuan every day as their holding cost according to the rent. They should pay 100 yuan as transport costs for each order. That is to say: c1 = 0.1, c3 = 100. Put these data into formula (156.1), we can get economic order period t* are 21 days and quantities listed in Table 156.1.

References

1. Wenping W (2010) Operations research. Science press, Beijing, p 233–237
2. Chuansheng X, Min Z (2002) The discussion of distribution concerned normal random variable's function. J Shandong Normal Univ (Nat Sci) 17(4):91–93
3. Yaowu L (1995) Probability theory and mathematical statistics. Xi'an jiao tong University Press, Xi'an, p 45–49
4. Xiaoxiao L, Peng W, Feng X, Yanfang X (2008) Application of fixed-quantity ordering method in the stock control of medical consumables. Inf Med Equip 23(12):61–62
5. Xian Z (2012) Commercial economic professional knowledge. China Personnel Publishing House, Beijing, p 145–147
6. Yun F, Jun Z, Jiaqin G, Yuanxing Z (2009) Optimization of the costly medicines management with activity-based costing inventory structure analysis and the order-point technology. Pharm Care Res 268–270
7. Qin Z, Qingli D (2005) Lot order policies based on lead time in supply chain. J SE Univ (Nat Sci Ed) 35(4):628–631
8. Chang HC (2004) An application of fuzzy sets theory to the EOQ model with imperfect quality items. Comput Oper Res 31(12):2079–2092
9. Monahan JP (1984) A quantitative discount pricing model to increase vendor's profits. Manage Sci 30(6):720–726
10. Cardenas Barron, LE (2001) The economic production quantity (EPQ) with shortage derived algebraically. Int J Prod Econ 70:289–292
11. Kim, CH, Hong, Y (1999) An optimal run length in deteriorating production process. Int J Prod Econ 58(2):183–189
12. Rosenblatt MJ, Lee HL (1985) Improving profitability with quantitative discounts under fixed demand. IIE Trans 17(4):388–395
13. Richter K (1996) The EOQ repair and waste disposal model with variable setup numbers. Eur J Oper Res 95(2):313–324

Chapter 157
Improve Effectiveness and Quality of Course Practices by Opening, Reusing and Sharing

Rao Lan and Xinjun Mao

Abstract This paper aims to investigate how to improve the effectiveness and quality of high-level education course practices based on novel strategy and information technologies. We observe and discuss several important properties of course practices for undergraduates of engineering disciplines such as inheritance, continuation, dependency, integration, etc. These properties, together with the several success cases in information area such as open source and crowd engineering, inspires us to innovate the way that the course practices to be performed. We propose that the course practices in high-level education should be opened, reused and shared across time, space and object. Such way is helpful to facilitate the course practices to be performed in an effective way and obtain higher quality. We have developed a software platform *PracStore* that enables undergraduates to browse, query, publish, reuse, and manage large scale course practice resources, interact and share their practice experiences of both success and failure.

Keywords Practice · Information technology · Reuse · Share

157.1 Introduction

In the past years, with the great advancement of high-level education and the rapid development of various technologies like information technology, biology, quantum computing, etc., there are great demands to improve the high-level

R. Lan (✉)
School of Humanities and Social Science, National University of Defense Technology, Changsha, China
e-mail: raolan21@21cn.com

X. Mao
Department of Computer Science and Technology, National University of Defense Technology, Changsha, China
e-mail: mao.xinjun@gmail.com

education quality to satisfy the society and industry requirements. Against the background, many efforts have been made to reform education, especially to enrich undergraduate's knowledge and capability, in a great number of universities and education organizations around the world. For example, in the area of computer science and technology, new version of computer science curriculum is to be revised by Association for Computing Machinery and IEEE Computer Society, etc., and will appear in 2013. The knowledge bodies of computer science and technology are re-arranged by deleting some obsolete knowledge and introducing some new knowledge based on the development of computer science and technology. The courses and their relationships are also reorganized to reflect the recent progresses and future trends of related areas.

Practices as an important and necessary part of course teaching play an increasingly important role in modern high-level education. It is an effective way to enrich the understanding of the knowledge that has been taught in the course and utilize the knowledge and skills to deal with problems. It is also an important link between the university education and future jobs. For example, an undergraduate can more quickly adapt to the job requirements if he once has made practices that are related with the working setting or the practices made in the university are helpful to deal with the problem in future work. Therefore, in recent years many attentions are increasing paid to reform and enforce the course practices, including: introducing more practices into course; investing on laboratory; buying and making more devices to support practices; designing and optimizing practice; managing laboratory based on information technology to support the practice activity 4. All of these efforts result in great progresses of course practices and enhancement of graduate's capability. Nowadays information technology especially Internet technology greatly changes the way with which we work, live and study. It provides an effective way to connect various persons, resources and data. It also influences immensely change the high-level education and course practices. Some new modes and their successes of information systems 12 (e.g., AppStore, open source community) inspire us to reform the course practices from the macro level and external viewpoint in order to take advantage of information technology to improve the effectiveness and quality of practices in high-level education. Especially we should change the way that practice is to be performed and facilitate the sharing and reusing of course practice cross different courses and curricula.

157.2 Characteristics of Course Practices

Though the knowledge body, curricula and education objectives are various for different disciplines, there are some common characteristics behinds the course practices, especially for the engineering disciplines. First, the knowledge body is often structural. Different knowledge body and courses are tightly related. Therefore, the courses and there relations in curricula can be modeled as a graph.

Some courses may depend on the knowledge body that is provided in other courses. Some practices should be made when specific practices have been made. Second, practices based on the knowledge body often take form of hierarchy, which means there are tight relationships between various practices. One practice may depend on another in term of knowledge, capability or experience. Some comprehensive practices should be performed when the constituent of the practices have been made. Third, knowledge is increasing growing and exploding. Any graduate can not obtain all of the knowledge in limited education duration. Therefore, it is a good way to practice and make experiment based on the existing fruits. According to the above analysis, we can identify some interesting and meaningful characteristics of the practices in high-level education.

- *Inheritance*
  A practice often needs elements (e.g., constituent, approach, experience) that are provided in other practices. In other words, a practice may inherit other practice. Therefore, it is not necessary for graduate to perform all elements or aspects of the practices, which means that if we can get a good experience or component to fulfill the practice, it is suggested to inherit these valuable constituents.
- *Dependency*
  There are tight dependencies between practices. For example, a practice is based on the output of another practice or depends on the component that is generated in another practice. Such dependency means the practices in curricula should be well-organized.
- *Continuation*
  A practice and corresponding constituents may be performed in multiple phases and across different courses or semesters. It can be continuously extended or revised to satisfy the practice requirements in different education phases. For example, for software engineering education, a practice of software requirement analysis can be further extended and continued to support the software design practice.
- *Integration*
  Practices may have different grains. Coarse-grain practices often comprise of fine-grain practices. Therefore, coarse-grain and high level practices can integrate a number of fine-grain and low level practice to satisfy the practice objectives.

157.3 Approach to Improving Course Practices

The above characteristics of practices in high-level education require us to consider the organization, management, arrangement and design of practices in a systematics way. Especially, we should seek method that is coherent with the characteristics of practices at a high level and from macro viewpoint to improve the effectiveness and quality of practices.

Some successful cases in formation areas give us inspirations of how to improve the effectiveness and quality of practices. We believe these approaches are meaningful and effective to reform the course practices. (1) The success of open source software. In the past years, open source obtains success and greatly changes the way with which software is developed. A typical sample is Linux. The essence of open source is that the source of software is opened and can be easily upgraded, extended and integrated by developers. Therefore, many software systems can integrate existing open sources and are not necessary to be developer from scratch123. (2) The success of crowding engineering. A typical sample is AppStore. It is imaginableness in traditional engineering way to develop millions of software systems in a comparative short time (e.g., 1–2 years). However, AppStore become successful and accumulates millions of software systems ranging from games to book reader. The essence of crowding engineering is to extensively make use of crowds (e.g., involving persons and their contributions) to jointly perform a task. (3) The wide application of Internet-based social media and interaction. The recent emergences of several new Internet applications such as WiKi, Blog, etc., greatly promote the interaction and cooperation among persons distributed in different geographical locations and inter-connected by Internet.

The above applications and experiences of Internet technology enlighten us to innovate the practice education and seek the new way to support the practice in order to improve the effectiveness and quality. In the past, more attentions are put on the design and arrangement of course practices. For example, we were more concerned about the contents, processes and device of practices. However in the future, as generating large amount of practice resources and the possibility that Internet technology provides to access these resources, we should focus on the accumulation, management, reuse and sharing of practice resources.

- Open practice resources (e.g., software, data, or even experiment). It will be an important and necessary activity in the process of course practices. All of practice resources can be opened for public so that they can be shared. The opened practice resources may come from open community (e.g., open source), or graduates that perform the practices, or third party. All of these resources can be organized as an open practice resource storage.
- Share practice resources. The resources in storage can be shared by graduates who have the authority to access the storage. Such share can be performed by in different practice stages and objects.
- Reuse practice resources. Before staring practices, graduates can query the practice resource storage to find the appropriate resources as the basis of practices. He can also refer to the associated resources to guide the practices. The new generated practice resources can be added into the storage.
- Monitor and Analyze practice situation. The practice elements can be further monitored and analyzed in off-line or on-line fashions so that some important information can be obtained, e.g., on-line number of practice elements, how many times a practice element to be reused, etc.

157.4 Conclusions

In order to support the openness, reuse and sharing of practice resource, and improve the effectiveness and quality of course practice, we have developed a software platform called PracStore that is deployed in network environment. It provides a number of following functionalities:

- Create practice project;
- Create and manage practice team;
- Support multiple interaction fashions in project members;
- Manage practice resource, including distribution, publication, etc.;
- Browse and query practice resources;
- Acquire and reuse practice resources in the storage;
- Statistic analysis of practice resources;
- On-line analysis of practice;
- Practice history analysis.

We have applied the above method and platform to support the course practices for undergraduates of software engineering discipline for one year. The result shows some interesting phenomena. First, it is helpful for course teacher to manage the practices in the whole practice process that may last for a long time. Second, it also provides an enabling way for undergraduates to manage large amount of course practices or comprehensive practices in their 4-year education. Especially, undergraduates are enthusiastic to open and publish their practices, and when their practices are used, they often feel successful. Third, the effectiveness and efficiency of practices are greatly improved as the support of various interactions in the platform and intense wills that their practices to be demonstrated and shared.

The future works consists of two parts. One is to enrich the resource storage and provide more practice resources. The other is to improve the platform to be easy-to-use and more friendly.

References

1. Weber Steven (2004) The Success of Open Source. Harvard University Press, Cambridge MA
2. Tsay JT, Dabbish L, Herbsleb J (2012) Social media and success in open source projects, Proceeding of the ACM 2012 conference on computer supported cooperative work companion, ACM Press, pp 223–226
3. Papadopoulos PM, Stamelos IG, Meiszner A (2012) Enhancing software engineering education through open source projects: four years of students' perspectives, education and information technologies, 677–678
4. Qian X, Hong T, Zeng Q, Wang X, Huang T (2012) The establishment of engineering education practice system and platform with feature specialty. In Kim H (ed): Advances in technology and management, AISC. 165, 531–537

Chapter 158
Application of PBL Teaching Method in the Experimental Teaching of Hematologic Examination

Min Sun, Ya Li Zhang, LiJun Gao and XinYu Cui

Abstract The PBL teaching method in the experimental teaching of hematologic examination was explored in this study. The experience on the application of PBL teaching method in the experimental teaching of hematologic examination reflected that the PBL teaching method had significant advantages in developing the students' learning ability, practical ability and cooperative spirits of group, and arousing their active learning motivations, indicating that the PBL teaching method should be a valuable teaching method to be spread.

Keywords Problem-based learning · Teaching method · Experimental teaching · Hematologic examination

158.1 Introduction

"Hematology and hematologic examination" is one of the major specialized courses in medical laboratory specialty. In this course, the students learn knowledge about the experimental diagnosis method and technology of hematology. As the students in this specialty, they are taught to achieve the purpose of mastering the c technology used for the correct diagnosis of diseases to provide some diagnostic evidences in laboratory for clinicians. In the former teaching, methods for the diagnosis of diseases in the course were simply introduced by the teachers to students one by one, and then the students just repeated the procedures to verify the methods and cognized the pathomorphology of given specimens which had been diagnosed definitely. Although the students could understand the basic skills and method of diagnosis in this way, they could not know how to comprehensively

M. Sun (✉) · Y. L. Zhang · L. Gao · X. Cui
Medical Laboratory College, Bei Hua University, Ji Lin city 132013 Ji Lin, China
e-mail: sunmin1964@qq.com

use or choose these methods to diagnose diseases correctly. PBL (problem-based learning) is a teaching–learning mode in which problems about the learning contents are taken as the focus to be discussed and studied by the students to achieve the purpose of solving problems. PBL was originated by Canadian McMaster University and has been known as an absolutely new teaching mode different from the traditional teaching method [1]. In order to take the disease diagnosis as the focus to improve the students' abilities in thinking and solving problems independently, and in clinical thinking, the teaching method was introduced to the teaching of hematology and hematologic examination. We thought that the method should simultaneously improve the students' ability of obtaining and evaluating information, and ability of teamwork and cooperation, shorten the gap between the basic medicine and clinical medicine, and make them become qualified clinical examination physicians soon after their leaving the school. This might make the teaching and the clinical work combined more closely and the result should be more likely to accord with the training objective. 1. Implementation of PBL teaching method.

This teaching method was implemented in a total of 256 students who were from medical examination specialty Grade 2005, Grade 2006 and Grade 2007. After the teaching of experimental diagnostic methods of hematology finished, the students were given 16-hour experimental courses when the students had mastered the basic methods. During the experimental courses, the students were assigned to complete a diagnosis of an unknown disease in groups independently.

158.2 Teaching Method

158.2.1 Analysis, Discussion, and Design of Experimental Scheme and Diagnostic Procedures by Students

The students discussed in groups, expounded their viewpoints, put forward the problems to be solved, referred to relevant material to select experiment method and designed the experimental scheme and steps. Mean wile, the teachers gave the guidance and instructional advices to them if it was needed.

158.2.2 Implement and Completion of the Various Experimental Projects by Students

Under the guidance of the teachers, the students performed the experimental procedures, analyzed the experimental results comprehensively, proposed the opinion on the diagnosis based on the experimental results, which were asked to be delivered in a form of experiment report and bone marrow report. At last, the guidance teachers summarized the experiments, evaluated the performance of the teams and marked for them according to the performance and the experiment reports. The teachers were asked to conduct the statistics on the accuracy of disease diagnosis, and then, the student symposium on it was held and the PBL teaching feedback questionnaires were distributed to the students.

158.3 Results of PBL Teaching Method Application

In this course, the PBL teaching method was carried out in 256 students from 3 grades. The effects of PBL were reflected through the students' performance in the class, experiment reports, conclusion of experimental diagnosis and questionnaire survey from the students. The results showed that, the students' memory and understanding of basic knowledge could be strengthened, and the students' thinking should be activated through setting problems; the students' abilities in the application of previous learned knowledge; since the whole teaching course proceeded focusing on the diagnosis of diseases, the students were encouraged to think by themselves all the time, conclude and sort out what they had learned, choose the diagnostic methods, even consult extracurricular material in order to solve the problems. In this way, the students could play a major role in their study and learn initiatively. On the other hand, the teachers could also have more opportunities to know about the students' personality, learning ability and motivation, etc. to achieve differential treatment in education. There was something we should pay attention to in the writing of the experimental report and the filling of the bone marrow report. On the one hand, the experimental report should reflect the design proposal, diagnostic program, experiment method and result; on the other hand, the bone marrow report in which the diagnostic conclusion was required was asked to be completed by the students to simulate the clinical practical situation, which might make the teaching more close to the clinical practice, arouse the students' learning interest, and integrate their nonsystematic knowledge into an organic whole to realize the aim that could be easily used after learning. The statistical data showed that the diagnostic accuracy by the students who were taught with the PBL method was 92.6 %, indicating that the students had not only mastered the learned knowledge basically, but also reflected the students' ability to utilize the knowledge. Finally, the questionnaire survey for PBL teaching was analyzed. The results showed that the students believed that PBL teaching method could make them clear the study goal, and stimulate their interests in the learning, which accounted for about 93 %; the PBL teaching method could help to break up the discipline boundary and cultivate their independent learning, accounting for 89.2 %; the students who thought that the PBL teaching method could help to update knowledge consciously and improve lifelong learning ability in the future accounted for 90.4 %; those who believed that the PBL teaching method could help to develop clinical thinking and improve their ability of searching relevant information and solving problems accounted for 95.3 %; those who considered that the PBL teaching method based on specific cases and students' independent self-study was superior to the traditional teaching methods accounted for 86 %; those who held an opinion that PBL teaching method could help to train and improve team cooperation ability accounted for 85.5 %. It could be understood from the results described above that the PBL teaching method might show some obvious advantages, such as promoting students' ability of learning new knowledge actively, cultivating and realizing the lifelong learning, breaking subject boundary, carrying out integrated teaching, fully reflecting medical integrity and so on.

158.4 Experience on the Application of the PBL Teaching Method

158.4.1 Advantages of the PBL Teaching Method

By applying PBL method to hematology and hematologic examination teaching, we find that the PBL method has lots of advantages compared with the traditional teaching method. One of the most prominent advantages is that the students study more initiatively. It is well known that the initiative in learning is in the side of students. The learning of the diagnosis of a disease is a process in which the students can be cultivated systematically in their clinical logical thinking, and could know how to use their own heads to reason and solve practical problems initiatively, which should be a real combination of theory and practice. The PBL method can realize the transfer from the existing knowledge to a new knowledge to make students understand the content learned by them toward a certain deep degree and realize that the acquisition of the new knowledge is a gradual process. [2] Moreover, the PBL teaching method may make students face to the specific clinical problems, in which all knowledge points of basic subjects and clinical subjects are applied throughout a real case to make different subjects infiltrate each other and easier for students to understand them. It can be deduced that the training in students' divergent thinking and lateral thinking abilities focusing on the diagnosis of a disease can improve greatly the students' ability in utilizing knowledge flexibly and make them possess the quality as a qualified doctor. In addition, the PBL teaching method is proved with a superior advantage in improving students' cooperation ability, communication skills, solving problem, working independently and communicative competence.

158.4.2 Relationship Between Teachers and Students in the PBL Teaching

In the PBL teaching mode, a corresponding change in the roles of teachers and students can takes place [3, 4]. The teachers are no longer ones who only transfer knowledge to their students as before, but change into the organizers, coordinator, directors and helper in students' learning activities, and they can fully bring into play the students' initiative, enthusiasm and innovative spirit by utilizing the situation, cooperation and exchange, to achieve the purpose that students effectively realize the meaning of the current knowledge [5, 6]. Through the application of PBL teaching method in the course, we think that teachers are positive builders of knowledge studying. In teaching activity, not only one single subject knowledge but also the training in students' learning abilities and their exploring spirits should be paid more attention to, students should actively construct their own knowledge through the interaction and personal thinking, each student should have his or her individual characteristics of creativity, and teachers' goal is to stimulate their students' potential and pay attention to each student's views and opinions [7, 8]. The relationship between teachers and students should be changed, the traditional idea that the students bow at teachers' word should also be changed, and a different teaching method adopted by teachers can result in a different relationship between teachers and students, so as to a different teaching effect [9–11]. PBL teaching mode focuses on students, pays attention to students' active exploration, and emphasizes students' subjective initiative, but it does not mean that the positive effect of teachers should be ignored. In the process of PBL teaching, the teachers should confirm the study direction, organize the learning activities, pay attention to mobilizing the students' learning initiative in the activities, sufficiently know about the students' individual differences, promote students' learning motivation, and provide assistance and guidance for the students, which should be the keys to improve the quality of teaching [12].

In summary, the PBL teaching model which is student-centered is different from the traditional teaching model which is teacher-centered. In the process of PBL teaching, the students play a main role, the teacher's job turns from single teaching to both teaching and guiding. This is not just a change in forms, but a change in both giving the students the knowledge in books, and abilities of analyzing and solving problems, and independent thinking and studying. Our results indicate that the method can improve students' abilities of solving problems and expressing themselves, and build a platform for the display of the students' creative thinking to fully confirm them and turn the boring study f to a interesting one, which may enhance the students self-confidence and enable them to adapt to their future works.

References

1. Zhu TH, Hua YJ et al (2005) Application of PBL teaching model in medical education. J Med Educ (5):48–50
2. Eshach H, Bitterman H (2003) From case-based reasoning to problem-based learning. J Acad Med 78(5):491–496
3. Bing YB, Ning YB, Rong WH et al (2006) Referring to advanced experience of exploring medical teaching mode conversion. High Educ Forum 2:30–32
4. Shan Kar PR (2008) Problem-based learning: the right direction for medical teaching. J Med Princ Pract 17:171–172
5. Koh GC, Khoo HE, Wong ML, et al (2008) The effects of problem-based learning during medical school on physician competency: a systematic review. CMAJ 178(1):34–41
6. Davis III TH, Wagner GS, Gleim G, et al (2006) Problem-based learning of research skills. J Electro cardiol 39(1):120–128
7. Hua SW (2000) The PBL model of medical education. J Med Philos 21(2):48–49
8. Fincham AG, Shuler CF (2001) The changing face of dental education: the impact of PBL. J Dent Educ 65(6):406–521
9. Sheng LZ, Qing XL, Xia ZY (2002) Advantage analysis and characteristics of graduate education mode based on issues. J Foreign Med Sci Med Educ 23(4):10–13
10. Jones RW (2007) Learning and teaching in small groups:characteristics, benefits, problems and approaches. Anaesth Intensive Care 35(4):587–592
11. Wun YT, Tse EY, Lam TP, Lam CL (2007) PBL curriculum improves medical students'participation in small—group tutorials. J Med Teach (29):1–6
12. Xiu PS, Hua HL, Pen CT (2006) Application of PBL in the diagnosis of experiment teaching. J Med Soc 19(5):49–50

Chapter 159
Study on Bilingual Teaching of Heat Transfer Curriculum Assisted by Distance Education

Shunyu Su, Chuanhui Zhou and Xiongbing Ruan

Abstract The development of information technology is of great benefit to modern education. Taking the heat transfer curriculum for example, which is a professional and foundational curriculum for building environment and equipment engineering speciality in our college, the results about the study of questionnaire on college bilingual teaching which is carried out both in English and Chinese for Chinese students were presented in this paper. Based on the outcome of 150 effective questionnaires for our bilingual teaching effect of heat transfer curriculum, the situation and common problems about the bilingual teaching of heat transfer curriculum were analyzed in this paper. And some proposes about bilingual teaching methods, such as promoting the development of distance education, were presented so as to improve the bilingual teaching level of college engineering science specialties.

Keywords Bilingual teaching · Distance education · Questionnaire · Individuation

159.1 Introduction

The aim to arrange bilingual teaching curriculum in Chinese college is to heighten students' whole English levels, especially professional English levels. Then the students can search English professional literatures to obtain latest scientific and technical information. Professional and foundational curricula are very suitable for bilingual teaching. Adding English–Chinese bilingual teaching properly in

S. Su (✉) · C. Zhou · X. Ruan
College of Urban Construction, Wuhan University of Science and Technology,
Wuhan 430070, China
e-mail: shunyusu@163.com

learning these curricula has benefit to the subsequent learning of professional English curriculum and collecting English literatures expertly [1].

The construction of college bilingual teaching curriculum faces many problems, such as suitable teachers, textbooks and reasonable teaching methods [2, 3]. In order to realize the situation and problems about heat transfer bilingual teaching curriculum clearly, the questionnaire survey for bilingual teaching effect of heat transfer curriculum was held in our college. The objects of this investigation are students who learn heat transfer bilingual teaching curriculum for building environment and equipment engineering speciality of our college in latest two years. There were 150 effective questionnaires in this survey. Based on the results of this questionnaire survey, the situation and common problems about heat transfer bilingual teaching curriculum in our college were analyzed in this paper. And some proposes such as online education on improving bilingual teaching were presented. It is helpful for promoting bilingual teaching effect.

159.2 Analysis of Bilingual Teaching Situation

Heat transfer curriculum is one of the professional and foundational courses which connect directly with speciality knowledge and skills for building environment and equipment engineering speciality in our college. It is the bridge and hinge between foundational curricula and speciality curricula [4, 5]. Since the setting of heat transfer bilingual teaching curriculum in our college in the year of 2006, bilingual teaching teacher has been making great efforts in the process of teaching speciality knowledge to create English language environment so as to promote students' speciality English language abilities effectively.

However, there are still some problems about bilingual teaching need to be solved. On the one hand, such as teacher, foreign teacher for bilingual teaching curriculum is more difficult to be obtained. Moreover, foreign teacher is only suitable for pure English teaching, but not suitable for bilingual teaching. Since English is not the native language for Chinese teacher, how to employ a suitable teacher is a big problem. Besides fluent English expressing ability and authentic spoken English, bilingual teaching teacher faces bidirectional thinking pressure between speaking English and Chinese. The frequent alternation of these two thinking methods will generate tension and affect teacher's ordinary teaching. It is a great challenge for bilingual teaching teacher.

On the other hand, such as students, they face double pressure of English language and speciality knowledge. English language includes the improvement of English speaking and listening abilities, and many fresh speciality English vocabularies. To master speciality knowledge is the final purpose for students. But heat transfer curriculum is a professional and foundational curriculum of building environment and equipment engineering speciality. Students didn't learn any speciality theory before and this curriculum is absolutely new to them. There are differences of learning abilities and situations among students. Some students even consider that heat transfer curriculum is difficult for them to be taught in Chinese, needless to say in English. How to arrange teaching contents is a great problem for bilingual teaching teacher. Therefore, there are many difficulties that the teacher and students may face.

159.3 Analysis of Common Problems

According to the survey results of 150 effective questionnaires for our bilingual teaching effect of heat transfer curriculum, some common problems were reflected from students' attitudes towards the bilingual teaching. They are as follows:

(1) Whether or not the bilingual teaching curriculum should be arranged. For this problem, nearly 50 % of the students approval but 20 % of them oppose, and the remainders abstain. If bilingual teaching will be pushed in order, students' learning and researching abilities of using English directly will be enhanced continuously. Since students' English levels are different, their attitudes towards the arrangement of bilingual teaching curriculum are also different.

(2) What kind of curriculum is suitable for bilingual teaching? According to the survey results, 32 % of the students consider professional and foundational curricula are suitable for bilingual teaching. 21 % of them consider professional curricula are suitable for bilingual teaching. 19 % of them consider public basic curricula are suitable for bilingual teaching. And the remainders abstain. But the practice of bilingual teaching shows it is suitable for bilingual teaching goals that choosing a professional and foundational curriculum as the bilingual teaching curriculum.

(3) How to choose bilingual teaching textbook and how to set English teaching proportion. The English original edition textbook of heat transfer written by American professor J. P. Holman is chosen as the textbook of heat transfer bilingual teaching curriculum in our college now [6]. And the Chinese edition textbook of heat transfer is the teaching reference book. According to the survey results, 63 % of the students consider it is moderate for bilingual teaching but 35 % of them consider it is difficult. And minority of them even considers it is easy. Most of the students consider it is suitable that the English teaching proportion is about 50 %. It is the regulation of our college that the textbook of bilingual teaching curriculum should be English edition. And except in Chinese the teacher should speak in English over 50 % in the classroom. The survey results show that our students have almost adapted to this teaching mode.

(4) How to adapt to learn bilingual teaching curriculum for students. According to the survey results, in order to learn heat transfer bilingual teaching curriculum better, 51 % of the students spent an hour each week learning this curriculum after class. 26.7 % of them spent two hours each week and 17.3 % of them spent three hours each week after class. 80 % of the students expect the teacher to tutor them and answer their questions after class once or twice each

week. Therefore, it needs the teacher and students to work hard together that improving teaching quality of bilingual teaching curriculum.

(5) What kind of test mode is suitable for bilingual teaching curriculum? The questionnaire was designed from two aspects of test questions mode and test answers mode. 52 % of the students consider it is suitable for bilingual teaching test paper that the test questions are in English and the test answers will be in Chinese. 37.5 % of the students consider it is suitable that the test questions are in English and the test answers could be written freely by students. And only 10.5 % of the students consider it is suitable that the test questions are in English and the test answers are also in English. It is very clear that the students' attitude towards the modes of test questions and test answers varies widely according to their English foundations.

159.4 Students' Demands to Bilingual Teaching

Except the necessary survey items, the questionnaire for bilingual teaching effect of heat transfer curriculum was designed some items that students could freely express their ideas and proposes to bilingual teaching. It will absolutely improve bilingual teaching level. These ideas and proposes are mainly as follows:

(1) The students expect the foundational knowledge will be taught slowly, and the extended knowledge will be taught quickly. It is better if the bilingual teaching textbook is both in English and Chinese at the beginning.
(2) The students suggest that professional English curriculum should be arranged ahead of bilingual teaching curriculum, or bilingual teaching should be combined with professional English in the class.
(3) English interacting activities between the teacher and students should be developed. The students expect the teacher will speak in English with them in the class as more as possible. They consider this is the convenient way to help them master professional English.
(4) The students suggest that the bilingual teaching textbook should be simple and easy to understand. The teacher should be excellent and suitable for bilingual teaching. That means the teacher can express any professional knowledge in English fluently.
(5) Many professional English vocabularies are initially contacted for students. But their English foundations are different. Therefore, the students obviously need help. They expect the teacher could strengthen helps to them after school, such as extracting and explaining new professional vocabularies for them.
(6) The learning platform should be provided for students with different foundations. Face-to-face education and exam-oriented teaching method are not enough for all students. There should be other measures of individualized education for bilingual teaching of heat transfer curriculum, such as online education.

These suggestions are different and even exactly opposite since their English foundations are different. Students with good English foundations expect the teacher to speak in English with them in the class as more as possible. But Students with poor English foundations expect the teacher to speak in Chinese with them in the class as more as possible. The conflict fact needs the teacher to make his choice and to arrange the content of the curriculum according to the specific situation.

159.5 Some Proposes on Bilingual Teaching

Some problems existing in bilingual teaching process were found and some suggestions were collected from students through this questionnaire survey. As a bilingual teaching teacher, the author wants to supply some suggestions here.

(1) The credits of bilingual teaching curriculum should be added properly so as to boost students' learning enthusiasm. The heat transfer curriculum carries 64 class hours and 3.5 credits before. And after it is executed bilingual teaching, we suggest that colleges which are in good conditions could execute different class teaching for the same curriculum at the same time, such as Chinese teaching class and Chinese–English bilingual teaching class. The credits in Chinese–English bilingual teaching class should be more than that in Chinese teaching class.

(2) The employed teacher for bilingual teaching curriculum should be trained and his spoken English should be enhanced. Bilingual teaching seminar of different levels and different subjects should be held on time. And teaching experiences should be summarized and exchanged on time so as to explore the approaches of how to improve teaching quality and teaching level.

(3) The teacher and students should act the performance of the bilingual teaching curriculum in class together. The teacher should be a good director of each class and let students participate in the classroom teaching so as to create an interactive atmosphere in class. While students participate in the classroom discussion, they could constantly improve their abilities of listening and speaking in English, and their professional English. Their abilities of thinking in English would also be brought up gradually.

(4) Open or distance education is the most important supplementary teaching method for the bilingual teaching of heat transfer curriculum. It is the result of modern information technology development. The difference between the teaching processes of distance education and traditional education is that the former has intenser feature of education informationization, which includes networking of teaching environment, multimedia of teaching resources, digitalization of communication and feedback, intelligence of process management and so on. As a new teaching mode, distance education separates teaching and learning in time and space. The network multimedia courseware provides a bran-new teaching mode. Teacher publishes the courseware online.

Students can access it in their flexible spare time. Therefore, the students' distinction of individuation will be considered and the abilities of learning by themselves will be fostered. This teaching method will also benefit to integrate resources and to share high-quality educational resources among different colleges.

159.6 Conclusions

The questionnaire survey, which is for bilingual teaching effect of heat transfer curriculum of building environment and equipment engineering speciality, was held in our college. The questionnaire contents relate to all aspects of bilingual teaching curriculum about which students generally concerned. According to the survey results, some common problems about bilingual teaching were reflected from students. Before the work of bilingual teaching is developed successfully, there are many difficulties that the teacher and students may face. The analysis of these problems will benefit future work of improving bilingual teaching quality and reaching bilingual teaching goal by taking corresponding measures. And some proposes are also presented in this paper, such as promoting the development of distance education.

Acknowledgments This work was supported by Teaching Research Project of Wuhan University of Science and Technology of China (2011× 041).

References

1. Chu SY, Zhang MX (2009) Grading assumption of bilingual teaching of professional foundation courses. China Electric Power Educ 5:226–227 (In Chinese)
2. Liu XY, Cao Y, Yang J (2010) Investigation on current situation of college bilingual teaching courses. China Electric Power Educ 34:112–114 (In Chinese)
3. Huang JH (2010) Analysis of difficulties and countermeasures of local college bilingual teaching. Sci Educ 6:1–3 (In Chinese)
4. Fu XZ, Sun CH, Jiang B (2009) Investigation and study on teaching content of building environment and equipment engineering in a university. High Archit Educ 18:57–60 (In Chinese)
5. Peng W (2006) Reform and practice on the curricula of building environment and equipment engineering specialty. High Educ Sci 1:52–53 (In Chinese)
6. Holman JP (2002) Heat transfer, 9th edn. McGraw–Hill, New York

Chapter 160
Nonlinear Analysis of Bioprosthetic Heart Valve on Suture Densities

Quan Yuan, Xia Zhang, Xu Huang and Hua Cong

Abstract In order to improve long term durability of bioprosthetic heart valve, we analyze and compare stress distribution of bioprosthetic heart valve leaflets with different shapes and suture density under the same load. The finite element analysis results are compared with each valve model. It shows that suture density has a significant effect on the dynamic behavior of the bioprosthetic heart valve, which lead to different stress peak values, different stress distributions and deformation. According to the finite element analysis results, we can conclude that the cylindric and spherical valve leaflet with 50 suture points has better dynamic properties. From the whole loading process, we can find that the dynamic mechanical performance of spherical valve leaflet with 50 suture points is better than the cylindrical valve leaflet with 50 suture points. The finite element analysis on the BHV could provide direct and useful information for the BHV designer.

Keywords Finite element method · Bioprosthetic heart valve · Stress distribution · Suture density

160.1 Introduction

Bioprosthetic heart valve has been widely used since 1965. During the 1980 s the scale of the bioprosthetic heart valve has been closed to the mechanical heart valve [1]. The use of bioprosthetic heart valves in replacing diseased natural valves has

---

Q. Yuan · X. Zhang (✉) · X. Huang
School of Mechanical Engineering Shandong University, Key Laboratory of High-efficiency and Clean Mechanical Manufacture (Shandong University) Ministry of Education, Jinan 250061, People's Republic of China
e-mail: 409041529@qq.com

Q. Yuan
e-mail: yuanquan66@sdu.edu.cn

H. Cong
School of Medicine Shandong University, Jinan 250061, People's Republic of China

become a routine procedure. Their long-term durability remains limited due to structural degradation of BHV tissue include mineraliaztion and associated leaflet damage, and mechanical damage independent of calcification [2, 3]. However these studies were mainly conducted on stress state of the valves, little attention has been devoted to the suture of the BHV [4]. In order to improve long-term durability of bioprosthetic heart valve, different suture density are analyzed and compared based on finite element method. This work could provide useful information for the bioprosthetic heart valve designer.

160.2 Method

160.2.1 Model of the BHV

The bioprosthetic heart valve is often made with porcine or bovine pericardial which belong to the hyperelastic material [5, 6]. Materials is a complex biological tissue, which has the differences in each direction of the mechanical and physical properties. Their stress–strain relationship shows the characteristic of nonlinear anisotropic. The analysis of anisotropic parameters in the following Table 160.1.

160.2.2 Finite Division

We use import the model of the cylindrical heart valve into the ANSYS software and the ANSYS software's subprogram-SHELL163 is used to analyze the stress distribution. We assume that the thickness of the valve leaflets is 0.5 mm. The solid model of the valve leaflets is divided into grid by subprogram of ANSYS software as shown in Fig. 160.1

Table 160.1 Orthogonal anisotropic parameters

Property	PET
Circumferential stress (Mpa)	4,600
Radial stress (Mpa)	4,600
Thickness direction stress (Mpa)	60,000
xy direction shear stress (Mpa)	15,862
yz direction of shear stress (Mpa)	4,252
xz direction of shear stress (Mpa)	4,252
xy direction poisson's ratio	0.45
yz direction poisson's ratio	0.0345
xz direction poisson's ratio	0.0345
Thickness (mm)	0.5
Density	1.01 e^{-9}

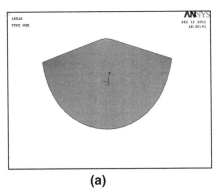
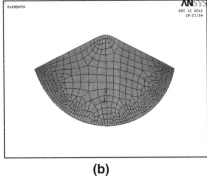

Fig. 160.1 a IGES file of valve leaflet, b Mesh division of valve leaflet

160.2.3 Boundary Condition of BHV

For rigid stent material, displacement vectors of every point in brim of a leaf is zero, so the boundary condition can be expressed as: $\{\delta\} = \{u, v, w, Qx, Qy, Qz\}^T = \{0, 0, 0, 0, 0, 0\}^T$ Fig. 160.2.

To represent loading during the bioprosthetic heart valve closing, the following pressure–time relationship is assumed in this work. The pressure on the bioprosthetic heart valve is modeled as to ramp, indicating an increase of pressure from 0 to 0.016 Mpa [7].

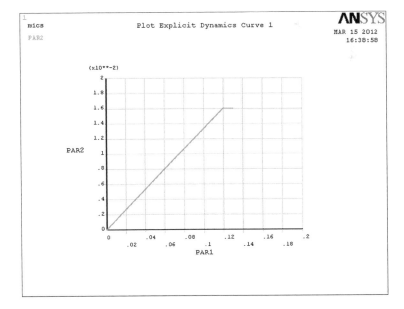

Fig. 160.2 Pressure loading curve for BHV

160.3 Result and Discussion

The finite element results of the cylinder and spherical heart valve are presented in Fig 160.3, 160.4, 160.5 and 160.6. We focus our attention on the peak stress and stress distribution of the valve leaflets.

160.3.1 Stress Distribution of Spherical Heart Valve

According to the finite element analysis results, we can conclude that the stress concentration mainly appears at the top of the attachment edge no matter what suture density. Non-uniform stress and deformation occurs at the top of the attachment edge of valve leaflets with 35 and 50 suture points, which indicates the suture density has more effect on the top of the attachment of the heart valve.

It can be seen from the Fig. 160.4 that the maximum peak von-Mises occurs at the top of the attachment edge no matter what the suture density is. The maximum stress with 35, 50 and 70 suture points is 9.42, 3.32 and 11.69 Mpa. The maximum stress with 70 suture points is much higher than that with 50 and 35 suture points. We can conclude that the 50 suture points has good dynamic mechanics performance.

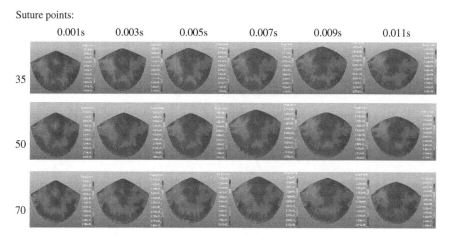

Fig. 160.3 Stress distribution of spherical valve leaflets with different suture density

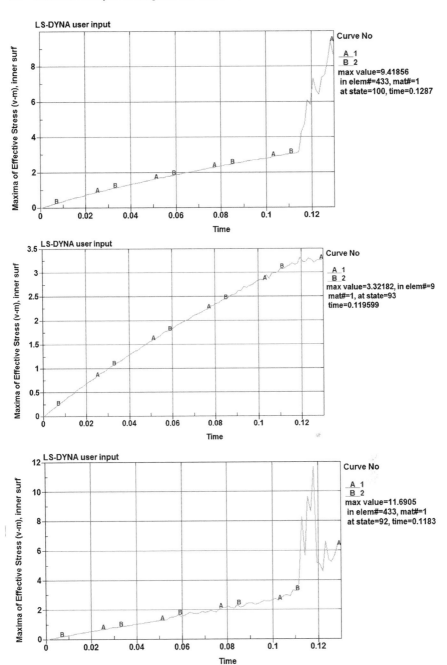

Fig. 160.4 Stress distribution of spherical valve leaflet

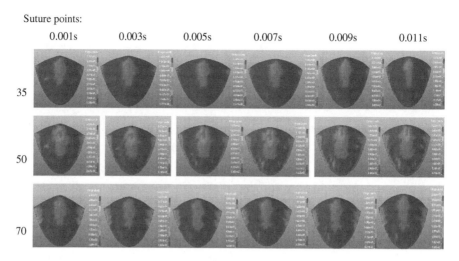

Fig. 160.5 Stress distribution of cylindrical valve leaflets with different suture density

160.3.2 Stress Distribution of Cylindrical Heart Valve

From the analysis results, we can know that the stress concentration appears at the top of the attachment edge and the abdomen of valve leaflets no matter what suture density. But the stress concentration appears at the abdomen of cylindrical valve leaflets with 50 suture density is more obvious. Non-uniform stress and deformation occurs at the top of the attachment edge of valve leaflets with 35 and 50 suture density.

From the results, we can conclude that the maximum stress of three kinds of suture density are approximate linear growth over time. The maximum stress with 35, 50 and 70 suture points is 3.87, 2.01 and 3.25 Mpa which all occur within 0.12 to 0.13 s. The stress with 50 suture points increases smoothly. Thus we can conclude that the cylindrical valve leaflet with 50 suture points has better dynamic properties.

160.3.3 Comparison

From the above analysis, we can find that no matter what suture density, the maximal stress always occurs at the top of the attachment edge on both the spherical and cylindrical valve leaflets. Non-uniform stress and deformation appears at this area which indicates the suture density has more effect on the top of the attachment of the heart valve. From the stress changing with time curve, valve leaflets all present the approximate linear growth under the suitable suture density. The maximum stress all occur within 0.12 to 0.13 s. The cylindric and spherical

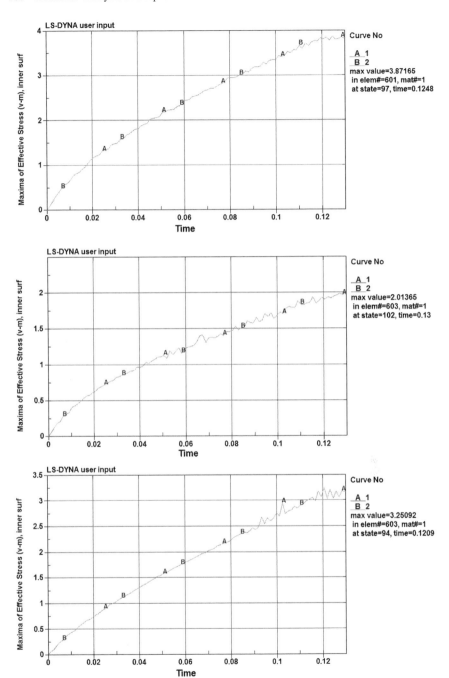

Fig. 160.6 Stress distribution of cylindrical valve leaflet

valve leaflet with 50 suture points has better dynamic properties. From the whole loading process, we can find that the dynamic mechanical performance of spherical valve leaflet with 50 suture points is better than the cylindrical valve leaflet with 50 suture points.

160.4 Summary

This paper constructs the parametric model of the spherical and cylindrical heart valve via computer aided design and the dynamic properties of the valve leaflet with different suture density is analyzed using the finite element method. The analysis results are compared and clearly show that the suture density has a significant effect on the mechanical properties of the valve leaflets. The peak von-Mises of the leaflet with different suture density is quite different. This work is helpful to optimize the value of the suture points and prolong the lifetime of the bioprosthetic heart valve.

Acknowledgments This work was supported by grants from Natural Science Foundation of State (No. 31170906) and Key Laboratory of High Efficiency and Clean Mechanical Manufacture (Shandong University) Ministry of Education.

References

1. Vongpatanasin W, Hillis LD, Lange RA (1996) Prosthetic heart valves. New Engl J Med
2. Turina J, Jamnicki B, Hug R, Turina MI (1999) Circulation 100
3. Li DY, Li LM, Peng YH (2011) Adv Sci Lett 4
4. Yuan Q, Zhang CR, Wang XW (2007) Int J Innov ComputI 3
5. Cox MAJ, Driessen NJB, Boerboorn RA, Bouten CVC, Baaijens FPT (2008) Mechanical characterization of anisotropic planar biological soft tissues using finite indentation: experimental feasibility. J Biomech 41:422–429
6. Pibarot P, Dumesnil JG (2003) Patient-prosthesis mismatch and the predictive use of indexed effective orifice area: is it relevant? Card Surg Today 2:43–51
7. Arcidiacono G, Corvi A, Severi T (2005) J Biomech 38

Chapter 161
Reflections on Primary Post Capacity-Oriented Integrated Practice Teaching of Oral Courses in Higher Vocational Colleges

Chun-feng Wang, Jin Ling, Jian-guo Yi, Min-jiang Huang and Guang-ye Zhao

Abstract Oriented with the primary job ability, the students in the experimental group were carried out integrated practice teaching of oral courses in Higher Vocational Colleges from the four aspects of target system, content system, security system and quality evaluation system of integrated practice teaching. The average scores of experimental group had significant difference compared with the traditional group ($P < 0.01$). The integrated practice teaching of oral courses not only Cultivated d students' job ability but also improved the quality of practice teaching.

Keywords Vocational education · Oral courses · Job ability · Integrated practice teaching of oral courses

With the continuous reform of health care system and the gradually development of health care service in the primary institutions, on the one hand, china's primary health care institutions need a large number of dentists [1], on the other hand, they took general model of diagnosis and treatment and provide general, full and comprehensive oral health care services for the primary people, which put forward new requirements and challenges to oral education in Higher Vocational Colleges and required that primary dentists must had solid primary skills, superb professional skills and comprehensive skills.

C. Wang (✉) · J. Ling · J. Yi · M. Huang · G. Zhao
The Clinical Department in Huaihua Medical College, Huaihua 418000, China
e-mail: wchf1723@126.com

161.1 The Current Situation and Problems of Practice Teaching of Oral Courses in Higher Vocational Colleges

Oral courses in higher vocational colleges was a very practical professional, which took the responsibility of training practical talents for the primary oral medical institutions [2]. As the main form of oral medicine education, oral practice teaching took improving students' job ability as the goal, helped students to master post practice elements and made more college graduates adapt to the primary dental post. At present, the primary oral medical talents in china were serious shortage and the existing oral talents could be difficult to meet the special needs of primary oral institutions, therefore, higher vocational education must strengthen the practice teaching and pay attention to the training of students' job ability for meeting the needs of primary job ability. But by the influence of environment and traditional mode of practice teaching, there was a big gap between the demand for qualified personnel in primary health care in china and the practice teaching of dentwasity in Higher Vocational Colleges [3].

161.1.1 Owing to the Lack of Systematic, the Current Practice Teaching of Oral Courses was not Connected with the Primary Skills Required by Primary General Medical Services

In verification experiments and demonstration experiments, the experimental teaching projects weren't really integrated according to the primary skills contents of oral medicine experiments, oral surgery experiments and prosthodontics experiments because of being organized and implemented by the different professional teachers. Therefore, the experimental projects like oral examination in oral medicine experiments, oral surgery experiments and prosthodontics experiments were repeated. Owing to the lack of systematic, the practice teaching could not culture students' primary skills required by primary general medicine [4].

161.1.2 Owing to the Lack of Consistency, the Current Practice Teaching of Oral Courses was not Connected with the Professional Skills Required by Primary Full Medical Services

The oral clinical operation was actually a continuous process, a physician must comprehensively examine patient's oral diseases and formulate a treatment plan and implement full treatment [5]. However, our practice teaching of oral course still used the traditional practice teaching mode of having experimental teaching after theoretical teaching according to the order of curriculum papers. So, the experimental teaching of the different courses or same courses was limited to simple mechanical imitation and was repeated verification of theoretical knowledge. Owing to the lack of consistency, the practice teaching could not culture students' professional skills required by primary full medicine services [6].

161.1.3 Owing to the Lack of Comprehensive, the Current Practice Teaching of Oral Course was not Connected with the Comprehensive Skills Required by Primary Comprehensive Medical Services

Comprehensive skills training was to let students learn to analysis and solve practical problems using theoretical knowledge, primary skills and professional skills in clinical practice. The traditional professional practice skills were respectively practiced in various courses accordance with the syllabus. Due to the lack of comprehensive treatment design and comprehensive skills training, coupled with students having no internship opportunities and taking turns in the hospital departments, which led to Students' lack of strong comprehensive skills, good humanistic quality and job skills.

161.2 The Idea of the Integrated Practice Teaching of Oral Courses in Higher Vocational Colleges

Stomatology mainly based on the clinical operation in the medical service industry was a strong practical clinical medicine. Oral practice teaching was a necessary stage from theoretical knowledge to oral clinical operation and was also the main form of oral medicine education. The practice teaching of oral courses in higher vocational colleges was difficult to play the overall advantages of practice teaching because of the lack of systematic, consistency and comprehensive. So, Higher vocational students had no the key ability of adapting to primary oral posts [7]. However the integrated practice teaching with integrity, progressive and integrated features had certain effect on overcoming traditional practice teaching mode with drawbacks of independence, fault and integration. Therefore, in order to adapt to the demand for primary post ability and meet the challenge, the integrated practice teaching system of oral courses in higher vocational colleges must be constructed.

161.2.1 Oriented with the Primary Job Ability, Established the Target System of Practice Teaching of Oral Courses in Higher Vocational Colleges

161.2.1.1 Established Total Target of Integrated Practice Teaching of Oral Courses in Higher Vocational Colleges: Cultivated D Students' Job Ability

We must carry out the research on the demand for urban and rural primary oral posts and master the demand for the knowledge, skills and quality of skilled personnel in primary hospital to determine the total target of practice teaching of oral courses.

161.2.1.2 Established the Subgoal of Integrated Practice Teaching of Oral Courses

1. Cultivated students' primary operation ability
2. Cultivated students' practical ability of professional technology
3. Cultivated students' Comprehensive practice ability

161.2.2 Based on Practice Teaching Target, Constructed Integrated Practice Teaching Content System

161.2.2.1 Constructed Integrated Practical Teaching Module According to the Three Subtarget of Practice Teaching of Oral Courses

1. Primary skills module: The primary skills module which job post need includes the history collection of oral common disease, the primary examination and auxiliary examination method about oral medicine, oral surgery and prosthodontics; the diagnosis and differential diagnosis and treatment principle of common diseases; hand washing and disinfection of oral mucosa; supragingival scaling; the block anesthesia of maxillary tuberosity and mandibular tubercles; the impression of maxillary and mandibular dentition, etc.
2. Professional skills module: The professional skills module which job posts need includes root canal therapy, periodontal surgery operation, reparations of fixed partial denture and removable partial denture and complete denture, cyst or tumor resection etc.

3. Comprehensive skills module: The Job ability, job quality and innovative ability module which job posts need. In a head phantom, the primary skills and professional skills about oral medicine, oral surgery and prosthodontics were formatted comprehensive training module and designed to three comprehensive experiments: (1) The diseases about anterior teeth trauma: in sequence, completed the IV cavity preparation of maxillary central incisor and resin filled, then root canal treatment, finally the tooth preparation and reparation of porcelain teeth and crown; (2) The diseases about molar apical periodontitis: first completed the preparation and filling of the class I cavity of the lower right first premolar and the class II cavity of the lower right first molar, then root canal treatments of the right first premolar and the first molar, and the extraction of right mandibular two premolar, finally the fixed bridge reparation of the right first premolar and the first molar; (3) The diseases about a large area of caries of posterior teeth: in sequence, completed class I cavity block preparation, root canal treatment, porcelain or metal full crown restoration and reparation of the left mandibular second premolar and the first molar.

161.2.2.2 Conducted Integrated Practical Teaching

Taking post jobs ability as the main thread, through the single training in the classroom, clinical practice, comprehensive professional skills training and comprehensive practice, the practice teaching contents not only interrelated but relatively independent with the theory teaching were reasonably allocated and conducted.

1. The single training in the classroom: The link was completed in the process of teaching. Teachers set the training programs according to teaching contents, students were required to complete the operation training in the classroom under the guidance of teachers. Through the single training in the classroom, Cultivated students'primary skills and professional skills.
2. Clinical practice: The link was completed in the process of teaching. According to the teaching contents, teachers organized students to the hospital internship, made students early familiar with medical environment, and shorten the distance between theoretical teaching and clinical practice. Through the clinical practice, Cultivated students' professional skills and job quality.
3. Comprehensive skills training: The link was completed after professional teaching. In accord with oral licensed assistant doctors' examination, training contents included primary skills and professional skills. Students were required to use tooth model in the head phantom to mimic the clinical operation procedure: first received patient and had doctor–patient communication and history collection, then had routine oral examination, conventional treatment, finally completed medical records, etc. Through comprehensive skills training, improved students' comprehensive skills before clinical, retaliated the "zero distance" docking between students learning and future post.

4. Comprehensive practice: In order to adapt to oral general, full, comprehensive treatment model in the primary hospital, we must take the traditional branch turns practice mode into two section type practice mode which was comprehensive practice after department practice. Interns were required to finish the examination and diagnosis, treatment planning, treatment operation, prognosis evaluation of the patient, and keep good communication with patients. In real job environment, systematic general clinical thinking was established and comprehensive skills for general clinic was obtained.

161.2.3 Supported with Books, Teaching Environment, Practice Base, Double-Quality Teachers and Teaching Methods, Constructed Integrated Practice Teaching Security System

161.2.3.1 Revise Practice Teaching Plans and Outline, Wrote the Integrated Practice Books of Primary Job Ability and Teaching Target

In order to ensure the implementation of integrated teaching mode from the content, teachers must merger or undo the repetitive experiments, increase comprehensive and design practice, highlight the characteristics of vocational education, strengthen skill training, revise the practice teaching plan and program, make the integrated school-based textbooks or lectures oriented with the primary job ability according to teaching goal.

161.2.3.2 Strengthened the Construction of the Integrated Practice Teaching Environment; Established the Integrated Practice Teaching Classroom of Oral Courses

The integrated practice teaching of oral courses required that the teaching places had not only experiment teaching equipment in sufficient quantities but also experimental teaching equipment with high quality. Constructing a good integrated practice teaching environment was the material guarantee of implementing integrated practice teaching.

161.2.3.3 Strengthened the Integration of Primary Health Care Institutions and Colleges, Established Hospitals and Schools Integrated Practice Base

Carried out cooperating with the hospital and established hospitals and schools integrated practice base according to the need of primary hospital oral posts ability and school teaching. Arranging students to primary hospital internship, inviting experts to give students lectures, training, teaching and medical guidance, and to participate in the construction of teaching materials, the revision of practice teaching outline and the edition of practical guide books, which made schools realized the integration of the post ability and teaching target in cooperation with the hospital.

161.2.3.4 Strengthened the Construction of Teaching Staff, Trained Double-Quality Teachers

Double-quality teachers were the fundamental guarantee for the integrated teaching practice of oral course [10], and played a decisive role in the integrated teaching process. In view of the oral professional courses with extremely strong practicality, oral teachers should practice in oral hospital more than 1 year and had received oral qualification, and were "double-quality teachers", who should not only had solid theoretical knowledge, but also had rich practical experience and the ability to implement integrated practice teaching of oral courses.

161.2.3.5 Strengthened the Fusion of Oral Professional Practice Knowledge; Implemented the Integrated Practice Teaching of Oral Courses

According to the oral practice teaching target of Higher Vocational Colleges, complying with the scientific, reasonable, practical and effective principles, oriented with the primary job ability, teachers and doctors were organized to repeatedly discuss how to break the boundaries of oral medicine, oral surgery, prosthodontics and orthodontics, and Construct a new course system of integrated practical teaching and implement integrated practice teaching of oral course.

161.2.4 Targeted on Teaching Quality, Constructed the Integrated Practice Teaching Quality Evaluation System

Evaluation on the quality of practice teaching was mainly the process one. Through the investigation and analysis, combined with the practice situation, first

Table 161.1 The score comparison of two groups [n (%)]

Group	Number of students	Excellent	Pass	Failing	χ^2	P
The experimental group	50	30 (60.0 %)	15 (30.0 %)	5 (10.0 %)		
The traditional group	52	25 (48.0 %)	20 (38.5 %)	7 (13.5 %)	30.8	2.05E- 07
Total	102	55 (53.9 %)	35 (34.3 %)	12 (11.8 %)		

determined the evaluation factors, then evaluated students' primary skills, professional skills and comprehensive ability. Indicators should be quantitative, human factors should be excluded as much as possible. On the base, set evaluation index and formatted systemic integrated practice teaching quality evaluation system.

161.3 The Effect of Integrated Practice Teaching of Oral Courses

The grade 2011 students were randomly divided into experimental group and traditional group. The students in experimental group were performed practice teaching of oral courses in higher vocational colleges, but the students in traditional group were performed traditional teaching method. Two years later, students' basic skills, professional skills and comprehensive skills were tested and compared in two groups. 80~100 scores were rated excellent, 60~79 scores were rated as pass, less than 60 points were failing. There was a significant difference between the experimental group and the traditional group ($P < 0.01$) (Table 161.1).

161.4 Summary

The current oral practice teaching couldn't provide high-quality medical service for primary dental patients because of lack of systematic, consistency and comprehensive. Graduates' primary skills, professional skills and comprehensive skills couldn't meet the needs of the post ability in china current primary health care institutions. Therefore, combined with the reform and development of china current primary health service system and the status of the independence, fault and dispersion of oral medicine specialty in traditional teaching mode in our college, oriented with the primary oral medical service and primary job ability, the students in the experimental group were carried out integrated practice teaching of oral courses in Higher Vocational Colleges from the four aspects of target system, content system, security system and quality evaluation system of integrated practice teaching. The practice teaching of oral courses had more advantages than traditional teaching (P < 0.01). On the one hand, it could cultivated student' primary skills, professional skills and comprehensive skills to adapt to the oral health care services and post ability, on the other hand, it could solve the weak links in the oral practice teaching in our school and enhance teaching quality, in addition, through the integrated practice teaching, teachers could grope for the experience of mutual participation, mutual benefits, complementary advantages, resource sharing between schools and primary institutions and provide a reference for the oral and other professional education teaching reform.

Acknowledgments Fund project: The teaching reform and research project of the Education Department of Hunan province, in 2012 (No. 604). The teaching reform and research project of Huaihua Medical College (No. 2010JG05).

References

1. Wu T, Chen Q, Li D (2010) A comparative study on higher education of stomatology in china and the united states. Fudan Educ Forum 8(6): 93–96
2. Wang S, Yu H, AO Q (2010) Reform and practice of stomatological experiment teaching. Northwest Med Educ 18(1):121–122
3. Wu J, Su J, Li S (2012) Personnel training methods in dental clinical practice. J Oral Maxillofac Surg 1(22):61–63
4. Zhang SK, Zheng Z, You H (2010) Founding the stomatological pre-clinical practical skill training platform Chinese. J Med Educ 5(30):744–745
5. Liu JY (2010) Teaching reform in oral medicine. Health Vocat Educ 28(3):58–59
6. Kang HY (2009) The teaching effect of three-in-one combination teaching approach in practice and training course in oral medicine health vocational education. China J Modern Med 27(7):71–72
7. Hu F (2009) Constructed ion of practice teaching system of ability standard in higher vocational education of dental technology. China High Med Educ 2009(5):18–19

Chapter 162
Excellent Man Marathon Runners and Plateau, Plateau Training Period Portion of the Blood in the Index Comparison Analysis

Zhang Sheng-lin

Abstract *Objective* Evaluate blood indexes of outstanding men's marathon athletes during training in sub-plateau and plateau areas, monitor the athlete's training load capability and physical function status; *Method* Based on the theories of experimental techniques and methods in sports physiology and sports biochemistry, use documentation method, measurement method and mathematical statistics; *Result* At different training stages of outstanding men's marathon athletes in sub-plateau and plateau areas, the athlete's hemoglobin (HB), serum values (CK), testosterone (T) have changed by the influence of training environment, the overall performance is that the blood index is on the rise from sub-plateau area to plateau area. The cortisol (C) value has decreased during training in sub-plateau area, and increased during training in plateau area; *Conclusion* At different training stages of outstanding men's marathon athletes in sub-plateau and plateau areas, the athlete's hemoglobin (HB), serum values (CK), testosterone (T) have changed by the influence of training environment, the overall performance is that the blood index is on the rise from sub-plateau area to plateau area. The C value has decreased during training in sub-plateau area, and increased during training in plateau area.

Keywords Blood index · Comparison · Marathon · Plateau · Sub-plateau

Biology is one of the important characteristics of metabolism [1]. The body through the different metabolic pathways can produce corresponding metabolites

Z. Sheng-lin (✉)
Lanzhou University of Science and Technology, Lanzhou 730050 Gansu Province, People's Republic of China
e-mail: zhangshl@lut.cn

in body fluids. Assays to all kinds of sports after the blood, urine and other body fluids of some biochemical components, can indirectly reveal the material movement characteristics and regularity of energy metabolism, and reflect the movement muscle energy balance, internal environment acidification, water and salt balance, tissue damage, nutritional status, etc., is an important content for functional evaluation of athletes [2].

162.1 Research Objects and Research Methods

162.1.1 Research Objects

In Gansu province team 12 excellent marathon athlete as the research object, training age 3.17 ± 1.32, mean age 16.67 ± 1.36 a, tall 1.64 ± 0.05 m, weight 56.0 ± 3.24 kg.

162.1.2 Research Methods

162.1.2.1 Literature

Refer to a lot of sports training and marathon and plateau, the plateau training biochemical indicator detection related literature.

162.1.2.2 Method of Measurement

Testing indexes, blood lactic acid, serum CK, serum testosterone (T), and Cortisol (C).

Testing requirements: sports training, after extracting the earlobe peripheral blood; Test equipment, fully automatic biochemical analyzer.

162.1.2.3 Mathematical Statistics

Data using Spss for Windows 12.0 package processing, the results with the average standard deviation of plus or minus ($\overline{X} \pm S$), according to data from the independent samples t test and one-way Anova, $P < 0.05$ indicates a significant difference, $P < 0.01$ indicates a highly significant difference [3].

162.2 The Results and Analysis

162.2.1 Twelve Excellent Marathon Athlete and Plateau, Plateau Training Arrangement

Men's marathon runner in Gansu province for the seventh national city games in 2011, improve athletes' aerobic endurance, and strengthens the special ability, starting in June 2011, geographical advantages, make full use of the plateau of Gansu and plateau for 4 months of intensive training. According to the arrangement of training plans and implementation: the first stage (2 weeks), the plateau environment) as the load adjustment period, objective to adapt to the plateau training gradually; The second stage (the plateau environment) for peak load, gradually achieve the large load training requirements; The third stage (plateau environment) for peak load intensity, make full use of the plateau geographical conditions increase the intensity of stimulation of athletes; The fourth stage (plateau environment) to replenish the adjustment period [4].

In each stage of the plateau, plateau training period blood indicators (Table 162.1).

162.2.2 The Plateau, Plateau Training Period of Hemoglobin (HB) Results and Analysis

Hemoglobin's main function is to transport oxygen and carbon dioxide, and participate in carbonate balance in the body and immune regulation. Athletes need to

Table 162.1 Twelve elite male marathoners and plateau and the plateau blood indexes in different stages of the training results ($X \pm S$, $N = 12$)

Phase indicators		The first phase (2 weeks)	The second stage (3 weeks)	The third stage (6 weeks)	The fourth stage (5 weeks)
HB (g/L)	$X \pm S$	160.11 ± 7.76	164.77 ± 9.939	170.17 ± 7.761	176.36 ± 12.477
	Max	176	184	176	204
	Min	153	146	145	158
CK (U/L)	$X \pm S$	547.55 ± 104.679	594.31 ± 113.668	634.50 ± 116.076	698.48 ± 152.801
	Max	652.20	707.90	740.57	851.28
	Min	442.70	481.80	580.51	545.20
C (nmol/L)	$X \pm S$	390.00 ± 34.059	360.16 ± 62.33	294.38 ± 30.640	366.70 ± 20.996
	Max	325.0	387.5	425.0	422.5
	Min	263.1	345.83	356.04	299.8
T (nmol/L)	$X \pm S$	18.016 ± 2.166	28.922 ± 5.279	15.297 ± 1.277	18.587 ± 1.80
	Max	16.78	20.979	20.629	34.965
	Min	13.636	16.434	15.240	22.132

Table 162.2 The plateau, the plateau stage four HB comparison results

(I) phase	(J) phase	Mean difference (I–J)	Std. error	Sig.
1	2	−0.366	0.3923	0.354
	3	0.611	0.4161	0.146
	4	−1.525*	0.3799	0.000
2	1	0.366	0.3923	0.354
	3	0.977*	0.3101	0.002
	4	−1.159*	0.2595	0.000
3	1	−0.611	0.4161	0.146
	2	−0.977*	0.3101	0.002
	4	−2.136*	0.2942	0.000
4	1	1.525*	0.3799	0.000
	2	1.159*	0.2595	0.000
	3	2.136*	0.2942	0.000

* The mean difference is significant at the 0.05 level

achieve ideal hemoglobin level, to show good results, male athletes normal 152 ± 13 g/L, altitude training is higher than normal levels [5], Table 162.1, according to the results of 12 elite male marathon athletes training in the first stage (plateau), hemoglobin is 160.11 ± 7.76 g/L, maximum 176 g/L, the minimum value of 153 g/L; The second phase (plateau), hemoglobin is 164.77 ± 9.939 g/L, maximum 184 g/L, a minimum value of 146 g/L; The third stage (plateau), hemoglobin is 170.17 ± 7.761 g/L, maximum 177 g/L, the minimum value of 145 g/L; The fourth stage (plateau), hemoglobin is 176.36 ± 12.477 g/L, maximum 204 g/L, the minimum value of 158 g/L. See from hemoglobin change results, athletes from plateau to plateau environment, hemoglobin is on the rise as a whole.

Using single factor analysis of variance method (LSD), four stages of the plateau, plateau (Table 162.2) (including: 1 the plateau stage; 2 high plateau; 3 the plateau stage; 4 plateau phase) can be seen from the comparison results (Table 162.2). The first stage (plateau) and the second (plateau), the third stage (plateau) HB changes there was no significant difference ($P > 0.05$), while the second and the third stage, the fourth stage and the first stage, second, third stage HB average there were significant differences ($P < 0.05$). That sports load arrangement is reasonable, the athlete to the plateau and adapt to altitude training.

162.2.3 The Plateau, Plateau Training Period of Serum Creatine Kinase (CK) Results and Analysis

After the great physiological load of exercise training, serum enzyme activity usually tend to rise, mainly reflect the exercise intensity and volume and the size of the body to adapt to the situation, male athletes of quiet normal between 10 and

Table 162.3 The plateau, plateau four stages CK multiple comparison results

(I) phase	(J) phase	Mean difference (I-J)	Std. error	Sig.
1	2	−47.6062	47.58684	0.320
	3	−108.3443*	47.58684	0.025
	4	−151.7704*	47.58684	0.002
2	1	47.6062	47.58684	0.320
	3	−60.7381	33.64898	0.075
	4	−104.1642*	33.64898	0.003
3	1	108.3443*	47.58684	0.025
	2	60.7381	33.64898	0.075
	4	−43.4261	33.64898	0.200
4	1	151.7704*	47.58684	0.002
	2	104.1642*	33.64898	0.003
	3	43.4261	33.64898	0.200

* The mean difference is significant at the 0.05 level

300 U/L, when big sports training intensity and volume, serum creatine kinase values tend to rise. See from Table 162.1, 12 men's marathon runners and plateau, plateau training stage 1 CK is 547.55 ± 104.679 U/L, maximum 652.20 U/L, the minimum value of 442.70 U/L; Phase 2 CK is 594.31 ± 113.668 U/L, maximum 707.90 U/L, minimum 481.80 U/L; The third phase of CK was 634.50 ± 116.076 U/L, maximum 740.57 U/L, the minimum 580.51 U/L; Phase 4 CK is 698.48 ± 152.801 U/L, maximum 851.28 U/L, the minimum 545.20 U/L. From the test results show that 12 men's marathon runners and plateau, plateau training serum CK value is on the rise.

Four stages on the plateau, plateau CK changes mean multiple comparison was carried out (Table 162.3).

It can be seen from the comparison results (Table 162.3), the first stage and second stage, the second and the third stage, third and fourth stage CK average change had no significant difference ($P > 0.05$), and the first and the third, fourth stage, the second and the fourth stage CK average change exists significant difference ($P < 0.05$). That is affected by the training environment and training load, the athlete's muscles stimulation and skeletal muscle injury in gradually deepened.

162.2.4 The Plateau, Plateau Training Period Cortisol (C) the Results and Analysis

Cortisol has certain regulation effect on the immune system, generally considered to be representative of how quickly the body catabolism, athletes in general between 165 and 720 nmol/l. See from Table 162.1, 12 excellent marathon athlete and plateau, plateau training first stage C 294.38 ± 30.640 nmol/l, 325.0 nmol/l, maximum minimum 263.1 nmol/l; Phase 2 C 366.70 ± 20.996 nmol/l, 387.5 nmol/l,

Table 162.4 The plateau, plateau four phases C indicators multiple comparison results

(I) phase	(J) phase	Mean difference (I–J)	Std. error	Sig.
1	2	−273.93*	42.431	0.000
	3	4.00	42.431	0.925
	4	−67.72	41.084	0.103
2	1	273.93*	42.431	0.000
	3	277.93*	30.003	0.000
	4	206.20*	28.066	0.000
3	1	−4.00	42.431	0.925
	2	−277.93*	30.003	0.000
	4	−71.72*	28.066	0.012
4	1	67.72	41.084	0.103
	2	−206.20*	28.066	0.000
	3	71.72*	28.066	0.012

* The mean difference is significant at the 0.05 level

maximum minimum 345.83 nmol/l; Third stage C390.00 ± 34.059 nmol/l, maximum 425.0 nmol/l, the minimum 356.04 nmol/l; Phase 4 C 360.16 ± 62.33 nmol/l, maximum 422.5 nmol/l, the minimum 299.8 nmol/l. Test results show that, in the land of the plateau, plateau training process, the athletes C of up–down–up trend, namely, the first and second stages, the third stage, the fourth stage, with the previous research reports are basically identical [5].

From Table 162.4 and the four stages plateau, plateau C values for multiple comparison results show that the second phase (plateau) serum C and the first phase (plateau) and the third stage (plateau) and the fourth stage (plateau) between the mean serum C there were significant difference ($P = 0.000 < 0.05$); The fourth stage (plateau) and the third stage (plateau) between the mean serum C there are significant difference ($P = 0.012 < 0.05$), suggesting the plateau and the plateau training on serum C effects of different athletes.

162.2.5 The Plateau, Plateau Training Period Blood Testosterone (T) Results and Analysis

Male athlete's influence on the performance of androgen plays an important role, when athletes blood testosterone increases, the body can be thought of synthetic metabolism, physical fitness enhancement [6], the male athlete of the Ref. [1] is between 9.5 and 35.0 nmol/l. Table 162.1, according to the results of 12 players and plateau, plateau training in the first stage of serum testosterone (T) was 15.297 ± 1.277 nmol/l, 16.78 nmol/l, maximum minimum 13.636 nmol/l; Phase 2 T ± 17.587 to 1.80 nmol/l, maximum 20.979 nmol/l, the minimum 15.434 nmol/l; Third stage T ± 17.016 to 2.166 nmol/l, maximum 20.629 nmol/l, the minimum

Table 162.5 The plateau, plateau four stages index T multiple comparison results

(I) 阶段	(J) 阶段	Mean difference (I–J)	Std. error	Sig.
1	2	−64.96	38.191	0.092
	3	−76.67*	38.191	0.048
	4	−245.28*	36.978	0.000
2	1	64.96	38.191	0.092
	3	−11.70	27.005	0.666
	4	−180.31*	25.261	0.000
3	1	76.67*)	38.191	0.048
	2	11.70	27.005	0.666
	4	−168.61*	25.261	0.000
4	1	245.28*	36.978	0.000
	2	180.31*	25.261	0.000
	3	168.61*	25.261	0.000

* The mean difference is significant at the 0.05 level

13.240 nmol/l; Phase 4 T ± 23.922 to 5.279 nmol/l, maximum 34.965 nmol/l, the minimum 17.132 nmol/l.

Four stages from Table 162.5 the plateau, plateau T measure multiple comparison results show that the fourth stage (plateau) serum testosterone (T) and the first phase (plateau), the second phase (plateau) and the third stage (plateau) between the mean serum testosterone (T) there were significant difference ($P = 0.000 < 0.05$); Instructions in the plateau and the plateau training stages of athletes serum testosterone were increased significantly, athletes are enhanced physical, but the plateau training athletes serum testosterone of seaborne improve significantly in the altitude training.

162.3 Summary

Twelve excellent marathon athletes in the plateau, plateau training phase, the hemoglobin (HB), serum (CK), testosterone (T) values of both exist significant difference ($P < 0.05$); C value for the altitude training phase decreased, and higher altitude training phase, and the plateau plateau training C there are significant differences between values ($P = 0.012 < 0.05$).

Twelve excellent marathon athletes in the plateau training body function, metabolism, can quickly adapt to, but in the plateau training function is still influenced by plateau environment, factors such as the training load, significant changes in blood indicators.

References

1. Feng L, Li K (2002) Athletes function evaluation of physiological and biochemical indexes commonly used testing method and application. People's sport publishing house, Beijing, 8:25–75
2. Wang Q (2004) Chinese excellent athletes competitive ability diagnosis and condition monitoring of research and establish. People's sport publishing house, Beijing, 2:5–10
3. Wang X (2002) Sports statistics and SPSS. People's sport publishing house, Beijing, 12:202–211
4. Dongliang Wang, Shenglin Zhang (2009) Marathoner Li Zhuhong the plateau training period and biochemical indicators monitoring. J Sport 6:98–101
5. Wang Q, Even the World, Feng WQZ (2007) Altitude training. People's sport publishing house, Beijing, 4:88–102
6. Zhang S (2007) Gansu province men middle-distance race athletes before the winter training HB, BUN and CK metrics evaluation. J Gansu Union Univ 7:112–114
7. Zhang S, Wang D, Li X (2008) Our excellent marathon athlete Li Zhuhong (2007) annual training cycle characteristics and exercise load analysis. J Shandong Sports Inst, 6:48–51

Chapter 163
The Implication of Collaborative Learning in College English

Yan Sufeng and Song Runjuan

Abstract Collaborative learning means two or more people learn or attempt to learn something together. In the classroom, students rarely communicate with each other due to the limited time. Therefore, this paper focuses on the collaborative learning of English for college students out of class. This thesis analyzes the features of collaborative learning and Chinese college English teaching first. Then I try to suggest ways to imply collaborative learning in college English. Problems about this issue are also mentioned at the end of the thesis.

Keywords Collaborative learning · College english · Teaching and learning · Strategies

163.1 Introduction

In Chinese college, students only have limited time to learn English, especially for non-English majors. They learn English as a tool to help them to improve their majors and also it is an important tool for them to know the latest development of their specialty all over the world. They need to read in English, speak English and listen to English, all these skills are essential for modern college students. In most universities, there are more than 60 students in one classroom. They can learn reading and listening pretty good. But it is not ideal for learning oral English and practice. The main factor is there is not enough time for them to practice. At the same time, it is really a huge task for teachers to manage such big classes if they want the students to practice English more during the class hours. Thus students need to practice English out of class. If the teachers can monitor or guide their

---
Y. Sufeng (✉) · S. Runjuan
College of Foreign languages, Shijiazhuang University of Economics, 136 Huai'an'dong'lu, Shijiazhuang, China
e-mail: 253583229@qq.com

learning out of class, that will be perfect. Thus, collaborative learning is just the right approach to apply to fulfill this.

163.2 Collaborative Learning

There is no well-received definition for the term Collaborative Learning [1]. Different researchers just focus on different aspects of it. He Kekang [2] defines it as the instruction method in which students are facilitated to learn and achieve a given learning goal collaboratively. Shu Dingfang [3] said that it is an instruction strategy by which instructors promote students to work in groups or communities.

No matter what the definitions are composed, this term has three main features: first, students learn in groups; second, they have a common aim; third, they support each other to create a facilitating environment of learning English.

There are basic theoretical principles under this approach [4]:

(1) Working together results in a greater understanding than would likely have occurred if one had worked independently.
(2) Spoken and written interactions contribute to this increased understanding.
(3) Opportunities are understood by students through classroom experiences of relationships between social interactions and increased understanding.
(4) Some elements of this increased understanding are idiosyncratic and unpredictable.
(5) Participation is voluntary and must be freely entered into.

There is a difference between collaborative learning and cooperative learning [5]. The cooperative learning deals exclusively with traditional knowledge while collaborative ties into the social constructivist movement. In cooperative learning, the authority remains with the instructor who retains ownership of the task. In collaborative learning, the instructor transfers all authority to the group.

163.3 Strategies Applicable to Collaborative Learning

163.3.1 The Information Gap

This is widely used strategy in collaborative learning. In this method, each member of the group has information which the others need in order to complete the same task or develop a complete report. A full preparation before the group discussion is necessary. They need to work on the topic to discuss the problem and obtain enough background knowledge of the topic. Thus, it will be possible to explain their information clearly to other people. At the same time, they will know what kind of information they need to know in order to complete the task.

163.3.2 Group Investigation

This involves the distribution of tasks across a classroom so that different groups study different aspects of the same topic for an extended period of time. These groups are responsible for doing their own planning, carrying out the study and presenting their finding to the class. They make their own study plans and task division. After the presentation of all groups, they need to work in their own groups and finish the whole task respectively. In order to apply this technique out of the classroom, teachers should give directions in the classroom and give more guidance during the process. The students finish their tasks mainly in groups out of the classroom, they just meet in the classroom to share their information and research result with each other and get what they need to complete the task. Thus, an out of class collaborative learning group is formed. During the process, students work together and communicate with each other and gain information from each other.

163.3.3 Learning Community

A learning community is a group of people who share common emotions, values or beliefs are actively engaged in learning together from each other, and by habituation. Such communities have become the template for a cohort-based, interdisciplinary approach to higher education. Experts frequently describe five basic nonresidential learning community models [6]:

(1) Linked courses: Students take two connected courses, usually one disciplinary course such as history or biology and one skills course such as writing, speech, or information literacy.
(2) Learning clusters: Students take three or more connected courses, usually with a common interdisciplinary theme uniting them.
(3) Freshman interest groups: Similar to learning clusters, but the students share the same major, and they often receive academic advising as part of the learning community.
(4) Federated learning communities: Similar to a learning cluster, but with an additional seminar course taught by a "Master Learner," a faculty member who enrolls in the other courses and takes them alongside the students. The Master Learner's course draws connections between the other courses.
(5) Coordinated studies: This model blurs the lines between individual courses. The learning community functions as a single, giant course that the students and faculty members work on full-time for an entire semester or academic year.

163.3.3.1 Writing Groups

In a writing group, all the students talk about their writing plans, read their own writings and others, rewrite their writings and edit their writings in the group [7]. Thus, there will be real communication. One benefit of writing groups is that it focuses not only on communication skills and collaborative learning, but also enforces their grammar. This is very important for foreign language learners.

163.4 Evaluation in Collaborative Learning

In collaborative learning, evaluation is not only made for teachers to evaluate students, but also for students to evaluate each other and themselves [8]. It is also a group evaluation. In this way, teachers can monitor students learning process and help them to get higher levels. Meanwhile, the group members can understand each other better in English learning process and provide advice for each other to improve the English of the whole group. The following are the main evaluation methods:

Peer evaluation Group members hand in reports on their own study and other student's performance. When they evaluate their partners, they get better understanding of their partners. That will facilitate their collaboration and help them to further their learning.

Teacher observation Teachers also need to pay more attention to the process of collaborative learning. It is better to use a portfolio for every student. All the documents resulted from their collaborative learning are kept in it. Thus, every progress they've made will be shown clearly in their documents.

163.5 Teachers and Students in Collaborative Learning

Students are no longer competing with each other. They collaborate with each other to reach a common goal. In the process, students participate in the activities voluntarily. They set the group's goal and make plans together. They negotiate to determine the concrete process of completing the task. They also evaluate each other. In such a way, they are involved in a relevantly fixed community. It is the students who are responsible for and take control of their own study.

The teachers are changing their roles too. Teachers are required to be an expert designer and competent facilitator. They design tasks for students out of class collaborative study. They also need to figure out ways to monitor students' learning out of the class. They should not simply give tests to students to evaluate them. They also need to find ways to encourage collaborative learning. They need to help students to participate in the collaboration give them guidance to ensure the smooth transition from the classroom to outside of the classroom. That is a real challenge for all teachers.

163.6 Conclusion

Collaborative learning is really good for college students to extend their learning time and train their communicative skills. At the same time, they also learn the spirit of collaboration which is necessary for social life. During the collaborative learning process, students negotiate with each other, make plans together, and work at their common goal together. They are in fact experiencing the society in the process of learning. That is what education should do. Thus, collaborative learning out of class is really good for college students. It has many benefits for both teachers and the students. A carefully planned collaborative learning is really a good way to improve students learning ability and communicative skills.

References

1. Hartley JR (1999) Effective pedagogies for managing collaborative learning in on line learning environments. Educ Technol Soc 2(2):12–19
2. He KK (1997) Constructivism—the fundamental theoretical base for the reform of traditional teaching. Elast Foreign Lang Teach 3:15–18
3. Shu DF (2004) Reorientation of the foreign language teaching. Foreign Lang Foreign Lang Teach 8
4. Panitz T (1997) Collaborative versus cooperative learning: a comparison of the two concepts which will help us understand the underlying nature of interactive learning. Office of Educational Research & Improvement, US Department of Education. http://home.cappecod.net/~tPanita/tedsartieles/coopdefinition.htm.
5. Rockwood R (1995) Cooperative and collaborative learning. Natl Teach Learn forum 6(4)
6. Smith BL (1993) Creating learning communities. Liberal Educ 79(4):32–39
7. Ye XM (2002) Applying research on the strategy of literacy community for english teaching in high schools. Unpublished post graduate degree thesis, Fujian Teachers University
8. Han J (2006) A study of collaborative learning out of class. Unpublished postgraduate thesis, Central South University

Chapter 164
Bilingual Teaching Efficiency of Prosthodontics in Different Teaching Methods

Liangjiao Chen, Ting Sun, Hua Fan, Yaokun Zhang, Ruoyu Liu and Longquan Shao

Abstract Objective to compare bilingual teaching efficiency of expository teaching method and PBL teaching method in Prosthodontics. Methods 120 students were randomly divided into 2 groups (n = 60), one group was taught by expository teaching method and the other group was taught by PBL teaching method. The t test was used to analyze the final scores and Chi square test was used to deal with the questionnaires. Results The average score of expository teaching group was 100.22 ± 7.82, with statistical differences in the score of PBL teaching group, which was 131.28 ± 7.12 ($P < 0.05$). 45.0 % of students understood the teaching content in expository group and 80.0 % in PBL group; 48.3 % of students were satisfied with the expository teaching method and 75.0 % in PBL group. There were statistical differences between two groups ($P < 0.05$). Conclusion PBL teaching method is more efficiency than expository teaching method. Students feel easy to understand the teaching content in PBL teaching method and satisfied with the PBL teaching method. PBL teaching method deserves popularization in bilingual class of Prosthodontics.

Keywords Prosthodontics · Bilingual teaching · PBL teaching method

---

L. Chen
The Stomatological Hospital of Guangzhou Medical University, Guangzhou 510140, China

T. Sun
The Medical Centre of Stomatology, The First Affiliated Hospital of Jinan University, Guangzhou 510630, China

H. Fan · Y. Zhang · R. Liu · L. Shao (✉)
Department of Stomatology, Nanfang Hospital, Southern Medical University, Guangzhou 510515, China
e-mail: shaolongquan@smu.edu.cn

164.1 Introduction

Prosthodontics is an important branch of dentistry and one of the main courses for dental students which deals with the replacement of missing teeth and related mouth or jaw structures by bridges, dentures, or other artificial devices. The purpose of bilingual teaching is to imparting professional knowledge, develop student's learning ability and open student's mind. Expository teaching method and PBL teaching method are commonly used in college teaching activity, but the efficiency of them in bilingual teaching of Prosthodontics is not well known. The present study was to compare bilingual teaching efficiency of expository teaching method and PBL teaching method in prosthodontics and acquire a better teaching method for prosthodontics.

164.2 Materials and Method

164.2.1 Materials

The study comprised 120 subjects who are dental students in same grade of Nanfang medical university (male 45, female 75).

164.2.2 Methods

120 subjects were randomly divided into 2 groups (n = 60), one group was expository teaching method group (EXP group) and the other group was PBL teaching method group (PBL group). This is a single-blind study.

164.2.3 The Questionnaire Collection and Arrangement

Made Standard for marking. The choice questions marked by machine. Short-answer question and clinical case analysis were marked by a same teacher. Statistical analyses were performed by SPSS 13.0. The t-test was used to deal with the final scores and Chi square test was used to deal with the questionnaires ($\alpha = 0.05$).

164.3 Results

All the subjects took part in examination and accepted questionnaire survey. The t-test result showed a significant difference in scores ($P < 0.05$). The score of EXP group was 100.22 ± 7.82 (mean $\pm$ SD) and PBL group was 131.28 ± 7.12

Table 164.1 Scores of EXP group and PBL group (x ± s) (n = 120)

Group	n	Score	F	P
EXP group	60	100.22 ± 7.82	1.2104	0.0000
PBL group	60	131.28 ± 7.12		

Table 164.2 Understanding rate of contents in EXP group and PBL group (%) (n = 120)

	Comprehension	Incomprehension	Total	Comprehension rate (%)	χ^2	P
EXP group	27	33	60	45.0	15.680	0.000
PBL gruop	48	12	60	80.0		
Total	75	45	120	62.5		

Table 164.3 Satisfaction rate of teaching method in EXP group and PBL group (%) (n = 120)

	Satisfaction	Unsatisfactory	Total	Satisfaction rate (%)	χ^2	P
EXP group	29	31	60	48.3	9.025	0.003
PBL gruop	45	15	60	75.0		
Total	74	46	120	61.7		

(mean ± SD) (Table 164.1). The comprehension rate of contents was 45.0 % in EXP group that lower than PBL group which was 80.0 %. The Chi square test showed a significant difference between two groups (P < 0.05) (Table 164.2). The satisfaction rate of teaching method was evaluated. The satisfaction rate of EXP group was 48.3 % that is lower than PBL group which was 75.0 %. The Chi square test showed a significant difference between two groups (P < 0.05) (Table 164.3).

164.4 Discussion

This study compared the examination score of Expository teaching method and PBL teaching method. The result indicated that the score of PBL group was higher than EXP group (Table 164.1) (P < 0.05). Why PBL group got higher scores? The possible reasons are followed. First, EXP group accept information passively, it is hard to focus on courses for a long time. It can not inspire student to explore knowledge actively. Second, Knowledge expansion is limited in EXP group. Students only acquire knowledge from textbook and lectures. In contrary, student must to explore information through variety of ways in PBL group. The process expand knowledge. Third, the contents of Prosthodontics is huge and hard to understand, only explain the information can not inspire students to thinking. Less thinking, less understanding. The questionnaire survey indicated the understanding rate was lower in EXP group. The pattern of PBL teaching is the lecturer present a clinical problem first, then students based on this question to explore the answer and to discuss in a small group. Last, the question discussed in class. In process of search answer, students must to collect many information and thinking. The process of discussion also improve the ability of information processing and expression ablitity. This teaching style inspire students to learning actively. Group discussion and class discussion cultivate the synthetical analysis ability and thinking ability. Thus, improving the understanding rate of contents and decreaseing the difficulties of learning that why PBL group students get higher scores. Wang [1] find that PBL teaching in bilingual class not only inspire student's interesting, but also improve synthetical analysis ability and increase comprehension rate. So the efficiency of PBL teaching may better than expository teaching in bilingual class.

The questionnaire survey showed that the comprehension rate of PBL group was higher than EXP group ($P < 0.05$) (Table 164.2). The comprehension rate in EXP group was 45.0 %, half of students do not understand the contents. The comprehension rate of PBL group reach to 80.0 %. This result indicated that the PBL teaching in bilingual class was benefical for students to understand and master the information. There are many professional words and difficult words in Prosthodontics, student feel hard to follow the lecturer in EXP group. Passively acceptance make students lose the interesting and passion. In contrary, PBL teaching is a step by step process. The first step is to master the professional words and general information. Students search the information themselves help them to understand the words and professional information. The second step is small group discussion. Students are asked to use professional words to express their viewpoints. It is helpful for students to thinking and to analysis. The third step is class discussion. In this step the questions are discussed deeply. These step by step process help students to understand the teaching contents easily. It is a active process. Previous research showed that PBL teaching is a active thinking process, it helps students to understand the teaching contents better [2]. Bilingual teaching is different from all-English teaching for foreign students [3].

The questionnaire survey indicated that the satisfaction rate of PBL group was higher than EXP group ($P < 0.05$). Students can not understand the teaching contents and can not feel the fun of learning cause the unsatisfied feeling to teaching methods. More than half of the students feel unsatisfied with the teaching method in EXP group. In contrary, most of students satisfied with the teaching method in PBL group because of they can involve themselves in learing process [4].

164.5 Conclusion

The bilingual class for Prosthodontics is to imparting professional knowledge, develop student's learning ability and thinking ability. The teaching methods effect the teaching efficiency directly. PBL teaching method may better than expository teaching method. It is worty of popularization in educational practice.

Acknowledgments This work was supported by the twelfth five-year plan of educational research of Guangdong province (2011tjk332), special nursery foster humanities and social science research fund of the southern medical university (2012–22), educational research subject of the nanfang hospital (10NJ-ZD01).

References

1. Wang L, He XL, Lu JG et al (2012) Application of PBL teaching combined with bilingual teaching to 8-years program medical students in general surgery. Hosp Adm J Chin People's Liberation Army 11(2):184–185
2. Qi DJ, Wang S, Yu XS et al (2012) Application of Problem-based Learning model in general practice teaching. Chin J Gen Pract 10(2):312–313
3. Shao LQ, Sun T, Liu DH (2011) Research of stomatology teaching for internationall medical students. Chin J Med Educ Res 10(7):858–860
4. Wang DJ, Wang HL Education (new edition), 4th edn. People's Education Press, Beijing, pp 36–38

Chapter 165
Practice of Paradigm Teaching on Circuit Theory

Yumin Ge and Baoshu Li

Abstract "Circuit Theory" is an important technical basic course for the college specialty of Electronics and Electrical Information. Students generally reflect that it is one of the most difficult courses. This article discusses an advanced teaching theory named "Paradigm Teaching" and gives an example which is about the "reciprocity theorem". The example proves that the teaching effect can be effectively improved by using "Paradigm Teaching" to "Circuit Theory".

Keywords Paradigm Teaching · Circuit theory · Reciprocity theorem

165.1 Introduction

"Circuit Theory" is an important technical basic course for the college specialty of Electronics and Electrical Information. It's the introductory course of circuit theory, as well as the bridge of learning follow-up specialized courses. Its importance is self-evident. In the teaching practice, how to further improve the quality of teaching to enhance students' comprehension is worthy to explorate.

With the continuous development and improvement of advanced teaching theory, many effective advanced teaching theories play an important role on teaching practice. These theories can make innovation on teaching ideas, methods, means, examine multiple perspectives, etc. It can greatly enrich teaching methods and teaching aids, reform examination method.

Y. Ge (✉) · B. Li
School of Electrical Engineering, North China Electric Power University, Bao Ding 071003 Hebei, China
e-mail: geyumin0505@sohu.com

165.2 Paradigm Teaching [1–5]

"Paradigm Teaching" is founded by a Germany educator named Martin Wagenschein. This education method is put forward to address the contradiction between knowledge expansion and limited study time. From another perspective, it reduces the burden of students.

Martin Wagenschein believes that "Paradigm Teaching" is "typical examples which hide nature, fundamental and underlying factors". Another representative of this genre named W. Klafki points out that "paradigm" must be good, classic and easily understood for students. They believe that the primitive phenomena of world can be explained through the individual examples which students can understand. Therefore, the center of "Paradigm Teaching" is typical examples. Students can master general examples by special ones and learning independently with the help of these general examples.

From the sense of teaching methodology, "Paradigm Teaching" firstly requires typical examples including basic concepts, theorems, theory and application that based on theoretical system. From the sense of teaching purpose, "Paradigm Teaching" requires students to get general, intrinsic and regularly things by limited typical examples objectively.

There are four unification in "Paradigm Teaching", which is shown as Fig. 165.1.

"Paradigm Teaching" may go on step by step in teaching process. The steps are shown in Fig. 165.2.

"Master individual" means that things can be explained through typical, specific and individual examples. "Master class" means that characteristics of this kind of thing can be gotten on the basis of first step. "Understand law" means that further regularity can be summarized on the basis of previous learning. "Get experience" means interpretation and students can improve the consciousness of solving problems with the application of knowledge.

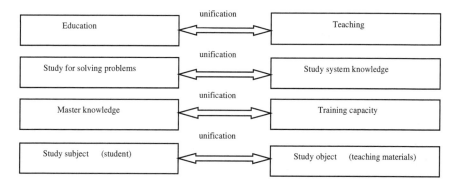

Fig. 165.1 Four unification in "Paradigm Teaching"

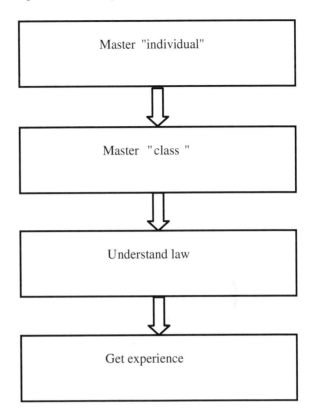

Fig. 165.2 Process in "Paradigm Teaching"

165.3 Application of "Paradigm Teaching" on "Circuit Theory"

165.3.1 Teaching Process

Though "Circuit Theory" puts emphasis on theoretical study, it has a close relationship with the engineering. Engineering projects will increase the vividness of classroom, inspire students' interest in learning and deepen students' understanding of the theory. Not all of the projects can serve as a "paradigm" except those have the following three characteristics: (1) basic; (2) foundation; (3) sample.

"Electromagnetic Measurement Technology" is one of the follow-up to "Circuit Theory" which puts focus on practical. Many measurement methods and principles can be explained by circuit theory. Also they may serve as "paradigm" of circuit class. "Voltage comparison" is one of the indirect measuring method of DC resistance, which can play a "paradigm" role in "Circuit Theory" when teaching "reciprocity theorem".

1. Step 1 of teaching: master "individual"

   First the question is put forward: A known standard resistor R_N and a resistor R_x to be measured connected in series with a constant voltage as power source, as shown in, how do you measure the value of R_x? Figure 165.3 shows the circuit diagram.

   Teacher proposes "voltage comparison" after students' discussion: measuring U_N (the voltage of R_N) and U_x (the voltage of R_x) with the same voltmeter, then according to

   $$\frac{U_N}{R_N} = \frac{U_x}{R_x} \qquad (165.1)$$

   the value of R_x can be gotten.

   Equation (165.1) is easy to be understood if the internal resistance of the above voltmeter is infinity. Actually voltmeter has limited internal resistance. The circuit diagrams of the former and later measuring are shown in Figs. 165.4 and 165.5.

   This "paradigm" has a directed relationship with practical problem and it can stimulate learning motivation of students. Students now have mastered this method to measuring resistance, that is, they have mastered "individual". But they cannot understand the following conclusion:

   $$I_x = I_N \qquad (165.2)$$

   So the measuring principle needs to be explained and the "reciprocity theorem" is put forward.

2. Step 2 of teaching: master "class"

   "Reciprocity theorem" points out that assuming the network NR, as shown in Fig. 165.6, only consists linear two-terminal resistors. When an independent voltage source works at port 1, the short circuit current at port 2 is equal to the short circuit current at port 1 when the voltage source works at port 2. That is $i_1 = i_2$.

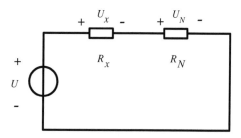

Fig. 165.3 Circuit diagram of "voltage comparison"

Fig. 165.4 Circuit diagram for measuring U_x

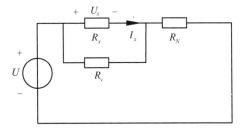

Fig. 165.5 Circuit diagram for measuring U_N

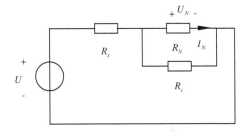

Figure 165.4 and Fig. 165.5 can respectively correspond with Fig. 165.6a, b. Then the NR can be expressed as Fig. 165.7. The port "ab" is port 1 and port "cd" is port 2. Now Eq. (165.2) is easy to gotten.

Teachers should focus on the essential characteristics of the "paradigm", combining with reciprocity theorem. In order to lead students from "individual" to "class", individual cases need to be classified. This phase requires students to think actively and proactively. Teachers can guide them to try more "individuals", Among these attempts they will explore the general.

3. Step 3 of teaching: understand law

   This part belongs to the deeper understanding of the stage. Some regularity hidden in "class" behind will be found based on the first two phases. Awareness of reciprocity theorem then goes to regularity. Therefore, the role of teachers is to guide students to take stock of the phenomenon, understand the general characteristics and rules of a particular class of things.

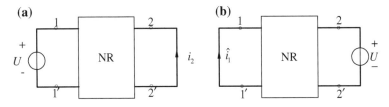

Fig. 165.6 Circuit diagram of "reciprocity theorem". **a** Circuit diagram before reciprocity. **b** Circuit diagram after reciprocity

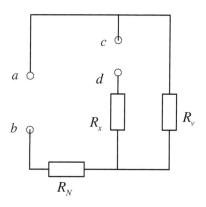

Fig. 165.7 Circuit diagram of NR

4. Step 4 of teaching: get experience
   This is the distillation of first three phases. It's the deduction after sum. Teaching focus shifts from objective knowledge to students' consciousness development. The aim is to make students understand not only objective theorem, but also the objects worked by the theory. The more important thing is to master the relationship between theorem and objects. Students now should transform objective knowledge to their own experience, which can become into their problem-solving skills. The purpose of education is realized.

165.3.2 Teaching Effects

"Reciprocity theorem" is one of the most difficult theorems for students to understand. Teaching practice has proved that students forget the theorem easily if teachers simply explain the certification process. But they are very easy to remember the theorem after using "Paradigm Teaching". Particularly they can use the theorem flexibly in the process of solving problems, and in the follow-up course, "Electromagnetic Measurement Technology", the related content becomes very receptive.

165.4 Conclusion

"Paradigm Teaching" emphasizes on the combination of "paradigm" and the reality of students' learning and life. It promotes the unity of teaching and education. It can arouse the students' learning motivation and initiative. Because it is no longer confined to a single discipline, the course structure in the past has been changed, which places too much emphasis on their own discipline and has a lack of integration. The course structure becomes balanced, comprehensive and selective, whish can training open horizon of students. It is in line with the current thinking of curriculum reform.

Of course, "Paradigm Teaching" also has some difficult problems to overcome. Firstly, it's difficult to choice a "paradigm" which is basic, foundational and sample. Secondly, it's hard to grasp the teaching process. Thirdly, it requires teachers to have a high teaching capacity because of the above two reasons.

The teaching process of "Circuit Theory" should be a comprehensive application of advanced teaching philosophy. "Paradigm Teaching" is just one of them. Only using different teaching methods at different stages can "Circuit Theory" be pushed to a new height.

References

1. Liu J (2009) Discussion on "Paradigm Teaching". China Educ Innov Herald 28:84–85
2. Li J (2011) Thoughts on "Paradigm Teaching" under the background of new curriculum reform. J Lvliang Educ Inst 6(28):108–109
3. Wu J (2010) Multidimensional analysis on the example teaching method. J Qinghai Natl Univ 3:89–92
4. Fan S (2009) Research on examples teaching methods in higher education. New West 8:227
5. Wang L, Ma A (2010) The rationality of modeling teaching and its era implication. Educ Teach Res 2:51–52

Chapter 166
The Study of Relationship Between the Nature and Other Properties of Traditional Chinese Medicines Based on Association Rules

Wang Zhe and Yu Hong-Yan

Abstract The association rule is an important branch of data mining, which reflects the correlation between the objects. In this paper, we use the technology of association rule to find frequent itemset between the nature and other properties of Traditional Chinese Medicines. Through many experiments, we have built the closely relationship of frequent itemset in Nature-Pharmacology, Nature-Indication, Nature-Western Medicine Name, Nature-Function, Nature-Flavour, Nature-Channel Tropism, Nature-Chemical Composition. etc., which provide valuable information for research the relationship between the nature and other properties of traditional Chinese medicines.

Keywords Association rule · Nature of traditional Chinese medicines · Relationship of properties · Frequent itemset

166.1 Introduction

The nature of traditional Chinese medicines is builded and summed up by actual efficacy and repeated verification, which was a highly condensed summary of a variety of medicines medical effects from the nature. Such as skullcap, Radix lsatidis has the effect of heat-clearing and detoxification to treat fever, thirst, sore throat, etc., which illustrate the two medicines with cold nature. On the contrary, if the medicines can reduce or eliminate the cold syndrome, then we can think that the medicines have more warmer nature, such as aconite, ginger has the effect of emitted cold temperature in belly cold pain and pulse to sink, which illustrate the two medicines with hot nature [1].

W. Zhe (✉) · Y. Hong-Yan
Henan University of Traditional Chinese Medicine, Jinshui Road No. 1, 450000 ZhengZhou, China
e-mail: wzhe_wz@126.com

With the development of the modernization of traditional Chinese medicine, the theory of nature and flavour of traditional Chinese medicine become the concerned hot, while it has few rules to follow in the research of nature and other properties of traditional Chinese medicine [2, 3]. We can't just stay with the traditional experience and theory, that we should reveals the scientific connotation by the data mining [4–6],which can mining the potential data, and it is the primary task to the research in the theory of traditional Chinese medicine nature.

Finding the relationship in the properties of Chinese medicine based on data mining, which not only promoting the quality standardization of Chinese medicine, but also helping reveal the principle of Chinese medicine multi-storey properties contact, which is the important part of the modernization of Chinese medicine. Mi Zhou, etc. [6], used data mining to find the lack nature of traditional Chinese medicine, he generated the association rules of "function"-"nature" though the decision tree algorithm. On the 20 flavour of traditional Chinese medicine which have functions, nature, flavour, but have not the data of channel tropism, he do the prediction of channel tropism. Er-xin Shang, etc. [7], used Apriori algorithm and improvement of association rules algorithm between datbases, which to find the valuable rules in the properties of nature, flavour, channel tropism and functions from the traditional Chinese medicine. It provides the data support for analysis the relationship in the composition of the internal medicine. A large number of experiment results showed that the technology of data mining can reveal the implicit knowledge of traditional Chinese medicine.

For the important role of natures in the properties of traditional Chinese medicine, in this paper, we collected information sources from books such as "Chinese Pharmacopoeia", "Traditional Chinese Pharmacology", "Pharmacy"(reference), "The Traditional Chinese Medicine Herbal Essence", "Pharmacology of Traditional Chinese Medicine" and "New Traditional Chinese Medicine", etc. Basis on the data of natures and other properties of traditional Chinese medicine, we builded the data model, and did lots of related work of mining. Would to find the valuable rules in the analysised properties of traditional Chinese medicine. We want to provided more comprehensive and reliable information platform for the researchers, and provide technical support for researching and applicating of traditional Chinese medicine.

166.2 Related Works

Association rule [8–10] is an important branch of data mining, it reflects the correlation between the things, and it can found the association or relationship between itemsets in the large amounts of data, these relationships are previously unknown or hidden.

Before data mining, first, we must determine the target of data mining, then we need to collect the data, do data pre-processing, data analysis and so on. Though the data of processing, we can mining the relationship in the natures and indications, function, pharmacology, western medicine name, flavour, channel tropism, chemical composition, etc.

166.2.1 Data Pre-processing of Traditional Chinese Medicine

Data processing is to reduce the inconsistency and incomplete of data, improving the data quality, which is the key stage to ensure the rational and effective of mining result. To discover the relationship in properties of Chinese medicine based on data mining, data processing is need to deal with the Chinese medicine data, and make the data meet the requirements of the algorithm.

In addition, to solve the problem of the same medicine with different name and the same name with different medicine, and part of medicine terms are inconsistent in function, indications, pharmacology. First, we need to do data preparing and data cleaning. Based on "Chinese Pharmacopoeia", "Traditional Chinese Pharmacology", "Pharmacy"(reference), "The Traditional Chinese Medicine Herbal Essence", "Pharmacology of Traditional Chinese Medicine", etc., and combined with the clinical treatment experiences, we collected, summarized, standard, and input data in Chinese medicine properties according to the principle of the same or similar mechanisms, provide a basis platform for the people who research the relationship in properties of Chinese medicine.

In this paper, we collected 717 kinds of commonly Chinese herbal medicine, and the property of nature include 13 kinds of values, such as "warm", "cold", "cool", "clam", etc. Moreover, for the indication of Chinese medicine, we collect 2,928 items, the content has "Dryness of cough", "Muscle atrophy weakness", "Chronic Cough", "Hemoptysis", etc. For the western medicine name, which include 3,289 items, the content has "Indigestion", "Dysentery", "Helopyra", "Chronic bronchitis", etc. For the pharmacology, which include 3,611 items, such as "Anti-allergy", "Anti-inflammatory", "Affect immune function", "insektizid", etc. For the functions, which include 3,023 items, such as "Zhixue", "Ziyin", "Xiaoji", "Huatan", etc. For the flavour, which include 1,110 items, the content has "pungent", "sweet", "bitter", "sour", etc. For the channel tropism, which include 1,610 items and the items content has "lung", "liver", "kidney", "spleen", "stomach", "heart", etc. For the chemical composition, which include 1,840 items, the content has "amino acid", "Glutin", "glucuronic acid", "organic acid", etc.

166.2.2 Related Methods of Data Mining

Apriori algorithm is developed by R. Agrawal [7] in 1994, its core is a set of ideas based on a two-stage frequency of recursive algorithm. The association rule belong to the rules of one-dimensional, single, boolean association. The algorithm use the iterative method of a layer search, and analysis the results to find interesting association rule through the "connect" and "prune" in the large amounts of data. And generated the strong association rules from the frequent itemsets according to the minimum confidence percent. However, Apriori algorithm may produce a large number of candidate itemsets, and may need to scan the database repeatedly.

In this paper, we improved the association rule based on Apriori algorithm, and build database based on the medical books of prior to mentioned. First, we need to divide Chinese medicine database into n parts, and generate a set of frequent itemsets for each section separately, then collect these itemsets to be a global candidate frequent itemsets. Based on the candidate frequent itemsets, "connecting" and "pruning" on the itemsets until generating the strong association rules. In addition, the program of data mining running on Matlab R2010a, and the system provides two ways of access.

166.3 Research Result

In this paper, we build the experimental environment with Microsoft SQL Server database and Matlab R2010a, which can analysis the database of traditional Chinese medicine, and mining the relationship between the nature and other properties.

In the 717 kinds of traditional Chinese medicines, For the property of nature, the value of "warm" appears most frequently. almost 189 herbs have the nature of "warm", such as "Ferula Asafoetida", "Folium Artemisiae Argyi", "star anise", etc. Followed is "cold" and "calm".

In the discovered rules, nature and flavour, channel tropism, and chemical composition appear together more frequently. Table 166.1 showed the maximum frequency itemsets in nature-flavour.

From the Table 166.1, we can find the maximum frequency itemsets of nature and flavour is "warm"-"pungent", the support is 117, and the support rate is 10.57 %, followed is "cold"-"bitter", "calm"-"sweet", "warm"-"sweet", "warm"- "bitter", "cold"-"sweet", "calm"-"bitter", etc.

For the nature and channel tropism, the value of "calm" and "liver" is most frequently, the support is 86, and the support rate is 5.35 %, Table 166.2 showed the maximum frequency itemsets in nature- channel tropism.

From the Table 166.2, we can find the maximum frequency itemsets of nature and channel tropism is "calm"-"liver", followed is "warm"-"liver", "warm"-"spleen", "cold"-"liver", "cold"-"lung", "warm"-"kidney", etc.

Table 166.1 Nature-flavour frequency itemsets

Num	Nature	Flavour	Support	Support rate (%)
1	Warm	Pungent	117	10.57
2	Cold	Bitter	107	9.67
3	Calm	Sweet	87	7.86
4	Warm	Sweet	61	5.51
5	Warm	Bitter	60	5.42
6	Cold	Sweet	60	5.42
7	Calm	Bitter	50	4.52
8	Micro-cold	Bitter	42	3.79
9	Calm	Pungent	32	2.89
10	Cool	Sweet	31	2.80

Table 166.2 Nature- channel tropism frequency itemsets

Num	Nature	Channel tropism	Support	Support rate (%)
1	Calm	Liver	86	5.35
2	Warm	Liver	84	5.22
3	Warm	Spleen	83	5.16
4	Cold	Liver	80	4.98
5	Cold	Lung	74	4.60

For the nature and chemical composition, the value of "warm" and "volatile oil" is most frequently, the support is 66, and the support rate is 3.60 %, followed is "cold"-"organic acid"," warm"-"esters"," cold"-"alkaloid", etc. Table 166.3 showed the maximum frequency itemsets in nature- chemical composition.

Similarly, for the nature and function of traditional Chinese medicines, the value of "cold" and "heat-clearing" is most frequently, the support is 91, and the support rate is 3.04 %, followed is "cold"-"detoxify", "warm"-"analgesics", "cold"-"cooling-blood", "micro-cold"-"heat-clearing", "cold"-"detumescence", "cool"-"heat-cleaning", etc. For the nature and pharmacology, the value of "warm" and "anti-inflammatory" is most frequently, the support is 57, and the support rate is 1.58 %, followed is "cold"-"antibiosis", "warm"-"antibiosis", "warm"-"analgesia", "cold"-"anti-inflammatory", "warm"-"affect the cardio-vascular system", etc. Moreover, through the experiment results, we find the maximum support rat in nature and the property of indication and western medicine name is 0.62 and 0.49 %.

Table 166.3 Nature- chemical composition frequency itemsets

Num	Nature	Chemical composition	Support	Support rate (%)
1	Warm	Volatile oil	66	3.60
2	Cold	Organic acid	48	2.62
3	Warm	Esters	47	2.57
4	Cold	Alkaloid	41	2.24
5	Calm	Saccharides	40	2.18

166.4 Conclusion

As a powerful tool of acquiring knowledge in a large number of data, association rule mining was used in all kinds of fields of Chinese medicine. While the complexity and uncertainties of the Chinese medicine make the data mining techniques exist some difficult problems in researching Chinese medicine.

In this paper, we do pre-processing for the collected data of nature and other related information, and build the experiment environment to find the relationship between the nature and other properties of traditional Chinese medicines. The experiment results can be analyzed stronger, and can be understood with the nature of traditional Chinese medicines, which have the worth of practical significance. In future, we plan to add more useful informations, to find the valuable relationship in the database for the people who studied in the field of traditional Chinese medicine.

References

1. Huang ZS (2012) Science of Chinese traditional medicine. People's Medical Publishing House, Beiging
2. Li MX, Fan Y (2008) Resarch on four properties of Chinese herb: current status,problems and countermeasures. Chin J Tradit Chin Med 23(7):565–568
3. Zhang B, Lin ZJ, Zhai HQ (2008) A research of traditional Chinese medicine property based on "three elements" hypothesis. Chin J Tradit Chin Med 33(2):221–223
4. Han JW, Micheline K (2010) Data mining: concepts and techniques (trans: Ming F, Xiaofeng M), 2nd edn. China Machine Press, Beijing
5. Tian L (2005) The application of data mining in the field of traditional Chinese medicine. Chin J Basic Med Tradit Chin Med 11:710–712
6. Zhou M, Wang Y, Qiao YJ (2008) Yanjiang: Predict the preliminary study of Chinese medicine lack of potency based on data mining. Chin J Inf Tradit Chin Med 93–94
7. Shang EX, Ye L, Fan XS (2010) Discovery of association rules between TCM properties in crude drug pairs by mining between datasets and probability test. World Sci Technol Mod Tradit Chin Med Materia Medica 12:377–382
8. Jin R, Lin Q, Zhang B (2011) A study of association rules in three-dimensional property-taste-effect data of Chinese herbal medicines based on apriori algorithm. J Chin Integr Med 9(7):794–803
9. Li ZH, Fan XS (2009) Research on association rules on asthma medication regularity between ancient and modern. Chin J Inf Tradit Chin Med 94–95
10. Chen SH, Lv JY (2008) The study on the nature of traditional chinese medicine based on nature flavor and combination meridian. Pharmacol Clin Chin Mater Med 58–62

Chapter 167
Usage of Turbine Airflow Sensor in Ventilator

Yaoyu Wu, Feng Chang and Dongmin Liu

Abstract *Objective* To reduce errors in measuring of the Tidal Volume of Ventilator by Turbine Airflow Sensor. *Methods* Describe the construction and principle and feature and discussed the flowrate characteristics of turbine airflow sensor, indicate that there is inertia at working by its construction. According to the working feature of Ventilator and analyzing flowrate curve, provide measuring and calibrating method of Tidal Volume of Ventilator. *Results* Improving the measuring accuracy by adjusting quantity of the Sensor pulse and measuring subsection of the capability coefficient. *Conclusion* The method is effective to reduce errors in measuring of the Tidal Volume and be inspected and verified well in product development.

Keywords Turbine airflow sensor · Ventilator · Vidal volume · Capability coefficient

167.1 Foreword

Ventilators are the clinical most commonly used first aid and the life support equipment. Along with microprocessor technology, high accuracy pressure and flowrate sensor technology; the rapid reaction valve system development and the application, caused ventilators to become one multily-disciplinary overlapping, the knowledge-intensive high-tech product, and gradually developed to the intellectualized direction [1]. But its key component airflow sensor and the application

---

Y. Wu (✉) · F. Chang · D. Liu
College of Engineering, Zhengzhou University Zhengzhou, Zhengzhou, China
e-mail: yaoyuwu2005@163.com

F. Chang
e-mail: zzdxoldchang@126.com

technology, is playing the very important role in ensuring Ventilators effective, safe, the comfortable aspect.

Separately introduced each kind of flowrate sensor principle, the characteristic and in Ventilators application in many literature [2–4]. In the practical application, with other several kinds (Differential pressure, thermal and ultrasonic wave) compares, the turbine airflow sensor by its structure simple, the non-zero creep, is affected slightly the stream condition, the price inexpensive applies universally in the domestically produced ventilators. This paper describe the construction and principle and feature and discussed the flowrate characteristics of turbine airflow sensor, according to the working feature of Ventilator and analyzing flowrate curve, provide measuring and calibrating method of Tidal Volume of Ventilator, have obtained the high quantity precision of the Tidal Volume.

167.2 Characteristics of Turbine Airflow Sensor

167.2.1 The Construction and Principle

The turbine airflow sensor by the shell, the flow diversion body, the turbine blade, the bearing and the photoelectricity signal detector is composed as shown in Fig. 167.1. The shell is the sensor main body part, be made of transparent plastic. The photoelectricity signal detector is composed by the light emitter diode and the photodiode, clamped center the shell the signal detector is loaded the center of the shell. The flow diversion body with the helix stator vane structure conduction is loaded at the sensor import and export. When gas through the flow diversion body, is forced the encompassment middle line to revolve intensely the swirl, thus impetus leaf blade high speed revolving. In certain current capacity (Reynold's number) in the scope, the leaf blade rotational speed with flow is proportional after the precession turbulent flowrate sensor place fluid rate of volume flowrate. When leaf blade revolving, thus can between the make-and-break signal detector light emitter diode and the photorectifier speed of light sends out the pulse signal,

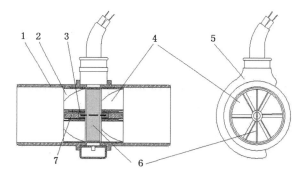

Fig. 167.1 Construction of turbine airflow sensor. *1* shell. *2* and *4* flow diversion body. *3* and *7* jewel bearing. *5* photoelectricity signal detector. *6* leaf blade

according to the electric eye signal make-and-break pulse frequency or the frequency, may convert for passes the sensor the current capacity or the gas flowrate.

As above, the Turbine Airflow Sensor is a kind of Speed type flowrate sensor. The output signal is the pulse frequency signal which is proportional with the current capacity, not the fluid temperature, the pressure ingredient, the viscosity and the density influence, has simply the structure, the duplication good, the stability high, the price inexpensive and so on the characteristics. But because has the leaf blade to transport the moving parts, its sensitivity, the frequency–response characteristic receives the leaf blade quality, the rotation inertia, the bearing friction force influence, thus creates this kind of sensor production "the inertia", causes responds "slowly" to the fast change air current. The main performance for starts when the air current, the pulse signal lag (so-called "effect starts to retard"), but has the pulse signal in the air current conclusion fashion (so-called to send out "effect stop rotation") [5]. Therefore, it is necessary to understand the turbine wheel airflow sensor the discharge characteristic.

167.2.2 Turbine Wheel Airflow Sensor Discharge Characteristic

The turbine wheel airflow sensor practical current capacity equation is:

$$Q_V = f/K \qquad (167.1)$$

In the formula Qv-the rate of volume flow, m³/s, f-the airflow sensor output signal frequency, Hz; K-the airflow sensor scaling factor, P/m^3 (P is pulse number).

Airflow sensor scaling factor K and current capacity Q (or pipeline Reynold's number) relational curve as shown in Fig. 167.2. The figure shows, the scaling factor may divide into two sections, namely linear section and non-linear section. Linear section approximately for work section 2/3, its characteristic and sensor structure size and fluid coherency related, can receive the patient secretion in the work process influence [5]. In the non-linear section, the characteristic the bearing friction force, the fluid viscous resistance influence is been big. When the current capacity is lower than the sensor current capacity lower limit also does not have the victory "the inertia", the scaling factor is a zero, then along with current capacity rapid change. In the measurable quantity scope, the K value change is small. When the current capacity surpasses the current capacity upper limit can change once more fierce and has the possibility to have the cavitation. The same structure turbine wheel airflow sensor characteristic curve shape is similar, the difference only lies in has the different system error level.

Fig. 167.2 Feature of turbine airflow sensor

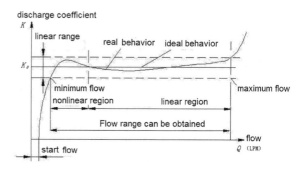

167.3 Ventilator Current Capacity Characteristic

167.3.1 Typical Current Capacity Curves

Figure 167.3 is typical Flowrate-time curve of Ventilator (constant discharge ventilation pattern) [6]. The horizontal axis represents the time, the ordinate axis represents the inspiration/expiration current capacity. 1: Transports the gas on behalf of the Ventilator the start, 2: Inspiration peak current capacity (PIF or PF), 3: Finished on behalf of the inspiration, the Ventilator stops the transportation gas. This time the humidity which supposes in advance to measure (VCV) has been completed or the designated pressure has attains (PCV), the transportation current capacity has completed (speed of flow changing-over), or the inspiration time has attained a designated standard (time changing-over), 4 → 5: On behalf of entire expiration time: Before including starts from the expiration to the next inspiration to start this period of time, indicated generally with t_E, 6: 1 → 4 is the inspiration

Fig. 167.3 Typical flowrate-time curve of ventilator

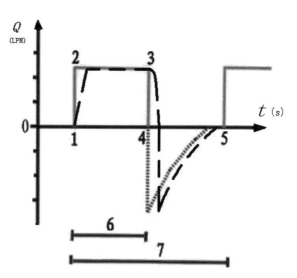

time, indicated generally with t_I, 7: On behalf of breath cycle time (t): $t = 60$ s/frequency.

167.3.2 Tidal Volume Calculation

The tidal volume is in the Ventilator ventilation process most important parameter, is directly affecting patient's vitality exchange effect. Under ideal ventilation condition, inspiration Tidal volume V_{t_I} with the current capacity Q_V relations is:

$$V_{t_I} = Q_V \times t_I \qquad (167.2)$$

But in the practical application, this kind ideal "the square-wave" is realizes with difficulty. In the gas channel stream velocity is not a constant speed, but is the dynamic change. In fact, in the gas transfer mechanism has certain intrinsic response time (including sensor response time), from 0 rises to the peak value speed of flow needs certain time. But after this response time has happen to created the inspiration air current outset rise slope, but when inspiration conclusion appears the micro negative slope deviation, as mentioned above, regarding this kind of turbine wheel airflow sensor is so. This phenomenon like chart 3 dashed line parts show. But inspiration Tidal volume for actual profile 1234 curve part area, namely for current capacity to inspiration time integral:

$$V_{t_I} = \int_0^{t_I} Q_V dt \qquad (167.3)$$

Formula (167.1) substitution formula (167.3):

$$V_{t_I} = \int_0^{t_I} \frac{f}{K} dt = f_{t_I} \int_0^{t_I} \frac{1}{K} dt = C_f \times f_{t_I} \qquad (167.4)$$

V_{t_I}-Inspiration tidal volume,ml; f_{t_I}-in inspiration time t_I airflow sensor output signal pulse number, frequency; C_f -airflow sensor measuring appliance volume efficiency, ml/time.

In summary, as a result of the Ventilator ventilation intermittence and the respiratory system air course resistance, elasticity and so on many factor influences, the Ventilator current capacity is the dynamic change. But uses this kind of turbine wheel airflow sensor to be possible to be possible to simplify the inspiration tidal volume as the pulse number and the volume efficiency product.

167.4 Pulse Number Survey and Compensating

167.4.1 Pulse Number Survey

Because the turbine wheel sensor has the movement part, therefore the Ventilator ventilation starts time, the pulse signal lag (so-called "effect starts to retard"), but has the pulse signal in the air current conclusion fashion (so-called to send out "effect stop rotation"). As shown in Fig. 167.4, starts when the inspiration, the sensor signal has the time delay Δt.

When ventilation conclusion (process inspiration time t_I), but also has the pulse signal to send out. If the pulse counts in inspiration time t_I, then in fact for in $t_I - \Delta t$ time actual pulse number, compares with the actual pulse number must be small, the tidal volume which calculates must be smaller than actually; Similarly, if the counting time in the entire ventilation cycle, namely in the $t_I + t_E$ time the pulse total quantity, has in fact contained "the false pulse signal" which creates as a result of the leaf blade inertia, calculates the tidal volume according to this to have the big error similarly. May know from the airflow sensor principle, "the effect starts to retard" and "the effect stop rotation" has certain relations, therefore, uses following two methods to carry on the pulse counting compensation: (a) The time will lengthen for $t_I + \Delta t$, soon counting time region t_I will translate in the time axis Δt, will take $t_I + \Delta t$ actual counting value f1; (b) The counting time and the counting region are invariable, in obtains the delay time Δt and counts f after the t_I actual pulse, the compensation pulse counts f_1 to carry on the computation according to the equation below:

$$f_1 = f \times \left(1 + \frac{\Delta t}{t_I}\right) \quad (167.5)$$

In the formula f_1-compensation pulse number, f-in inspiration time t_I airflow sensor output signal pulse number, time; $\Delta t - t_I$ starts to the airflow sensor to send out the pulse signal the delay time, s.

Through actual indicated that, both compensation precision error basic consistent, the second way is easier through the programming to realize, therefore uses the second pulse counting compensating process.

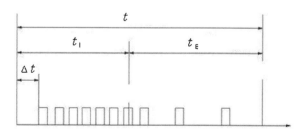

Fig. 167.4 Pulse counting of turbine airflow sensor

167.4.2 Volume Efficiency Calibration

By the Fig. 167.2 and the formula (167.1) may see, in scaling factor K and the gas channel the current capacity becomes the approximate linear relations in certain speed of flow scope, but is not the constant, but is in certain undulation scope. Moreover, the different operating mode condition influence, the airflow sensor can have under the different respiratory system air course condition the different performance, therefore, the different speed of flow Q_V correspondence has different scaling factor K. But volume efficiency C_f and the K existence correspondence relations, we may affirm, in inspiration time t_I, different pulse number correspondence different volume efficiency C_f. In order to guarantee the tidal volume the accurate survey, we install the airflow sensor in the actual respiratory system air course, through stipulation certain inspiration time t_I. From small to big gradually adjusts the inspiration speed of flow, obtains the pulse to count f (process to revise) with the tidal volume corresponding relations curve, as shown in Fig. 167.5. May regards as the tidal volume and the pulse number the partition linearity relations. The partition recovers the regulation actual precision to be higher, but consumes the microcomputer chip controller limited resources are also bigger. Therefore, guaranteed the survey tidal volume error in ±8 % is a principle. Through different airflow sensor actual survey, just like this article in 1.2 states, its capacity—pulse curve basic consistent, but has the different system error. Therefore, when volume production when reads in the computer chip procedure, consideration system error corrected value.

167.4.3 The Tidal Volume Calculates with the Compensating Process

According to the formula (167.4, 167.5), and experiment actual result, the Ventilator inspiration tidal volume uses the following formula in the procedure:

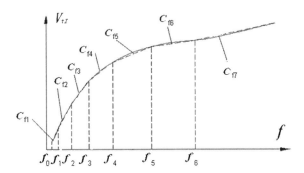

Fig. 167.5 Rating curve of capacity coefficient

$$V_{t_l i} = V_{t_l 0} + C_{fi} \times f_i \times \left(1 + \frac{\Delta t}{t_{Ii}}\right) \qquad (167.6)$$

$V_{t_l 0}$-the tidal volume compensation value, ml; C_{fi}-corresponds the different pulse number corresponding volume efficiency, ml/time; f_i-in inspiration time tI airflow sensor output signal pulse number, time; $\Delta t - t_I$ starts to the airflow sensor to send out the pulse signal the delay time, s.

At the same time, establishes two forms, one is f value and V_{t_l} corresponding relations when the actual pulse number is smaller than f_0, selects the table look-up method to discover Vt_I the value; One is works as when $f_i \leq f < f_{i+1}$, corresponds C_{fi}. Through the micro controller in inspiration time t_I, the judgment examination delay time Δt, the pulse measures f, the revision pulse counts the volume efficiency value sector after the compensation pulse which f_I judges its is at, withdraws the corresponding volume efficiency, finally substitutes the formula (167.6) then to obtain in inspiration time t_I the tidal volume. After development ventilator estimated data and measured data contrast, tidal volume quantity error scope between $-7\ \%$ and $+4\ \%$.

167.5 Conclusion

Turbine wheel airflow sensor its unique feature has the time hysteresis quality, and regarding the different ventilator system and the speed of flow gas, has the different volume efficiency. Compensates through the pulse counting and partitions the demarcation airflow sensor volume efficiency method to be possible to increase the tidal volume measuring accuracy, and obtained the very good confirmation in the product development, has obtained the satisfactory measuring accuracy in the actual product development.

References

1. Yu H, Wei H (2003) Ventilator intelligentized machinery ventilation. China Med Instr Mag 27(1):47–50
2. Yang D, Liu M (2004) Medical airflow sensor technical characteristic as well as in ventilator application. China Med Equip 1(13):42–43
3. Fan X, Tao S, Xue X (2003) New airflow sensor on Ventilator application. Shandong Univ Sci Technol Nat Sci 17(2):72–75
4. Lin H, Lin K (2005) Gas flowrate sensor structure, principle and in ventilator application. Med Equip 18(3):24–25
5. Fang G, Chen X (2004) Yang tiande ohmeda anaesthesia ventilator tidal volume error the influence factor analysis. Chinese Med Equip J 06:47–48
6. Yu S (2000) Modern mechanical ventilation monitoring and clinical application. China Union Medical University Press, Beijing, p 41

Chapter 168
Study on the Model of Double Tutors System in Postgraduate Education

Jian Wang and Zhongyan Han

Abstract Double tutors system is a new cultured mode for the innovation and practicality of postgraduates. The purpose of this paper is started with the introduction of the education of postgraduates majoring in basic medical science (BMS), comprehensively introduces the advantages, management and evaluation of double tutors system for medical postgraduates, explores the role and significance of the double tutors model in medical postgraduate education, and seeks a new way to improve the quality of postgraduate education to meet the needs posed by the expansion of enrollment.

Keywords Double tutors system · Medical postgraduate · Cultivation model

168.1 Introduction

Double tutors system, as a new postgraduate training mode, is aimed at the cultivation of a large number of innovative and practical talents in order to meet the needs of social development. One tutor is from the university, the other tutor is from the cooperative departments or units such as research institutes, hospitals, etc. or expert in this field. In order to satisfy the demands of the society for innovative and practical talents with comprehensive capabilities [1], and to better explore social education resources, we have adopted double tutors system in postgraduate education and achieved better results.

J. Wang (✉) · Z. Han
Department of Aetiology and Immunology, Medical College, Anhui University of Science and Technology, Huainan 232001 Anhui, China
e-mail: wangjian8237@sina.com

168.2 The Establishment and Development of the Double Tutors System

Double tutors system refers to the practice of assigning a postgraduate one in-school tutor and one out-school tutor. The guidance of the postgraduate on preliminary courses and basic research is in the charge of the in-school tutor, while the latter guidance related to clinical researches is in the charge of the out-school tutor. With the joint and complementary supervision of the two tutors, their respective advantages can be best applied and the comprehensive innovative abilities and research proficiencies can be remarkably improved [2]. The first tutor (in-school tutor) works in the school into which the postgraduate is admitted and supervises the postgraduate on relevant major courses. The second tutor (out-school tutor), a part-timer invited to the school, is usually one with profound work experiences and sound professional skills. In the course of the joint supervision of postgraduates, it is usually the first tutor who chooses the second tutor.

In this document, it is stated that in addition to the number of students planned in the postgraduate plan of the Ministry of Education in 2009, a further 50,000 full time professional degree postgraduates will be enrolled. How to educate these full time professional degree postgraduates has become a hot topic in the circle of education. In order to cultivate a higher quality of medical postgraduate students and to satisfy the needs of the society, the double tutors system has been gradually applied in graduate education in many medical colleges.

168.3 Advantage of Double Tutors System

The main duties of the school tutor are to develop the ability of students to learn, to enhance the development potential of students, to gradually influence them with the ethics of the teacher so as to cultivate the students' good learning style and methods, and to improve their academic performance and to cultivate the professional skills of the students. In the beginning period of the supervision, it is difficult for the students to understand the major courses well because they haven't studied them long. School instructors should provide a variety of guidance for students under the credit system not only in course selection and professional knowledge, but also in learning methods and professional development. As the students learn more and more specialized courses and professional knowledge, the instructor should continue to provide a variety of guidance for students, such as understanding of the specialized knowledge, the relationship among the various professional courses, and how to use professional knowledge in practice. In the later learning stages, the school tutor must supervise the students on dissertations, thesis writing, and academic ethics.

The main responsibilities of the outside school tutor is to cultivate the students' professional ethics, to improve the students clinical skills, and to improve the ability of the students to solve practical problems, to enable the students to form the initial professional judgment, so as to meet the needs of the future work. The out-school tutor is also supposed to engage in the supervision of the students in graduation practice, degree thesis and graduation design.

The in-school and out-school tutors have their respective merits, which, when combined, can lead to further advantages. (1) Better professional understanding and further space of development. Medical postgraduates need a broader and deeper scope of knowledge, broader horizon, as well as the original insights in science research. (2) Individualized teaching can be achieved. Findings of psychological researches have shown that there are individual differences in personal qualities, therefore the education mode which ignores the difference of individual medical students will yield poor results. The double tutors system has its unique advantages compared with the traditional supervision system. For example, under this system, reasonable attention is paid to individual students. (3) Knowledge of medical theory and clinical ability can be combined. One experience is shared by many medical students, which is their feeling at a loss when conducting clinical practice even after long time spent on medical theories. The problem lies in the big gap between theoretical knowledge and clinical practice and the students' inability to convert theoretical knowledge to clinical abilities. With the help of two tutors from campus and off-campus, the students can participate in clinical clerkships and internships following the off-campus mentors in extracurricular time. In the course of practice, the students will not only increase the perceptual knowledge, also deepen the understanding and application of the theoretical knowledge in practice after frequent diagnosis and treatment of puzzling and difficult cases. After a period of training, the ability to combine theoretical knowledge and clinical practice will be gradually improved.

168.4 Management of Double Tutors System

168.4.1 The Qualifications of Tutors

Both the in-school tutors and out-school tutors play an authoritative role in guiding the students in areas of ideological education, daily living and studies. The ideological attitude and demeanor of the tutors may have a direct impact on students, so the licensing of tutor qualifications must be very strict. To guarantee the smooth implementation of double tutor system and to demonstrate the advantages of the tutors, all aspects of the double tutor system should be improved, for example, double tutor selection, appointment, management, supervision and quality evaluation. The selection of out-school tutors must satisfy the following conditions. The first, the out-school tutors should have extensive practical experiences and sound theoretical level. The second, the out-school tutors can provide the postgraduates with opportunities of social practice. The out-school tutors selection and the licensing of qualifications are organized and completed by the graduate department of universities, and the joint supervision agreements should be signed in which the respective rights and obligations should be listed. The third, in the appointment process of out-school tutors, the combination of the theories from in-school tutors and the practice from outside school tutors should be given full consideration, so as to avoid significant gap between theoretical learning and actual demands the students may confront. The fourth, during the process of postgraduate training, the in-school and out-school tutors must complete the guidance in cooperation and design plans of supervision, discuss the researches the students should take part in, get involved in the guidance of the degree thesis, provide professional courses and academic lectures for graduate students. The fifth, in the course of supervision, importance should be attached to social practices. It is important to make good use of social resources, and to create an environment which is conducive to the harmonious combination of theories and practices. The experiences should be constantly summed up, the problems that crop up gradually being solved, so as to establish and improve the double tutors system. The sixth, the high-level papers can be published during postgraduate study.

168.4.2 The Management of the Double Tutors System

Tutors, as the promoters and practitioners of the double tutors system play a decisive role in the implementation of the double tutors system. Double tutors system needs the protection of a scientific management system, and the unnecessary interferences and mandatory provisions imposed on the in-school and out-school tutors must be reduced. For example, the very common enforced regulation which forces the tutors to successfully apply for a certain number of projects and to hold a certain number of meetings with the students, which is highly likely to lead to the tutors' perfunctory behavior and low-yielding performances. Thus the traditional process-oriented management should be changed to an objective-oriented style. The responsibility pledges between the school and the instructors must be signed and the reasonable evaluation systems should also be established simultaneously. The work and living style of the tutors as well as the actual needs of the students should be to the largest extent respected, and an environment should be created conducive to the equal and open communication between the supervisors and the students. In order to improve the political and ideological quality of the tutors and the level of professional skills, the tutors popular among the students should be given extra bonus through performance assessment.

The basic course instructors rigorous scientific attitude and excellence in learning style, indomitable perseverance, diligent study, constant innovation, will all have subtle influence on student life [3]. When instructors undertake research projects and set up research guidance group, the personal experiences, the researches, the individual abilities and interests of students all should be given full consideration. The purpose is to train students to have research quality and ability in literature review, research design, data processing and summary report, so as to create a solid and generous foundation for the students in future clinical practice and scientific research. A research article or a literature review must be finished by the student as the first author.

168.4.3 To Improve the Postgraduates' Identifying with the Tutors

Graduate students are the main body of education. Double tutors system as a new and humane education mode centering upon the students, must ensure two-way choice. By extensive publicity and education, the students completely understand double tutors system and change the long-held concepts in the teaching of academic postgraduates, and simultaneously improve the postgraduates' identifying with the tutors. Only when the students really accept and cooperate with the two tutors in theoretical researches and practices, can the double tutors system be smoothly implemented. If the students believe that a mentor is not suitable for himself, the mentor can be replaced through the normal channels. In addition, the combination of best in-school and out-school tutors should be encouraged. The top tutors may supervise the top students, which is conducive to the emergence of outstanding talents.

In summary, the model of double tutorial system is useful exploration for training graduate students in the new situation.

Acknowledgments This research was supported by the grants from Educational Science Foundation of Anhui Province (2012jyxm209), China, and also supported by the key grants from Educational Science Foundation of Anhui University of Science and Technology (No: 2012–27).

References

1. Du J, Ge Y, Gu L (2007) Reflect on cultivation of clinical skills and research capacity in eight-academic year medical students. Acta Univ Med Nanjing Sci 3:78–80
2. Yang Z, Zhou Q, Dong W et al (2010) Analysis on the application of double tutorial system in the training of medical graduate students. Chin J Edu 30:624–625
3. Yi S, Liu X, Tao W et al (2009) Practice and exploration of applying basic-tutor in eight-year medical education. China High Med Educ 9:118

Chapter 169
Research on the Mobile Learning Resources Based on Cellphone

Huang Lehui and Xing Ruonan

Abstract Mobile learning is a new way of digital learning. Learning at any time, any place and in any way has became a trend. With the continuous development of wireless network technology, increasingly perfect phone functions and declining civilian prices, mobile learning has gradually in popularity. Learning resources is one of the two research areas of education technology. Mobile learning resources is an important foundation to start M-learning, while the design of learning content is the core of resources construction. This article focused on the design of learning resources, the construction of learning delivery systems and its content presentation to analysis and discuss, hope to provide greater reference to develop mobile learning resources.

Keywords Mobile learning · Learning resources · Content presentation

169.1 Introduction

Mobile technology has led to a new style of mobile learning. At the same time, mobile learning has also changed people's learning way which from formal extends to informal, and provides a new form to serve our lifelong learning. Mobile learning needs to consider learning resources problems at first. The characteristics of mobile learning demand course content clear and learners in the informal learning pursuit of practical knowledge requires point dapper. So the

H. Lehui (✉)
Education School, Jiangxi Science and Technology Normal University,
Nanchang 330000, China
e-mail: yjgnie@163.com

X. Ruonan
Xing Ruonan, Communication School, Jiangxi Normal University, Nanchang 330000, China

design of learning resources, the construction of learning delivery systems and its content presentation will play a decisive role in implementation status of mobile learning.

169.2 What is Mobile Learning Resources?

Learning resources has been received much concerns from some educational technology researchers. By use of the system process view, people connect the media to other elements of teaching process, and form a new teaching method, that is, promote effective teaching through use resources [1]. More far-reaching impacts on our educational technology community are the definition of learning resources determined in 1994. Learning resources is anything that can help individuals learn and operate effectively [2]. Mobile learning resources [3] is a kind of digital information resources, which is designed for reflect some specific learning content and teaching strategies, and support some certain mobile learning activities. It is the source of knowledge construction, and is the basis for building mobile learning, including mobile services platform and its supporting learning content.

169.3 Content Presentation of Mobile Learning Resources

After determined learning content and planned learning components, people should make the appropriate decision to present learning content. The presentation of learning content must be by means of a delivery system. When faced with specific learning terminal and special learning content, it is a problem that we need to explore, how to select the appropriate media presentation.

169.3.1 Introduction of Mobile Learning Delivery System based on Cell-Phones

169.3.1.1 Learning Delivery System

Educational Communication [4] is a kind of communicational activity, through effective media channel, educators complied with certain purposes and selected suitable information content, sent specific educational objects knowledge, skills, ideas, concepts, etc.

In any formal educational process, it is called delivery system [5] that is a basic method of management and delivery of teaching and learning activities. in the mobile phone learning environment, the phone is a learning delivery system.

169.3.1.2 Construction of Mobile Learning Delivery System

Mobile phone learning delivery system is a behavior or process that regards the mobile wireless network as the carrier to pass or exchange information. A complete and effective mobile learning delivery system should include four aspects, for example, the mobile learning resources library, the information transmission channel, the mobile learning terminal and learners. The general model shows as Fig 169.1.

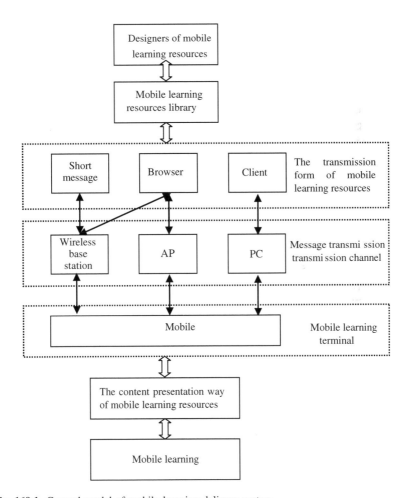

Fig. 169.1 General model of mobile learning delivery system

169.3.2 Content Presentation Way of Mobile Learning Delivery System based on Cell-Phones

169.3.2.1 Existing Form of Mobile Media

The phone functions gradually becoming powerful and rich, from the original phone to SMS, MMS, and then to the mobile newspaper, the mass media status has gradually established. The existing form of mobile media is colourful, on the basis of Refs. [6, 7], we summarized the existing forms of mobile media are Table 169.1.

Table 169.1 Existing forms of mobile media

Existing form	Media types	Advantages	Disadvantages
Phone	Sound	Message convey timely, accurate and have a good communication	Mobile callers are usually one-to-one, not one-to-many. The conversation quality is affected by the signal strength
Short message	Text	The information transmission has not effect on our normal life, and the short message can be stored	The communication characters are restricted by small capacity. The presentation form of SMS is more single
Multimedia messaging service	Text; Picture; sound; Animation	The multimedia have a good effect and can interact with others	Have a low-speed communication and need to open the GPRS function
Cell phone broadcast	Sound	He dissemination of information close to life	The dissemination of information is vulnerable to signal interference, and need to build FM broadcast regulator into cell phone
Cell phone TV	Sound; Video	Have a vivid and authentic picture, easy for the public to accept, and also have a great potential for development	Cell phone TV has a low-speed communication and is vulnerable to network transmission quality impacts. At the same time, it is required to install the client software to receive image
Mobile video	Sound; Video	Support multi-user involvement, interactive	More paid products, and need mobile phone to install the third-party software
Web browser	Text; Picture; sound; Video; Animation	To support thematic learning, can accept the large amount of information	By the impact of network transmission quality, the function needs to open GPRS services, and all services cost much money
E-book	Text; Picture	Text-based, larger capacity, more practical	Support restricted file formats; poor content is not easy to organize

169.3.2.2 Type and Characteristics of Mobile Media

The famous Canadian communication scholar Marshall McLuhan has point out, the media is an extension of the human body functions. Under the guidance of the micro-learning theory, the mobile learning resources are designed by a variety of multimedia. Some studies have point out that if the media are poorly designed, may lost the media characteristics and discount learning outcomes. Because of the restrictions in the foot of the screen, storage capacity, display format and data processing capabilities, the ordinary learning resources are difficult to apply on the phone. Therefore, in design resources process, it is necessary that people accord to the characteristics of mobile learning and the functions of mobile learning terminal, and combined with the law of media presentation and application characteristics for different learning content, designed reasonable and effective media present form, making the resources presentation optimized.

169.4 Conclusion

With the view of lifelong learning has been proposed, the importance of mobile learning is becoming increasingly apparent, and its advantages in the process of educational information are obvious to all. As a typical way of informal learning, the root of the differences between mobile learning and traditional learning is that the introduction of a new technology. In terms of mobile learning, studying the design of M-learning resources content is a complex and meaningful work. From the perspective of the learning content presentation, this article analysis the content designs of mobile phone learning resources. The presentation of learning content must be by means of certain delivery system. How to select an appropriate media presentation is the key link of content design? Hope that the research will provide some information and reference for the future development of quality mobile learning resources.

References

1. He K, Li W (2002) Education technology. Beijing Normal University Press, Beijing
2. Barbara BS, Rita CR(1999) Educational technology: the definition and category of field, translate by Wu M, Liu Y. The Central Radio and Television University Press, Beijing
3. Huang R, Jyri S (2008) Mobile learning—theory• status• trend. Science Press, Beijing
4. Zhang J (2006) Modern education technology—theory and application. Higher Education Press, Beijing
5. Dick W, Lou C (2004) Instruction system design, translated by Wang Q. Higher Education Press, Beijing
6. Bing H, Lei W (2009) Analysis on forms of mobile media and research on its foreground. Press Circles 02:74–75
7. Fu J (2010) Research and development strategy of domestic mobile learning. Jilin University, Jilin

Chapter 170
Data Structure Teaching Practice: Discussion on Non-recursive Algorithms for the Depth-First Traversal of a Binary Tree

Zhong-wei Xu

Abstract The recursive algorithms for depth-first traversal of a binary tree are widely expatiated upon in data structure textbooks. There are three depth-first traversal sequences for a binary tree, preorder, inorder, and postorder traversal sequences. My literature survey indicates the most references present the depth-first traversals algorithms as recursive ones. Some literatures have introduced the non-recursive algorithms only for one of these three traversal sequences of a binary tree. In this paper a general non-recursive algorithm for the depth-first traversal of a binary tree is proposed. This general non-recursive algorithm can visit every nodes of a binary tree in preorder, inorder, or postorder traversal sequence. The algorithm analysis shows that this new algorithm is efficient and easy to understand. The implementation of this new algorithm was done in C and the complete algorithm was tested.

Keywords Binary tree · Depth-first traversal · Non-recursive

170.1 Introduction

A binary tree traversal require that each node of the tree be processed once and only once in a predetermined sequence. There are two general approaches to the traversal sequence, depth first and breadth first [1]. In a breadth-first traversal, each level is completely processed before the next level is started. The algorithm for the breadth-first traversal has been introduced in many literatures [1, 2]. In a depth-first traversal, all of the descendents of a child are processed before the next child. Most textbooks and reference books present the traversal algorithm as a recursive

Z. Xu (✉)
School of Mechanical, Electrical and Information Engineering,
Shandong University at Weihai, Weihai, Shandong Province, China
e-mail: xuzhongwei@sdu.edu.cn

algorithm. The recursive formulation allows us to write compact and easy to understand algorithms to manipulate trees. But it is also meaningful to study corresponding non-recursive algorithms. On one hand, this study could deepen the comprehension about how recursion work, on the other hand, in the non-recursive algorithms programmers could operate the recursion stack in order to trace the recursion process. Some literatures have introduced the non-recursive algorithms only for one of the three traversal sequences of a binary tree [3, 4]. Reference [2] has presented two versions of non-recursive algorithm for the inorder traversal of a binary tree. The author of this paper has designed a general non-recursive algorithm for the depth-first traversal of a binary tree based on an analysis on the control flow of binary tree depth-first traversal. This general non-recursive algorithm can visit every nodes of a binary tree in preorder, inorder, or postorder traversal sequence.

170.2 The Basic Idea of the Algorithm

The non-recursive depth-first traversal algorithms are loosely analog to recursive ones by defining a recursive stack frame explicitly. As a general non-recursive algorithm for the three depth-first traversals, it must be based on the common factors, i.e. the control flow of depth-first travel illustrated by Fig. 170.1.

We inspect a node in the binary tree and treat it as the "current node". If the control flow has not yet flowed into its left subtree, then the control flow will flow into its left child, and this left child will become the "current node". If the control flow has returned from its left subtree, then the control flow will flow into its right child node, and this right child node will become the "current node". If the control flow has returned from its right subtree, then the control flow will flow back into its parent node, and this parent node will become the "current node". As the transformation of the "current node" role proceeds in the binary tree in order, the control flow will pass all the nodes in the binary tree in depth-first traversal order. In the process of depth-first traversal, if the "current node" is visited before the control flow gets into its left subtree, the traversal sequence will be preorder; if the

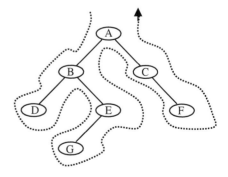

Fig. 170.1 Shows a way to visualize the depth-first traversal of the binary tree. Imagine that you are walking around the tree, starting on the left of the root and keeping as close to the nodes as possible. The footmarks would form the path along witch the processing proceeds in the depth-first traversal

"current node" is visited before the control flow gets into its right subtree but after the control flow returns from its left subtree, the traversal sequence will be inorder; if the "current node" is visited after the control flow returns from its right subtree, the traversal sequence will be postorder.

170.3 The Auxiliary Data Structure

When the control flow has returned from the right subtree of the "current node", it will go back by the save route to its parent node. So a stackframe is a necessary auxiliary data structure in the non-recursive depth-first traversal algorithm, and the element at the stack top serves always as the "current node".

Standing on the "current node", there are three statuses must be distinguished in order to select a node the control flow will go into in the next step. The first is that the control flow will go into the "current node" for the first time, the second is that the control flow has just returned form the left subtree and will go into the "current node" for the second time, the third is that the control flow has just returned from the right subtree and will go into the "current node" for the third time. Hencc it is feasible to introduce two Boolean items into each stack elements to identify these three status.

The structure of the linked binary tree and the recursion stack defined in C are shown in Table 170.1.

170.4 The Algorithm Description

The algorithm shown in Table 170.2 is a general non-recursive depth-first algorithm for preorder, inorder, postorder traversal of a binary tree. The parameter "T"

Table 170.1 The structure of the linked binary tree and the recursion stack

```
#define STACK_SIZE 100
typedefine struct biNode
{   biElemType data;
    struct biNode *lchild;    // left child pointer
    struct biNode *rchild;    // right child pointer
} biNode, *biTree;
typedefne struct
{   biTree ptr;
    bool lchB, rchB;          //be used to distingush the three status.
} stElemtype, stackType[STACK_SIZE];
```

Table 170.2 A new general non-recursive algorithm for the depth-first traversal of a binary tree

```
void GeneralTraverse(BiTree T, char mode ) {
    InitStack(S);   t = {T, false, false};   Push(S,t);
    while (!StackEmpty(S))  {
    GetTop(S, t);
    switch {
    case !t.curPtr:
            Pop(S, t);  break;
    case t.lchTraveled && t.rchTraveled:
            if(mode == 'L') visit(t.curPtr->data); // postorder
            Pop(S, t);          break;
    case !t.lchTraveled:
            if(mode == 'F') visit(t.curPtr->data); // preorder
            Pop(S, t);  t.lchTraveled = true;
            Push(S, t);    //take down footprint
            t = { t.curPtr->lchild, false, false};
            Push(S, t);    //go into left subtree
            break;
    case !t.rchTraveled:
            if(mode == 'I') visit(t.curPtr->data); //inorder
            Pop(S, t);  t.rchTraveled = true;
            Push(S, t);    //take down footprint
            t = { t.curPtr->rchild, false, false};
            Push(S, t);    //go into right subtree
    } // switch
  } //while
} //GeneralTraverse
```

is a pointer that points to the root node of the binary tree to be traversed. The values of the parameter "mode" could be 'L', 'I', and 'P'. These values are corresponding to preorder traversal, inorder traversal, and postorder traversal respectively.

170.5 Experiment

The implementation for the general non-recursive algorithm shown in Table 170.2 was done in C and the complete algorithm was tested, and a function that creates a binary tree in preorder, a function that visits a node of the binary tree are also included. The execution process of the C implementation is listed below.

Please input the value of every nodes in preorder (the blank is corresponding to a NULL tree): ABD□□EG□□□C□F□□<CR>

The preorder traversal sequence is: ABEGCF
The inorder traversal sequence is: DBGEACF
The postorder traversal sequence is: DGEBFCA

. The binary tree created above is same as that illustrated in Fig. 170.1. The results of the experiment are right apparently.

170.6 Summary

Some literatures have present non-algorithms only for preorder traversal or last-order traversal. All these non-recursive algorithms apply to only one of the three traversal orders, and these algorithms itself are difficult to read. The idea of the non-recursive algorithm presented in this paper is in accordance with control flow of depth-first traversal of a binary tree. This algorithm is clear and fluent; it is of generality without additions of complexity in space and time. Hence it is worthy to adopt the algorithm presented in this paper in data structure teaching.

References

1. Gilberg RF, Forouzan BA (1998) Data Structures: A Pseudocode A pproach with C. PWS Publishing Company, Boston
2. Yan Wei-min and Wu Wei-min Wu (2007) Data Structure (in Chinese). Tsinghua University press, Beijing
3. AI-Rawi A, Lansari A, and Bouslama F (2003) "A new non-recursive algorithm for binary search tree traversal". In: Proceedings of the 2003 10th IEEE international conference on electronics, circuits and systems, ICECS 2003, vol 2, pp 770–773
4. Liu Zhong-hua and Zhang Ying-chao (2010) Depth-first Search and Non-recursive Algorithm. Sci & Technol Inf (in Chinese) 25:160–161
5. Weiss MA (1993) Data Structures and Algorithm Analysis in C++. The Benjamin/Cummings Publishing Company, Redwood City
6. Wang M (2011) Non-recursive simulation on the recursive algorithm of binary tree reverting to its corresponding forest in intelligent materials. Appl Mech and Mater 63–64:222–225
7. Vinu V Das (2010) A new non-recursive algorithm for reconstructing a binary tree from its traversals. In: Proceedings of the 2010 2nd international conference on advances in recent technologies in communication and computing, ARTCom 2010, pp 261–263

Chapter 171
Contrast Analysis of Standardized Patients and Real Patients in Clinical Medical Teaching

Zhang Yali, Xi Bo, Zhou Rui, Chunli Wu, Feng Jie, Jiping Sun, Jing Lv, Qingzhi Long and Bingyin Shi

Abstract *Objective* To investigate the role and characteristics of Standardized Patients (SP) in clinical medical teaching. *Methods* The differences were analyzed between SP and real patients through the questionnaire survey. *Results* ① There were no significant differences on the teaching effect between these two methods ($P > 0.05$). ② The effect of SP is better than that of the real patients in compliance, cooperation ($P < 0.05$). ③ SP were not impacted by time and season. *Conclusion* SP have the same clinical teaching effect as real patients, while SP were better than real patients in compliance and cooperation, and SP were more suitable for clinical practice.

Keywords SP · Real patients · Clinical medicine students with 8-years program

Categorization: G642 Identification code: A

Clinical skills training plays a vital part in the training of qualified medical workers. But there are many problems in the teaching process, such as difficulties finding typical cases, or some diseases being limited by season or time. In addition, there are fewer patients and more students, resulting in students obtaining the history repeatedly from the same patient. Because of this, poor compliance of patients can affect clinical teaching greatly [1]. In response to this situation many hospitals have put forward and trained Standardized Patients (SP) to meet the learning needs of medical students in recent years. The effect of SP on clinical skills training was compared to the effect of traditional patients among the medical students in our hospital's 8-years program.

Z. Yali (✉) · X. Bo · Z. Rui · C. Wu · F. Jie · J. Sun · J. Lv · Q. Long · B. Shi
Department of Nephrology, Xi'an Jiaotong University, Shaanxi 710061, People's Republic of China
e-mail: zhangyali516@sohu.com

171.1 Materials and Methods

There were 27 5th year medical students of the 2008 8-year medical program in our hospital. SPs were the qualified "patients" who completed a comprehensive training and examination in 2011. The control group was the hospitalized patients whose conditions were stable.

171.1.1 Methods

Problems in the clinical practice learning process were divided into five aspects. Each item was subsequently divided into three grades (very good, average, and poor grade) and was quantified from bad to good (from four to ten points). The scores were acquired through a questionnaire survey by the SP and ward patients (the patients of clinical inquiry).

171.1.2 Statistics Processing

SPSS 17.0 software was used for statistical analysis. Count material was presented as percentage, and grade material was analyzed with a Wilcoxon rank test. Measurement data was analyzed by normality test. If it was normality, $\bar{x} \pm s$ was used. Random material was compared using a t-test. If it was not normality, the data were presented as median and interquartile range and analyzed by Wilcoxon rank test. $P < 0.05$ shows that the difference was statistically significant.

171.2 Results

2.1 Compliance between two groups
   As shown in Table 171.1, the compliance of the SP group was more excellent than that of the control group.

Table 171.1 Comparison of compliance

Group	Excellent n (%)	Good n (%)	Bad n (%)	score	
				M	$Q_1 \sim Q_3$
SP	26 (100.0)	0 (0.0)	0 (0.0)	10.0	10.0 ~ 10.0
control	10 (38.5)	14 (53.9)	2 (7.7)	7.0	7.0 ~ 10.0
Z value	−4.726				−4.712
P value	0.000				0.000

Table 171.2 Language competence with regard to diseases

Group	Excellent n (%)	Good n (%)	Bad n (%)	Score ($\bar{x} \pm s$)
SP	18 (69.2)	7 (26.9)	1 (3.9)	9.0 ± 1.6
control	7 (26.9)	14 (53.9)	5 (19.2)	7.5 ± 1.9
Z(t) value	−3.099*			−3.219▲
P value	0.002			0.002

* presented as Wilcoxon. ▲ presented as t-test

2.2 Language competence: the language competence of the SP group was better than that of the control group (Table 171.2).

2.3 Disease comprehension: There were no significant differences in the understanding of their own diseases between the two groups (Table 171.3).

2.4 There were no significant differences between the integrity of the illness narrated by the two groups (Table 171.4).

2.5 As shown in Table 171.5, the relationship between doctors and patients was compared.

Table 71.3 Disease comprehension between the two groups

Group	Excellent n (%)	Good n (%)	Bad n (%)	Score ($\bar{x} \pm s$)
SP	9 (34.6)	16 (61.5)	1 (3.9)	7.9 ± 1.7
control	12 (46.2)	12 (46.2)	2 (7.7)	8.2 ± 1.8
Z(t) value	−1.215*			0.648▲
P value	0.0.224			0.520

* presented as Wilcoxon. ▲ presented as t-test

Table 171.4 Comparison of the integrity in two groups

Group	Excellent n (%)	Good n (%)	Bad n (%)	Score	
				M	$Q_1 \sim Q_3$
SP	12 (46.2)	14 (53.9)	0 (0.0)	7.0	7.0 ~ 10.0
control	6 (23.1)	19 (73.1)	1 (3.9)	7.0	7.0 ~ 9.3
Z value	−0.602*			−0.877▲	
P value	0.547			0.381	

Table 171.5 Comparison of doctor-patient relationship

Group	Excellent n (%)	Good n (%)	Bad n (%)	Score	
				M	$Q_1 \sim Q_3$
SP	25 (96.2)	1 (3.9)	0 (0.0)	10.0	10.0 ~ 10.0
control	10 (38.5)	15 (57.7)	1 (3.9)	7.0	7.0 ~ 10.0
Z value	−4.354			−4.546	
P value	0.000			0.000	

171.3 Discussion

Standardized Patients (SP), also known as simulated patients, refer to relatively healthy adults who, after standardized and systematic training, not only can display the clinical symptoms and signs of actual patients but also can undergo clinical examination. SPs can provide opportunities for medical students to practice their clinical skills. In addition, SPs can provide reliable feedback information for student evaluation [2]. They also serve three different roles: patient, evaluator and instructor.

Clinical skills training is a practical subject. It is necessary to practice and reinforce medical knowledge repetitively during the learning process. Due to the enhanced consciousness of patients self-protection, lack of patient cooperation with medical students, or the seasonal nature of some diseases, there is an increasing lack of clinical resources for the training of clinical skills, which influences teaching quality greatly. In early 1964, American scholars put forward the idea to train standardized patients, and subsequently this was developed rapidly in the American medical colleges. SPs are used not only in teaching and evaluation, but also in the examination for medical licensure [3]. In recent years, SPs were carried out in many universities in China. This kind of pioneering spirit has been very important for medical students and will impact the diagnosis and treatment of disease [4]. In recent years, it was reported that SPs play a very important role in diagnostic teaching [5], clinical skills, and clinical assessment in our country [6]. However, the effect of SPs in clinical teaching remained unknown.

We found that there were significant difference in compliance, language competence, and establishment of doctor-patient relationships between SPs and real patients through questionnaire surveys from students, while there were no differences on understanding of state of the illness and the integrity of the illness narrated by the two groups. Our results showed that SPs could achieve the same effect as real patients in medical teaching, while SPs had a greater advantage in compliance and establishment of the doctor-patient relationship. In addition, SPs had other distinct advantages, such as the ability to evaluate the history taking skills and physical examination skills of interns. They also are not influenced by time and season. The well repeatable characteristics of SPs could satisfy the need of clinical medical teaching. Thus, SPs will provide a favorable model of clinical medical teaching [7]. According to our experience, the following aspects should be considered: 1. Selection Criteria of SPs: SPs should have good language competence, understanding power, communication skills, physical strength, and memory. In addition, SPs should love doing their work and have adequate time to do it. 2. SPs should be trained systematically. Only after passing the examination should they engage in clinical medical teaching. 3. The learning done through an SP should be incorporated with the learning on the wards.

In summary, SPs have a very good effect in clinical medical teaching, and they have many advantages over real patients. And because there are more advantages over ordinary patients, SPs should be widely used in clinical medical education.

References

1. Rethans JJ, Grosfeld FJ, Aper L et al (2012) Six formats in simulated and standardized patients use, based on experiences of 13 undergraduate medical curricula in Belgium and the Netherlands. Med Teach 34(9):710–716
2. Petrusa ER (2004) Taking standardized patients based examinations to the next level. Teach Learn Med 16(1):98–110
3. Mary W et al (writer), Wang Q (editor-translator) (2009) .A 10-year Review of literature on the use of standardized patients in teaching and learning. Fudan Educ Forum 7(6):92–94
4. Yuan Y, Chen X (2007) The peculiarity and countermeasure of medical students' innovative diagnosis. Res Med Edu 6(7):629–630
5. Chen ZX, Xiao J (2008) The importance of the clinic skill learning center in diagnostics teaching. Res Med Edu 7(2):155–174
6. Liu XW, Duan XF, Xue WX, et al (2008) Practice and research of SP on cultivation of skills in Chinese medical science. J Yunnan Univ Tradit Chin Med 31(4):60–64
7. Swiggart WH, Ghulyan MV, Dewey CM (2012) Using standardized patients in continuing medical education courses on proper prescribing of controlled substances. Subst Abus 33(2):182–185

Chapter 172
Effect of Jiangtang Fonglong Capsule on Expressions of Insulin of Deaf Animal Models of Diabetes

Ruiyu Li, Kaoshan Guo, Lizhen Tang, Yanzhuo Zhang, Meng Li and Bin Li

Abstract Objective: To observe the influence of jiangtang fanglong capsule to hearing impairment in deaf diabetes animal models. 50 Wistar rats randomly selected from 60 Wistar rats. The other 10 rats were normal control group (group A). 50 Wistar rats with experimental deaf diabetic, induced by 55 mg/kg streptozotocin (STZ) once intraperitoneal, were randomly divided into five groups. And the five groups contain model control group (group B), lower density (3.3 g/kg. d) jiangtang fanglong capsule was administrated (group C), middle density (310 g/kg. d) jiangtang fanglong capsule was administrated (group D), high density (3.3 g/kg. d) jiangtang fanglong capsule was administrated (group E) and yuquanwan (25 g/kg. d) was administrated (group F). After 60 days, test the fasting blood glucose (FBG), body weight (BW) and fasting insulin (FINS) of the wistar rats. Calculate the HO-MA-IR and HOMA-B, insulin was measured by radioimmunoassay. Tests showed that compared with model group, jiangtang fanglong capsule in middle and high dose groups reduce the index of the animal models in a dose-dependent manner ($P < 0.05$, $P > 0.01$), the HOMA-β shrink as the dose increased ($P < 0.05$, $P > 0.01$), improve the insulin expression in pancreatic islets ($P < 0.05, P > 0.01$), compare group E to B, it doesn't make any sense ($P > 0.05$). Our results suggest that jiangtang fanglong capsule could improve the pancreatic β-cell's function of the diabetic deaf animal model.

R. Li (✉)
Institute of Integrated Traditional and Western Medicine, Second Affiliated Hospital, Xingtai Medical College, No. 618 Gangtiebei Road, Xingtai, Hebei, China
e-mail: Liruiyu651021@163.com

K. Guo · L. Tang · Y. Zhang
Second Affiliated Hospital of Xingtai Medical College, No. 618 Gangtiebei Road, Xingtai, Hebei, China

M. Li
Health Team of Hotan Prefecture Detachment of Chinese Armed Police Force in Xinjiang, Hotan, China

B. Li
Department of Biochemistry, Hebei Medical University, Shijiazhuang, Hebei, China

Keywords Jiangtang Fanglong capsule · Diabetic · Deafness · Wistar rats · Streptozocin

172.1 Introduction

Diabetes may be lead to the sensorineural deafness, which mechanism research didn't yet definitely now, we once used Jiangtang Fanglong capsule to treat diabetes and deafness patients, also had some effects [1–4]. To further explore the therapeutic mechanism, this experiment observed the influence of diabetic deaf animal model with streptozotocin (STZ) by Jiangtang Fanglong capsule. The preliminary report is as follows.

172.2 Material and Methods

172.2.1 Drug

The important ingredient of Jiangtang Fanglong capsule (come from our team) were kudzuvine, red sage root, rhizome of Sichuan lovage, fox glove, chinese wam, indianbread, alismatis rhizome, dogwood fruit, magnetite, etc. All drugs were bought in the Shijiazhang Le Ren Tang, which were identified as geo-authentic Chinese medicinal materials and were made to Jiangtang Fanglong capsule suspension.

172.2.2 Animal

The healthy adult male Wistar rats (200–250 g) was 60, without voice exposed history.

172.2.3 Animal Model

We selected Wistar rats 50 randomly form the 60. According to Wang Shi-Li, Yu De-Min, ect paper, we replicated the experimental diabetic deaf animal model [5, 6]. 50 Wistar rats with experimental deaf diabetic, every rat were fasting 12 h, every rat were given 55 mg/kg streptozotocin (Sigma Company) by intraperitoneal injection, which were diluted by 0.1 mg/L natrium citricum buffer solution (pH 4.2). The levels of blood glucose and urine glucose were measured after 1 week of medication. When blood glucose >14.2 mmol/L and urine glucose > (+++), building diabetic model was success. After 2 months of medication, we took auditory brainstem response (ABR) detection to every rat. When ABR threshold value was significantly increased, it was diabetic deaf animal model, we got into our experiment observation.

172.2.4 Grouping and Using Medicine

Ten Wistar rats randomly selected from 60 Wistar rats before modeled as normal control group (group A), was feed with normal fodder, give saline the same as the other group. 50 Wistar rats with experimental deaf diabetic, induced by 55 mg/kg streptozotocin (STZ) once intraperitoneal, were randomly divided into five groups. And the five groups contain model control group (group B), lower density (3.3 g/kg. d) jiangtang fanglong capsule was administrated (group C), middle density (10 g/kg. d) jiangtang fanglong capsule was administrated (group D), high density (3.3 g/kg. d) jiangtang fanglong capsule was administrated (group E) and yuquanwan (25 g/kg. d) was administrated (group F) with 10 in each group. After 60 days, test the fasting blood glucose (FBGO), body weight (BW) and fasting insulin (FINS) of the wistar rats.

172.2.5 The ABR Examination Tests

The rats were administered intraperitoneal injection with pentobarbitale sodium (45 mg/kg) before test. After anaesthesia, Traveler Express E type ABR detection apparatus was performed to examine ABR threshold value. Needle form electrode, record electrode were placed at parietal bone external periosteum of the junction middle point of the two pinna superior border, reference electrode were placed at contralateral pinna, grounding electrode were placed at ipsilateral pinna, the TDH-39p type Earphone was used to give voice, the Earphone was placed at the point of 2 cm from external auditory meatus, the bandpass filters with 100–3000 Hz, the routine measurement was performed in a sound shielding room. We recorded ABR threshold value (wave II), the change of the latency and inter period of each wave of ABR of every group rats.

172.2.6 Determination of Index

(1) The determination of FBG and Fins: 7080 autobiochemical analyzer (Hitachi Ltd.) test the fasting blood glucose (FBG); Serum insulin was measured by

radioimmunoassay, and the kits offered by Ltd. Nanjing. (2) HOMA formula [7] was used to estimate IR and secreting function of islet beta cell. Calculating the status of insulin resistance (HOMA-IR) and function of islet beta cell (HOMA-β). (3) Islet was analyzed by immunohistochemical method: kill rats, pancreatic acinar cells were isolated, paraffin-embedded, dehydrate using graded ethanol, be sliced continuously in 5 μm. After immunohistochemical stains, select five from every group randomly. Light microscope slices in each of 10 randomly selected high power field. Image-pro plus Graphics Analysis tool was used.

172.2.7 Statistical Analysis

Statistics analysis adopted SPSS 11.0 statistical package, measurement data are expressed as the mean ± SEM ($\bar{\chi} \pm s$), The t test was adopted for comparison between groups. Values of $P < 0.05$ were taken to indicate statistical significance.

172.3 Results

172.3.1 The Impacting of Jiangtang Fanglong Capsule on the Fasting Blood Glucose (FBG), Body Weight (BW), Fasting Insulin (FINS), HOMA-IR and HOMA-β of the Wistar Rats

Compare with group B, Jiangtang Fanglong capsule in middle and high dose groups reduce the index of the animal models in a dose-dependent manner. ($P < 0.05$, $P > 0.01$). But the HOMA-β shrink as the dose increased. ($P < 0.05$, $P > 0.01$); Let me compare group E to B, it doesn't make any sense ($P > 0.05$) (Table 172.1).

172.3.2 The Change of Islets on Immunohistochemistry

The enhanced expression of the Ins in rats' Islet cell in the group D group E and group F, it manifests itself as significantly improve on the average optical density and positive cells on the percentage of the total area ($P < 0.05$, $P > 0.01$). But the the average gray dropped dramatically ($P < 0.05$, $P > 0.01$). Compared group E to F, it doesn't make any sense ($P > 0.05$) (Table 172.2).

Table 172.1 Changes of FBG, BW, Ln HOM-IA and HOMA-β after treatment ($\bar{\chi} \pm s$)

Group	n	FBG (mmol/L)	Body weight (g)	Ln Fins (mmol/L)	Ln (HOMA-IR)	Ln (HOMA-β)
A	10	4.95 ± 1.40 # ☆	416.89 ± 22.42 # ☆	2.43 ± 0.19 # ☆	1.08 ± 0.35 # ☆	4.63 ± 0.20 # ☆
B	10	21.19 ± 3.22	469.03 ± 17.73✕	3.36 ± 0.18	3.32 ± 0.20	3.50 ± 0.14
C	10	19.24 ± 2.60 ☆	455.74 ± 25.26	3.22 ± 0.19 ☆	2.99 ± 0.25 ☆	3.67 ± 0.15 ☆
D	10	16.69 ± 2.14 #	445.18 ± 22.45✕	3.10 ± 0.23✕	2.69 ± 0.35✕ △	3.73 ± 0.17✕ △
E	10	14.78 ± 3.29 #	436.60 ± 20.63 #	2.99 ± 0.19 #	2.48 ± 0.34 #	3.84 ± 0.12 #
F	10	13.47 ± 2.32 #	444.74 ± 17.09✕	2.85 ± 0.21 #	2.25 ± 0.30 #	3.95 ± 0.18 #

A Normal; B Diabets in no-treatment; C Low dose of turbid; D Middle dose of extract; E High dose of extract; F Yu Quan Wan
Us B group, ✕$P < 0.05$ # $P < 0.01$; Us F group, △ $P < 0.05$, ☆ $P < 0.01$

Table 172.2 Changes of the insulin expression level of islet β-cells after treatment ($\bar{\chi} \pm s$)

Group	n	Average optical density	Average gray
A	10	0.49 ± 0.09 # ☆	94.99 ± 18.66 # ☆
B	10	0.24 ± 0.07	160.59 ± 15.75
C	10	0.28 ± 0.07 ☆	149.36 ± 15.89 △
D	10	0.31 ± 0.09※	136.18 ± 17.29※
E	10	0.39 ± 0.08 #	112.70 ± 16.64 #
F	10	0.35 ± 0.09 #	126.09 ± 10.556 #

Us B group, ※$P < 0.05$ # $P < 0.01$; Us F group, △ $P < 0.05$, ☆ $P < 0.01$

172.4 Discussion

Diabetes may be lead to the sensorineural deafness, which mechanism research didn't yet definitely now, but it is very important to control the development of diabetes. Isletβ cell plays a key role in insulin production. Insulin and osteocalcin have a close relation. Animal studies have shown that increase the dose of osteocalcin bring the gene expression raise of the insulin and Isletβ cell proliferation [8, 9]. Kidney-tonifying traditional Chinese drugs can stimulate the proliferation, differentiation and maturation of osteoblasts. It could correct the disorder and lower function in the system of "nerve-endocrine-immunity network" and "nerve-endocrine-bone metabolism" [10]. Some evidence has showed that jiangtang fanglong capsule play an adjusting role on the osteocalcin of sensorineural deafness patients that leaded by the Diabetes on the different type [11]. So this essay attempts deeply analyzes the insulin expression in pancre after the rats was given by jingtang fanglong capsule. It provides an objective basis.

The important ingredient of Jiangtang Fanglong capsule (come from our team) were kudzuvine, red sage root, rhizome of Sichuan lovage, fox glove, chinese wam, indianbread, alismatis rhizome, dogwood fruit, magnetite, etc. In which rhizome of Sichuan lovage go through the twelve regular meridians, with Red sage root, rhizome of Sichuan lovage also have the action of activating circulation to remove blood stasis, kudzuvine raise send up the lucid yang and guide medicine, it is all right for to go ahead, fox glove softly enrich the blood and nourish kidney and replenish essence, chinese wam invigorate the spleen and stomach and help digest, indianbread waterlog and damp spleen, alismatis rhizome of promoting dampness, dogwood fruit nourish the liver and kidney, heavy magnetite (Main ingredient: FeO_4) can firm kidney-Yin deficiency, "the people with Kidney deficiency and deafness and blurred vision all do use that" recorded in Amplification on Canon of Materia Medica. Jiangtang Fanglong capsule have the action of activating circulation to remove blood stasis. Jiangtang Fanglong capsule not only improve hearing of the patients that leaded by the Diabetes, but also improves the whole body situation. So it is worth to apply to clinical use.

Tests showed that compared with model group, Jiangtang Fanglong capsule in middle and high dose groups reduce the index of the animal models in a dose-dependent manner. ($P < 0.05$, $P > 0.01$), and significantly reduces with dose increased. But the HOMA-β shrink as the dose increased. ($P < 0.05$, $P > 0.01$). Jiangtang Fanglong capsule improve the insulin expression obviously ($P < 0.05$, $P > 0.01$). It showed that Jiangtang Fanglong capsule could improve the pancreatic β-cell's function of the diabetic deaf animal model. We can speculate that it matters the way Jiangtang Fanglong capsule increase the secretion of osteocalcin. These are some of hypothesis topics about "kidney-bone-diabetic network" a waiting be verified.

References

1. Li RY, Guo KS, Guo WY (2012) The influence of Jiangtang Fanglong capsule on diabetes accompanied with deafness in different syndrome on the hypothalamic-pituitary-adrenal axis. Int J Tradit Chin Med 34(2):1117–1118
2. Li RY, Wu LP, Song N et al (2000) TCM treatment of diabetic hearing loss-an audiological and rheological observation. J Tradit Chin Med 20(3):176–179
3. Li RY, Li M, Wang R, Li B et al (2008) Jiang Tang Fang Long Jiao Nang in treating non-insulin dependent Diabetes Mellitus with hearing loss. J Otol 3(1):45–50
4. Li RY, Guo YL, Liu JW (2011) The effect of Chinese kidney-tonifying drugs on diabetes deafness. Mod J Integr Tradit Chin West Med 20(6):654–656
5. Wang SL, Chen XM, Bi DZ (2004) Study on preparation of experimental hearing impaired diabetes animal model induced by Streptozotocin. J Audiol Speech Pathol 12(6):402–403
6. Yu DM, Wu Y, Yin H (1995) A study on experimental diabetes an imalmodels induced by streptozotoein. Chin J Diab 3(2):105
7. Hanffer SM, Kennedy E, Gonzalez C et al (1996) A prospective analysis of the HOMA model: the mexico city diabetes study. Diabetes Care 19:1138–1141
8. Lee NK, Sowa H, Hinoi E et al (2007) Endocine regulation of energy metabolism by the skeleton. Cell 130(3):409–411
9. Ferron M, Hinoi E, Karsenty G et al (2008) Osteocalcin differentially regulates beta cell and adipocyte gene expression and affects the development of metabolic diseases in wild-type mice. Proc Natl Acad Sci USA 105(13):5266–5270
10. Shen ZY, Chen Y, Huang JH (2006) Syndrome differentiation through drug effects in mapping the two regulatory pathway of gene networks in Shen deficiency syndrome. Chin J Integr Tradit West Med 26(6):521–525
11. Li RY, Li M, Guo YL (2011) The influence of Jiangtang Fanglong capsule on diabetes accompanied with deafness in different syndrome on the osteocalcin. J New Chin Med 43(2):32–33

Chapter 173
The Discussion for the Existence of Nontrivial Solutions About a Kind of Quasi-Linear Elliptic Equations

Bingyu Kou, Lei Mao, Xinghu Teng, Huaren Zhou and Chun Zhang

Abstract The paper is concerned with the follow problems:

$$\begin{cases} -\text{div}\left(|x|^{\alpha}|\nabla u|^{p-2}\nabla u\right) = |x|^{\beta}u^{p(\alpha,\beta)-1} - \lambda|x|^{\gamma}u^{p-1} + |x|^{\mu}u^{q-1} & u(x) > 0, x \in \Omega \\ |\nabla u|^{p-2}\frac{\partial u}{\partial n} = 0 & x \in \partial\Omega \end{cases}$$

It is the kind of the problem with Neumann boundary. Let Ω be a bounded domain with a smooth C^2 boundary in $R^N (N \geq 3)$, $0 \in \Omega$, and n denote the unit outward normal to $\partial\Omega$, and $1 < p < N$, and $\alpha < 0, \beta < 0$, such that

$$p(\alpha, \beta) \triangleq \frac{p(N+\beta)}{N-p+\alpha} > p, \gamma > \alpha - p, \ p < q < p(\alpha, \mu),$$

For various parameters α, β, γ and μ, we establish some existence results of the solutions in the case of $0 \in \Omega$. The novelty of the paper is that the scopes of the parameters α, β, γ and μ, play an important role in the existence of solutions, because of the singularity and the non-compactness.

Keywords Quasi-linear elliptic equations · Caffarelli-Kohn-Nirenberg inequalities · Critical exponents · Nontrivial solutions

173.1 Introduction

Quasi-linear elliptic equations are broadly applied in many subjects, it is not only applied in quantum mechanics, celestial mechanics, thermodynamics, and it is also closely associated with many mathematics branches. Therefore many scientists

B. Kou (✉) · L. Mao · X. Teng · H. Zhou · C. Zhang
College of science, PLA university of Science and Technology,
Nanjing 211101 Jiangsu, People's Republic of China
e-mail: koubei@163.com

pay close attention to the kind of the equations. The equation we research comes from rotational structure of astrosphere in astrophysics. The result of the research can explain some physical phenomenon of celestial body, and stimulate the development of the mathematic.

We consider the following quasi-linear elliptic problems with Neumann boundary and singular coefficient:

$$\begin{cases} -\text{div}\left(|x|^{\alpha}|\nabla u|^{p-2}\nabla u\right) = |x|^{\beta}u^{p(\alpha,\beta)-1} - \lambda|x|^{\gamma}u^{p-1} + |x|^{\mu}u^{q-1} & u(x) > 0, x \in \Omega \\ |\nabla u|^{p-2}\frac{\partial u}{\partial n} = 0 & x \in \partial\Omega \end{cases}$$

(173.1)

where $\Omega \subset R^N (N \geq 3)$ is a bounded domain with C^2 boundary, $0 \in \Omega$, and $1 < p < N, \alpha < 0, \beta < 0$, such that $p(\alpha,\beta) \triangleq \frac{p(N+\beta)}{N-p+\alpha} > p, \gamma > \alpha - p, p < q < p(\alpha,\mu)$. n denote the unit outward normal to $\partial\Omega$.

After the pioneering paper by Brezis and Nirenberg (See [1]), a large number of papers appeared concerning the Dirichlet problems with critical exponents. The corresponding problems with Neumann boundary condition have also been extensively studied in recent years. In 2000 (See [2]), Ghoussoub and Yuan obtained positive solutions of (173.1) with Dirichlet boundary condition in the case $\alpha = 0$. In [3], problem (173.1) with $\alpha = 0$ was studied in various domains or with various boundary conditions. In [4], Bartsch, Zhang and Shuangjie Peng consider problem (173.1) in a cone or some other domains with Dirichlet or Neumann boundary conditions for the case $0 \in \partial\Omega$ and $p = 2$, and obtained some existence and nonexistence results of positive solutions.

For this type of problem, the following well-known Caffare-Kohn-Nirenberg inequalities (See [5]) have played an important role in many applications by virtue of the complete knowledge about the best constant $S_{\alpha,\beta}$ and the extremal functions (See [6]):

$$\left(\int_{R^N} |x|^{\beta}|u|^{p(\alpha,\beta)}\right)^{\frac{p}{p(\alpha,\beta)}} \leq S_{\alpha,\beta}^{-1} \int_{R^N} |x|^{\alpha}|\nabla u|^p \; \forall u \in C_0^{\infty}(R^N) \quad (173.2)$$

where[1]

$$1 < p < N, \alpha > -N + p, \frac{\alpha}{p} \geq \frac{\beta}{p(\alpha,\beta)}, \beta \geq \alpha - p \quad (173.3)$$

$p(\alpha,\beta)$ is called the critical Sobolev-Hardy exponent, since when $\alpha = \beta = 0$ and $\alpha = 0, \beta = -p$, (173.2) are classical Sobolev and Hardy inequalities respectively. Moreover, the sharp constant $S_{\alpha,\beta}$ can be achieved except $\beta \neq \alpha - p$.

To prove our main results, we first construct a Palais-Smale sequence $\{u_i\}$ by using the Mountain Pass Lemma and then give a threshhold value under which the

---

[1] For simplification of sign, we omit dx, which is the mark of element of the integral.

173 The Discussion for the Existence of Nontrivial Solutions

Palais-Smale sequence $\{u_i\}$ is pre-compact. To verify that the energy corresponding to the Palais-Smale sequence $\{u_i\}$ is lower than the threshold, we use the function $u_\varepsilon(x)$ (defined by (173.1)) which can achieve $S_{\alpha,\beta}$ in R^N as a test function to estimate the energy $J(u_i)$.

173.2 Preliminary Results

Define a weighted Sobolev space $W_\alpha^{1,P}(\Omega)$ by:

$$\left\{ u \in L^p(|x|^\gamma, \Omega) : \int_\Omega |x|^\alpha |\nabla u|^p + \int_\Omega |x|^\gamma |u|^p < \infty \right\}$$

With the norm $\|u\|_{W_\alpha^{1,p}}^p = \int_\Omega |x|^\alpha |\nabla u|^p + \int_\Omega |x|^\gamma |u|^p$, where $L^p(|x|^\gamma, \Omega)$ denotes the usual weighted $L^p(\Omega)$ space with the right $|x|^\gamma$.

Define the following functional which corresponds to problem (173.1):

$$J(u) = \frac{1}{p} \int_\Omega (|x|^\alpha |\nabla u|^p + |x|^\gamma |u|^p) - \frac{1}{p(\alpha,\beta)} \int_\Omega |x|^\beta u_+^{p(\alpha,\beta)} - \frac{1}{q} \int_\Omega |x|^\mu u_+^q, u$$
$$\in W_\alpha^{1,p}(\Omega)$$

To prove our main results, we will first give the following preliminary lemmas, which can be found in [4]:

Lemma 2.1 For $1 \leq q < p(\alpha, \beta)$, the imbedding $W_\alpha^{1,P}(\Omega) \longrightarrow$ imbedding $L_\beta^q(\Omega)$ is compact.

Lemma 2.2 Let $S_{\alpha,\beta}$ be defined as in (173.2). For all $\delta > 0$, and when $0 \in \Omega$, there exists a constant $C(\delta)$ depending on δ such that: if $0 \in \Omega$

$$\left(\int_\Omega |x|^\beta u_+^{p(\alpha,\beta)} \right)^{\frac{p}{p(\alpha,\beta)}} \leq \left(S_{\alpha,\beta}^{-1} + \delta \right) \int_\Omega |x|^\alpha |\nabla u|^p + C(\delta) \int_\Omega |x|^\alpha |u|^p \, \forall u \in W_\alpha^{1,p}(\Omega),$$

Lemma 2.3 Let $\{u_i\}$ be a sequence in $W_\alpha^{1,p}(\Omega)$ satisfying that $J(u_i) \to c$ and $J'(u_i) \to 0$ In $(W_\alpha^{1,p}(\Omega))'$ as $i \to \infty$. If

$$c < \frac{\beta + p - \alpha}{p(N+\beta)} S_{\alpha,\beta}^{\frac{N+\beta}{\beta+p-\alpha}}$$

Then the problem (173.1) has a solution $u \in W_\alpha^{1,p}(\Omega)$ which satisfies $J(u) \leq c$.

Lemma 2.4 Assume α, β and $p(\alpha, \beta)$ satisfy (173.3) and $\gamma > \beta - p, \alpha \leq 0$. Then the norm $\left(\int_\Omega |x|^\alpha |\nabla u|^p + \int_\Omega |x|^\alpha |u|^p \right)^{\frac{1}{p}}$ is equivalent to the norm $\left(\int_\Omega |x|^\alpha |\nabla u|^p + \int_\Omega |x|^\gamma |u|^p \right)^{\frac{1}{p}}$.

By Lemma 2.2 and Lemma 2.4, we have $W_\alpha^{1,p}(\Omega) \longrightarrow \text{imbedding} L^{p(\alpha,\beta)} \left(|x|^\beta, \Omega\right)$, but the imbedding $W_\alpha^{1,p}(\Omega) \longrightarrow \text{imbedding} L^{p(\alpha,\beta)}\left(|x|^\beta, \Omega\right)$ is not compact due to the invariance of $\int_\Omega |x|^\alpha |\nabla \cdot|^p$ and the norm $\|\cdot\|_{L^{p(\alpha,\beta)}(|x|^\beta, \Omega)}$ under the dilation $u(\cdot) \to \varepsilon^{\frac{N+\alpha-p}{p}} u(\varepsilon \cdot)$ $(\forall \varepsilon > 0)$. Therefore, the ranges of the parameters play very important role in the existence of the solutions for the problem (173.1). Since $W_\alpha^{1,p}(\Omega) \longrightarrow \text{imbedding } L^{p(\alpha,\beta)}\left(|x|^\beta, \Omega\right)$, the functional J is well defined, and by the Lemma 2.2 and the Lemma 2.4, the functional J is also C^1-smooth in $W_\alpha^{1,p}(\Omega)$, and hence by the strong maximum principle (See Proposition 3.1 in [7]), its critical point is a weak solution to problem (173.1). We will employ the mini-max theory to find the nontrivial critical points of J. The main difficulty is that, owing to the non-compact embedding $W_\alpha^{1,p}(\Omega) \longrightarrow \text{imbedding } L^{p(\alpha,\beta)}(|x|^\beta, \Omega)$, J does not satisfy the Palais-Smale compactness condition.

173.3 Main Results

Theorem 3.1 Suppose $0 \in \Omega$ and (173.3) holds. Let $1 < p < N, \lambda > 0$, $\alpha < 0, \beta > \alpha - p, \mu > \alpha - p, \gamma > \alpha - p, p < q < p(\alpha, \mu)$. Then problem (173.1) has a nontrivial solution in one of the following cases:

(1)
$$\alpha - p < \mu \leq \frac{N - p^2 + p\alpha}{p-1}, \mu < \beta, \gamma \geq \frac{N - p^2 + p\alpha}{p-1}, p < q < p(\alpha, \mu);$$

(2)
$$\alpha - p < \mu \leq \frac{N - p^2 + p\alpha}{p-1}, \mu > \beta, \gamma \geq \frac{N - p^2 + p\alpha}{p-1}, p(\alpha, \mu) - \frac{p}{p-1} < q < p(\alpha, \beta);$$

(3)
$$\frac{N - p^2 + p\alpha}{p-1} < \mu \leq \frac{(q-p+1)N - pq + q\alpha}{p-1}, \mu > \beta, \gamma \geq \frac{N - p^2 + p\alpha}{p-1}, p(\alpha, \mu) - \frac{p}{p-1} < q < p(\alpha, \beta);$$

(4)
$$\alpha - p < \mu \leq \gamma, \mu < \beta, \alpha - p < \gamma < \frac{N - p^2 + p\alpha}{p - 1}, p < q < p(\alpha, \mu);$$

(5)
$$\alpha - p < \mu \leq \gamma, \mu > \beta, \alpha - p < \gamma < \frac{N - p^2 + p\alpha}{p - 1}, p < q < p(\alpha, \beta);$$

(6)
$$\gamma < \mu < \frac{(q - p + 1)N - pq + q\alpha}{p - 1}, \mu < \beta, \alpha - p < \gamma < \frac{N - p^2 + p\alpha}{p - 1},$$
$$p(\alpha, \mu) - \frac{p(p + \gamma - \alpha)}{N - p + \alpha} < q < p(\alpha, \mu);$$

(7)
$$\gamma < \mu < \frac{(q - p + 1)N - pq + q\alpha}{p - 1}, \mu > \beta, \alpha - p < \gamma < \frac{N - p^2 + p\alpha}{p - 1},$$
$$p(\alpha, \mu) - \frac{p(p + \gamma - \alpha)}{N - p + \alpha} < q < p(\alpha, \beta)$$

173.4 The Proof of the Main Results

In this section, we try to prove Theorem 3.1.
Set

$$c^* = \inf_{u \in W_\alpha^{1,p}} \left\{ \sup_{t > 0} J(tu); u \geq 0, u \not\equiv 0 \right\}.$$

We can easily check that $c^* \geq c$, where c is the mountain-pass level defined as

$$c = \inf_{\psi \in \Psi} \sup_{t \in (0,1)} J(\psi(t)),$$

In which

$$\Psi = \left\{ 0 \not\equiv \psi \in C([0, 1], W_\alpha^{1,p}(\Omega)) : \psi(0) = 0, J(\psi(1)) \leq 0 \right\}.$$

Using a standard argument (See [7] for example), we only need to check that

$$c^* < \frac{\beta+p-\alpha}{p(N+\beta)} S_{\alpha,\beta}^{\frac{N+\beta}{\beta+p-\alpha}},$$

From [8], we find that the following form of the extremal function u_ε achieves the best constant $S_{\alpha,\beta}$ in Caffare-Kohn-Nirenberg inequalities under the condition $\alpha \leq 0$:

$$u_\varepsilon(x) = \frac{\varepsilon^{\frac{N-p+\alpha}{p(p-\alpha+\beta)}}}{(\varepsilon + |x|^{\frac{p-\alpha+\beta}{p-1}})^{\frac{N-p+\alpha}{p-\alpha+\beta}}} \qquad (173.4)$$

In the following we shall show that for ε small enough there holds:

$$\sup_{t>0} J(tu_\varepsilon) < \frac{\beta+p-\alpha}{p(N+\beta)} S_{\alpha,\beta}^{\frac{N+\beta}{\beta+p-\alpha}}$$

Denote $B_r = B_r(0)$ is an open ball of radius r centered at 0. Set $\Omega_1 = \Omega - B_r(0)$, $\Omega_2 = R^N - B_r(0)$.

By direct calculation, we see:

$$\int_\Omega |x|^\alpha |\nabla u_\varepsilon|^p = \int_{\Omega_1} |x|^\alpha |\nabla u_\varepsilon|^p - \int_{\Omega_2} |x|^\alpha |\nabla u_\varepsilon|^p + \int_{R^N} |x|^\alpha |\nabla u_\varepsilon|^p$$

$$= O(\varepsilon^{\frac{N-p+\alpha}{p-\alpha+\beta}}) + S_{\alpha,\beta}^{\frac{N+\beta}{p-\alpha+\beta}}$$

And

$$\int_\Omega |x|^\beta |\nabla u_\varepsilon|^{p(\alpha,\beta)} = \int_{\Omega_1} |x|^\beta |\nabla u_\varepsilon|^{p(\alpha,\beta)} - \int_{\Omega_2} |x|^\beta |\nabla u_\varepsilon|^{p(\alpha,\beta)} + \int_{R^N} |x|^\beta |\nabla u_\varepsilon|^{p(\alpha,\beta)}$$

$$= O(\varepsilon^{\frac{N+\beta}{p-\alpha+\beta}}) + S_{\alpha,\beta}^{\frac{N+\beta}{p-\alpha+\beta}}$$

We can obtain the following results by direct calculation (See [1]):

$$\int_\Omega |x|^\gamma u_\varepsilon^p = \int_\Omega \frac{\varepsilon^{\frac{N-p+\alpha}{p-\alpha+\beta}} |x|^\gamma}{(\varepsilon+|x|^{\frac{p-\alpha+\beta}{p-1}})^{\frac{p(N-p+\alpha)}{p-\alpha+\beta}}} = \varepsilon^{\frac{p(p-1)+\gamma(p-1)-\alpha(p-1)}{p-\alpha+\beta}} \int_\Omega \frac{|x|^\gamma}{(1+|x|^{\frac{p-\alpha+\beta}{p-1}})^{\frac{p(N-p+\alpha)}{p-\alpha+\beta}}}$$

$$= \begin{cases} O\left(\varepsilon^{\frac{p(p-1)+\gamma(p-1)-\alpha(p-1)}{p-\alpha+\beta}}\right) & \alpha - p < \gamma < \frac{N-p^2+p\alpha}{p-1} \\ O\left(\varepsilon^{\frac{p(p-1)+\gamma(p-1)-\alpha(p-1)}{p-\alpha+\beta}} |\ln \varepsilon|\right) & \gamma = \frac{N-p^2+p\alpha}{p-1} \\ O\left(\varepsilon^{\frac{N-p+\alpha}{p-\alpha+\beta}}\right) & \gamma > \frac{N-p^2+p\alpha}{p-1} \end{cases}$$

And it is easy to check that

$$\int_\Omega |x|^\mu u_\varepsilon^q = \begin{cases} O(\varepsilon^{\frac{p(p-1)\mu+p(p-1)N+q(1-p)(N-p+\alpha)}{p(p-\alpha+\beta)}}) & \text{if } \alpha-p<\mu<\frac{N(q-p+1)-pq+q\alpha}{p-1} \\ O(\varepsilon^{\frac{p(p-1)\mu+p(p-1)N+q(1-p)(N-p+\alpha)}{p(p-\alpha+\beta)}}|\ln\varepsilon|) & \text{if } \mu=\frac{N(q-p+1)-pq+q\alpha}{p-1} \\ O(\varepsilon^{\frac{q(N-p+\alpha)}{p(p-\alpha+\beta)}}) & \text{if } \mu>\frac{N(q-p+1)-pq+q\alpha}{p-1} \end{cases}$$

By $\alpha > -N+p$ and $\beta \geq \alpha - p$, we know

$$p\alpha > -N+p^2+p\beta - \beta > -N+p(p+\beta) - \beta \geq p\alpha - (N+\beta)$$

So we have $\alpha - p < \beta < \frac{N-p^2+p\alpha}{p-1}$. Moreover, from $\alpha - p < \mu \leq \frac{N(q-p+1)-pq+q\alpha}{p-1}$, We can also obtain:

$$\frac{p(p-1)\mu+p(p-1)N+q(1-p)(N-p+\alpha)}{p(p-\alpha+\beta)} < \frac{q(N-p+\alpha)}{p(p-\alpha+\beta)} < \frac{N+\beta}{p-\alpha+\beta}$$

On the other hand, $q > p$ implies

$$\frac{N(q-p+1)-pq+q\alpha}{p-1} > \frac{N-p^2+p\alpha}{p-1}.$$

Hence, for the case (1), (2), (3) in the Theorem 3.1, the following inequality holds:

$$\sup_{t>0} J(tu_\varepsilon) \leq (\frac{1}{p} - \frac{1}{p(\alpha,\beta)}) S_{\alpha,\beta}^{\frac{N+\beta}{p-\alpha+\beta}} + O(\varepsilon^{\frac{N-p+\alpha}{p-\alpha+\beta}}) - O(\varepsilon^{\frac{p(p-1)\mu+p(p-1)N+q(1-p)(N-p+\alpha)}{p(p-\alpha+\beta)}})$$

$$= \frac{p+\beta-\alpha}{p(N+\beta)} S_{\alpha,\beta}^{\frac{N+\beta}{p-\alpha+\beta}} - O(\varepsilon^{\frac{p(p-1)\mu+p(p-1)N+q(1-p)(N-p+\alpha)}{p(p-\alpha+\beta)}})$$

$$\leq \frac{p+\beta-\alpha}{p(N+\beta)} S_{\alpha,\beta}^{\frac{N+\beta}{p-\alpha+\beta}}$$

For the four cases of (4), (5), (6), (7) in the Theorem 3.1, the following inequality holds:

$$\sup_{t>0} J(tu_\varepsilon) \leq (\frac{1}{p} - \frac{1}{p(\alpha,\beta)}) S_{\alpha,\beta}^{\frac{N+\beta}{p-\alpha+\beta}} + O(\varepsilon^{\frac{p(p-1)+\gamma(p-1)-\alpha(p-1)}{p-\alpha+\beta}}) - O(\varepsilon^{\frac{p(p-1)\mu+p(p-1)N+q(1-p)(N-p+\alpha)}{p(p-\alpha+\beta)}})$$

$$= \frac{p+\beta-\alpha}{p(N+\beta)} S_{\alpha,\beta}^{\frac{N+\beta}{p-\alpha+\beta}} - O(\varepsilon^{\frac{p(p-1)\mu+p(p-1)N+q(1-p)(N-p+\alpha)}{p(p-\alpha+\beta)}})$$

$$\leq \frac{p+\beta-\alpha}{p(N+\beta)} S_{\alpha,\beta}^{\frac{N+\beta}{p-\alpha+\beta}}$$

Consequently, the compactness condition is verified, and we complete the proof.

References

1. Brezis H, Nirenberg L (1983) Positive solutions of nonlinear elliptic equations involving critical Sobolev exponents. Comm Pure Appl Math 36:437–477
2. Ghoussoub N, Yuan C (2000) Multiple solutions for quasi-linear PDE involving the critical sobolev and hardy exponents. Trans Amer Math Soc 352:5703–5743
3. Ghoussoub N, Kang X (2004) Hardy-sobolev critical elliptic equations with boundary singularities. Ann Inst H Poincaré Anal Non Linéaire 21:767–793
4. Bartsch T, Peng S, Zhang Z (2007) Existence and non-existence of solutions to elliptic equations related to the Caffarelli-Kohn-Nirenberg inequalities. Calc Var Partial Differential Equations 30:113–136
5. Caffarelli L, Kohn R, Nirenberg L (1984) First order interpolation inequalities with weights. Compos Math 53:259–275
6. Catrina F, Wang Z-Q (2001) On the Caffarelli-Kohn-Nirenberg inequalities: sharp constants, existence (and nonexistence), and symmetry of extermal functions. Comm Pure Appl Math 54:229–258
7. Wang X-J (1991) Neumann problem of semi-linear elliptic equations involving critical sobolev exponents. J Differ Equ 93:283–310
8. Horiuchi T (1997) Best constant in weighted sobolev inequality with weights being powers of distance from the origin. J In-equal Appl 1:275–292

Chapter 174
A Team-Learning of Strategies to Increase Students' Physical Activity and Motivation in Sports Community

Hongyv Wu, Xiabing Fan and Dinghong Mou

Abstract The Physical Activity (PA) levels of many college students in China are currently in sufficient to promote health benefits. Sport governors may influence students' motivation to be physically active in PE lessons, but few intervention studies have examined motivational strategies in sports clubs. The purpose of this study was to compare the effect of three motivational strategies, each based on Team-Learning Theory (TLT), on PA levels, and their hypothesized antecedents, over a period of 6 months. A modified TBL method was used in two periods of the sports club: acrobics and a more challenging hip pop. Individual and group answers to all questions were recorded, and a motivation form was collected for each period. Students provided positive feedback. Group performance was better than individual performance during the TBL exercises. TBL was more successful when the tasks were very difficult. Performance of the group on the hip pop period showed significant motivation over that in the aerobics part. Conclusion: The results suggest that TBL provides increasing students' physical activity and motivation, and provide insight into appropriate design of TBL practices.

Keywords Physical activity · Youth · Team-learning theory · Sports clubs

---

This work was supported by a grant from Educational Commission of Jiangxi Province, China (Grant No. JXJG-11-8-10).

H. Wu (✉) · X. Fan · D. Mou
East China Institute of Technology, Xuefu Road.56, Fuzhou, Jiangxi Province, People's Republic of China
e-mail: hywu44@yahoo.cn

X. Fan
e-mail: 1021301256@qq.com

D. Mou
e-mail: hywu44@gmail.com

174.1 Background

Physical inactivity is one of the leading modifiable causes of death and disease all over the world. Regular Physical Activity (PA) decreases the risk of developing cardiovascular disease, diabetes, some cancers, obesity, osteoporosis, and other chronic conditions, but many adolescents and youth in China are not sufficiently active to accrue associated health benefits. Youth who lack motivation in PE often report negative experiences and relationships with their Sport clubs, which is why it is imperative for researchers to examine strategies for sport governors to motivate their students more effectively toward achievement of higher levels of PA.

174.2 Methods

We elected to incorporate the newly acquired TBL method into two sessions in order to introduce a technique that enhances student centered and active practicing, and fosters deep understanding of game presented. Our choice was based on the fact that over the years, the sport club sessions without any instruction, rather than interactive developments between sport clubs and students, because the students seldom came due to the aforementioned congestion. The two laboratory sessions during which we applied the TBL method were (1) aerobics and yoga session and (2) a hip pop/Pilates (HP/P) session. Both sessions were held 2–3 days after the relevant faculty member delivered two didactic power point presentations about each topic. Learning objectives were listed upfront for all of the club sessions, including these, and distributed to all students at the beginning of the session. It is important to note that while the students had a good background for aerobics and hip pop, in that they had encountered these principles in the sport clubs in their 1st year.

Table 174.1 shows the flow of the modified TBL activity. Weinte grated phase 2 into phase 3 since we believed that the current highly congested curriculum, would not allow proper implementation of TBL, which depends on self-learning in phase 1. We wanted to apply the well-described four S's of the TBL procedure whereby individuals and groups worked on the 'same and significant problem'. First the students understand the tasks and answered the questions individually; following this, they were practiced to freely form their own groups, after a period of 6 months the students were provided one set of answers per group. The questions were formulated as either true/false or multiple choice single best answer questions. Finally, small groups performed together. There were 12 groups of 3–5 students each.

Note that both individual and group answers were not graded, and we did not perform any peer evaluation. At the end of each session, the students filled a session evaluation form consisting of seven questions to be answered on a five

Table 174.1 Implementation of the modified TBL in sport club

Time	Activity
	Phrase 1 modified
100	Two Aerobics and yoga lectures followed by a brief explanation of the proposed TBL method
100	Phases 2 and 3 combined
5	Introduction to the tasks and review of the proposed TBL method
3 months	Individual work on the self-learning part
3 months	Free small groups formation
60 m	Whole class performance of the tasks one group by one

items Likert-like scale (Table 174.2). Finally, we compared the level of students' physical activity at the end of this first section of the phase 1 with the performance of students during the past 6 months on the same quiz.

Since the quiz covered several topics, we were able to examine the differences in the level of students' physical activity in the HP/P part of the quiz, as well as that in the general fitness principles. This comparison was done in two ways: one considered all questions related to the topic in different years and the other considered only those questions that were repeated from year to year (Table 174.3).

The latter analysis would be a more reliable indicator of changes in student performance being a function of changes in student comprehension rather than question difficulty. We did not analyze the part of the test dealing with aerobics and hip pop because in this part was taught by a new instructor, in addition, there had been no aerobics and yoga experience in previous years. In contrast, the other parts, including hip pop and Pilates, had been given by the same coach for the previous 15 years. It should also be noted that while the exercises in aerobics and yoga were completely novel, the cases used in hip pop/Pilates had been given to previous classes; the only difference being that TBL was not used in previous years, led by the same instructor.

Table 174.2 Frequency distribution (%) of the answer to the questions

	Answers					
	Yes	No	No Certain	Yes	No	No Certain
Doing physical exercises is more than 50 times	37	63	0	85.2[a]	14.8	0
Doing physical activity each week more than two times	50.6	46.9	2.5	88.3[a]	11.7	0
Doing physical activity last more than 1 hour	79	6.2	14.8	78.6	21.4	0
Exercise intensity more than before	90.1	8.6	1.2	88.1	11.9	0
Improve the level of skill	33.3	44.9	21.9	75	8.3	16.7
Improve the level of abilities	74.4	7.7	17.9	75	25	0
Your health is better	16.7	71.8	11.5	91.7[a]	8.3	0

[a] $p < 0.05$ using Z-test for comparison of two proportions

Table 174.3 Number of students responding to the motivation questionnaire for the two TBL parts

Evaluation questions	Likert scale						Likert scale					
	1	2	3	4	5	Mean(SD)	1	2	3	4	5	Mean(SD)
The period was well organized	20*	26	5	1	0	1.75(0.711)	63	17	0	0	0	1.21(0.421)
The programmers were suitable	24*	17	8	3	0	1.81(0.908)	54	26	0	0	0	1.32(0.47)
The arrangement was well paced	17*	23	10	2	0	1.94(0.865)	57	18	5	0	0	1.35(0.597)
I benefited from this method of learning	18*	20	9	4	1	2.04(1.009)	58	18	2	2	0	1.35(0.685)
I would like other future workout to be in the TBL format	26*	12	11	2	1	1.85(0.865)	50	21	4	1	1	1.45(0.761)
I benefited from the small group workout	21*	13	12	6	0	2.06(1.056)	56	15	3	2	4	1.54(1.046)
I benefited from the traditional workout	22	18	8	3	1	1.90(0.995)	48	19	9	2	2	1.65(0.961)
I like having to work in a group	20*	18	9	4	1	2.00(1.025)	47	19	5	7	22	1.72(0.709)

*$p < 0.05$ using Z-test for comparison of two proportions

174.3 Results

All 2nd year the students attended the aerobics club (N = 81) and most of them participated in the hip pop club (N = 78). Students formed their own groups; nevertheless, there was a fair diversity in gender and sports abilities distributions within these groups. Participation in the performances was broad within the teams and comparable among them.

As expected from TBL, and despite using a modified TBL approach, group performance was better than individual performance in both TBL exercises (Table 174.2). In the aerobics club, only five students from different teams had a high level upon individual testing, whereas after teamwork all levels of physical activity increased. The improvement in the frequency of 'yes' answer was significant for questions in which the frequency of 'yes' on the individual responses was below 68 %, the lowest being 37 %. For questions answered more by 74 % of students, group work did not significantly improve performance, although the response rate became 100 %. As for the hip pop part, the performance of the groups was not as remarkably improved with only one question answered 'no' by all groups. Two questions reached statistically significant difference when comparing individual to group performance. These questions were correctly answered by 44.9 and 33.3 % of the club following individual responses. Individual students scored 19.2, 16.7, and 0 % 'Y' answers on three questions, and group performance was not significantly improved over individual performance. Only one question was considered 'easy' and did not reach statistical significance when comparing the individual 'Y' (74.4 %) to the group 'Y' (86 %). Finally, all questions in the hip pop had a relatively high incidence of 'No' answer for individual and/or group.

Table 174.3 displays the comparison between the motivations for both periods. Note that most students evaluated the aerobics period (80 out of 81) while only 52 out of 78 evaluated the hip pop period. The students in this club thought that the second period was better organized and better paced, the tasks were more suitable, and students benefited more from the TBL method of practicing in the hip pop part when compared to the first one. Furthermore, after the hip pop, students were more enthusiastic about working in small groups compared with their attitude after the aerobics part. Interestingly, students benefited from the whole class discussion in both part, while the hip pop attendees did not benefit much from the small group practice. Finally, after both periods, students indicated that they would like future workout to be formatted as TBL.

174.4 Conclusion

This article describes our initial experience with modified TBL in two periods of the sports club for college students at the ECIT in China. Students provided positive feedback and the process was rewarding and much more interactive than usual traditional condition. Performance of the students on the end of this study was improved in students who took TBL relative to those in previous classes, who were instructed in a more traditional manner. This study also provides some insight about designing more appropriate cases and problems for TBL, so that the experience is beneficial, successful and well-received by students. We believe that with time and experience, TBL will prove to be an effective and highly rated innovative learning technique in physical education, thus providing more active workout and deeper understanding for our students.

Chapter 175
Research on Feet Health of College Students

Pan Meili

Abstract The feet of 606 people were measured with the natural sample survey to get all students footprint and size. *Results* In the number of subjects, the standard No. of girls was between 36 and 37 yards, the length of plantar was concentrated in one type; the standard No. of boys was about 40 yards, the length of plantar was concentrated between one-half and two type. Flat foot was 8.17 %, the normal foot 70.26 %, high arch foot 21.57 %. *Conclusion* The feet in all parts of the size of young people at South were different from the north, the regional differences was considered in the standard last design and production, standard No. and so on.

Keywords Students · Health · Flat foot · High arch foot

175.1 Introduction

Chinese medicine believes that foot is the root for people. In twelve meridians of the human body, six meridians contact with foot. Therefore, the foot is usually referred as the second heart, which plays a vital power role in the blood circulation. In general, foot discomfort reflects a part of the body in different degrees of lesions, foot health can't be ignored! So this paper surveyed foot health status of 606 students, which a theoretical basis for the promotion of the healthy development.

P. Meili (✉)
Guangzhou College of South China University of Technology, Guangzhou 510800, China
e-mail: 2beautypan@163.com

175.2 Experimental

175.2.1 Experimental Subject

Students of Guangzhou College of South China University of Technology are the experimental subject. A total of 606, girls of 388, boys of 218, mainly from Guangdong. Age is mainly distributed in the 20–24-year-old. The weight of girls are at 45–49 kg; the boys are at 60–69 kg. The height of girls is between 155 and 165 mm; the boy's height is between 165 and 175 mm.

175.2.2 Experimental Contents

Ball girth, instep girth and foot width of subjects were measured. The arch form was observed by footprints. Other basic information, including weight, sports form, wear shoes and so on, were surveyed by questionnaire.

175.2.3 Experimental Methods

175.2.3.1 Footprint Measurement

With bilateral barefoot, pigments were covered in the feet of subjects, and then standing up on the on A4 paper prepared in advance, which showed the different color footprints.

Measuring the length of "ab" and "bc", according to the ratio between ab and bc, the arch was divided into three types, including flat, normal and high arch. The

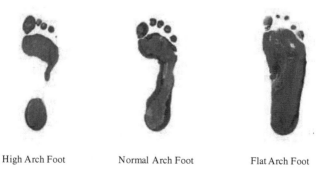

High Arch Foot   Normal Arch Foot   Flat Arch Foot

Fig. 175.1 The different arch foot

Fig. 175.2 The different arch foot of footprint measurement

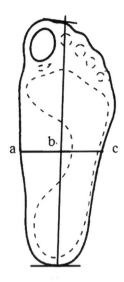

ratio of 1:0 was high arch, 1:1 was normal, 1:3 was flat. Shown in Figs. 175.1 and 175.2.

175.2.3.2 Measurement of Foot Width

The internal width of first metatarsophalangeal joint (ab) was the length from axis of last underside to the first metatarsophalangeal joint. The outer width of fifth metatarsophalangeal joint (cd) was the length from axis of last underside to fifth

Fig. 175.3 The measurement of foot width

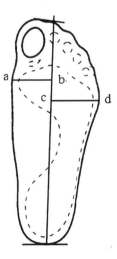

metatarsophalangeal joint. The foot width was the sum of both. Shown in Fig. 175.3.

175.2.3.3 Measurement of Ball Girth

Ball girth is the length along metatarsophalangeal joint. Shown in Fig. 175.4.

175.2.3.4 Measurement of Instep Girth

Instep girth is the length along the bump of instep point. Shown in Fig. 175.5.

175.2.3.5 Method of Data Analysis

The method of natural sampling was used in this research.

175.3 Results and Discussions

175.3.1 Size Code

Shoe size is a reflection of foot characteristics and laws for a region or a country. The standards of shoes size are different from the country. The shoe size range of adult female is between 35 and 39, adult man is between 38 and 45. Shoe size involves a wider scope, if each shoe size should cut pattern, undoubtedly it will increase the workload, therefore, middle size code is a a benchmark in our country.

Seen from Table 175.1, shoes size of girls were from No. 35 to No. 39, the majority of which were between No. 36 and No. 37. Therefore, middle of size code should be between No. 36 and No. 37.

Seen from Table 175.2, shoes size of boys were from No. 38 to No. 44, the majority of which were No. 40. Therefore, middle of size code should be No. 40.

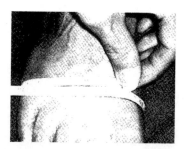

Fig. 175.4 The measurement of ball girth

Fig. 175.5 The measurement of instep girth

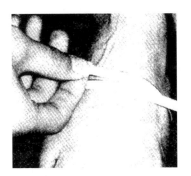

Table 175.1 Statistics about size code of girls

Size code	35	36	37	38	39
Proportion (%)	9.3	28.7	30	15	17

Table 175.2 Statistics about size code of boys

Size code	38	39	40	41	42	43	44
Proportion (%)	2	6	42	20	14	7	9

175.3.2 Arch

Seen from Table 175.3, among 606 students, the proportion of high arch feet was 21.57 %, flat foot was 8.17 %, and normal foot was 70.26 %. In the high arch feet, the proportion of girls was 98 %, the ratio of boys was 2 %. In the flat feet, the proportion of girls was 5 %, which were congenital. The ratio of boys was 95 %, parts of which were caused by strenuous exercise.

175.3.3 Ball Girth

Seen from Table 175.4, among 388 students, the proportion of ball girth in one type was 60 %. Therefore, most of which were in slim type. The subjects basically come from the southern city of Guangzhou and Guangxi. So the last process should take into account differences between South and North for the average age of the 22-year-old.

Table 175.3 Statistics about proportion of arch

Arch	High arch	Normal arch	Flat arch
Proportion (%)	21.57	70.26	8.17

Table 175.4 Statistics about ball girth data of girls

Type of ball girth	1	1 1/2	2	2 1/2	3
Proportion (%)	60	19	11	5	5

For example, the middle size was No. 36, the length of ball girth (one type) was about 218.5 mm.

Seen from Table 175.5, among 218 students, the proportion of ball girth was between one half type and two type. Therefore, most of which were between slim and standard type.

For example, the middle size was No. 40, the length of ball girth (one and half type, two type) was between 236 and 239.5 mm.

175.3.4 Instep Girth

According to statistics, the instep girth = 100 % ball girth. Seen from Table 175.6, the length of girls ball girth mainly concentrated between 211 and 220 mm. However, the middle size of girl was No. 36, most of ball girth were in one type, the length of which was 218.5 mm, so that was 1:1 between the middle of ball girth and instep girth, which meet the aforementioned formula.

Seen from Table 175.7, the length of boy instep girth mainly concentrated between 231 and 250 mm. However, the middle size of boy was No. 40, most of ball girth were in one half and two type, the length of which was between 236 and 239.5 mm, so that was 1:1 between the middle of ball girth and instep girth, which meet the aforementioned formula.

175.3.5 Foot Width

According to the formula, the foot width = the internal width of first metatarsophalangeal joint + the outer width of fifth metatarsophalangeal joint. Seen from Table 175.8, the foot width of the subjects girls were mainly between 86 and 95 mm. Seen from Table 175.9, the foot width of the subjects boys were mainly between 96 and 110 mm. Therefore, both belonged to the standard.

Table 175.5 Statistics about ball girth data of boys

Type of ball girth	1	1 1/2	2	2 1/2	3
Proportion (%)	10	39	30	11	10

Table 175.6 Statistics about instep girth data of girls

Instep girth (mm)	190–200	201–210	211–220	221–230	231–240	241–250
Proportion (%)	8.33	21.53	34.72	24.31	9.72	1.39

Table 175.7 Statistics about instep girth data of boys

Instep girth (mm)	210–230	231–250	251–270	271–290	291–310	311–330
Proportion (%)	4.35	36.52	33.9	16.53	7.83	0.87

Table 175.8 Statistics about foot width of girls

Foot width (mm)	75–80	81–85	86–90	91–95	96–100	101–105
Proportion (%)	1.5	13.5	27.9	36	15.8	5.3

Table 175.9 Statistics about foot width of boys

Foot width (mm)	86–90	91–95	96–100	101–105	106–110	111–116
Proportion (%)	2.6	8.6	29.3	30.2	23.3	6

175.4 Conclusions

Through the above study, the following results can be obtained.

1. Among 606 subjects, the middle size of girls was between No. 36 and No. 37, of which boys was about No. 40.
2. Among 606 students, the proportion of high arch feet was 21.57 %, flat foot was 8.17 %, and normal foot was 70.26 %. In the high arch feet, the proportion of girls was 98 %, the ratio of boys was 2 %. In the flat feet, the proportion of girls was 5 %, which were congenital. The ratio of boys was 95 %, parts of which were caused by strenuous exercise.
3. The proportion of ball girth in one type was 60 %. Therefore, most of which were in slim type. The proportion of ball girth was between one half type and two type. Therefore, most of which were between slim and standard type.
4. The length of girl ball girth mainly concentrated between 211 and 220 mm, and the length of boy instep girth mainly concentrated between 231 and 250 mm.
5. The foot width of the subjects girls were mainly between 86 and 95 mm. The foot width of the subjects boys were mainly between 96 and 110 mm. Therefore, both belonged to the standard.

In conclusion, the feet in all parts of the size of young people at South were different from the north, the regional differences were considered in the standard last design and production, standard No. and so on.

Acknowledgments Financial support by the Guangzhou College of South China University of Technology. Authors also thank every student who participate this program.

References

1. Guojian P (2005) Analysis on the arch [J]. Chinese J Rehabil Med 20(10):759–760
2. Shixiu L, Bining L (2000) Report on the arch development of preschoolers [J]. Mod Prev Med 27(2):186
3. Changjie L, Raoxun G (2000) Arch type about teenagers [J]. J Branch Campus First Mil Med Univ 23(1):15–17
4. Shigang G (2012) Principle of last design [M]. China Light Industry Press, pp 20–21

Chapter 176
Uncertain Life

Shao-lin Wang and Dian-ming Jiang

Abstract *Objective* To studying human apparent death and discover and propose the concept of uncertain life; meanwhile briefly describe experimental evidence such as *the third state of matter*. *Method* Define the concept of apparent death; meanwhile combine clinical cases to analyze and study the status of apparent death of human being. *Results* Uncertain lifes exist in a superposition status of "being dead and being alive," in other words apparent death is uncertain life, also is intermediate state of life: in a state between life and non-life, also known as the third state of matter. Until a doctor pronounces a uncertain life to be dead or saved, the person takes one certain status of death or life. *Conclusion* We proposed that a uncertain life is a person in the state of apparent death, and that a uncertain life stays in a superposition state of being dead and being alive; in other words a uncertain life exists in the uncertain status of being dead and being alive. After a doctor pronounces a uncertain life dead or alive, the uncertain life becomes one certain status of being dead or being alive.

Keywords Life · CPR · Apparent death · Death

176.1 Introduction

Cardiopulmonary resuscitation, CPR. We carefully and thoroughly studied the state of apparent death, which is a state that life floats in and out of the human body, and is a moment that life and death mixed together inside a human body. This is a unique and valuable period, and it's of great significance for studying medicine, and exploring other mysteries of human life.

S. Wang (✉) · D. Jiang
312 First Zhonshan Road, Yuzhong District 400013 Chongqing, China
e-mail: 782480307@qq.com

176.2 Materials and Methods

176.2.1 Clinical Data

Case information:
 The patient, male, 35 years of age, Hospital number: 140516, Orthopedic 2–5 bed.
 Diagnosis: cervical C6 spondylolisthesis combined with top digit paraplegia.
 Main complaint: admitted to the hospital because of "neck injury caused by a fall from a height associated with a loss of function for a month, symptoms worsened for a week."
 At 15:30 on August 13, 2010, the patient's breathing and heartbeat stopped, blood pressure and oxygen saturation can not be measured, consciousness was lost, pupillary light reflex disappeared, and heart electrical activity stopped. After immediate chest cardiac massage, Cardiopulmonary resuscitation [1, 8]; at 15:41 the patient restore breathing 22 times/min, heart rate 162 beats/min, blood pressure 192/125 mmHg, blood oxygen saturation 90 %. The patient didn't respond when his name was called, but the pressure orbital reflex still existed, the patient continued to inhale oxygen, dopamine was used to maintain blood pressure, at 16:10 the patient gradually regained conscious.
 At 9:10 am on November 3, 2010, the patient's breathing stopped again; he didn't respond when his name was called, his bilateral pupillary light reflex was lost, his artery pulse was no palpable, and his blood pressure and oxygen saturation could not be measured. Cardiopulmonary resuscitation including chest compressions and other measures was immediately performed, at 9:40 his heart rate, respiration, blood pressure, and blood oxygen saturation were all 0, he lost his bilateral pupillary light reflex, his pupils dilated, his aortic pulse (groin area, neck, arm pits, top of the feet, etc.) couldn't be felt, and he was then pronounced dead.

176.2.2 Treatment Methods

Definition of the status of apparent death: from the moment a patient's heartbeat, breathing, and cardiac and electrical activity stop to the moment the patient's heartbeat, breathing, and cardiac electrical activity restart, or the patient is pronounced to be dead [5], the status of the patient during this period.
 When the patient enters into a status of apparent death, chest compressions were immediately performed until the patient's cardiopulmonary activity restarted; an oxygen mask was then put on the patient, epinephrine was injected, an endotracheal tube was inserted, and dopamine was injected to maintain blood pressure. After the vital signs were stable, the patient was transferred to the ICU care and to receive further treatment.

176.2.3 Study Methods

We analyzed and studied the above clinical information according to the principles and equations of quantum mechanics and quantum medicine.

176.3 Results

A uncertain life exists in a superposition status of "being dead and being alive," in other words he or she is in the eigenstatus of "death and life." Until a doctor pronounces a uncertain life to be dead [10] or save, the uncertain life takes one of the eigenstatus of "death and life."

176.4 Discussion

176.4.1 Analyses of the Two Apparent Death

The first "apparent death": from the patient's breathing, heartbeat, and cardiac and electrical activity stopped to 11 min later he was saved (resuscitation: breathing, spontaneous cardiac rhythm, and electrical activity of the heart restarted).

The second "apparent death": (occurred 80 days after the first "apparent death") the patient's breathing and heartbeat stopped and the electrical activity of the heart disappeared. Despite of all the rescue attempts, the patient was not saved and he was pronounced dead half an hour after the apparent death started.

The first "apparent death" lasted 11 min, and the second "apparent death" lasted 30 min.

We'd like to ask: apparent death is death or life? At this time, is the patient a dead person or a live person? I got three answers, but all the three answers are wrong.

The first answer: some people told me that during the first apparent death the patient was a live person whereas during the second apparent death the patient was a dead person. Their reasons were as follows: after first apparent death, the patient was successfully rescued and therefore he was not dead during the first apparent death. And during the 11 min of the apparent death, the patient was indeed alive. After the second apparent death, the patient was not saved after 30 min of rescue attempts, and therefore the patient was dead during the second apparent death. The rational of this answer was based on whether or not the patient was saved after the apparent death. In other words, the results of the rescue attempts were used to determine the previous status of the patient was death or alive. Essentially the later results of life or death were used to decide the earlier status of life or death? However, the universal law of the development of things is that history determines reality, history cannot be changed, and reality can neither change nor determine history!

Take the patient as an example, and I would like to ask you the status of the patient 10 min after each of the two apparent deaths. At this time, the results of the two apparent deaths were not yet out, and it was thus not clear whether the patient was dead or alive, os which status was this patient in? A dead person or a live person? Can you give me an answer? To be more accurate, I should ask you this question twice at different time: the first time is at 10 min after the first apparent death, your answer will be recorded, and the patient will be save 1 min later; the second time is at 10 min after the second apparent death, your answer will also be recorded, and death will be pronounced 10 min later. Neither of your two answers can be used to determine whether the result of the rescue attempts is death or life.

The second answer: the patient was alive during the apparent deaths. Most people hold this view. These people believe that before a doctor pronounces death all patients should be considered being alive and they should be saved by all means. This view is widely accepted by society and the medical community, and it's both sensible and legal.

But this view is not reasonable, and it is not in agreement with scientific laws and the truth. According to scientific reasoning, the above view is contradictory. I would like to ask those who hold this view, the patient is dead only after the doctor pronounces he or she is dead? For example, currently the most common view is that one can only be pronounced death after at least half an hour rescue attempts [1]. I want to ask, are there any essential differences in the patient's life or death status between 5, 29, or 31 min (at this time the patient has already be pronounced dead) after the apparent death? The patient's vital signs are the same at 5, 29, and 31 min after the apparent death. The differences between these time frames are absolutely not as big as the difference between one minute before and after the apparent death. Therefore, this view is not correct. The more obvious contradiction and mistake of this view is: people who hold this view think that when a patient enters into the status of apparent death, the patient should be treated like an alive person because at this time the status of apparent death is "life"; But if the rescue attempts fail and the patient is pronounced dead, the death time must be considered starting from the beginning of the apparent death, which essentially means that the patient was already dead when the apparent death took place, meaning the status of the apparent death is "death". This life and death itself is contradictory! However, this contradiction in fact indicates an exciting answer, and the contradiction itself hints that the phenomenon of apparent death is a phenomenon of both life and death. Combining with the principles of quantum mechanics, we naturally think that at this time the apparent death is the superposition of "life" and "death"!

The third view: the patient had no signs of life during the apparent deaths, thus the patient was already dead; if the patient was saved later, he or she was "resurrected." This cannot be right because it's common knowledge that dead people [7] cannot be resurrected.

Based on the above analyses, it's not correct to say that the status of the patient during apparent death is alive or dead.

Meaning it's not correct to consider the patient either as a dead person or a live person.

This is a big problem, a big difficult problem.

We think, the status of the patient during apparent deaths [9] is both life and death. In other words, at this time the patient is both a dead person and a live person. The patient is in the superposition of both "life and death."

176.4.2 Status of Apparent Death is the Superposition Status of "Life and Death," the Status of Uncertain Life

From a person's (e.g., a hospitalized patient) heart and breathing stop–no life signs such as cardiac electrical activity–until a doctor pronounces that the patient is dead or successfully saved, the person exists in a superposition status [11] of "life and death." If we define this status as apparent death or apparent death (Fig. 176.1), then the status of apparent death is the superposition of "death and life."

We define that a uncertain life is a person who is in the status of apparent death. A uncertain life exists in a superposition status of "being dead and being alive," in other words he or she is in a state between life and non-life, also known as the third state of matter. Afterward, the situation may develop towards "life," meaning the rescue is successful and the patient regains consciousness; the situation may also develop towards "death," meaning the rescue fails and the patient dies; In quantum mechanical [6] terms, at the moment the patient takes one of the eigenvalues of "death or life." Definition of the status of apparent death: the status of a patient between the patient's heartbeat, breathing, and cardiac and electrical activity stop and the patient's heartbeat, breathing, and cardiac electrical activity restart, or the patient is pronounced to be dead.

We think that the state of the patient during apparent deaths was both life and death, or uncertain state. In other words, during that time the patient was both a dead person and a live person. The patient was in the superposition of life and death. Or uncertain state of being dead and being alive.

We therefore propose that a uncertain life is a person who is in the state of apparent death, and that a uncertain life exists in a superposition state of being

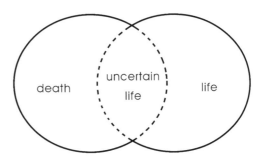

Fig. 176.1 Schema of apparent death (uncertain life)

dead and being alive. In other words, he or she is in the uncertain state one of death and life. Afterward, the situation may develop towards life, meaning the resuscitation efforts are successful and the patient regains consciousness; the situation may also develop towards death, meaning the resuscitation efforts fail and the patient dies; at the moment the patient takes one of the certain status of death and life.

References

1. American Heart Association (2005) American Heart Association Guidelines for cardiopulmonary resuscitation and emergency cardiovascular care [J]. Circulation 112(Suppl):IV1–46, IV133–135
2. Gribbin J (2009) In search of Schrodinger's Cat [M], 2nd edn. Hainan Publication House; Hainan, pp 167–177
3. Hey PW (2005) The New Quantum Universe [M], 1st edn. Scientific and Technical Publisher of Hunan Province; Hunan, pp 33
4. Holger B, Franz G (2002) Diagnosing brain death without a neurologist [J]. BMJ 324(22):1471—1472
5. Hsieh ST (2002) Brain death worldwide: accepted fact but no global consensus in diagnostic criteria [J]. Neurology 58(1):20—25
6. Ke S-Z, Ju G-X et al (2007) Quantum Mechanics [M], 1st edn. Scientific Publisher; Beijing
7. Rünitz K, Thornberg K, Wanscher M (2009) Resuscitation of severely hypothermic and multitraumatised female following long-term cardiac arrest [J]. Ugeskr Laeger 171(5):328–329
8. Sam D, Christopher D, Philip B (2003) Advancing toward a modem death: the path from severe brain injury to neurological determination of death [J]. CMAJ 168(8):993—995
9. Sasson C, Kellermann AL, McNally BF (2009) Termination of cardiopulmonary resuscitation for out-of-hospital cardiac [J]. JAMA 301(7):722–723
10. Swash M, Beresford R (2002) Brain death: Still—unresolved issues worldwide [J].Neurology 58(1):9—10
11. Zou B-Y (ed) (2004) Thermodynamics and molecular biology [M], 1st edn. Central China Normal School; Wuhan, pp 348

Chapter 177
Large-Scale Clinical Data Management and Analysis System Based on Cloud Computing

Ye Wang, Lin Wang, Hong Liu and Changhai Lei

Abstract With the exponential increase of Electronic Health Record systems in China, large-scale clinical data management and analysis have become big challenges. This paper depicts a novel system named Clinical Data Managing and Analyzing System, which uses hybrid XML database, and HBase/Hadoop infrastructure to handle big amount of heart disease clinical data analysis online. Using standardized format of Clinical Document Architecture, the system now has integrated more than 50,000 valvular heart disease clinical documents and provided efficient distributed data mining tools as well as data managing tools for doctor users from multi heart clinical centers in six different 3A hospitals of China.

Keywords CDA · EHR · Data management · Data mining · HBase · Hadoop

177.1 Introduction

Recently, Electronic Health Record (EHR) in China is increasingly regarded as the most important data basic for enhancing the quality of nation-wide health care. More and more paper based medical records are now being converted and archived as EHR documents and being shared across the nation on the Internet [1]. As a major part of EHR documents, clinical data and the related medical follow-up data are increasing explosively as well. In China, these electrical documents are often inputted, stored and managed by appointed nurses in the hospitals. However, there are too many different kinds of standards, protocols and applications in different

Y. Wang · H. Liu · C. Lei (✉)
Information Center, Second Military Medical University, Shanghai, China
e-mail: lei@smmu.edu.cn

L. Wang
The 85th Hospital of PLA, Shanghai, China

hospitals and different fields. It is still hard to manage and share the clinical data on Internet among doctors or nurse users from all over China.

From 2010, working for the project "Standardized Surgical Treatment of Valvular Heart Disease" funded by Chinese Ministry of Health (MOH), our research group helped six 3A hospitals' departments of Cardiothoracic Surgery in three major cities of China collaborate to establish a heart disease clinical documents managing, sharing and analyzing platform. These six hospitals are Changhai Hospital and Zhongshan Hospital in Shanghai, Fuwai Hospital, Anzhen Hospital and PLA 301 Hospital in Beijing, and People's Hospital in Guangzhou. Our working group now has gathered more than 50,000 valvular heart disease clinical documents and the related follow-up data forms for more than 20 years (from 1991–2012), and these data are still increasing rapidly every day. When we were designing and implementing this Clinical Data Managing and Analyzing System (CDMAS), we focused on three major concerns as below.

1. **Standardized data format:** Different hospitals have different forms of clinical data. How to standardize and integrate these unstructured paper-based documents or semi-structured Electronic Medical Records (EMR) is a big problem first of all.
2. **Data analyzing:** This clinical data managing and sharing system is also designed for scientific research purposes. In addition to several basic managing and querying tools, it should also provide some data analysis functionalities and should be user-friendly.
3. **Scalability for large amount of data:** Most clinical documents have rich content of information, such as **Patients basic information**: name, date of birth, blood type, allergies, family history information; **Progress notes**: Admitting diagnosis, medical order, discharge diagnosis; **Nursing Records**: temperature, pulse and respiration chart; **Inspection records**: the survey report, computed tomography (CT or CAT) images, magnetic resonance images (MRI), the DR image, the DSA videos, X-rays, ultrasound images, etc.; **Operation record**: preoperative, intra-operative, and post-operative records. Each capacity of a clinical document file could reach 1–50 MB. If we are aiming to build a nationwide heart disease clinical data managing system, which could maintain over 500,000–1,000,000 clinical documents, the system must be able to scale up to 500 GB–50 TB levels. Querying, searching and analyzing over such a big amount of data will be a tough challenge we shall handle.

177.2 Background

Cloud Computing has become an academic and industry hot spot which has brought new opportunities to various fields or applications while the cloud provides perfect scalability and an alternative to expensive data center infrastructure [2, 3]. Cloud Computing is a promising parallel processing solution to the computation challenges on health care and bio-informatical data analyze [4]. In recent years many researches focus on electronic health care data managing and processing using Cloud Computing techniques [5]. In the paper [6], Jeff Dean proposed an efficient distributed programming model called MapReduce used by many Google systems. It is a powerful beginning mechanism for Cloud Computing kernel. And according to [7], MapReduce has become a highly effective and efficient tool for large-scale fault-tolerant data analysis. Begun as part of Nutch (an open source search engine) by Doug Cutting, Hadoop is an open source implementation of Google MapReduce framework [8]. It is now a popular tool and platform designed for deep analysis and transformation of very large data sets. Nowadays, many well known distributed systems and databases are based on Hadoop. In the paper [9], authors used traditional relational database and Hadoop to develop a hybrid distributed XML database (XBase) for XML-based health care documents. And they evaluated the research prototype with a large scale of data on a massive computing facility.

In the paper [10] presented on 2011 ICDM workshop, the authors investigate the deployment of Medical Markup Language (MML) to store and analyze patient data worldwide in conjunction with SaaS (Software as a Service) cloud services for cost savings and energy efficiency. They also discussed about privacy concerns and security aspects. They used public cloud to store these data. But they did not give a detailed data-analyzing framework. Paper [11] presented a distributed architecture for sharing electronic health records utilizing public and private clouds, which overcomes some of the security issues inherent in cloud systems. This system, called HCX (Health Cloud eXchange), allows for health records and related healthcare services to be dynamically discovered and interactively used by client programs accessing services within a cloud. And paper [12] also proposes an EHR sharing and integration system in healthcare clouds. The authors also analyzed the security and privacy issues in access and management of big amount of EHR documents.

We have studied related work about using Cloud Computing techniques to handle big amount of health records or clinical documents. Most of these works focus on efficiency of distributed medical data storage and querying (especially on HL7 XML documents), and some of them pay attention on security and privacy while implementing the whole system. However, none of these works presented a secure data mining and analysis framework for medical data based on Cloud Computing infrastructure, and applies it into a real clinical data management and analysis system.

177.3 Standardized Data Format

The six 3A hospitals involved in our project have different formats of valvular heart disease clinical documents, which are totally non-structured (paper based) or semi-structured. To standardize the data format in this multi center project, our working group took use of the Clinical Document Architecture (CDA) standard. In

October of 2000, Health Level 7 (HL7) organization developed CDA which is an XML based markup criteria intended to specify the encoding, structure and semantics of clinical documents for exchange, as a part of the HL7 version 3rd standard. Today in the U.S. the CDA standard is the basis for the Continuity of Care Document (CCD) specification, which has been selected by the U.S. Healthcare Information Technology Standards Panel as one of its standards [13]. A CDA document is a defined and complete information object that can exist outside of a HL7 message. It is an XML document consisting of a header and a body while the header identifies the patient, provider, document type, etc. and the body has a mandatory human-readable part with an optional encoded part for software processing. As well as text, it can include images, animations, sounds, videos and other multimedia content [14].

In 2003 HIMSS Conference, Microsoft presented its InfoPath based CDA V2.0 which could be a visualized editor and standard for CDA XML documents. In CDMAS project, we developed an electronic clinical document template of valvular heart disease based on Microsoft InfoPath CDA standard. This template contains 14 different kinds of data sections, which are described in Table 177.1. And we designed more than 1,000 different attributes for this valvular heart

Table 177.1 Data sections in valvular heart disease CDA document

Name	Includes
Patient's essential information	Name, ID, gender, date of birth, etc.
Contact information	Living address, Email, mobile phone, etc.
Preoperative basic records	Past medical history like hypertension, diabetes, asthma, gout, thyroid disease, etc.
Preoperative heart state descriptions	NYHA, arrhythmia, myocardial infarction, tracheal intubation, etc.
Preoperative inspection records	Echocardiography, lung function, renal function, liver function, blood, BNP, etc.
Medication administration record (MAR)	Dopamine, epinephrine, digitalis, diuretics, phosphodiesterase inhibitors, etc.
Surgery basic records	Date, doctor, incision, artificial lung, IABP, VAD, ECMO, cardiopulmonary bypass, etc.
Surgery for valvular heart disease	Mitral, initiative flap, tricuspid, pulmonary valve, paravalvular leak repair, etc.
Other surgeries simultaneously	Major vascular surgery, coronary artery bypass grafting, deformity correction of congenital heart, atrial fibrillation, etc.
Post-operative records	Stay time in ICU, ventilation time, pleural fluid drainage in 12 h, pulmonary artery pressure, medicine, blood used, etc.
Post-operative complications	Low cardiac output syndrome, pericardial tamponade, serious arrhythmia, ARDS, tracheotomy, lung infection, etc.
Sequelae	Surgery results descriptions, healthy or death, cause of death, etc.
Discharge instructions	Digoxigenin, antisterone, aspirin, warfarin, furosemide tablets, amiodarone, etc.
Follow-up records	Date, recorder, living state, heart function, drug use, ECG, echocardiography, postoperative complications, etc.

disease CDA template. Since a single patient has multi medical follow-up records and could have more than once surgery in a clinical document, we use iterative XML trees and nodes to describe. Hence the total amount of attributes for each individual's CDA document would be a dynamic number.

Using this electronic clinical document template, doctor and nurse users from hospitals could create and edit clinical documents both offline and online. Our working group developed an ASPX website using XML FormViewer (a Microsoft ActiveX control used in Web forms to create, delete or edit Infopath document) based on Microsoft SharePoint server for online users. They can login the website and directly create, delete or edit CDA Infopath documents on web pages and then store the CDA Infopath files into the SharePoint server. For offline users, we provide a Web Service API to import or export bulks of the CDA Infopath documents. Offline users could both use a special user defined client or use a normal Microsoft InfoPath client to communicate with the CDMAS system when they get online.

177.4 Querying CDA XML

Creating, deleting and editing CDA documents are basic data managing tools for CDMAS system. However, once the clinical documents were saved into the platform, searching and querying on the big dataset would be a more frequent job for doctor and nurse users. As described above, CDA documents are tree-structured XML files with hierarchical information. XML (eXtensible Markup

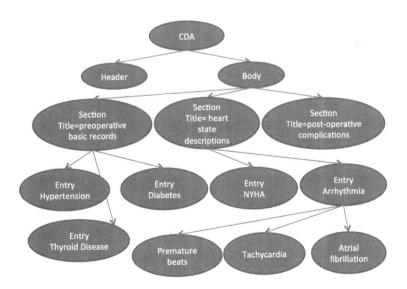

Fig. 177.1 Tree-structured CDA document

Language) is a de facto standard for information exchange among different health care applications. Figure 177.1 illustrates an example XML tree-structured CDA document.

The most frequent queries over clinical data have some certain patterns. CDMAS now support four basic types of interactive queries as following:

1. Boolean queries, such as node (for example: //section [title = "preoperative basic records"]/Diabetes) value = true or false
2. Range queries, such as node value is in a certain range or not (for example: $2011.01.01 < date\ of\ surgery < 2012.01.01.$ or $10 < age < 20$)
3. In set queries, such as one or more complications after surgery are in the set of {pericardial tamponade, serious arrhythmia, ARDS, tracheotomy, lung infection}?
4. Aggregation queries, such as MIN, MAX, or AVERAGE weight of patient.

To implement these XML queries efficiently, we choose Microsoft SQL Server 2008 as a hybrid XML database. It provides XPath, XQuery and SQL-XQuery hybrid querying methods. We store CDA XML files both in Microsoft SharePoint server and SQL Server 2008 database. The original CDA XML files are stored in the SharePoint Server including the image and video content. And all the XML text based content, which could be queried and indexed, is stored in the SQL Server XML database. We build both XML content and structure index in SQL Server to improve the efficiency of XML querying. For different clients (including Inforpath client, user-defined client and browser based client) usage, we also implement an application layer using WCF (Windows Communication Foundation) Web Service as the data storage system interface for CDA documents creating, editing, deleting and querying. It is a system service application which host secured Web Service, which works above the SQL Server and SharePoint Server.

177.5 Data Analysis Over Large Amount of Data

CDMAS system also provides data analysis tools, as well as data managing and querying tools. For medical research, 3 types of statistic and data mining algorithms listed here are often used on EHR data, which are 1. Clustering, 2. Classification, and 3. Frequent Pattern Mining. CDMAS has large data sets to be analyzed by these algorithms. Simple querying problems could be solved by centralized database system, however data mining and analysis tasks are much more complicated. As we discussed above, each capacity of a clinical document file could reach 1–50 MB. CDMAS system should be able to handle 500 GB–50 TB clinical data. Hence traditional centralized client–server model cannot solve data mining and analysis problems over such big amount of XML data. Based on efficiency and scalability consideration, we chose using Hadoop based distributed system to implement data analysis module in CDMAS. So we build a hybrid system, which is based on an HBase/Hadoop NOSQL system integrated with an SQL Server relational database. Data analysis system in CDMAS is composed of three major parts as below.

1. The first part is a JAVA Tomcat application uses SQL Server as the underlying relational database. We use Apache Axis to implement a SOAP ("Simple Object Access Protocol") Web Service interface communicating with user API. Some basic health information is stored in SQL Server such as username, ID, phone number, XML CDA file (in a XML column) and so on for basic query and analysis. It has complete replications in different hospital servers and would synchronize all the data periodically.
2. More complicated CDA data is stored in HBase. XML based CDA document has a big amount of attributes and many blank values. For example, in our system most of the CDA documents have more than 1,500 attributes, while many of them have blank values. Built on top of Hadoop/HDFS, HBase provides a distributed, column-oriented data store model as Google's Bigtable, which fit for XML based CDA or EHR data storage. And HBase has already implemented the low-level distributed storage of the HBase table data and nodes fault-tolerant processing [3, 22]. In HBase system, HRegion is the smallest unit for distributed storage, which is maintained in HRegionServers (Data Nodes in Hadoop system). And the HMaster server is responsible to assign the HRegions to each HRegionServer and balance the workload. In our system, HMaster server also acts as the Hadoop Name Node. We also have a Zookeeper clusters used for coordinating the whole distributed system in CDMAS. Zookeeper is an open source Apache project, which is a centralized service for maintaining configuration information, naming, providing distributed synchronization, and providing group services. We model CDA documents into a big table, using user ID as the row key. When CDA table size reaches the threshold, HRegion split will be automatically triggered and data will be automatically distributed in HRegionServers (DataNodes) by the load balancing of HMaster. As long as new HRegionServer (DataNode server) is added in, the storage capacity and the read-write throughput of the system will be increased as well.
3. On the top this hybrid database system, we built a data analysis interface leveraging Apache Mahout data-mining library. Mahout is an open source data mining and machine-learning tool, which is scalable to "reasonable large" datasets. Mahout library provides core algorithms for clustering, classification and batch based collaborative filtering are implemented on top of Apache Hadoop using the MapReduce paradigm, which could take HBase data as input. We use Mahout to implement an efficient distributed data mining and analysis interface for different clients in the system of CDMAS. Doctors could make different data analysis using this interface easily.

In summary, we built CDMAS an efficient distributed clinical data managing and analysis system for multi hospital data centers. Figure 177.2 shows the CDMAS system architecture.

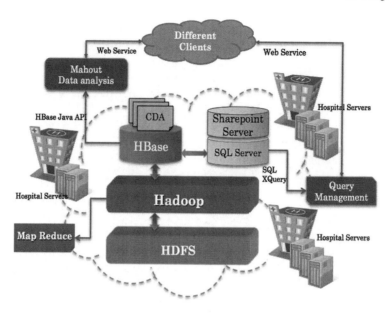

Fig. 177.2 CDMAS system architecture

177.6 Conclusions

Electrical clinical documents managing and analyzing has recently become a rising hot topic of health care research. This paper depicts a novel distributed system called CDMAS, which manage and analysis large-scale clinical data. In this system, CDA based valvular heart disease clinical documents are stored and managed in a hybrid XML database and a distributed HBase system. CDMAS system now has already integrated more than 50,000 valvular heart disease clinical documents and provided efficient distributed data mining tools as well as data managing tools for doctor users from multi heart clinical centers in six different 3A hospitals of China. XML database used in CDMAS provided managing, indexing and querying features. Using Mahout library based on Hadoop, CDMAS provided efficient data mining and analysis tools over big amount of data. To protect privacy and security of the patients' sensitive information, strong encryption methods and security mechanisms are implemented in the system. Furthermore, CDMAS established a standard large-scale CDA based clinical documents managing and analyzing system, not only for valvular heart disease, but also for all kinds of XML based health care documents.

References

1. Kahn S, Sheshadri V (2008) Medical record privacy and security in a digital environment. IT Prof 10(2):46–52
2. Taylor R (2010) An overview of the hadoop/mapreduce/hbase framework and its current applications in bioinformatics. BMC Bioinformatics 11(12):S1
3. Sarathy V, Narayan P, Mikkilineni R (2010) Next generation cloud computing architecture: enabling real-time dynamism for shared distributed physical infrastructure. In: 2010 19th IEEE international workshop on enabling technologies: infrastructures for collaborative enterprises (WETICE), June 2010, pp 48–53
4. Wang Z, Wang Y, Tan K-L, Wong L, Agrawal D (2011) ECEO: an efficient cloud epistasis computing model in genome-wide association study. Bioinformatics 27(8):1045–1051
5. Fernández-Cardeñosa G, de la Torre-Díez I, López-Coronado M, Rodrigues J (2012) Analysis of cloud-based solutions on EHRs systems in different scenarios. J Med Syst 36:3777–3782. doi: 10.1007/s10916-012-9850-2
6. Dean J, Ghemawat S (2008) Mapreduce: simplified data processing on large clusters. Commun ACM 51(1):107–113
7. Dean J, Ghemawat S (2010) Mapreduce: a flexible data processing tool. Commun ACM 53(1):72–77
8. White T (2010) Hadoop: the definitive guide. Yahoo! Press, New York
9. Li W-S, Yan J, Yan Y, Zhang J (2010) Xbase: cloud-enabled information appliance for healthcare. In: Proceedings of the 13th international conference on extending database technology, EDBT'10, ACM, New York, USA, pp 675–680
10. Tancer J, Varde AS (2011) The deployment of mml for data analytics over the cloud. In: 2011 IEEE 11th international conference on data mining workshops (ICDMW), Dec 2011, pp 188–195
11. Mohammed S, Servos D, Fiaidhi J, Kamel M, Karray F, Gueaieb W, Khamis A (2011) Developing a secure distributed OSGi cloud computing infrastructure for sharing health records, vol 6752. Springer, Berlin, pp 241–252
12. Chen Y-Y, Lu J-C, Jan J-K (2012) A secure ehr system based on hybrid clouds. J Med Syst 36:3375–3384. doi: 10.1007/s10916-012-98306
13. Ferranti JM, Clayton Musser R, Kawamoto K, Hammond EW (2006) The clinical document architecture and the continuity of care record: a critical analysis. J Am Med Inform Assoc 13(3):245–252
14. Dolin RH, Alschuler L, Beebe C, Biron PV, Boyer, D Essin SL, Kimber E, Lincoln T, Mattison JE (2001) The hl7 clinical document architecture. J Am Med Inform Assoc 8(6):552–569

Chapter 178
Satisfaction Changes Over Time Among Dentists with Outpatient Electronic Medical Record

Hong-wei Cai, Yu Cao, Hong-bo Peng, Bo Zhao and Wan-hui Ye

Abstract Objective: To evaluate the changes of dentists' satisfaction with newly deployed outpatient Electronic Medical Record (EMR) system over time in a large teaching hospital in China. **Design**: A repeated cross-sectional survey was conducted with two rounds of data collection: 2 months post-EMR implementation and 8 months post-EMR implementation. Questionnaires were distributed to dentists working on dental chair and filled out anonymously. The mean and standard deviation (SD) of the satisfaction scores between two round surveys were analyzed. **Results**: 74 respondents from 81 filled out the survey at the first round, and 48 respondents from 52 filled out at the second round. The mean satisfaction scores from the second round were significantly higher than those from the first one. There were also differences among different types of departments. **Conclusion and Discussion**: The results suggested that there was a tough time at the initial stage of outpatient EMR implementation. We also found that end-user satisfaction with outpatient EMR improved over time.

Keywords Outpatient EMR · Dental · Satisfaction · Questionnaire

178.1 Introduction

There is a widespread recognition that Electronic Medical Record (EMR) systems have significant potential in improving the quality of care, increasing efficiency of medical staff and reduce overall costs at the same time. EMR systems are increasingly deployed in hospitals nowadays due to the push of governments [1]. However, EMR systems' implementation had been proved time consuming and

H. Cai (✉) · Y. Cao · H. Peng · B. Zhao · W. Ye
Information Center, Stomatological Hospital, Fourth Military Medical University,
Xi'an 710032, China
e-mail: hwcai@fmmu.edu.cn

challenging [2], few had reached the expectations as they originally planned. There are too many barriers involved in the implementing of a new EMR system, such as physicians' resistance, lack of IT support staff and interoperability [3]. Some studies suggest that overall satisfaction with EMR among physicians after implementation tend to be significantly lower than their pre-implementation expectations [4]. Some attempts to implement Information technology to healthcare have failed [5]. The satisfaction of end-users, undoubtedly, is an important factor contributing to the successful implementation of EMR systems. And few studies have examined end-user satisfaction with EMR in the short term (e.g., 2 months after EMR implementation) and longer term (e.g., 8 months after EMR implementation). We deployed our new outpatient EMR system in May, 2012. In this study, dentists' satisfactions and attitudes on outpatient EMR system were surveyed in two time points in terms of template, writing speed, reliability, training, expectations and totally satisfaction.

178.2 Design

The study was performed in a stomatological teaching hospital with 280 dental chairs in the middle of China. We used a repeated cross-sectional study design with two rounds of data collection: 2 months post-EMR implementation and 8 months post-EMR implementation. Dentists working on dental chairs were asked to fill out the same survey for both rounds of data collection. All departments were divided into 4 types, "oral surgery, oral orthopedic, oral medicine and oral general". We compared dentists' satisfaction scores with outpatient EMR between two round surveys.

We created a questionnaire to assess the effects of EMR implementation and dentists' satisfactions. The design of the questionnaire was informed by the existing literature surrounding customer satisfaction and information technology (IT) implementations in healthcare fields [6, 7], together with professional advices. There were six categories and 12 items in the questionnaire, including "Template of EMR", "Writing Speed of EMR", "Reliability", "Training", "Expectations" and "Totally Satisfaction". Each item was ranked on a scale from 0 (worst or lowest satisfaction) to 10 (best or highest satisfaction). Table 178.1 describes the items and standards of grading in the questionnaire.

Researchers distributed paper questionnaires to dentists working on dental chair. Therefore not all dentists had a chance to fill out the survey if they were not present when surveys were distributed. After 1–2 days, questionnaires were collected by researchers. The questionnaires were filled out anonymously.

Table 178.1 Satisfaction questionnaire for outpatient EMR

Categories	Items	Symbols	Score 0	Score 10	Your score
Template of EMR	Number of template	a_1	No template	Plenty of templates for all common diseases in specialized field	
	Classification of template	a_2	Too chaos to find the template needed	Classification is clear and easy to find	
	Writing style of EMR	a_3	Writing EMR all by typing	Writing EMR all by clicking on a mouse	
	Satisfaction for specialized fields template	a_4	Very disappointed	Very satisfied	
Writing speed of EMR	Mean writing time for first visit patient	b_1	More than 1 h	Less than 3 min	
	Mean writing time for subsequent visit patient	b_2	More than 0.5 h	Less than 1 min	
Reliability	System error	c_1	Too many system errors to use	Never experienced system errors	
	System halt	c_2	Too much occurred, hardly can use	Never experienced system halt	
Training	Training from EMR software company	d_1	Received no training	Received systematic training	
	Training by colleagues in the same section	d_2	Received no training	Received systematic training	
Expectations	The gap from reality to ideality	e	Far from ideality	Too good to be true	
Totally satisfaction		f	Would rather go back to old system	Very satisfied	

178.3 Results

SAS 9.1 were used to analyze the survey data. The means and standard deviations of scores for each item were calculated and compared. Two-group t test was used to compare the differences of scores between two-round surveys. Table 178.2 describes end-user satisfaction with outpatient EMR for four types of departments (oral surgery, oral orthopedic, oral medicine and oral general) in two-round of surveys.

The results of Table 178.2 reveal that:

(1) In the first round of survey, the average scores of all items were less than 8, except for $a_1(1)$, which was 8.09. $e(1)$ and $f(1)$ were scored less than 7. This shows that at the first round of survey, the satisfaction level of outpatient EMR among dentists was fairly low.

Table 178.2 End-user satisfaction with outpatient EMR in two-round of surveys

Symbol[a]	Mean scores and SDs for oral surgery	Mean scores and SDs for oral orthopedic	Mean scores and SDs for oral medicine	Mean scores and SDs for oral general	Total mean scores	P value
$a_1(1)$	7.67 ± 1.97	7.90 ± 1.55	8.83 ± 1.49	7.59 ± 1.50	8.09 ± 1.65	0.0007
$a_1(2)$	8.78 ± 1.30	7.86 ± 1.21	9.00 ± 0.87	9.07 ± 0.70	8.81 ± 1.02	
$a_2(1)$	7.42 ± 2.39	8.00 ± 1.70	7.75 ± 2.21	7.18 ± 2.07	7.64 ± 2.06	0.0001
$a_2(2)$	8.67 ± 1.32	8.00 ± 1.41	8.94 ± 1.20	9.13 ± 0.92	8.81 ± 1.20	
$a_3(1)$	7.33 ± 2.42	7.24 ± 1.26	7.33 ± 1.93	6.94 ± 1.71	7.22 ± 1.78	0.3821[b]
$a_3(2)$	8.22 ± 1.86	7.43 ± 1.27	7.88 ± 2.03	8.47 ± 0.74	8.06 ± 1.58	
$a_4(1)$	7.83 ± 2.04	8.00 ± 1.18	7.67 ± 1.83	7.29 ± 1.79	7.70 ± 1.69	0.0574[b]
$a_4(2)$	8.89 ± 1.76	7.57 ± 1.62	8.71 ± 1.05	8.87 ± 0.92	8.63 ± 1.30	
$b_1(1)$	7.67 ± 2.67	7.76 ± 1.30	6.67 ± 1.55	6.65 ± 1.84	7.14 ± 1.82	0.0446
$b_1(2)$	9.00 ± 1.58	7.86 ± 1.86	8.29 ± 1.05	8.87 ± 1.30	8.54 ± 1.38	
$b_2(1)$	7.92 ± 2.68	8.81 ± 0.81	7.17 ± 1.69	7.59 ± 1.37	7.85 ± 1.73	0.0336
$b_2(2)$	9.56 ± 0.73	8.00 ± 1.63	8.65 ± 1.17	9.00 ± 1.36	8.83 ± 1.29	
$c_1(1)$	7.83 ± 1.70	7.86 ± 1.11	6.22 ± 2.13	6.06 ± 2.25	6.92 ± 2.01	0.0014
$c_1(2)$	7.67 ± 1.58	7.86 ± 1.35	8.06 ± 1.20	7.80 ± 1.26	7.88 ± 1.28	
$c_2(1)$	8.08 ± 1.73	7.76 ± 1.58	5.65 ± 2.50	5.53 ± 2.15	6.63 ± 2.32	0.0002
$c_2(2)$	7.89 ± 1.54	8.00 ± 1.29	7.82 ± 1.51	8.27 ± 1.28	8.00 ± 1.38	
$d_1(1)$	7.67 ± 2.19	7.05 ± 3.22	8.04 ± 1.83	7.00 ± 2.62	7.46 ± 2.52	0.0575[b]
$d_1(2)$	8.56 ± 1.24	6.43 ± 2.44	8.00 ± 1.50	7.87 ± 2.29	7.83 ± 1.94	
$d_2(1)$	7.08 ± 3.09	8.00 ± 2.30	7.42 ± 3.05	8.47 ± 1.07	7.77 ± 2.51	<0.001
$d_2(2)$	9.44 ± 0.73	7.14 ± 1.77	9.06 ± 1.20	8.93 ± 1.33	8.81 ± 1.42	
$e(1)$	7.42 ± 2.35	7.24 ± 2.05	6.04 ± 1.85	6.00 ± 2.65	6.59 ± 2.24	0.0021
$e(2)$	8.22 ± 1.64	6.86 ± 1.46	7.76 ± 1.52	8.40 ± 1.06	7.92 ± 1.46	
$f(1)$	7.58 ± 2.39	7.57 ± 1.25	6.08 ± 1.98	6.18 ± 2.48	6.77 ± 2.10	0.0020
$f(2)$	8.11 ± 1.76	7.71 ± 1.38	8.06 ± 1.39	8.40 ± 1.12	8.13 ± 1.36	

[a] $x(1)$ stands for the first round of survey, while $x(2)$ stands for the second round of survey. The meaning of each x is in Table 178.1
[b] P values were bigger than 0.05

(2) In the first round of survey, the average scores of $c_1(1)$ and $c_2(1)$, which are related to the reliability of the system, were less than 7. It suggests that in the first time of survey, the most pressing problem about the outpatient EMR system was its poor reliability.
(3) In the second round of survey, the average scores of almost all items were more than 8, except for $c_1(2)$ and $e(2)$. It implies that stability of the system remained a problem.
(4) P values of "a_1, a_2, b_1, b_2, c_1, c_2, d_2, e and f" between two round of surveys were all less than 0.05, which stands for statistically significant. And "f" is the totally indicator of satisfaction in this study. The P value of "f" was 0.002 (8.13 ± 1.36 in the second round compared with 6.77 ± 2.10 in the first round). The results suggest that at the second survey time, the end-user satisfaction about the outpatient EMR improves greatly.
(5) The SDs of scores in the second survey were narrower than those in the first one, which implies that after another 6 months' training and use, dental staff had reached a convergent and higher level of utilization of the outpatient EMR system.
(6) In addition, the scores of "oral orthopedics" departments between the first and the second round of survey were roughly the same, which is very different from other types of departments. We learnt from these sections that though they were required to use EMR by hospital regulations, they also wrote a paper record for each patient, where much detail information was collected. Outpatient EMR exists only as an auxiliary for paper medical records for them. In other words, they are not fully use the outpatient EMR.

According to the statistical data from outpatient EMR system, outpatient EMR utilization ratio in Jan, 2013(at the second survey time) reached 92.6 % (39550/42707) compared with 60.1 % (27549/45784) in July, 2012 (at the first survey time).

178.4 Discussion

Despite the potential benefits, the implementation of outpatient EMR systems has been proved challenging. Though there is no commonly accepted evaluation standard of the successfulness of outpatient EMR implementation [4, 8], user perceptions and attitudes are thought to be critical factors.

In our study, dentists' satisfaction level towards newly employed outpatient EMR were fairly low at the first round of survey, which is consistent with Vishwanath's research results for outpatient EMR [4]. In our study, end-user satisfaction improved remarkably at the second round of survey, which is in consistent with Hoonakker's study about the changes satisfaction of ICU nurses over time in CPOE (Computerized Provider Order Entry) system [5].

The results suggested that there had been a tough time at the initial stage of outpatient EMR implementation. IT teams should make good preparation for the big challenges in this stage.

There are some limitations in this study. The sample size is relatively small. The quality of EMR is not included in the questionnaire, due to the heterogeneity among different types of dental departments. And same dentists may have filled out the questionnaire in both rounds of data collection, which means that the way some dentists have responded to the questionnaire survey in second round, can have been influenced by the way they responded to the questionnaire in the first time. In the second round, a small number of respondents such as medical students or refresher doctors may have not been working with the outpatient EMR for 8 months.

The implementation of the EMR system is so complex a process, some may even last for several years, that there is no commonly accepted standard to assess the effect. User satisfaction, from another point of view, can reflect the effect of the system and applications. It is a good indicator of whether the system implemented successfully. More longitudinal studies should be conducted to study the end-use satisfaction curve for IT system implemented in healthcare fields.

References

1. Sheikh A, Cornford T, Barber N, Avery A, Takian A, Lichtner V, Petrakaki D, Crowe S, Marsden K, Robertson A, Morrison Z, Klecun E, Prescott R, Quinn C, Jani Y, Ficociello M, Voutsina K, Paton J, Fernando B, Jacklin A, Cresswell K (2011) Implementation and adoption of nationwide electronic health records in secondary care in England: final qualitative results from prospective national evaluation in "early adopter" hospitals. BMJ 343:d6054
2. Robertson A, Cresswell K, Takian A, Petrakaki D, Crowe S, Cornford T, Barber N, Avery A, Fernando B, Jacklin A, Prescott R, Klecun E, Paton J, Lichtner V, Quinn C, Ali M, Morrison Z, Jani Y, Waring J, Marsden K, Sheikh A (2010) Implementation and adoption of nationwide electronic health records in secondary care in England: qualitative analysis of interim results from a prospective national evaluation. BMJ 341:c4564
3. Jha AK, DesRoches CM, Campbell EG, Donelan K, Rao SR, Ferris TG, Shields A, Rosenbaum S, Blumenthal D (2009) Use of electronic health records in U.S. hospitals. N Engl J Med 360:1628–1638
4. Vishwanath A, Singh SR, Winkelstein P (2010) The impact of electronic medical record systems on outpatient workflows: a longitudinal evaluation of its workflow effects. Int J Med Inform 79:778–791
5. Hoonakker PL, Carayon P, Brown RL, Cartmill RS, Wetterneck TB, Walker JM (2013) Changes in end-user satisfaction with computerized provider order entry over time among nurses and providers in intensive care units. J Am Med Inform Assoc 20:252–259
6. Wakefield DS, Halbesleben JR, Ward MM, Qiu Q, Brokel J, Crandall D (2007) Development of a measure of clinical information systems expectations and experiences. Med Care 45:884–890
7. Fornell C, Johnson MD, Anderson EW, Cha J, Bryant BE (1996) The American customer satisfaction index: nature, purpose, and findings. J Mark 60:7–18
8. Kazley AS, Diana ML, Menachemi N (2011) The agreement and internal consistency of national hospital EMR measures. Health Care Manag Sci 14:307–313

Chapter 179
Discussion on English Collaborative Learning Mode in Vocational Schools Under the IT-Based Network Environment

X. Yang and H. H. Tan

Abstract The application of IT into teaching has become a hot topic in current teaching filed; Benefiting from the development of IT, collaborative learning is involved in many new elements and is forward developed,which provides a new opening to the reform of English teaching. This paper introduces the theories of collaborative learning, and analyzes the necessity of integrating collaborative learning in IT-based environment into English teaching. It aims at exploring the way of English teaching reform in higher vocational schools from the perspective of collaborative learning in IT-based network environment.

Keywords Collaborative learning · IT-based network environment · Teaching mode · Vocational school

179.1 Introduction

With the rapid increasing needs for higher vocational and technical talents in current society, higher vocational and technical education has already made many reforms and gotten a large number of achievements. The specialty, complexity and biodiversity of English teaching in higher vocational schools have attracted more and more attention from experts in related realm. The guidance of English teaching in higher vocational schools is that practice is priority; sufficiency is degree, proposed the aim of cultivating students' English application ability, underlined the application and specialty of teaching context, and thus promoted English

---

X. Yang (✉)
Hubei College of Chinese Medicine, Ren Min Road 4th, Jing Zhou 434020, China
e-mail: yangxiananna@yahoo.com.cn

H. H. Tan
Schools of Foreign Studies Yangtze University, Jing Mi Road 88th, Jing Zhou 434025, China
e-mail: tanhonghui@yangtzeu.edu.cn

teaching in higher vocational schools to a scientific system. Fortunately, the fast development of network teaching brought new vital force for English teaching reform in higher vocational schools. For these reasons, this essay is going to explore the way of English teaching reform in higher vocational schools from the perspective of collaborative learning in IT-based network environment.

179.2 Necessity of Collaborative Learning

179.2.1 Current Study on English Teaching in Vocational Schools

Since the situation of students' resource of higher vocational schools is complex so there are many difficulties needed to be solved to achieve the aim of cultivating vocational and technical talents with higher English application ability that most of students' English is poor; The traditional English teaching mode with teacher-centeredness could not satisfy the aims and needs of English teaching now. Under these situations, we should explore the new special English teaching mode in higher vocational schools based on students' English level and social needs.

179.2.2 Interaction in English Teaching in Network Environment

Network-based English teaching differs from the traditional English teaching fundamentally in teaching environment. Network integrates sound, text, video, flash, image and other multimedia into a unit which provides a user-friendly, more vivid and more vigorous interacting environment to English teaching, which helps students explore initiatively and discover by themselves. Consequently, it is considerably helpful for students to form and upgrade their cognitive structure. Network-based English teaching not only has advantages in showing and passing target knowledge but also helps students and teachers make best use of contents, dialogues, and make students fully understand and initiatively build the construction of English messages.

179.3 Collaborative Learning in the Network Environment

179.3.1 Definition of Collaborative Learning

Collaborative learning is a team process where members support and rely on each other to achieve an agreed-on goal. The classroom is an excellent place to develop team-building skills you will need later in life. There is an organized relation among learners' individual activities. On one side, students should complete their work independently; on the other side, students should co-work with each other, share the resources and information and have the common responsibility to complete the unitary tasks. In this process, individuals could fully argue the issues through face to face talking, discussing, debating and other forms to find out the best way to achieve the learning goal. Therefore, collaborative learning helps students upgrade their thinking ability and cognitive ability, has benefit to enhance students' communicating ability and tolerance of others' different opinions and helps students keep healthy emotional state.

179.3.2 Basic Theories of Collaborative Learning Mode

Collaborative learning mode is based on constructive and humanistic education theories.

Constructivism is a theory of knowledge which argues that humans generate knowledge and meaning from an interaction between their experiences and their ideas and takes context, collaboration, dialogues and meaningful cognitive structure as four factors in the learning environment.

Humanistic theory focuses on human-centered curriculum, emphasizing on exploring human's creative potential and processing emotional education. It proposed that teachers should make the guiding roles based on the students-centeredness, which mainly focuses on students' individual differences and individual values.

All in all, the two theories all focus on student-centeredness, emphasize students' cognitive structure, stress on creating real, specific and vivid teaching and learning environment, require full use of various learning resources and information, pursuit the open learning process, advocate collaborative learning and enforce emotional exchange between students and teachers.

179.4 Design the English Collaborative Learning Mode in Vocational Schools in Network Environment

This essay takes *New Century English* II, Unit Six, Sino-American Relationship as an example of collaborative learning mode in vocational schools in IT-based network environment.

179.4.1 Collaborative Objects

Collaborative objects are the specific learning tasks which should be solved in the collaborative learning. As the guider of the collaborative learning, English teachers should assign several tasks according to studying objectives of each unit, which could motivate students' inner learning needs and stimulate their learning interests. In this unit, we set the several mini objectives related with the overall goal "Sino-American Relationship" as the main four following topics: Sino-US diplomatic relations, trade issues, Taiwan issues and area security issues.

179.4.2 Collaborative Learning Environment

Collaborative learning environment includes two parts: one is learning environment; the other is resource environment. The learning environment is mainly based on the usage of multi-media classroom provided by BBS, message board, e-mail and chat room. Resource environment mainly refers to resources in the network. Teachers provide students with the websites according to unit topic such as http://www.fmprc.gov.cn/eng/index.he, http://ww.nixonfoundation.org digital books, digital magazines, personal page.

179.4.3 Implementation of collaborative Activities

Implementation of collaborative activities is the key step to achieve the final success of collaborative learning. In this unit studying process, learning activities can alternate with each other or be in the order. Take Sino-US diplomatic relations as an example. It contains following steps: collecting information—primary accumulation of information—gaining of structure of material and information—discussions among members in each group—getting the deeper understanding and knowledge structure.

179.4.4 Evaluation of Collaborative Work

The assessments include three parts: self-assessment, peer feedback and teacher's assessment. The factors in evaluating process include rationality of division of task, property of cooperating way and involvement of members. The factors in evaluating works include refinement of tasks and completion degree of tasks. Combing these two sides, teacher proposes corresponding suggestions and advice.

179.5 Conclusions

Collaborative learning has become an important teaching mode, which has a great influence on English teaching. This mode not only provides students with colorful communicating activities, making up deficiencies in traditional English teaching reform but also cultivates students' learning enthusiasm, initiatives and cooperating abilities. What we mention here is that collaborative learning mode is just an effective way, which makes it possible to fully explore students' potentials and only if teachers and students actively and effectively navigate the pace and make the best of this mode integrating every network function into learning process, could the reform be a sound success. Hopefully, network can play an enormously positive role in students' learning and personality development.

References

1. Hao Z (2004) Discussion on the mode of vocational college network teaching. Liaoning Higher Vocational Technical Institute Journal, Fushun
2. Jianhua Z, Kedong L (2004) Teaching design based on cooperative learning under IT. E-Education Research, Lanzhou
3. Ping L (2005) The study of the instructional design and application about collaborative learning under network. Journal of Further Education of Shaanxi Normal University, Xian
4. Ruiqing D (2008) Teaching design based on cooperative learning under IT. China Educational Technique & Equipment, Beijing
5. Shuxiao X, Jingpei L (2002) The research and application of collaborative problem-based learning under network environment. E-Education Research, Lanzhou
6. Wanchun L (2005) Research on IT-based instructional design competencies of teachers. China Economist, Shanxi

Chapter 180
The Design of Learner-Centered College Teaching Resource Libraries

Cui Wei, Liang Lijing and Hua Wei

Abstract The teaching-centered construction of the traditional teaching resource libraries makes students unable to customize resources for autonomous learning, and meanwhile gives rise to problems such as shortage of resources, slow updating and lack of resource evaluation mechanism. This paper presents a learner-centered college teaching resource libraries based on Web 2.0 technology, which takes learners into the production, maintenance and management of resources to achieve the aggregation and push of customized resources, so that it can better solve the problems faced by the traditional teaching resource libraries.

Keywords Teaching resource library · Web 2.0 · Resource aggregation · Resources push · Customized learning · Autonomous learning

180.1 Introduction

With the development of educational informationization, the college teaching gradually walks from traditional classrooms to networks. In recent years many colleges have constructed college teaching resource libraries such as network courses, excellent courses, discipline resource platforms and teaching resource

---

C. Wei (✉) · H. Wei
Information Engineering Department, Luzhou Vocational and Technical College,
35 Wayaoba Road, Luzhou, Sichuan, China
e-mail: cccpmig29@gmail.com

H. Wei
e-mail: 183107549@qq.com

L. Lijing
Business School, Luzhou Vocational and Technical College, 35 Wayaoba Road, Luzhou,
Sichuan, China
e-mail: 43228795@qq.com

platforms to meet the needs of students' autonomous learning and help them build a lifelong learning system. These teaching resource libraries have solved the problems of storing and sharing teaching resources, and relieve the thirst of college teachers and students for teaching resources in the context of networks. But the existing teaching resource libraries are usually the network version of traditional classrooms, which are constructed still with teaching as their center to offer students unidirectional aid of teaching process, so gradually they can't meet the requirements of college teachers and students for customized and autonomous learning.

180.2 Limitations of Traditional Teaching Resource Libraries

The teaching-centered content of resources: The construction of traditional teaching resource libraries focuses on teaching and reproduces traditional class teaching in the network. The resources in the system only have such a single flow in which "teachers upload resources for students to view", and can't support the applied requirements of the learner-centered autonomous and customized learning. Therefore, the main service targets of teaching resource libraries—college students, lack enough enthusiasm to learn by applying the teaching resource libraries. This results in the low actual utilization rate of teaching resource libraries of various colleges and universities, and the aim of aiding the teaching can't be achieved very well [1].

Deficient and slowly-updated teaching resources: The lack of teaching resources is one of the major problems in the teaching resource library construction [2]. The main reason is that releasing resources in the system heavily depends on a small number of resource providers (usually just teachers) and fails to give full play to resource users (mainly students).

In the traditional teaching resource libraries, the management of resources is based on the classification system which was defined at the beginning of construction, and appropriate resources can be filled in a relatively pre-fixed mode [3]. This way lacks flexibility, and the updating of resources also heavily depends on resource providers, which inevitably leads to the problem that the resources can't be updated timely. On the other hand, as time goes on, the relatively fixed classification system results in the problem that the resources with new storage formats and presentation ways as their carriers are also hard to join the traditional teaching resource libraries [4].

180.3 Construction Thoughts on Learner-Centered Teaching Resource Libraries

Breaking the construction pattern of teaching-centered teaching resource libraries is the key to solve the problems that exist in traditional teaching resource libraries. Transforming a large number of users of the teaching resources (mainly learners) from the single role of consumers of teaching resources into the role of producers, maintainers, consumers and evaluators of the teaching resources can solve the problems that resources are deficient and updated slowly. Transforming the usage of resources from the unidirectional uploading and viewing into a multidimensional interactive manner including uploading, associating, customizing, pushing, assessing and discussing can effectively support autonomous and customized learning.

The standardization of resources: The premise to build teaching resource libraries based on Web 2.0 technology is to realize the standardization of resources stored in libraries. Only on this basis can the construction, storage, aggregation and push of resources be realized by means of RSS, Wiki and so on. The resources supported by the teaching resource libraries should cover all the knowledge, wisdom, tool and material resources in the whole teaching process. From the perspective of standardization, any stored resources should be abstracted into the metadata including the resource's name, type, classification, keyword, description, attachment, grade and evaluation. Any resource must be transformed into the resource metadata according to the standard so that it can be shared after it is put into the library.

The management and organization of resources: Tag on the basis of the resource classification can be used to solve this problem. Each user can make multiple Tags on the released and accessed resources according to his interest and need. The tags of a resource made by broad users can constitute a description set of the resource, and then reflect the system of the resource library. The association relationship can be also established between the resources with the same Tag. By comprehensive use of traditional resource classification manner and Tag, users can not only seek resources level by level in the resource library but also get all the resources in which they're interested by searching tags, thus the personal resource sharing can be achieved.

On this basis Blog technology is introduced to create a personal portal for each teacher or student in the teaching resource library. A teacher can upload all the related resources in his own personal portal and set proper tags to classify his resources into different courses. A student can transship interesting resources into his own personal portal and classify them or set tags according to his own requirement, for sure he can also release his own resources. Through the personal portal, a user can carry out the unified management over the resources that he has released or he is interested in by using three dimensions of time, classification and using group, so as to realize his customized autonomous learning.

Co-construction of resources: As the traditional producers of teaching resources, teachers have limited personal power, so they usually can't track the usage of the resources and it's also hard for them to timely maintain the resources and amend the defects of the resources. This is one of the root causes for the low quality of teaching resources.

Actually, as the major consumers of teaching resources, students can also make contributions to the production of teaching resources in the process of their learning, such as pointing out the slips in the courseware, offering their class notes and sharing the test questions obtained from other channels.

Wiki is a collaborative resource co-construction platform on which multiple users can collaboratively create, browse and modify the resources. After the teacher creates a resource in his own personal portal, students can directly edit the imperfections they find in the process of browsing the resource and save the revised resource into a new version, thus follow-up users can view various versions of the resource. Through this collaboration, the co-construction of resources can be realized to insure the authority and perfectness of resources and improve the quality of resources fundamentally.

The aggregation and push of resources: The traditional teaching resource libraries can just passively wait for users to browse but can't actively push the latest resources in which users may have interest. It's of great important for the users' autonomous learning to aggregate the related resources and actively push them to users and make users get the latest resources in real time according to the users' personal customization.

180.4 The Basic Design of Learner-Centered Teaching Resource Libraries

With Web 2.0's "User as Center" as the basic principle, we make use of Blog to accumulate resources, make use of Wiki to co-construct resources, make use of Tag to associate and aggregate resources, make use of RSS to customize and push resources, and finally realize a learner-centered teaching resource library for users' autonomous learning that supports teachers and students to co-construct teaching resources.

Navigation and retrieval: The navigation system is constructed by comprehensively applying traditional classification of courses and Web2.0's Tag technology. On the one hand, resources are classified according to the level of departments, majors and courses, and different subcategories are set under each course according to the users' actual requirements. For example, classification can be done either according to the file type of the media resources or according to the related documents in Technical Specifications of Modern Distance Education. Users can browse downward level by level through the classification system, till they find the resources they need. On the other hand, through Tag classification, users can view all the resources under a certain Tag. The retrieval of resources is done mainly by using keywords to do the fuzzy search in resource titles, descriptions and Tags and all the related resources are given to users for reference.

Personal portals and public resources: Individual users are the core of the system. Every user releases his resources through his personal portal, and each resource is synchronically released to the personal portal and the system's public resource library. A user can enter the personal portal of others (such as teachers) through the navigation to find the resource he needs, can make use of the functions such as transshipment and RSS push to integrate the resources into his own person portal, and can co-construct the resources through Wiki. The customized teaching resources obtained in this way constitute the user's personal learning space. The resource released in the user's personal portal will be synchronically released to the public resource library according to its category. According to the resource customization rules defined by the administrator, the public resource library can be obtained in real time through RSS to update the resources in personal portals.

References

1. Yuanyuan Q (2012) Discussion on construction strategies for college teaching resource libraries. Mech Vocat Educ (5)
2. Xiaojun Jiang, Qiang Han (2008) Several major problems and countermeasure analysis in the construciton of teaching resource libraries. China's Adult Educ 11:132–133
3. Xiangdong C (2007) The construction of network educational resources based on Web 2.0. China's Educ Inform 4:58–60
4. Shichuan W (2007) Thoughts on some problems in the construction of college teaching resource libraries. J Jiangnan Univ (Educational Science Edition) 3:78–81

Chapter 181
Research on Practice Teaching of Software Engineering

Lianying Sun, Chang Liu, Baosen Zhang, Tao Peng and Yuting Chen

Abstract Software engineering talent needs knowledge of computer systems as well as software development capabilities. To achieve this goal, a training program and reformed practical curriculum was developed. This paper, taking Subject Perception course as an example, introduces reform and innovation in teaching of software engineering professional practice courses. In the reformed course, six hardware experiments covering from basic logic to combined logic were devised, and a circuit experimental platform developed by teachers was employed. Emphasizing practice, the reformed course deepens understanding by students of 1st year of the relationship between computer hardware systems and software instructions. The teaching reform will stimulate students' interest in learning and lay the foundation for students to engage in embedded software development.

Keywords Subject perception · Practical teaching · Experimental platform · Circuit board making

Software industry is flourishing and software engineering talents is strong demand. What are the characteristics of software engineering talents? What are the requirements of the enterprise software engineering talents? To address these issues, we conducted a lot of research into the literature and the industry. Based on these researches and our analysis, we believe that software engineering talents are required to master the basics of computer science [1, 2] and be capable of software engineering practices [3, 4]. The basics of Computer science is the knowledge of

---

Support funding: Talents Support Project of Talents Enhancing University Development Plan in Beijing Union University (BPHR2011A04, BPHR2012F01).

L. Sun (✉) · C. Liu · B. Zhang · T. Peng · Y. Chen
College of Information Technology, Beijing Union University, No. 97 Beisihuan East Road, Beijing 100101, Chao Yang District, People's Republic of China
e-mail: xxtlianying@buu.edu.cn

computer hardware, and is abbreviated as "hard" aspect in this paper. Software engineering practice capability means that students will be able to engage in the development of software, and is abbreviated as "soft" aspect in this paper. For the purpose of training a qualified software engineering talent, we have developed a training program combined with "both soft aspect and hard aspect". Subject Perception course, which is scheduled into the first semester of college training program, is a new practical course and best reflects the new curriculum training program idea. Taking Subject Perception course as an example, this paper introduces how the "soft and hard" idea is realized in a professional practical course.

Subject Perception course is a basic professional course, aimed at improving low graders' professional awareness, stimulating their interests in learning the expertise. In 2009, College of Information Technology of Beijing Union University started this course [5]. With nearly 4 years of teaching, we have accumulated experiences and developed a new experimental platform. The experimental platform consists of six groups of experiments, with gradually increasing difficulties so as to ease digestion by target students. With such designed course, students can more readily comprehend the operating mechanism of computer instructions, and master the basic methods of problem-solving and methodology. Through practices, this course develops students' ability of understanding and following the "way of thinking" of a computer system in problem-solving. This practice will lay the foundation for students to engage in embedded software development.

181.1 Course Objectives

Computer science is an important basis of software engineering [6]. Subject Perception course introduces basic knowledge of computer systems and helps students to understand how computer hardware processes and implements instructions. The teaching content includes basic gate circuits, combinational logic circuit and solder experiments. Through practices, students will fully understand the internal operation mechanism of computer system, which paves the way for learning follow-up courses, such as C programming, computer organization principles and other professional courses, at the same time it will build the base for working on embedded software development in the future. In the end, we will achieve the aim "Perceive profession, practice and innovation".

181.2 Practical Contents Design

The course targets at undergraduate students, looks to increase the understanding by students of professional knowledge, with sub-modules and task-driven methods being used [7]. The course includes six sets of basic experiments, which are

On–off circuit, AND gate circuit, OR gate circuit, counter circuit, storage circuit and arithmetic unit circuit. It will introduce internal operation mechanism of computer system step by step. Details are shown in Table 181.1.

According to the contents of experiments, teachers develop circuit boards, which are shown in Fig. 181.1. Students should weld the experiments and accomplish circuit boards under the basis of circuit working principles.

Taking 'and' gate circuit as an example, it introduces the design principle of experiment platform. The aim of experiment is to make students master the concept of logic 'and', and know how to use hardware to achieve 'and' operation. The 'and' gate circuits consists of diode or integrated circuits (See Fig. 181.2). The platform, using reusing technologies, combines these two shorts together. Remove integrated circuits U1A and then they become 'and' gate circuits formed by diodes; remove two diodes D1, D2 and then they become integrated circuits 'and' gate. When switches 1 and 2 are on high level, the voltage of the resistor R2 is high, the triode T1 will be nonconductive and the luminous diode L12 glows. Either switch 1 or switch 2 being on low level will result in T1 nonconductive and L27 not glowing. By solder and verifying experiments, students can fully experience different ways of achieving hardware 'and' operation.

Meanwhile, comparing the 'and' operation and '&&' statement in C programming, students will understand that some assignments can be accomplished with either hardware or software.

181.3 Teaching Effectiveness

From 2012, Subject Perception course began to be implemented in accordance with the new program. Students were very interested in the solder practice, and considerably stimulated and highly enthusiastic for learning.

Before the experiment, teachers need to do a lot of preparation work. Experimental tools include: multimeter, electric iron, chromium frame, soldering and tweezers, etc. Experiment materials are resistors, capacitors, luminous diode, triode and integrated circuits. In addition, teachers should explain in detail each experiment circuit principle, so that students understand the theoretical basis of the operation. Students should get acquainted with each component, know polarity and other physical characteristics of components and use multimeter skillfully. As students are from lower grade, precautions, basic steps, concrete technique and other aspects should be introduced to assure success of the experiments.

When experimental content, materials, principles of knowledge are ready, students can proceed to do the welding experiments. They will be divided into several groups, with two to three students in one group using one common circuit board, but every member gets his or her part of work specifically. Students weld the digital components to the correct position according to circuit diagram. The complete effect of circuit manufacture is shown in Fig. 181.3.

Table 181.1 Practical contents and training objectives

Practical topic	Content	Training objectives
On–off circuit	Make on–off circuits	Know diode, triode and other components
		Understand the working principles of components
AND gate circuit	Make diode 'and' gate circuits from integrated circuits	Understand and building logic 'and' relationship
		Understand accomplishment of 'and' hardware
OR gate circuit	Make diode 'or' gate circuits from integrated circuits	Understand and building logic 'or' relationship
		Understand accomplishment of 'or' hardware
Counter circuit	Make four bit binary counter circuits made up by integrated circuits	Know digital signal pulse
		Understand binary
		Understand data plus/minus carry principles
		Understand hexadecimal principle
		Understand the relationship among binary, decimal system and hexadecimal
Storage circuit	Make storage circuits made up by eight bit latch	Understand the storage principle of digital signals
		Understand 'read' and 'write' realization of hardware
Arithmetic unit circuit	Make four bit binary add/subtract arithmetic unit	Master relationship between binary and hexadecimal
	Shown by hexadecimal principle	Understand add operation
		Understand subtraction operation

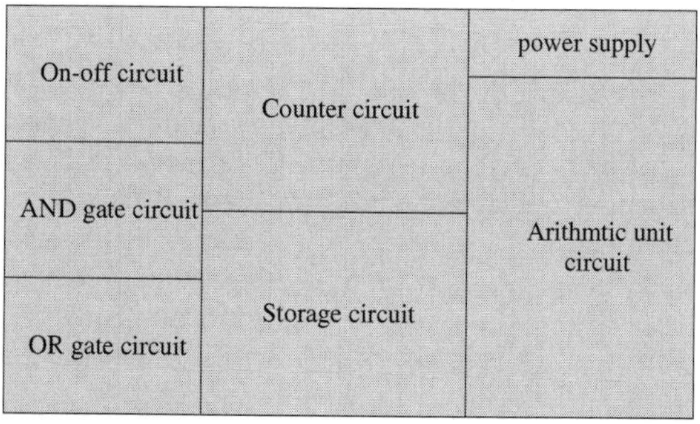

Fig. 181.1 Circuit board structure

[Circuit board layout showing: On-off circuit, Counter circuit, power supply, AND gate circuit, Arithmetic unit circuit, OR gate circuit, Storage circuit]

The application of experimental platform has high operability, which arouses students' interests and improves the learning of profession. In experiments, students operate carefully and help each other. Their enthusiasm is aroused and team work spirit cultivated. The experiment platforms help students understand basic

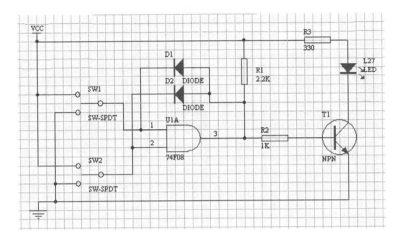

Fig. 181.2 AND gate circuit diagram

Fig. 181.3 Complete circuit

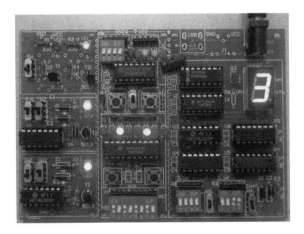

knowledge of computer system, such as digital logic, machine notation, number system conversion, storage principles, instruction execution, and so on. Especially binary, of which the conception of carry and overflow is not clear to students, is the fundamental of computer system. In the platform, the counter circuits and operation circuits turn binary plus/minus operation, carry, overflow, storage, conversions of number system and so on, from design principles to hardware realization, giving students direct performance and helping them gain full understanding, which offer support to subsequent learning programming basis,computer organization principles.

Compared to traditional textbook-teaching methods, understanding basic knowledge and theories from vivid specific operation experiments is more efficient. With stimulated interests, students become more active in operating and thinking, and this helps the cultivation of innovation ability and sets good basis to learning major.

181.4 Conclusion

Subject Perception course is the practice of software engineering in first semester. It is based on the idea of "soft and hard combination". The course has six hardware welding experiments from basic logic to combined logic. Through operation, students understand the relationship between computer hardware systems and software instructions. Subject Perception is a novel practice and exploration of the way of cultivating software engineering talents who got a background of computer systems knowledge, and will hopefully lead to new ideas for similar practical teaching.

References

1. Xiong W, Hong M (2010) Exploration and practice of construction on software engineering. J High Edu Sci Technol 29(1):59–61
2. Wang W (2008) Research on software engineering undergraduate education. Comput Educ 2008(24):96–97
3. Li H, Zhang H, Lu W (2009) Research and practice on the practical teaching system of software engineering based on ability training. Res High Educ Eng 2009(2):84–87
4. Ma Y, Zhang G, Wang W (2006) Reform and practice of software engineering experimental teaching mode. Educ Career 2006(36):149–150
5. Liu C, Sun L, Shang X (2012) Subject perception teaching research and practice in application-oriented university. J Beijing Union Univ (Nat Sci) 26(2):71–73
6. Teaching Steering Committee of the Ministry of Education of Software Engineering (2011) Colleges software engineering specification. Higher Education Press, Beijing, p 6
7. Peng Y, Shen X, Zhang Q (2012) Study and practice on experimental teaching method of computer software course. Exp Technol Manag 2012(4):173–175

Chapter 182
Construction of Transportation Professional Virtual Internship Platform

Zhao Jianguang and Lui Ruijun

Abstract The rapid development and wide application of network technology is to lay a solid foundation for the college the virtual internship platform. The literature and logical analysis method was used in this article. The establishment of the virtual internship model is proposed in the transportation professional in the text. The framework structure and main contents of the virtual internship platform for building were discussed in-depth on the basis of analysis of the characteristics and advantages of the virtual internship platform.

Keywords Transportation professionals · The virtual internship · Internship platform · Construction

182.1 Introduction

Transportation is a very strong practical subjects, to better reflect the professional characteristics of the transportation specialized courses through practice teaching. Colleges and universities transportation professional practice teaching in China lags behind the theoretical teaching to a large extent. The theoretical knowledge alone can not meet the actual needs of students after graduation to adapt to the field of transportation to the demand of the complex talent under the conditions of market economy. The production internship is Important practical teaching link in the transportation professional and can deepen and objective factors from outside influence, causing to the traditional practical teaching methods are faced with unprecedented difficulties and challenges, only opening up new ideas, building new practice teaching mode to adapt to the new situation, but to enhance

Z. Jianguang · L. Ruijun (✉)
College of Transportation Beihua University, 132011 Jilin, China
e-mail: z7811232005@yahoo.com.cn

constantly the student practice ability, and meet the needs of the unit of choose and employ persons. For this, this article puts forward the idea of virtual practice, that is to establish virtual practice platform by using computer simulation technology, organize students to participate in virtual internships, let users interact with virtual environment. Although the existence of the virtual practice form is virtual, but the value and function is real, the reform is of great significance.

182.2 The Role of Virtual Training Platform

The convenient conditions that network technology provides for the application and development of the virtual practice mode, has a good application prospect in the education of colleges and universities.

182.2.1 Flexible Training Way, Make up for the Inadequacy of Companies in Practice

Virtual practice mode is different from the traditional practice teaching mode, it can provide students with different teaching content, students determine the learning content and learning process according to the actual situation, to satisfy the different needs of students. In the business field practice of some very complex procedure, long period, high risk business, these phenomena can be simulated by virtual reality technology and used to practice in the virtual environment, students can go deep into the various scenes in the enterprise that is not caused by the two sides have any risk, also can experience different work scene, transform a variety of roles. By establishing virtual practice bases on the computer simulation experiment and practice environment, access to the real world practice teaching effect.

182.2.2 Broke Through the Time and Geographical Limitations, can be Repeated Many Times, System, Coherent Situation Simulation Practice

In virtual reality breakthrough the limitation of time and space, organization can unbridled repetition practice drills for many times, still can go deep into the object that the real world cannot look inside to experiment (practice), showing any time experimental progress or internship phase of the scene from different angles, to ensure the system and continuous of simulation internship project.

182.2.3 The Sharing of Resources, Reflects the Low Cost Advantage of Virtual Practice

The virtual internship platform sharing of educational resources through the computer network, thus saving the repeated introduction of many low-level redundant construction of the infrastructure and equipment funding, and is conducive to improving the overall school conditions and raise the standard of teaching. Virtual reality technology to establish the experimental practice environment is virtual, when requiring update or upgrade to a new laboratory equipment, practice base, only in the virtual reality of the computer hardware and software environment to regenerate can, so as to ensure that the practice of teaching be able to keep up with the needs of teaching and technology development.

182.3 Virtual Practice Platform Construction of Transportation Professional

182.3.1 Transportation Professional Overall Construction Framework of Virtual Training Platform

Transportation professional virtual practice is mainly composed of virtual practice platform, virtual libraries and open laboratory management system of subjects of three parts, with the help of a graphic/image, simulation and virtual reality technology, to create a visualization on computer network virtual training environment. Through the combination of virtual practice and field practice, solve the problem that the systemic production internship is not strong, but also learners develop autonomous learning in the practice teaching link according to their own need.

According to transportation professional personnel training mode and training requirements, combined with the professional reality condition, put forward the overall frame of transportation professional virtual training platform construction, its content covers transportation professional cognition practice and virtual production practice. As shown in Fig. 182.1

182.3.2 Transportation Professional Virtual Practice Platform Frame Function Introduction

The virtual practice platform of transportation specialty in our college, including five module practice content of the transportation and logistics, transportation

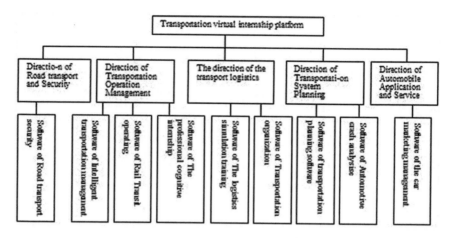

Fig. 182.1 The frame of virtual practice platform of transportation major

management, transportation planning, the road traffic safety and automobile use, the function of each module includes practice requirements, safety education, training modules according to the corresponding direction, such as: Table as shown in Fig. 182.1, Table 182.1. The whole system is a common platform based on the hardware platform, unified organization and management of information, in the form of software outsourcing. Students can carry out vehicle driving simulation training, testing and evaluation of the road safety, intelligent traffic system cognition in a variety of road traffic environment, practice content simulated sales service car. Detailed module functions are as follows:

Including the internship program, internship report, internship evaluation form module. The internship program provides current transportation professional "production internship implementation details", internship report; internship evaluation form provides a report, appraisal form template that "the production internship Implementing Rules" require students to complete.

Safety education is often ignored in the virtual practice, in order to highlight its important role, in the platform design, the safety education is as an independent module to be set, Including safety education, safety code specification, process guidance module. Each module has a safety education for the software system and the scene of the actual work to ensure the correct cognition and operations of students.

The virtual internship module content includes five professional direction and nine training internship module. The virtual internship module firstly show items flow through intuitive picture (photo) and simple instructions and further provide students with interactive and immersive virtual internship feelings with multiple ikonic flash animation and field record video. Following a brief function of several software should have.

Table 182.1 Transportation professional virtual practice platform introduced frame function

Building objectives	Transportation professional virtual internship platform				
Building functional modules	Direction of transportation logistics	Direction of transportation operation management	Direction of road transport and security	Direction of transportation system planning	Direction of automobile application and service
Sub modules — Base modules	Internship requirements: internship program, internship report, internship evaluation form safety education; for the software system, and in the actual work scenarios				
Sub modules — Functional modules	Simulation training of professional understanding etc.	Operation management of the intelligent etc.	The road traffic simulation	Transportation system planning software	Automotive marketing management
Software source	Purchase				

182.4 Conclusion

1. Transportation professional virtual internship platform, breaking through the limitations of the traditional practice pattern, that is an effective solution to inadequate funding for student internships, systemic series of problems, and improve the quality and efficiency of the professional internship, is great significance for the formation of a new training model and method.
2. The development Virtual technology is a product of the information age, and has broad application prospects in the fields of education, scientific research, is a new direction of development of experiment and practice teaching, that will promote the teaching concepts, teaching style and teaching content to change, and is mainstream and trend of the development of higher education.

References

1. Liu Y (2004) The research and practice of transportation professional adaptable talents cultivating mode[J]. Tech Coll Edu 3:42–44
2. Qu Z (2007) Functions and characteristics of the virtual laboratory. Changsha Univ 5:105–106
3. Liu W (2007) Transportation practical teaching reform exploration. China Metall Edu 2:32–33
4. Bernardo W (1999) 29th ASEE/IEEE Frontiers in education conference; 10:13d6–6–13d6–10
5. Chen S H et al (1999) Proceedings IEEE Hong Kong Symposium. Robot Contr 7:756–760

Chapter 183
Chronic Suppurative Otitis Media Bacteriology Culturing and Drug Sensitive Experiment of Er Yannig

Wu Liping, Hu Xiaoqian, Li Meng, Hou Jinjie and Li Ruiyu

Abstract *Objective* to study the chronic suppurative otitis media relations with bacterial infection and drug sensitivity test of Er yannig. *Methods* 55 cases of different type according to the regulation method of ear cavity samples of patients with chronic suppurative otitis media, test their anaerobic bacteria, aerobic bacteria respectively, and at the same time observe ear drug sensitive test. *Results* 55 pathogens of chronic suppurative otitis media patients 52 strains, including aerobic bacterium infection nine strains, accounting for 36.5 %. 18 strains of anaerobic bacteria infection accounted for 34.6 %, mixed aerobic and anaerobic bacteria infection 15 strains, accounting for 28.8 %; Er yanning drug sensitive test, the bacteriostasis of aerobic bacteria rate was 67.7–94.4 %, is sensitive to all anaerobic bacteria. *Conclusion* chronic suppurative otitis media by anaerobic bacteria and aerobic bacteria mixed infection, Er yanning has a dual antibacterial effect.

Keywords Chronic suppurative otitis media · Er yanning drug sensitive test

Chronic suppurative otitis media is ent common disease, the effect of inner ear function and complications in inflammatory process increasingly cause the attention of both at home and abroad [1–4]. Topical or oral application of antibiotic resistant bacteria and mutation bacteria cause of ototoxic also increased year

---

W. Liping · H. Xiaoqian
Hebei Medical University Affiliated Xingtai People's Hospital Clinical Laboratory, Xingtai, Hebei, China

L. Meng
Health Team of Hotan Prefecture Detachment of Chinese Armed Police Force in Xinjiang, Xinjiang, China

H. Jinjie
Xingtai Medical College, No. 618 Gangtiebei Road, Xingtai City, Hebei Province, China

L. Ruiyu (✉)
Second Affiliated Hospital of Xingtai Medical College, No. 618 Gangtiebei Road, Xingtai City, Hebei Province, China
e-mail: liruiyu651021@163.com

by year. Therefore systematic research for the disease has important clinical significance, this paper carried out a chronic suppurative otitis media bacteria culture and Chinese traditional medicine is given priority to Er Yanning ear drops drug sensitive experiment observation, the results reported below.

183.1 Data and Methods

183.1.1 Clinical Data

This group of 46 cases, male 27 cases, female 19 cases, minimum 2 years of age, maximum 58, in 3–31 to see more. Clinical classification: simplex 36 cases (42 total), caries type 3 cases (5 total), cholesteatoma type 7 cases (8 total). Career: staff 5 people, 9 workers, 1 farmers, students and other 21 people.

183.1.2 Drugs and Methods

Er yanning ear drops (consist of rhubarb, cortex phellodendri, etc.) provided by the Er yanning team, see the article [6], acquisition methods according to the rules extraction, middle ear cavity secretion specimens to minimize the exposure time in the air, the extraction of sample immediately to restore blood AGAR and normal blood AGAR, respectively for anaerobe and aerobe training, at the same time will smear, gram's staining microscopy specimens aerobic blood AGAR at 37 °C, anaerobic bacteria cultivation, the ventilation method is adopted, the specimen after inoculation, anaerobic bacteria tank at 37 °C, in addition to the use of conventional anaerobic bacteria assay method (morphological staining, culture characteristic, biochemical reaction and drug susceptibility evaluation, the necessary time to use 3650 A UV fluorescent analyzer to observe colony), some species are also applied AP 120-20 A series of medium, the numerical method for anaerobic bacteria identification, aerobe determination of minimum inhibitory concentrations (MICS) by double broth dilution method, bacteria to Er yanning ear drops 4/L or less as sensitive, sensitive bacteriostatic ratio = Sensitive to number/strains by 100 %.

183.2 Results

55 specimens isolated pathogenic bacteria strains 52 strains, positive rate was 95 %, including 19 strains of aerobic bacteria, accounting for 34.5 %, mainly for *Staphylococcus aureus*, *Escherichia coli*, proteus, *Pseudomonas aeruginosa*, 18 strains of anaerobic bacteria accounted for 32.7 %, mainly bacteroides fragilis, corrosion of bacteroides, melanin production such as bacteroides, anaerobic bacterium and aerobic bacteria mixed infection 15 strains, accounting for 27.2 %.

Table 183.1 Chronic suppurative otitis media secretions germiculture results (%)

Type	Aerobic bacteria	Anaerobic bacterium	Anaerobic and aerobic bacteria mixed infection
Pure 42	17 (40.48)	16 (38.0)	7 (16.6)
Caries 5	0 (0)	1 (20)	3 (60)
Cholesteatoma 8	2 (25)	1 (12.5)	5 (62.5)

Table 183.2 Er yanning ear drops of aerobe in vitro antibacterial activity

Bacterial species	MIC range	MIC50/MIC90	Antibacterial rate (%)
E. coli	0.125 ~ ≥ 64	0.25/2	93.75
Proteus	0.125 ~ ≥ 64	0.5/2	94.44
Pseudomonas aeruginosa	0.25 ~ ≥ 64	2/8	85.0
Staphylococcus aureus	0.5 ~ ≥ 64	2/8	67.74

Table 183.3 Er yanning ear drops of 4 kinds of drugs on drug sensitive test of anaerobic bacteria

Medicine	Bacteroides fragilis (8)			Corrosion of bacteroidetes (4)			Produce melanin bacteroidetes (3)			Generation of streptococcus (3)		
	S	M	R	S	M	R	S	M	R	S	M	R
Er yanning	8			3	1		3			3		
Metronidazole	8			3	1		3			3		
Erythromycin	3	3	2	2	2		2	1		2	1	
Carbenicillin	8			4			2	1		3		

S: sensitive M: medium sensitivity R: resident

Chronic suppurative otitis media secretions bacterial culture results are shown in Table 183.1.

Er yanning ear drops of aerobe in vitro antimicrobial activity are shown in Table 183.2.

Chronic suppurative otitis media anaerobic bacteria culture results in bacteroides fragilis is relatively rare, in order to observe ear rather antimicrobial range of ear drops, at the same time, choose the other four kinds of antimicrobial agents to do comparison, The Er yanning ear drops, metronidazole, carboxy benzyl penicillin of anaerobic bacteria is the most sensitive, detailed in Table 183.3.

183.3 Discuss

In recent years, the main treatment of chronic suppurative otitis media by oral or local application of antibiotics, but antibiotics ototoxicity caused more and more attention both at home and abroad, as well as increasing along with the modern medical science examination methods for chronic suppurative otitis media bacterial infections. This paper, taking the bacterial culture results show that the aerobic bacteria (34.5 %), anaerobic bacteria accounted for 32.7 %, the anaerobe and aerobe mixed infection (27.2 %), therefore selects ototoxicity and anti anaerobe and aerobe are important principles of treatment of this disease.

Chronic suppurative otitis media bacterial infection is regarded as the objective basis of pathogenic bacteria in aerobic bacterium infection, but higher medical colleges and universities teaching material (otolaryngology) has not yet been explains the relationship between chronic suppurative otitis media and anaerobic bacteria infection.

According to statistics at home and abroad in chronic suppurative otitis media, proteus and *Pseudomonas aeruginosa* infection, account for important position. For anaerobic bacteria infection, with the method of hospital routine bacterial culture results cannot be checked out, to conventional antibiotics are often invalid. According to the statistics in 1977, about 60 % of clinical infection specimens of anaerobic bacteria can be detected. Of course, chronic suppurative otitis media in delay is painless and break out repeatedly and pathogenic anaerobic bacteria have close relationship. For its mechanism abroad Fulgum after think tissue injury may release enzyme, causes of middle ear fluid oxygen tension is reduced, some anaerobic bacteria and protected. When aerobic bacterium infection also consume oxygen content of the middle ear fluid, so fluid of chronic suppurative otitis media, otitis media for anaerobe is an excellent growing conditions. Others think problems of anaerobic bacteria pathogenic under certain conditions, such as the body's normal immune function decline, local its entirely caused by trauma of skin mucous membrane damage, or improper use of some antibiotics and dysbacteriosis caused by making some conditional pathogenic bacteria colonization, these general conditions do not cause disease or weak virulence of bacteria on the basis of the possible formation of endogenous infection. This study suggests that chronic suppurative otitis media by aerobic bacteria, anaerobic bacteria infection alone, and often mixed infection, the mixed infection may be associated with bacterial pathogenic collaborative, its mechanism remains to be further discussed in detail.

References

1. Wang I, Dai CF, Chi FL (2007) The etiology of chronic inflammation sex around with facial nerve paralysis. Middle Ear Chin. Otolaryngol. J. 42:889–892
2. I KM, N H, Onod, et al (2006) Differentiated bi-facial nerve Paralysiscnused by middle ear Cholesteatoma and effects of surgicalintervention. Acta. Otloaryngol 126: 95–100
3. Fang L, Liu JL (2008) The influence factors of chronic suppurative otitis media bone conduction hearing loss analysis. Audiol. Speech Dis. J. 6:513–514
4. Feng HY, Chen YJ (2004) The correlation between chronic suppurative otitis media and sensorineural deafness. J. Clin. Otolaryngol. Dept. 579
5. Wei NR (1989) Otolaryngology science second edition. People's Medical Publishing House,Beijing, p 298–302
6. Li RY, Li WJ, Hui JQ (1994) Er yanning ear drops for the treatment of chronic suppurative otitis media clinical observation. Intermed. Should 29(11):48–49

Chapter 184
Research Hotspots Analysis of Hypertension Receptor by PubMed

Chaopeng Li, Qinting Zhang, Yang Liu, Shuangping Wei, Jungai Li,
Jinjie Hou, Ruijuan Zhang, Weiya Guo, Lijun Wang, Yuhong Liu
and Ruiyu Li

Abstract The papers about hypertension in Pubmed were retrieved, and Medical Subject Headings (MeSH) in retrieved papers were analyzed (word frequency analysis, clustering analysis, co-word network graph), it suggested that the current hypertension receptor research hotspots had focus on Angiotensin receptor, adrenergic β receptor, endothelin receptor, mineralocorticoid receptor, also the most importance of which was the angiotensin receptor.

Keywords Hypertension · Receptor · Word frequency analysis · Clustering analysis · Co-word network graph · Angiotensin receptor

184.1 Introduction

Hypertension is a major public health problem worldwide, there are approximately 1 billion individuals suffer from high blood pressure worldwide [1], at present the fundamental research of hypertension is mainly related to the research of receptor and ligand, it has a great significance to pathogenesis and treatment of hypertension. We hope that through this research the analysis of the Medical Subject Headings (MeSH) can draw the outline of hypertension receptors research hotspot.

C. Li · S. Wei · J. Li · J. Hou
Xingtai Medical College, No. 618 Gangtiebei Road, Xingtai, Hebei, China
e-mail: wein871@sohu.com

Q. Zhang · R. Zhang
Civil Administration General Hospital of Hebei Province, Xingtai, Hebei, China

Y. Liu · W. Guo · L. Wang · Y. Liu · R. Li (✉)
Second Affiliated Hospital of Xingtai Medical College, No. 618 Gangtiebei Road, Xingtai, Hebei, China
e-mail: liruiyu651021@163.com

Therefore this research retrieved the hypertension papers of PubMed (http://www.ncbi.nlm.nih.gov/pubmed) within recent 5 years, got 79,825 papers, and analyzed MeSH of above papers using co-word Analysis [2].

184.2 Materials and Methods

First, we retrieved PubMed papers with publication dates between 1 January 2008 and 15 November 2012. Second, search terms was "hypertension" [MeSH Terms] OR "hypertension" [All Fields] OR "high blood pressure" [All Fields]. Third, using Microsoft Excel we recorded All MeSH terms of above papers, and sort and filter the terms, and looked for the high frequency terms (occurrences), and we also counted occurrences of two high frequency terms together in the same paper, setting up the original co-word matrix. Fourth, the statistical analysis: we made MeSH term's clustering analysis using SPSS13.0 statistical software, draw the co-word network graph of the high frequency terms using Cytoscape software [3].

184.3 MeSH Terms Analysis of Papers about Hypertension

184.3.1 MeSH Terms Word Frequency Analysis

We retrieved 79,825 papers, among them we got 68, 183 papers with MeSH terms, we extracted MeSH terms and established the MeSH terms database. We got 13 MeSH terms of receptor which occurrences frequency was over 130 (including 130), We also got 13 MeSH terms of ligand which occurrences frequency was over 669 (including 669), which self and which derivatives may do ligand, and was a specific chemical or drug name). From Table 184.1, we can inferred some ideas: the relevant research of receptor hotspots mainly concentrated in the angiotensin receptor, adrenergic receptor beta, endothelin receptor and mineralocorticoid receptors, etc., it also suggests that angiotensin receptor has become hypertension receptors most major research hotspots (Table 184.2).

184.3.2 Clustering Analysis of the High Frequency MeSH Terms

This research used hierarchical clustering analysis which is one of the most commonly used Classify analysis to analyze the above 26 MeSH terms, drew a dendrogram, and the results were shown in Fig. 184.1.

Table 184.1 The top 13 MeSH terms about receptor

Ranking	MeSH terms	Occurrences frequency (times)
1	Angiotensin II Type 1 Receptor Blockers	1,611
2	Adrenergic beta-Antagonists	909
3	Receptor, Angiotensin, Type 1	564
4	Angiotensin Receptor Antagonists	390
5	Receptors, Endothelin	294
6	Receptors, Mineralocorticoid	229
7	Receptor, Angiotensin, Type 2	168
8	Receptor, Endothelin A	159
9	Receptors, Cell Surface	153
10	Bone Morphogenetic Protein Receptors, Type II	144
11	Receptors, G-Protein-Coupled	142
12	Adrenergic alpha-Antagonists	132
13	Vascular Endothelial Growth Factor Receptor-1	130

Table 184.2 The top 13 MeSH terms about ligand

Ranking	MeSH terms	Occurrences frequency(times)
1	Blood Glucose	1,636
2	Nitric Oxide	1,436
3	Angiotensin II	1,267
4	Creatinine	1,083
5	Tetrazoles	1,036
6	Renin	979
7	C-Reactive Protein	898
8	Aldosterone	811
9	Triglycerides	784
10	Insulin	752
11	Cholesterol	731
12	Nitric Oxide Synthase Type III	700
13	Reactive Oxygen Species	669

From the Fig. 184.1, in addition to individual MeSH term as "Receptors, the G-Protein-Coupled", we could seen the other high frequency MeSH terms could be divided into the following eight groups. Group 1 contains MeSH terms (Angiotensin II Type 1 Receptor Blockers; Receptor, Angiotensin, Type 1; Receptor, Angiotensin, Type 2; Angiotensin II), one group with multiple MeSH terms of angiotensin receptor suggests angiotensin receptor is the research hotspot now [4], MTT method (methylthiazolyl tetFazolium) is a kind of chemical experiment method, used in the research of angiotensin receptor [5]. Group 2 contains MeSH terms (Renin; Aldosterone; Receptors, Mineralocorticoid), it suggests that aldosterone is a mineralocorticoid, it also is important component of RAAS (renin-angiotensin-aldosterone system). Group 3 contains MeSH terms (Nitric Oxide; Nitric Oxide Synthase Type III; Reactive Oxygen Species), it

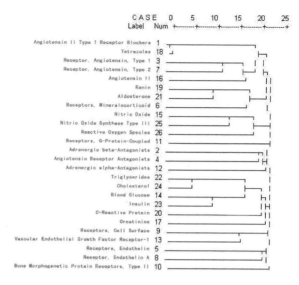

Fig. 184.1 Hierarchical clustering analysis dendrogram of MeSH terms

suggests that uncoupling of Endothelial nitric oxide synthase is the important mechanism to the decrease of the level of nitric oxide and the increase of the level of reactive oxygen [6]. Group 4 contains MeSH terms (Adrenergic beta-Antagonists; Angiotensin Receptor Antagonists; Adrenergic alpha-Antagonists), it suggests that they have certain relevance in biological processes. Group 5 contains MeSH terms (Triglycerides; Cholesterol; Blood Glucose; Insulin; C-Reactive Protein; Creatinine), it suggests that they have certain relevance in biological processes. Group 6 contains MeSH terms (Receptors, Cell Surface; Vascular Endothelial Growth Factor Receptor-1), it suggests that Vascular Endothelial Growth Factor Receptor-1 is one of vascular endothelial growth factor [7]. Group 7 contains MeSH terms (Receptors, Endothelin; Receptor, Endothelin A; Bone Morphogenetic Protein Receptors, Type II), it suggests that endothelin receptor and Bone Morphogenetic Protein type II receptor have certain relevance in biological processes.The above clustering results suggest that several MeSH terms within one group have certain inherent logic connection between each other; If there are no known correlation between the MeSH terms, it indicates we find a new research hotspot.

184.3.3 Co-word Network Graph of the High Frequency MeSH Pair

By analyzing receptor MeSH terms of the top 10 (word frequency) and ligand MeSH terms of the top 10 (word frequency),which totaled 20, we got the top 6 MeSH terms pair (A and B, see Table 184.3) and co-word network graph of the

Table 184.3 The top 6 MeSH terms pair

Ranking	MeSH terms A	MeSH terms B	Co-word occurrences frequency (times)
1	Angiotensin II Type 1 Receptor Blockers	Tetrazoles	1,168
2	Blood Glucose	Insulin	718
3	Renin	Aldosterone	542
4	Blood Glucose	Triglycerides	524
5	Receptor, Angiotensin, Type 1	Angiotensin II	428
6	Angiotensin II Type 1 Receptor Blockers	Angiotensin II	344

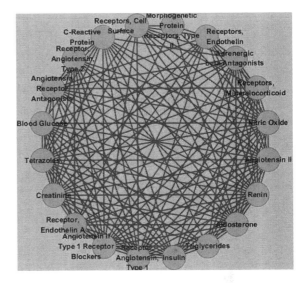

Fig. 184.2 Co-word network graph of the high frequency MeSH terms pair

MeSH terms pair (see Fig. 184.2). Especially the first MeSH terms pair of Angiotensin II Type 1 Receptor Blockers and Tetrazoles appeared 1,168 times in the same paper, it was far higher than that of the second MeSH terms pair (718 times, blood sugar and insulin).

In Fig. 184.2 the edge represents the concurrence relationship between MeSH terms pair and if the edge between one MeSH term to other MeSH term, it suggests that the one MeSH term is more important, it is in the center of the research hotspots. So we could infer that angiotensin receptor is current research hotspot in the field of hypertension receptors, and MTT method (methylthiazolyl tetFazolium) is usually used in the research of angiotensin receptor.

184.4 Concluding Remarks

By analyzing MeSH terms (word frequency analysis, clustering analysis, co-word network graph) of PubMed papers about hypertension, we could infer that the current hypertension receptor research hotspots had focus on Angiotensin receptor, adrenergic β receptor, endothelin receptor, mineralocorticoid receptor, also the most importance of which was the angiotensin receptor.

References

1. Chobanian AV, Bakris GL, Black HR et al (2003) The seventh report of the joint national committee on prevention, detection, evaluation, and treatment of high blood pressure: the JNC 7 report. JAMA 289(19):2560–2572
2. Viedma-Del-Jesus MI, Perakakis P, Muñoz MÁ et al (2011) Sketching the first 45 years of the journal psychophysiology (1964–2008): a co-word-based analysis. Psychophysiology 48(8):1029–1036
3. Lopes CT, Franz M, Kazi F et al (2010) Cytoscape web: an interactive web-based network browser. Bioinformatics 26(18):2347–2348
4. Oprisiu R, Fournier A, Achard JM et al (2013) Association between Angiotensin receptor blockers and better cognitive outcome: urgent need for a randomized trial. JAMA Neurol 70(3):413–414
5. Han YS, Lan L, Chu J et al (2013) Epigallocatechin gallate attenuated the activation of rat cardiac fibroblasts induced by angiotensin II via regulating β-arrestin 1. Cell Physiol Biochem 31(2–3):338–346
6. Chan SH, Chan JY (2013) Brain stem NOS and ROS in neural mechanisms of hypertension. Antioxid. Redox Signal [Epub ahead of print]
7. Ohuchi SP, Shibuya M, Nakamura Y (2013) The RNA aptamer inhibiting human vesicular endothelial growth factor receptor 1 without affecting the cytokine binding. Biochemistry 52(13):2274–2279. doi:10.1021/bi301669p

Chapter 185
Creative Approaches Combined with Computer Simulation Technology in Teaching Pharmacology

Chuang Wang and Jiejie Guo

Abstract Pharmacology is a key course among a number of preclinical courses in the schools of medicine, nursing, preventive medicine, dentistry, pharmacy, etc., and deals with the study of drugs regarding their sources, uses, metabolism excretion, dosages, adverse effects, interactions, and contraindications. To date, more and more traditional teaching methods in pharmacology are introduced, mainly including lecture based learning (LBL), problem based learning (PBL) mode, computer assisted teaching (CAT), computer assisted learning (CAL) experimental skills training in pharmacology and so on. In addition, these teaching methods above still focus on drugs not the relationship between with drugs and diseases of patients. Moreover, traditional pharmacology teachings focus more on drugs instead of therapeutics, such that although pharmacological knowledge is acquired, practical skills in prescribing remain weak. However, although teaching pharmacology to medical students has long been seen as a challenge and one to which a number of innovative approaches have been taken. The aim of this present article is to provide those who are interested in teaching of pharmacology to be acquainted with the teaching of pharmacology, including the traditional teaching methods and also the application of new one teaching method combined with computer simulation technology in pharmacology.

Keywords Pharmacology · Drug targets · Computer simulation technology

C. Wang (✉) · J. Guo
Ningbo University School of Medicine, 818 Fenghua Road, Ningbo 315211, China
e-mail: wangchuang@nbu.edu.cn

J. Guo
e-mail: 307276490@qq.com

185.1 The Role of Pharmacology in Medicine Education

185.1.1 The Characteristics, Goal and Mission of Pharmacology

Pharmacology is an essential course that contributes basic theory, elementary knowledge and scientific principals to diseases prevention and rational use of drug. It is also a double bridge that links medicine and pharmacy, basic medicine and clinical medicine. The scope of pharmacology involves function sciences (physiology, pathology, biochemistry and molecular biology), morphology (human anatomy, embryology, and parasitology) and clinic (internal medicine, surgery, gynecology, pediatrics) and many other disciplines. Pharmacology is characterized by wide range of contents and profound theories, making it an indispensable course for medical and pharmaceutical research as well as clinical and production practice. The goal of pharmacology includes: (1) to clarify the action of drug and underlying mechanism, support rational use of drug, maximization of drug effect and avoidance from adverse effect; (2) to develop new drug and novel purpose of existing drug; (3) to provide supports and methods for other life science researches. The theory of pharmacology has its vertical extent and connections with other parallel disciplines. Learning of pharmacology theory should be on the basis of knowledge on physiology, biochemistry, microbiology, immunology, physiopathology, etc. Its close relationship with clinical practice extends the width and depth of pharmacology [1].

185.1.2 How to Teach Pharmacology?

Pharmacology is a key course among a number of preclinical courses in the schools of medicine, nursing, preventive medicine, dentistry, pharmacy, etc., in China. Through half-year study, students can acquire the basic knowledge of the fundamental principles of pharmacology and its clinical applications, the basic skills in doing pharmacology experiments, know the professional knowledge of the laws and regulations of drug administration. And students could have the basic ability to perform scientific research in pharmacology. While in the traditional teaching the students were taught in a series of preplanned pharmacology lectures, that was teacher centered teaching [2]. This is the problem faced by many of us pharmacology teachers in a medical school setting. This problem arises because many of us who are basic scientists do not understand the role pharmacology plays in medical practice. To date, how to help students understand the knowledge of drugs and to use drugs correctly in patients may be an important project to be demonstrated.

185.2 Traditional Methods in Teaching Pharmacology

Traditional methods of pharmacology training for most medical students concentrates more on theory than on practice. The material is often drugs centred and focuses on indications and side effects of different drugs. However, in clinical practice the reverse approach has to be taken, from the diagnosis to the drugs. In addition, most patients vary in age, gender, size and sociocultural characteristics, all of which may affect treatment choices. Moreover, patients also have their own perception of appropriate treatment and should be fully informed partners in therapy. All of this is not always taught in medical schools, where the number of hours spent on therapeutics may be low compared to traditional pharmacology teaching. Although the students whose taught by traditional teaching methods acquired the basic pharmacological knowledge, practical skills remain weak. For example, the traditional teaching methods induced undergraduate students in many medical schools, learn little about the therapeutic use of drugs and even when them became doctors after graduation rely too much on the promotional efforts and information from the pharmaceutical industry. In order to solve these problems, the teaching methods in pharmacology need to be rethink. In this section, we focus on the application of some traditional teaching methods of pharmacology, although there are many deficiencies in helping students to understand the relationship between drugs, diseases and patients.

As we know, medical education is being performed either in "classical" way (lecture based learning, LBL) or in a more advanced form incorporating other teaching approaches, such as problem based learning (PBL) [3–6]. In the classical way of education, the teacher has a leading position and students passively accept information offered (The traditional teaching method is shown in Fig. 185.1). Thus, various teaching methods are furnished in pharmacology lectures. Compared with LBL, the PBL provides the opportunities for students to participate in the teaching and learning activities. The core of PBL is group discussion, with a typical group of 25 students. The teacher will give a case briefing and then a question is forwarded. The students will speak in turn to address the question. PBL puts emphasis on self study and there after training in discussions on drug choice and treatment of the patient described in the case during seminars. Teacher plays the role of a discussion facilitator and coordination in making up a pharmacotherapeutical plans. Additionally, animations are also used to illustrate the mechanism of drugs, making the abstracts lively and easy to understand.

Furthermore, computer-aided multimedia teaching is extensively used in all aspects in pharmacology teaching. By the help of computer technology, e-resources on pharmacology are increasingly to support or replace traditional teaching methods. By the help of information, general strategies about how teachers can get information from web sites and how to use the information successfully have been provided in some universities. However, multimedia courseware in aid of blackboard is the common way of teaching with lower involvement of student creativity.

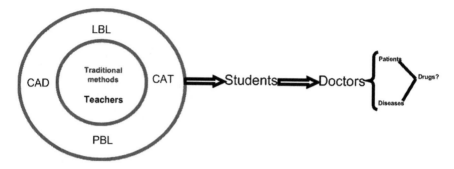

Fig. 185.1 Traditional teaching method in pharmacology. *LBL* lecture based learning; *PBL* problem based learning; *CAT* computer assisted teaching; *CAD* computer assisted learning

All in all, in the last two decades a number of educational programs have been developed to improve the teaching and learning of pharmacology and therapeutics. The World Health Organization (WHO) action programme on essential drugs has developed a manual for undergraduate medical students on the principles of rational prescribing [7]. Students are taught about a standard pharmacotherapeutic approach to common disorders resulting in a set of first choice drugs, called personal or P-drugs. They are also taught how to personalize the set of P-Drugs to specific patients. The student should also be able to solve therapeutic problems, prescribe appropriate drugs for disease conditions and communicate meaningfully with the patients. These methods provide us the new ideas in our novel pharmacology teaching methods.

185.3 Creative Approaches in Teaching Pharmacology

Gaining knowledge and at the same time applying this knowledge in practice is essential for learning in general and, presumably, also for the development of treatment scripts by medical students. This so-called context-learning seems to be more effective in many ways than sequential learning, in which learning and applying knowledge is separated. The positive effect can be explained by theories from cognitive psychology and medical problem-solving. These theories suggest that the way in which knowledge is stored in the brain is essential for its recall and application. Therefore, storing pharmacotherapeutic knowledge in combination with the situation in which this knowledge will be applied benefits the speed and quality with which the information is recalled. However, our traditional teaching methods could not solve above problems effectively. The innovation and reform of the teaching methods of pharmacology in countries around the world is continuing to explore.

In short, our students could not use pharmacology knowledge effectively in clinical application because of traditional teaching methods excessively emphasized the basic theories and knowledge of medicine. In theory, with the continuous progress of drug synthesis, screening technology, new drugs continue to emerge, so medicine theory and its pharmacology knowledge update are very rapidly. To be sure, the drugs targets of human diseases and drugs are constant in a certain period of time. Our creative teaching methods in present study guided students focusing on the diseases and typical drugs targets and helped them to finding a link "bridge" between from numerous drugs and their complex interactions with diseases. While, this "bridge" is the drugs targets which are regulated by drugs and are constant in a certain period of time.

Therefore, the aim of our creative method is to help students learning drugs targets and their pharmacological theories in teaching, and to guide students to classify the drugs targets according to the similar effects and distribution in body, to let more students be inspired and encouraged to learning pharmacology knowledge. Since the computer is a useful tool for both teaching and learning in medical education. Furthermore, we will cooperate with Institute of Information Science and Technology of Ningbo University in China to development a computer controlled diseases simulation (including male and female models respectively). This computer simulation will show different manifestations and characteristics of clinical diseases and automatic program of computer will automatically analyze what drugs targets may relate to these diseases, which typical drugs will be selected and also including the administration methods, dosage, and matters needing attention of these drugs. Our current creative teaching methods in pharmacology are shown in Fig. 185.2.

Similarly, in order to adapt to this new teaching methods, our evaluation system and examination activities will also be carried out reforms. We will provide the patients information from the hospital as the test, to ask the students making decision what drugs should be treatment on these patients, why use it, how to use it and what is the matters needing attention? So our examination will guide students from diseases, to search drug targets and find out the appropriate drugs according to the drug targets. In order to compare the teaching effects between traditional methods and our present creative methods in teaching pharmacology. Our study was carried out among the third semester medical students at Ningbo University Medical School. Twenty male students were randomly divided into two groups,

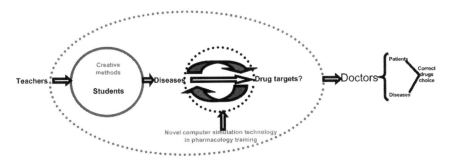

Fig. 185.2 Our current creative teaching method in pharmacology

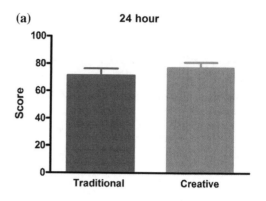
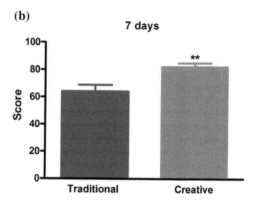

Fig. 185.3 Compare with traditional and creative teaching methods in pharmacology

they were taught by using the traditional teaching methods and our innovative teaching methods the chapter of antihypertensive drugs respectively. 24 h later the traditional pharmacology exam was conducted and the creative exam which including a large number of application knowledge was also performed 7 days later. As shown in Fig. 185.3, the mean subject score in traditional exam was no significantly difference between two groups (Students t-test, $P > 0.05$) indicating both these two teaching methods showed similar effects in helping students to learn basic knowledge of pharmacology. However, the mean subject score treated by our novel teaching methods was significantly higher compared to the students taught by traditional methods (Students t-test, $P < 0.01$, Fig. 185.3). Our present data demonstrated that our creative teaching methods in pharmacology can improve the long-term memory of knowledge and also the application ability in students. In addition, compared with our novel evaluation system, traditional testing methods limited the scope of testing student learning, and equally important, is of limited value for guiding student learning. Our current examination activities may be one the promising approaches to measure student's application of pharmacology knowledge in clinical treatments.

Given that problem-oriented teaching can help students appreciate the relevance of the acquired information for appropriate prescribing and problem-based learning (PBL) has been gaining ground in medical education. Our novel teaching methods in pharmacology dose not negate these traditional teaching methods. Correspondingly, traditional teaching methods will also be selectively adopted when using the novel teaching approaches. We believe that this comprehensive teaching methods will make up for the defects of traditional teaching methods cannot guide the clinical application effectively.

Acknowledgments This work was supported by Teaching Research Project of Ningbo University (To Dr. Chuang Wang in 2013).This project also sponsored by K. C. Wong Magna funded at Ningbo University.

References

1. Joshi A, Trivedi M (2010) Innovations in pharmacology teaching. Int J Pharm Biomed Res 1(2):62–64
2. Li W, Zhang Y, Zhang C, Zhang X (2004) Pharmacology teaching and its reform in China. Acta Pharmacol Sin 25(9):1233–1238
3. Barrows HS (1985) How to design a problem-based curriculum for the preclinical years. Springer, New York
4. Michel MC, Bischoff A, Heringdrof MZ, Newmann D, Jokobs KH (2002) Problem versus lecture based pharmacology teaching in a German medical school. Naunyn Schmiedbergs Arch Pharmacol 366:64–68
5. Feng GQ, Fu RF, Wang ZJ (2003) Preliminary study and application in pharmacology teaching with learning oriented method. Chin Pharmacol 20:16
6. Barrows HS (1994) Practice-based learning: problem-based learning applied to medical education. Southern Illinois University School of Medicine, Springfield, p 145
7. De Vries TGPM, Henning RH, Hogerze HV, Fersle DF (1994) Guide to good prescribin. World Health Organization, Geneva

Chapter 186
Problems and Counterplans of College English Independent Study Under Network Environment

Zhai Fengjie

Abstract Since the teaching reform of college English, English teaching in Chinese universities has been challenged by many new problems which are now compelling Chinese universities to carry out student-oriented independent network environment English study models. Through the methodology of comparative study, this article intends to analyze the existing problems and the corresponding reasons in the network environment college English independent study process, and to offer practical counterplans for the problems to enhance the English learning ability of Chinese college students.

Keywords Network environment · College english · Independent study · Counter plans

Independent network environment English learning plays a significant role in college English teaching of Chinese universities, the enormous information flow generated by which could make available more round-way teacher-to-student communication opportunities and timely feedback channels for college English teachers. But it has been a well accepted fact that the students' independent learning efficiency is generally below expectation in the practices of independent learning and teaching in recent years. To analyze the reasons of these problems and take appropriate measures to help improve the application of independent network Environment College English learning is, therefore, of great significance for Chinese universities.

Z. Fengjie (✉)
International College, Tianjin University of Technology and Education,
No.1310, Dagunan Road, Tianjin, Hexi District 300222, China
e-mail: zhaifengjie@yahoo.com.cn

186.1 The Importance of Network Independent Learning

Network independent learning in college English teaching and application is a huge change to the way of college English teaching in China. This is embodied not only in students' English learning styles and learning ability, but also in performance on the changes in the way of teachers' English teaching. This function displays in the following respects.

186.1.1 Network Independent Learning Stimulates Learning Motivation and Enhance Efficacy

Self-efficacy refers that the individual believes that he has the ability to complete some or certain kinds of tasks, which is the concrete embodiment of individual ability and the confidence in certain activities. It is firstly put forward by American psychologist Bandura, it is the important motivated factor which affects independent learning. It affects not only students' academic target selection, but also their learning strategy choice, thus having an important impact on their academic performance. Traditional ways of English teaching make students in a passive knowledge receiver location, which is difficult to arouse the enthusiasm and initiative of students learning, so it not only cause students to lose interest in learning English, but also affects the enthusiasm of learning English. It also causes students to regard English learning goal orientation as the examination, therefore, leading students to loss self-efficacy of English learning. Under the network of English independent learning, students are learning initiative and executors and they need to monitor the whole process of their own learning activities, thus arousing the students' learning initiative and enthusiasm.

186.1.2 Network Independent Learning Optimizes Learning Methods and Improves Efficiency

As a foreign language, English learning means mastering not only the vocabulary, grammar and some basic declarative knowledge learning, but also comprehensive mastery of procedural knowledge such as oral English, reading comprehension, listening comprehension, and writing. Compared with the traditional English teaching methods, network independent learning can fully combines the dual advantages which are independent learning and networked computer learning center, providing the new learning environment and conditions, and provides the way and method of teaching and learning to reform the current college English study mode, which develops the new learning mode of English learning declarative knowledge such as vocabulary, grammar and oral English, listening and writing and other comprehensive procedural knowledge to a comprehensive development.

186.1.3 The Network Independent Learning can Change the Role of Teachers in Teaching

In the traditional way of teaching, teachers' role is to teach, supervise and guide the students' learning management. Because the network independent learning requires the independence of the learners to learn under network and intelligent teaching of teachers, thus, it makes teachers free from teaching and management in English language teaching, but focusing more on guiding and advising of students learning. And this kind of work center of gravity change promotes the specialization of teachers and the transformation of teacher's role.

186.2 The Problems Existing in the Network Independent Learning Mode

186.2.1 The Low Time Utilization Rate of Students Learning

Under the premise of guaranteeing the Internet time, during the practice it is found that students don't have much time for effective learning on the Internet, some students often watch online courses, chatting or watching video program in systems. In the long run, learning goals cannot be completed and learning quality cannot be guaranteed.

186.2.2 Low Rate of Learning Resources Utilization

In the network independent learning, the learning resources mainly refers to the network courses, courseware, online teaching information, online training, and other network resources, including teachers review submissions, face-to-face tutoring, etc. Therefore, network independent learning can be regarded as "controlled" independent learning. Many students cannot adapt to this way, they treat the network course learning as traditional classroom lectures, which only focus on facts and conclusions, but not good at using a variety of learning tools.

186.2.3 Low Self Evaluation of Learners

The network learners in their learning evaluation is not high, some students think network independent learning is equal to the traditional teaching mode of interaction between teachers and students, study pressure is not obvious and they are vulnerable to outside interference. Because of the bigger allure of network, the less learning support they can get, the quality of their learning progress and learning is not satisfactory.

The reason of unsatisfactory network independent learning effect of some students is because of the lack of metacognition and learning strategies. Metacognitive processing is learners' internal information, it is learners' awareness of their own thinking, it plays planning, monitoring and regulating role in learning and is the key to acquire and improve learning skills. It is also strategies of any set of specific learning process, collectively known as metacognitive learning strategy, which generally includes self-monitoring, self-directed, self assessment and self adjusting, etc.

Self-monitoring strategies is the process of learners to use some standards to assess their learning, in order to adjust learning method and ability to achieve goals. Network learners generally lack the ability in reality. The richness of network information and the convenience to access, on the one hand, provides convenience for learners, on the other hand, brings difficulties to those learners who have poor self-control. Poor self-control ability makes them out of the direction of the study, reducing the efficiency of learning. Meanwhile under the influence of the bad information of network, they are lost in the network virtual space and can't help themselves, resulting in a decline of thinking ability and weaker resolution on their information consciousness and ability.

Self-directed strategy is that learners use written or oral forms to present the learning process or method, in order to instruct, guide, supervise and urge their learning. Network learning has less class tension or teachers' supervise and check. Facing more electronic data easily makes learners to ignore self-direction, thus reducing the learning efficiency.

Self-assessment strategy is the ability of learners to evaluate their own learning and feedback ability, which is one of the keys to the ongoing of the independent learning. The traditional face-to-face teaching is usually examined and evaluated by school. In independent learning, learners are completely responsible for their own learning and to evaluate the learning process and results. Due to the former traditional education mode and the habit of relying on others for a long time to assess the effects, most network learners are not good at independent self-study and not active in learning every sector of self assessment, which leads to the result that study cannot verified timely, and the difficulties and problems in study could not be found and solved in time, thus influencing the learning efficiency.

186.3 Strategies to Improve the Ability of Network Independent Learning of College Students

Analyses by synthesis, to solve these problems hindering the development of the networked independent English learning, improving the college English independent learning ability should strive to do the following.

186.3.1 To Strengthen Independent Learning Consciousness and Improve Learning Ability

For network independent English learning, students should master the methods of independent learning and resolve all sorts of problems hindering the independent learning by themselves. The core of independent learning is democracy, and it relies on the self-reflection, the ability of self monitoring and self evaluation during their self independent learning. To improve the ability, the first is to create independent learning environment, let students have the perception of success and happiness from English learning, and fully mobilize students' learning initiative and enthusiasm, thus strengthening students' independent learning awareness, dispelling the fear of learning from psychological angle which students focus on the traditional teaching mode, and improving the students' self-efficacy.

To improve students' English independent learning ability is a long-term project, which not only builds a correct understanding of English learning for students, but also improves learning self-efficacy. It also needs the students to fully understand their learning ability, on the basis of the efforts to strengthen their learning ability. Under the guidance of teachers and network independent learning system, students need to master the basic knowledge and skills of English learning, gain the strategy of English independent learning, on the basis of self reflection, self monitoring and self evaluation and improve their learning of metacognitive level.

186.3.2 To Strengthen the Guidance and Management of Students' Independent Learning

The improvement of student's independent learning ability requires not only the students' hard-working, but also the supervision and guidance of teachers. Students' English learning under the network environment and their acquisition of learning strategies usually depends on the initial supervision and guidance of teachers. To be specific, in the network of English independent learning, teachers should make full use of computer multimedia interaction and networked characteristics, and ask students to combine their actual level and interest to choose corresponding information into the study. Monitor student's learning in their study and fully play the auxiliary role of solving students' problems and difficulties. Organize students to conduct effect evaluation after learning, self evaluate firstly, and then communicate the learning experience to produce symbiotic effect. Advocate on the basis of independent learning to strengthen extensive exchanges and cooperation between students, between teachers and students. Learn the excellent experience from others under the condition of network independent learning and change the incorrect study method in order to provide necessary conditions and power for improving the whole English learning results.

186.3.3 To Improve the Course Content and Optimize Software and Hardware Facilities

For the course editor of independent learning, to revise and improve network course is their responsibility in the network independent learning. Specifically, it requires giving priority to student-orientation in curriculum design and teaching materials model, which should be from the learner's psychological characteristics and conform to the guiding ideology of independent learning, be simple and readable. At the same time, universities should gradually establish and improve the support service system of independent learning to provide support services to meet the needs of the students' independent learning by the forms of telephone, E-mail, audio-visual reading rooms.

Finally, it is critical to strengthen system construction and complete the teaching support service work, because any teaching reform requires the support of entire school teaching system. In order to successfully implement independent learning mode, universities should establish the perfect teaching support service system, teaching management system and quality assurance system with a corresponding of evaluation system, rewarding and punishment system. By comparison, achieve the implementation of teaching management and teaching support scientific institutionalization, standardization and ensure the coordinated and orderly work manner of all departments.

References

1. Gu yueguo M (2004) Network education study. Foreign Language Teaching and Research Press, Beijing
2. Tian Zhihui C (2001) College english teaching proceeding. Beijing Broadcasting Institute Press, Beijing
3. Wu Jinye M (2001) Contemporary chinese language teaching methodology. Henan University Press, Henan
4. Xiang Erlan J (2009) Network independent learning and college oral english classroom teaching. J North China Electr Power Univ
5. Xu Jinfen M (2007) Theory and practice of college foreign language independent learning. China Social Science Press, Beijing

Chapter 187
Integrity Verification of Cloud Data

Fan-xin Kong and Li Liu

Abstract This paper proposes a new program on the integrity of the data to the probabilistic methods when the number of documents inserted the pseudo-tuple becomes large. In this program, pseudo-tuple inserted in accordance with different particle size were signed. And a user constructs a new type of data structure. In order to ensure normal conversation between the user and the cloud at the same time, this paper uses a challenge-response mechanism. Then a user uses this new data structure to verify its integrity in the client.

Keywords Cloud computing · Pseudo-tuple · Data integrity · Signature

187.1 Introduction

With the rapid development of the information industry, more and more enterprise and users like to put data to the third party for save and management. Cloud computing is generated with this requirement because it can solve the rising costs of storage. Cloud computing is a new computing model, which enables users to easily access on-demand data resources. In the case of high storage devices, the data update rate is also rising. In addition to reducing storage costs, we reduce the maintenance costs of the data. To the data stored in the data center by the user, you can enjoy high-quality applications and services. This can bring the following benefits: (1) reducing the burden of storage; (2) access to data from geographic

---

F. Kong (✉) · L. Liu
School of Information Science and Engineering, China Shandong Provincial Key Laboratory for Novel Distributed Computer Software Technology, Shandong Normal University, Jinan, China
e-mail: xiaoshantianzi@163.com

L. Liu
e-mail: liuli_790209@163.com

space constraints; (3) reduction of maintenance costs [1]. However, due to the special nature of the cloud environment, the user can not manage their own data stored directly, resulting a series of security problems. For example, security issues of confidentiality, availability and integrity, and so on, where Integrity is the most basic problem of theirs [2]. The data integrity is to ensure that the real data from the data owner.

Currently, many researchers have done a lot of work on the integrity of the data. For example,[1] Sion put forward a challenge to the agreement to ensure that the service providers to perform user query [3]. But its security and correctness can not be guaranteed, because the service provider can modify the return results. Ateniese G proposed the POR method for testing data integrity [4]. Shachamd et al improved the POR and they put forward the Minato-POR program using BLS signatures gathered to generate a constant the certification value [5].

Xie Min et al. put forward integrity verification program of outsourced database based on probability [6]. To some special tuples mixed in data, when queried, these monitoring tuples will be returned with a certain probability in program. However, for many applications, it has an obvious deficiency: audit on the integrity of the data, it must be stored in the client with all of these insertion of pseudo-tuple. With the increase in the data file stored in the cloud, pseudo-tuple that will increase result in occupying a lot of space in the client. To address this issue, this paper designs a new program of cloud data integrity testing. First, overall pseudo-tuple is signed. Then its re-grouping is signed. Client sends the challenge value for querying to the tuple that are needed to verify. Its validate the results returned in the structure of the new data structure. Their returned results will be validated in new data structure we construct in this paper.

187.2 Program Introduction

187.2.1 Related Concepts

Homomorphism certification: the nature of Homomorphism certified: the data blocks that are m_i and m_j are signed, then we obtain their signature that are P_{m_i} and P_{m_j}. We obtain $P_{m_i+m_j}$ of the data blocks $m_i + m_j$ by P_{m_i} and P_{m_j} calculated.

In this paper, the pseudo-tuple of each file will be signed, then its signature T_{m_i} is obtained. At last, overall pseudo-tuple is signed. We obtain its signature T_0. When the tasks of authentication are doing, user sends a challenge value (i, h_i) that is random to cloud. However, this challenge value is used to challenge the tuples of file. Here, i is a random value, h_i is corresponding to i.

Bilinear map: $G_1 \times G_2 \rightarrow G_T$, here, G_1 and G_2 is additive group. G_T is multiplicative cyclic group. The map has (1) efficient computational; (2) bilinear $e(h_1^a, h_2^b) = e(h_1, h_2)^{ab}$; (3) non-degenerate $e(g_1, g_2) \neq 1$, $g_1 \in G_1$, $g_1 \in G_1$.

187.2.2 Construction of the Data Structure

Merkel hash tree is a balanced binary tree. The depth of tree is very high and cost of construction and inquiry is large. Li et al. combine *Merkle* with $B+$ (MB) to improve verification efficiency. This paper will use this data structure. But we do not begin from the whole tree for verification, but from partial validation. This partial validation is similar to MB that is built. All pseudo-tuple signature (total signatures) is stored in root node. The branch node store its signature when file is cut many blocks. Technology of homomorphism authentication is used for this data structure.

Service providers will only return the query results and the corresponding node value when the user queries. When the verification begins, we query from the root. If the value of the root node is the same to the return to the values, we believe the data integrity. Otherwise, we believe the data that is incomplete. The signature value of the pseudo-tuple that is inserted into all the files is stored in root node. In the query process, when we want to query the minimum validation tree, we do not need to traverse the entire tree. That is right what we only traverse the smallest tree.

187.2.3 Initialization

When user inserted pseudo-tuple in file, user puts pseudo-tuple signed. We take all pseudo-tuple as a single file F_0. We take the signature of pseudo-tuple inserted into each small file as a single file m_i. Then are shown in formula (187.1).

$$F_0 = (m_1, m_2, \ldots \ldots m_i, \ldots m_n) \quad (187.1)$$

We send their signature and tuple to cloud. Then client delete pseudo-tuple. We only store the signature of pseudo-tuple. According to the nature of the homomorphic certified, we cut file blocks. They are shown in formula (187.2).

$$F_0 = (F_{11}, F_{12}, \ldots \ldots F_{1n}) \quad (187.2)$$

n of the formula (187.2) is different from the formula (187.1).

Then, we cut file that has been cut into blocks step by step. For example:

$$F_{1i} = (F_{2i1}, F_{2i2}, \ldots \ldots F_{2in}) \quad (187.3)$$

and so on.

187.2.4 Integrity Test

The verification's process of data integrity is actually a complete chain of trust. In this scheme, it is divided into three phases: the preparation phase, the session stage, validation phase.

Preparation phase: A user uses a algorithm of key generation to generate a key and a private key. This algorithm of key generation is $KeyGen(\cdot)$. Their keys are (pk, sk). User signs the pseudo-tuple of each file. They are shown in formula (187.4).

$$t = F_{id}^{//} \, SSign_{sk}(F_{id}) \qquad (187.4)$$

Users run algorithm of validation tag that a verification value φ_i is generated by for each file.

When users send tuples to the cloud server, a user puts the collection of signature and verification value together to the server. And at the same time, a user deletes the pseudo tuple of the local and validation tag.

Session Stage: When we transfer data between cloud an integrity verification also is needed. Before the establishment of this process, we must firstly ensure consistent that data packet and signature is between users and DSP. In this process, the cloud needs to provide proof of query execution query for the data submitted by the user.

Firstly, a user submits a query Q, then we calculate its hash value $H(Q(m_i))$. Because the hash value has unidirectional and irreversibility. i is a challenge value of the query process.

Secondly, when DSP returns query results after DSP receives query a user submitted, DSP returns the corresponding response of i at the same time. To verify the data information will be also returned in session stage. Cloud server uses the public key for validation. If successful, F_{id} will be recovered. Otherwise, the validation is out. After receiving the challenge value, the server will use *Genproof* to generate evidence of replies.

Again, DSP returns query results user needs. This can be based on the return value of the response to determine whether the DSP is correctly execute the query or return the correct results.

Validation phase: During the session, the overall signature of the all files will be the first returned. When verification is running, according to a traversal method, the client start with the root node. If they are consistent, we believe that the data is complete. Otherwise, we return the session stage again for the next value of node. The client start verification from the child node of the root node again. And so on.

187.3 Performance Analysis

This paper will analyze the following aspects of the program.

Storage: First the client store the signature of the pseudo-tuple, not stored pseudo-tuples. The amount of storage became smaller than that we store pseudo tuple. At the same time, the pseudo-tuple is signed. So it is more safe that client stores signature of the pseudo-tuple than that client stores pseudo-tuple. The security of the data will been assured.

Communications: In this paper, a challenge—response mechanism is used in session between the user and the cloud. In addition to return the correct results in the query, traffic and bandwidth is relatively small. This is because its validation is not all tuples. The possession of the challenge value and their results of returning is not great and they are fixed constant value bits.

Verification: When validation begins, that is right that we only construct a minimum of a tree that based on need. We have no need to construct the whole tree. This will not only reduce the cost of storage but also improve the efficiency of query validation. When verification begins, we start from the root. It is not necessary to verify the whole tree. Even if a large number of files that are needed are large, its time of consumption is not great.

Computational complexity: In the conversation stage, the computational complexity between the customers and the server of challenges is $O(1)$. And the number of the file that the response of sever for challenge require is $O(1)$. In addition, the cost of the communication for a single challenge is $O(1)$. The complexity of the data block depending on the number of files is $O(n)$.

187.4 Conclusion

To ensure data integrity in the cloud computing, the program is put forward for insertion pseudo-tuple case. The program is for mass data, however, it is is not practical for the insertion of a single data file. This scheme can support the integrity of the data for testing with higher verification efficiency and lower the amount of storage. But the program also has shortcomings, for example, is only how to verify the integrity of data, not how to recover its integrity for the incomplete data.

Acknowledgments This work is supported by the National Science Foundation of China (No. 61170145), the Specialized Research Fund for the Doctoral Program of Higher Education of China (No. 20113704110001), the Natural Science Foundation of Shandong (No. ZR2010FM021) and the Taishan Scholar Project of Shandong, China.

References

1. Wang C, Ren K, LOU W et al (2010) Toward publicly auditable secuer cloud data storage services. IEEE Netw 24(4):19–24
2. Feng DG, Zhang M, Zhang Y et al (2011) Cloud computing security research. J Softw 22(1):71–83
3. Sion R (2005) Query execution assurance for outsourced databases. In: Proceedings of the 31st international conference on Very Large Data Bases (VLDB'05), Trondheim 30 Aug– 2 Sep 2005, pp 601–602
4. Ateniese G, Burns R, Curtmola R et al (2007) Provable data possession at untrusted stores. In: Proceedings of the 2007 ACM conference on computer and communications security, Whistler, pp 598–609
5. Shacham H, Waters B (2008) Compact proofs of retrievability. In: Proceedings of Asiacrypt 2008, Melbourne, pp 90–107
6. Xie M, Wang H, Yin J et al (2007) Integrity auditing of outsourced data. In: Proceedings of the 33rd international conference on Very Large Data Bases (VLDB07), Vienna, Austria, pp 782-793, 23–27 Sep 2007
7. Li FF, Hadjieleftheriou M, Kollios G et al (2006) Dynamic authenticated index structures for outsourced databases. In: Proceedings of ACM SIGMOD conference, pp 121–132

Chapter 188
Establishing Automotive Engineering School-Enterprise Practice Training Model Based on Excellent Engineer Plan

Geng Guo-qing, Zhu Mao-tao and Xu Xing

Abstract "Excellent Engineer Education and Training Plan" of the Ministry of Education is specially aimed at cultivating the students' capability of engineering practice and innovation. Aiming at the current situation of the engineering teaching, colleges should establish the modern engineering-practice center and cooperate with the major-related enterprises, and establish a series of teaching systems which serve the students through their entire learning period. This article explains the characteristics of the college-enterprise practice training center established by JiangSu University and NanJing Automobile Groups, pointing out that engineering elements and training projects should be mixed together in the process of practice base construction in order to completely improve students' engineering quality and engineering practice ability.

Keywords Excellent engineer · College-enterprise cooperation · Engineering practice · Automobile engineering

Introduction

"Excellent Engineer Education and Training Plan" of the Ministry of Education is aimed at fostering a large number of high-quality, innovative and various types of engineering and technical talents who are adaptive to the economic and social development, facing the industry, the world and the future. However, with the rapid growth of the domestic economy, higher education, especially, the engineering education cannot adjust itself to the economy development and the cultivated technical talents cannot meet the demands of the modern enterprises, which is bounded to the practice education of the engineering education [1, 2].

According to the survey and analysis, there are problems as follows existing in the current practice teaching:

G. Guo-qing (✉) · Z. Mao-tao · X. Xing
School of Automobile and Traffic Engineering, Jiangsu University, Zhengjinag 212013, China
e-mail: genguoqing1978@163.com

1. The uncertainties of practice bases and the decline of company's involvement. These years, companies are reluctant to receive college interns whose internship, they think, will disrupt the pace of normal producing, which leads to the frequent changes of interning bases and hinders the deep practice-teaching. This frustrates students' enthusiasm for interning and the students can hardly have a chance to take a deep practice [3].
2. Students 'enthusiasm for internship declines. Most of the internship, basically, centers in visiting and attending lectures. Because of the changing modes of students 'employment, this sort of internship reduces their enthusiasm for internship [4].
3. The disadvantages of interning in large group. The traditional way of internship is intensified internships, the advantage of which is conducive to management and the disadvantage of which is discouraging individualistic characteristics and reduces students' passion of improving the certain major-studying through internship.
4. The insufficient fund. Because of the increasing living cost and the low increase.

188.1 Excellent Engineer Training

"Excellent Engineer Plan" basically consists of three factors [5]:

1. Enterprises to participate deeply in the training;
2. To cultivate engineering talents according to general standards and industry standards;
3. To boost students' engineering and innovative abilities. This plan is focused on developing students' engineering practice and creative ability.

Jiangsu University was identified as the first batch of pilot colleges for the "Excellent Engineer Plan". Over years of exploring and practice, to carryout the plan has been deemed as a vital important chance to its development and application of teaching method. In terms of the current situation of practice teaching in higher education, the Jiangsu local economy and social development, Jiangsu University has regulated the teaching contents and the teaching method based on realities of our auto major development in order to boost students' engineering practice abilities, creative abilities and global competence. We also have built practice centers for the outstanding engineering talents to explore the new approaches.

188.2 Enterprise Engineering Practice

The enterprise engineering practice needs the participation of college, enterprise and college student. In order to minimize the gap between talent-cultivating in tertiary education and enterprises' demands, Jiangsu University and NanJing Auto enterprise have established a complete set of experimenting and teaching project with its own strength so as to develop high-quality and comprehensive engineering people who have an extensive of knowledge. This project is aimed at strengthening engineering practice capability, engineering designing capability and engineering creative capability. With all these means, a new mode will be carried out that enterprise play a major role, supplemented by colleges. Based on the general standards and industry standards, college reforms its teaching methods and, finally, strengthens students' engineering ability and innovation.

188.2.1 Objectives of the Engineering Practice Center

According to the objectives: sharing, mutual interaction, quality priority", the plan of outstanding talents-cultivating should be given the priority and we should work hard to make this center become the first class one for the cultivation of engineering talents.

Sharing—engineering practice educational center is built by Jiangsu University and NanJing auto enterprise. We work together to build the center, establish the quality-supervision systems, write the textbooks, construct the teaching staff and so on. The built center will not only for the cultivation of engineering practice educational center but also for further improvements and opening up to the world.

Mutual interaction—college and enterprise take the best of their advantages and resources to compensate the other side's weakness. College uses its researching staff to provide the needed technologies and talents while the enterprise assists in the cultivation of more creative young teaching staff that has a strong ability in practice.

Quality priority—the best educational secrecies from both should be given priority in the construction of the center. College send the best students and the best teaching staff for the training and researching while the enterprise primarily supplies the best accommodations, studying surroundings and the first-class teaching facilities and field.

188.2.2 Excellent Engineer Training Practice in Enterprise

188.2.2.1 Construct the Multi-Function and Enterprise-College Platforms for the Automobile Engineering Practice Education

Guided by the instruction of large-scale engineering education and the improvements of students' engineering practice capability, along with the comprehensive capability, we build the new training system of open higher education based on college-enterprise cooperation. The system is characterized by its multi-education styles, which help the students to reach the top of their researching field.

188.2.2.2 Creat Combined-Training Mechanism for College and Enterprise

The connotation for college-enterprise cooperation training students is to set training goals, build course-teaching system, carry out training procedures, assess talent-cultivating quality all together. It may take undergraduate about one year to study in enterprises, learning the advanced technologies and company cultures, carrying out engineering practice, participating in the technology reforms and engineering-developing, which develop their occupational spirit and moral.

188.2.2.3 Build High Level Engineering Teaching Staff

In order to achieve the goal, the teaching faculties are required to have experiences of engineering practice, some of who should be qualified with certain working years in enterprise. We invite engineers with rich practical and management experience as part-time teachers from NanJin Automobile Group, professional courses teaching task; Or as a tutor to guide the graduations' design tasks.

188.2.2.4 Create the Practice-Teaching Condition

Instructed by the idea that what we are practicing now is what we are facing in the future work, we are exploring the new mode of college-enterprise cooperation to construct an engineering internship center that has the best equipments of auto major, the high quality resource-sharing platform and closely follows the main trend of technology-developing. The center is also aimed at teaching, scientific researching, training, technology-development and we believe by importing enterprise technology, introducing talents, capita and management, can the students' engineering practice be ensured.

188.2.2.5 Reform Curriculum System and Teaching Method

According to the standards, the curriculum system and teaching contents should be reformed to boost students' engineering designing capability and engineering creating capability, along with the cultivation of multi-talents. Based on the study of existing problems, projects and cases, their innovative ability should be improved and they are capable of writing essays all by themselves. Five types of curriculums and eight types of characteristic textbooks and their supporting courseware will be done during the vital construction of the vehicle engineering, forming a platform for resources-sharing.

188.2.2.6 Design Standard System and Assessing System for Excellent Engineering Plan

Combined with the college-running orientation, college's characteristic specialties, talent-cultivating objectives, and the demands of the outstanding talent plan, our college' cultivating system will be based on the general criterion and industry criterion.

The systems and plans will be open to the whole society, providing information and receiving supervision. The quality-assessing system of the center will refer to the global general practice and global criterion to assess the quality of involved majors.

188.3 Conclusion

China's tertiary education, especially, the engineering education, has failed to keep pace with the economy-developing, but with the implementation of the "excellent engineer plan", students' engineering practice ability, creating ability and international competence will surely be improved, boosting the development of higher engineering education. As the first batch of pilot colleges, University of JiangSu will continuously explore and perfect this new mode of cultivating engineering-teaching talents by deep cooperation between college and enterprise, which fosters a great many engineering talents in different fields who are innovative and adaptive to the development of economy and society.

Through years of exploration and practice, as well as the work of "class of the outstanding engineers" in grade 2008 and 2009, we have built the structure of practice-teaching for vehicle major and achieved good results. Students trained in the center are warmly welcomed by the society and companies because of their basic individual qualities, solid foundation of theoretical knowledge, and practical ability. So this new mode is indeed an excellent approach to develop students' engineering practice and creative capability, making student foster a good sense of professionalism, engineering quality, a correct concept of self-value and employment, which shuts the needed-capability gap between graduates and skilled workers.

References

1. Hui J-Z, Cao J, et al (2010) Modern engineering training center of innovation experimental area of exploration and practice. Res Explor Lab 29(3):111–113
2. Ye Z-P ,Jin P-H (2007) China engineering education practical teaching research. High Eng Educ Res 4:74–77
3. Zhang G-L , Gao J-J, et al (2007) Necessity of engineering education reform based on engineering graduate status and enterprise needs. Exp Technol Manage 24(8):112–114

4. Luo Z-X (2008) Engineering education professional certification and its impact on practice teaching in colleges and universities. Res Explor Lab 27(6):1–3
5. Ji F, Gao F, et al (2009) Improve the "automobile structure", quality of teaching. High Educ Forum 9(9):67–69

Chapter 189
Mechanical Finite Element Analysis to Two Years Old Children's Orbital-Bone Based on CT

Jing liu, He Jin, Tingting Ning, Beilei Yang, Juying Huang and Weiyuan Lu

Abstract It is common that children whose one eyeball is smaller than the other or with one eyeball missing develop facial asymmetry at the Clinical Ophthalmology. In order to seek effective intervention strategies for the children, we study the developmental enginery of children's orbital-bone and the influence factor of biomechanics. We set up the model which based on 2-year-old children's orbital-bone CT images. The model is prepared for further biomechanics analysis. There are several reports for orbital-bone nowadays. However, most of them are concerned about adults instead of children who are in period of blooming growth, especially 2-year-old.

Keywords Children's orbital · Mechanics parameter · Establishment

189.1 Introduction

Nowadays, it frequently occurs in the clinics of ophthalmology that a child becomes malformed in his/her face because of the smallness in one eye or the lack of one eyeball. This malformation severely affects the appearance of the subject. Research data shows that the normal development of maxillofacial region has close positive correlation with orbital development [1]. Anson Chau et al. pointed out that the size of the eyeball affects the development of the orbital volume, and the effect is far more significant in children in development stage than in adults [1].

T. Ning · B. Yang · J. Huang · W. Lu (✉)
Institute of biological medicine engineering, Capital Medical University, Beijing 100069, China
e-mail: lusnow@ccmu.edu.cn

J. liu · H. Jin
Institute of Basic Medicine, Capital Medical University, Beijing 100069, China

Besides, more investigations showed that the development of orbital volume also relates to the age. The study by Robert et. al. showed that the orbital volume of 0–15 years old children and adolescents increase with age, and the speed attains its maximum during the age of 0–5 [1–4]. Therefore, effective intervention should be applied when the children's orbital part is at its peak development. For this purpose, we use software Mimics to build a model based on CT images, aiming at the orbital–bone of 2-year-old healthy children, and use finite element analysis (FEA) package ANSYS to do some biomechanical analysis.

Presently, there are several reports on orbital modeling and mechanical FEA, most of them, however, are pertaining to adults instead of children, especially 2-year-old, who are in period of rapid growth.

189.2 Modeling

Mimics is an interactive medical image control system developed by Materialise. It is a highly integrated and easy-to-use 3D image generating and editing software, which can import various scanning data (CT, MRI), build and edit 3D models, and export them in generic CAD (Computer Aided Design), FEA or RP (Rapid Prototyping) formats. With Mimics, large scale of data conversion can be made on a PC [5].

189.2.1 Materials

CT images of a two years old child that contain the orbital parts are provided by TongRen Hospital. This data comes from the CT scan of the subject head with a Philips Brilliance 64 CT scanner. The acquisition setup is as follows: tube voltage 140 kV, MAS 256 mA·s^{-1}, slice thickness 0.313 mm, window width 4,000 Hu, window center 700 Hu. In total, 515 coronal images, 515 sagittal images and 150 axial images are acquired. The resolution is 512×512. The data output is stored in DICOM (Digital Imaging and Communications in Medicine) format and recorded in CD-Rom.

The Mimics software is purchased by School of Biological medicine engineering, Capital Medical University.

189.2.2 Modeling

- The following rules have been observed in the modeling:

    1. Accuracy: the model matches the actual physiological structure.

2. Simplicity: some minor structures that do not pose significant influence on the analysis are abandoned for the convenience of subsequent mechanical analysis.
3. Intactness: no holes should exist in the model, thus, the sclerotin in the ethmoidal plate of the orbital wall is thickened a little bit in the modeling. The reason is that the output from Mimics should be a complete closed surface. However, the sclerotin in the ethmoidal plate of the orbital wall is extremely thin and with lots of holes which are difficult to process, may emerge when reconstructed. Therefore, the sclerotin of this part is slightly thickened to avoid the generation of holes in the process of smoothing.

- Selected proper thresholds (the default lower and upper thresholds for bone are 226 and 2796, respectively). Data are imported after noise is eliminated using region growth.
- The 3D model is built [6–8].

189.3 Settings of the Mechanical Parameters in ANSYS Analysis

The ANSYS package is a multi-purpose computer design program for FEA, which can be used for the problems of structure, fluid, electricity, electromagnetic field and collision. The package provides interface to most CAD software and data communication & exchange is easy to accomplish. The first thing to use ANSYS package to perform biomechanical analysis for the two-year-old healthy child's orbital part after the modeling with Mimics is to set proper mechanical parameters. But the relevant mechanical parameter was hard to find, so a lot of work had be done on finding proper parameters. Then we used ANSYS package to do preliminary mechanics FEA.

189.3.1 Settings of Mechanical Parameters

After surveying, we found that there was no available relevant mechanical parameter of analysis for this particular type of subject. It is necessary to do iterative trials to find out the settings step by step [4, 8, 9]. The details are provided below.

1. Create a block in ANSYS whose length, width, and height are 3, 3, and 1, respectively. After query and exploration, we finally set the elastic modulus to $1.37 * 10^{10}$ Pa, and Poisson's ratio to 0.35. Constraints for all directions are applied to the underside of the block, and a 10 Pa pressure is applied from the above. After these, we enter the solver.

2. Double the height of the model, and then calculate the stress and strain on the surface points of the block.
3. Decrease the elastic modulus and observe the resulting stress and strain.
4. Set different Poisson's ratio, and observe the stress on the surface points of the block.
5. Input different pressure, and observe the stress and strain on the surface points of the block.

189.3.2 Progress of Mechanical Analysis

1. Import the ANSYS area files (*.lis) which exported from Mimics into ANSYS. Now, the model is a closed surface. Set up the type of analysis as structure analysis.
2. Set model material. This experiment ideally see orbit as uniform linear elastic material, setting unit types for solid45, elastic modulus for 13.7×10^9 Pa, Poisson's ratio of 0.2, density of 1.233 g·cm^{-3}. Due to the lack of children's data, the parameters comes from adult's which have been processed.
3. Body the closed surface.
4. Due to the complex and irregular model structure, we use intelligent method to meshing it into 73,600 units. As shown in Fig. 189.1.
5. According to the references, infant's orbital pressure is about 9.5 kPa. We exerted a 9.5 kPa surface pressure on the inner surface of the orbit, and applied constraints for all directions to the marginal points of the front and the back pole. As shown in Fig. 189.2.
6. Entering the solver.

189.3.3 Result

Make out the orbit-stress circle. As shown in Fig. 189.3.

From the picture, we can see that the stress differences between points are very small.

In order to find out the distinction between different areas of the orbital internal surface, we choose several points in different areas of the orbit, respectively, to observe the stress. It can be seen that the stress and strain of the inside area is slightly greater than the outside area, generally. And it is greater in the back area. All of them can be seen as sensitive areas.

189 Mechanical Finite Element Analysis

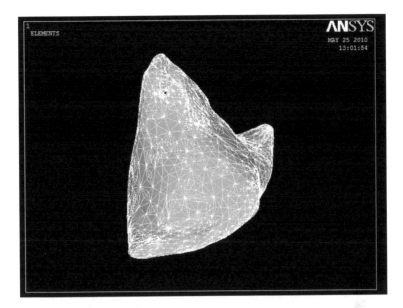

Fig. 189.1 Orbital model after meshing

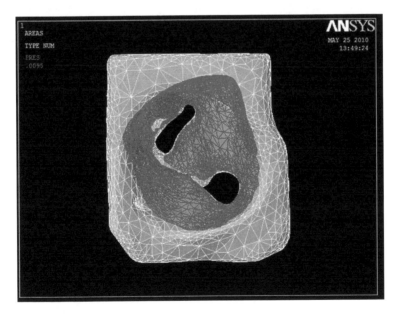

Fig. 189.2 Orbital models after meshing and applying constraints

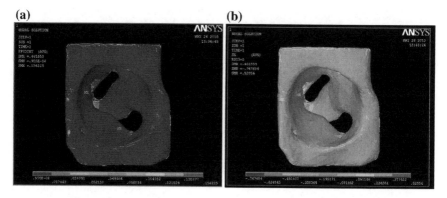

Fig. 189.3 The orbit-stress circle

189.4 Discussions and Analysis

Currently, there are reports on the modeling and mechanical FEA of adults' orbital region based on CT images, but no reports on children are presented before. The modeling of orbital region for children in the early stage of development is difficult because the sclerotin of some parts is extremely thin according to the structure of the orbital region, and no relevant mechanical parameters is available for reference. However, based on the iterative trials and exploration described above, it proves that they could be determined after the modeling with Mimics, which paves the way for later study.

During the analysis of 2 years old children's orbit by ANSYS, the stress differences between points in the image are pretty small, it is hard to show the sensitive area directly. This problem is maintained to be solved.

Acknowledgements He Jin is a coordinate first author. This work is supported by National Natural Science Foundation of China (Grant No.: 30900288), Funding Program for Academic Human Resources Development in Institutions of Advanced Education of Beijing (Grant No. PHR20100898), and Basic-Clinical Scientific Collaboration Fund of Capital Medical University (Grant No.: 2009JL06).

References

1. Uchio E, Ohno S, Kudoh K, Kadonosono K, Andoh K, KisielewiczL T (2001) Simulation of airbag impact on post-radial keratotomy eye using finite element analysis. J Cataract Refract Surg VOL 27 (11) : 1847–1853
2. Zhang G-d1, Tao S-x2, Mao W-y3, Chen J-q3, Luan X-g2, Zheng X-h4, Liao W-j1 (2010) Measurement of bone density based on three-dimensional reconstruction and finite element analysis. J Clinl Rehabilitative Tissue Eng Res Vol.14, No.9
3. Ge Li, et al. (2010) tThree-dimensional finite element analysis of the subtalar joint by mimics and ANSYS. J Math Med Vol. 23 No. 2

4. Zeng Pan (2007) Fundamentals of Finite Element Analysis. Tsinghua University Press, Beijing
5. Chen ZB, Wan L (2007) Modelling approaches for medical finite elements. J Clin Rehabilitative Tissue Eng Res Vol.11, No.31
6. Uchio E, Watanabe Y, Kadonosono K, Ma tsuoka Y, Goto S (2003) Simulation of airbag impact on eyes after photo refractive keratecto-my by finite element analysis method. Graefes Arch Clin Exp Ophthalmol 241(6):497–504
7. Tao L, Liangxian X, Wenbing T, Yubin C, Zhen T, Yinghui T (2012) Blast injuries to the human mandible: development of a finite element model and a preliminary finite element analysis. Injury, Int. J. Care Injured 43:1850–1855
8. AI-Sukhun J, Lindqvist C, Kontio R (2006) Modelling of orbital deformation using fnite element analysis. J R Soc Interface 3(7):255–2262
9. Escott EJ. Rubinstein D (2003) Free DICOM image viewing and processing software for your desktop computer:what's available and what it can do for you. Radiographics:A Review Publication of the Radiological Society of North America,Inc (5)

Chapter 190
Study on Digitalized 3D Specimen Making of Pathologic Gross Specimen Basing on Object Panorama

Ran Hua-quan, Jiang Jun and Zeng Zhao-fang

Abstract In order to solve the problem that traditional medical pathologic specimens are not convenient for preserving or teaching, this study proposes a new method of constructing digitalized 3D model of pathologic gross specimen with object panorama. This method firstly applies high-definition camera to shoot the photo of pathologic gross specimen in 360°, then processes the photos with software to achieve the digitalized 3D interactive display of the specimen. Research shows that this digital pathologic specimen can effectively retain the important medical information of the original specimen, and is very convenient for classroom teaching as well as E-learning.

Keywords Object panorama · Pathologic gross specimen · E-learning

190.1 Introduction

Pathological specimen derived from human tissue or organ is often used as an important source for medical teaching, medical treatment and scientific research. Especially in medical teaching, the pathological specimen has irreplaceable effect on pathological exhibition. As most pathological specimens are required from human beings, it produces large difficulties in obtaining them. Moreover, it takes heavy work and very long time to manufacture the specimens and makes serious loss of quantities of specimens during processing. Therefore, how to take fully advantage of specimen is always a thorny question for the pathology workers [1].

R. Hua-quan · J. Jun
Modern Education Technology Center, Chongqing Medical University, Chongqing 400016, China

Z. Zhao-fang (✉)
No.3, Yi Xue Yuan Road, Yuan Jia Gan, Yu Zhong Area, Chongqing 400016, People's Republic of China
e-mail: zeng000@126.com

At present, the traditional method is to take images of pathological gross specimen using photography technique and then digitize these images to store, thereby achieving the preliminary storage and transmission of pathological specimen [2, 3]. Yet, this method is limited as the photography displays merely the sites which are significant lesions rather than the overall view of the specimen, resulting in lose of some important information. Thus, we develop the method which can take images circularly in 360° by Object Panorama technique and can provide the simulation interactive features. We assume that this new method may effectively reduce the limitations of individual photography and largely improve the value-in-use of pathologic gross specimens.

190.2 Object Panorama Technique

As one of the panoramic techniques, Object Panorama Technique is also called Object VR. Panoramic Technique is a kind of virtual reality technology to generate realistic images using image-based rendering technology, which accomplishes the scene sweeping and object 3D display by piecing the images or photos together. Panoramic photography is one of the fastest growing image technologies on the Internet, although it cannot be called full 3D image technology, but it has been widely used based on that the on-site images are close to the real, the simulation camera panning can be dragged by mouse, and it has the virtual scene roaming function.

Object Panorama technique is mainly used to show the 3D images of the object, when taking the image, the camera targets on the object, turns the object rather than turn the camera, after rotates one angle, takes one image, and completes the images respectively. Object panorama software is used to process the images, and the level 360° rotation can be done by mouse drag to show the object's 3D panorama. At present, object panorama technique is mainly used in electronic commerce on the Internet for 3D display of goods such as handicrafts and electronic products, also it can be used for cultural relics and artwork appreciation [4, 5], but it has not yet been reported in the medical field in China. Regarding its characteristics, we can put the object panorama technique for object three-dimensional digital display in medical morphology.

190.3 3D Digital Production of Pathologic Gross Specimen

190.3.1 The Specimen Image Shooting Process

Materials: Camera with macro lenses (Canon 5D Mark II, 36×24 mm^2 CMOS, 21.1 million pixels), tripod (lifting and rotating tripod), scale (15 cm measurement), 2 illuminating lamps (500 W), background cloth (1 m^2 cotton cloth, strong contrast colors with specimen such as red, blue, cyan), pathologic gross specimen, special rotating table.

Primary treatment of specimen: blood stain or blot on the fresh specimen can be gently removed by gauze, the curing process can be used to make sure the specimen in the fixed location if the specimen was too soft, and the curing process was the same as the pathological gross specimen making process. The glass jar with specimen must be cleanly to ensure the transparency. When taking out of the pathological specimen and taking image, it cannot be squeezed to avoid damage. First removed the soak solution and absorbed the excessive water to avoid reflective phenomenon during shooting process.

Light source: the indoor photography was adopted in order to guarantee the stable light ray. Two illuminating lamps with 400–500 W were selected as light source, which can guarantee the specimen get enough light brightness and the light brightness in different points was no difference.

Shooting process: the specimen was placed in the special rotating table according to the human body normal anatomic position and fixed into the appropriate location by calibrated scale, and the dark cotton clot was taken as background. Set up dynamic close-up mode, fine image quality, resolution 4080 × 2720, JPEG format before taking images; According to the size of the pathological specimen, the specimen camera occupied the whole camera aperture by digital zoom, and the distance between lens and specimen was 40–70 cm in most cases; During the shooting process, first half pressed the shutter and then pressed to the bottom to avoid camera shake resulting in blurred images if quick pressed. The initial position of turn table was recorded during first shooting process, after taking one image, rotated the specimen 15° by turn table and continued taking images, and after rotating one cycle, total 24 images were taken, in other words, the specimen shooting process was finished. Consistent exposure should be noticed during shooting process [6, 7]. Figure 190.1 was a sequence of images.

190.3.2 Image Processing

Copied the photos into the computer, used the Photoshop software to modify the image resolution to be 800 × 600, then adjusted the brightness, contrast, hue etc. to ensure that the color effect of each photo was consistent to avoid the jumping view during image play. The lesion sites were marked with arrow on the images as required, then saved the images and set up the image quality to be "high". The original image files were about 2000 KB size, after software processing, the images were compressed to be 100 KB, because the compressed images were more easily to be transmitted on the Internet. But the compressed images should be guaranteed the basic read effect.

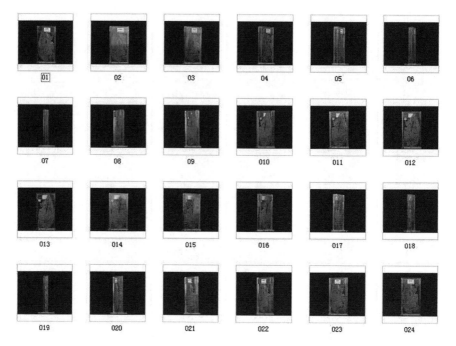

Fig. 190.1 Sequence pictures of nutmeg liver gross specimen

190.3.3 The Making Process of Object Panorama Product

The key of the panoramic work was how to regularly arrange the images. At present, there were plenty of professional panoramic softwares, and among which the appropriate one for the object panorama product fabrication is the Jietusoft and Object2vr etc. The Object2vr has more overall characters than Jietusoft, which can easily create a single-layer or multi-layer object images, and in this research, Object2vr was mainly used.

Basic process: Imported the image files into Object2vr according to the shooting orders, and then in the "view parameter", the typical lesion images or pathological images were set up as the default view; The hotspot editor was used to add interactive elements to the object images, including hot links, information prompt dialog box, website skip links and other commands, besides, action hotspot editor can contribute to lesion features dynamic display; If added specific function button such as animation and sound, the images will be more lively. Domain locking and time setting were added on the "Locking" interface which can restrict the products at the specified site use or control use limitation to protect the copyright. Finally output the images.

Object2vr supports 3 kinds of output modes including Flash, Html 5 and QTVR. Flash and the QTVR are common unified output file formats, thus the special player and plug-in are required. Html 5 output as a set of file combination, the actual application combination includes HTML, CSS, and JavaScript, also the plug-in is not required in browser play, therefore, the customer service is very convenient, but because the documents which Html 5 file outputs are numerous, it is not applicable as teaching materials while applicable as virtual simulation platform for the clients to browse. Flash is the most widely format, and most video players support Flash file playback. Also the Flash play plug-in—Adobe Flash player is the most common plug-in on the browser, when browsing panorama product by Flash, the plug-in is not required to install, besides, Flash can be embedded in PowerPoint which can effectively assist the teachers for PPT lectures.

For the convenience of teachers' independent teaching application and online browsing, the object panorama products of pathological gross specimen were all used Flash format. Figure 190.2 is the object panorama product of nutmeg liver pathological gross specimen. In this product, we can use the mouse to drag the object for level 360° rotation to show the object's 3D images, also we can dynamically view the annotation notes on object, and the bottom toolbar can make the image amplification, mitigation, rotation and full screen view etc.

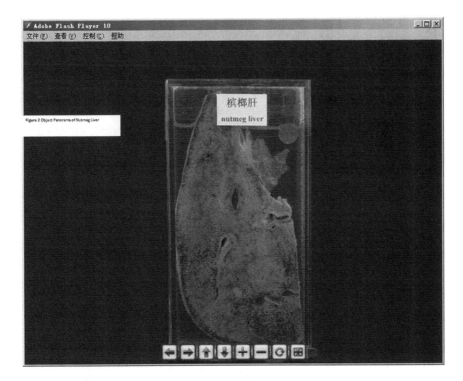

Fig. 190.2 Object panorama of nutmeg liver

Table 190.1 Comparison of several digital methods for pathologic specimens

Method	Processing period	Realistic	Interactive	Play device requirement	Plug-in
Object panorama	Short	Best	Yes	Low	Yes
Picture taking	Very short	Medium	No	Low	No
Virtual reality	Long	Good	Yes	High	Yes

190.4 Results

Object panoramic product has the characters of strong authenticity to view object, high image quality, high definition and full screen of the scene, which makes the perfect detail display. The data size is small, for example, the size of 800 × 600 pixels with 24 images is about 2400 KB, which is convenient for network transmission and online browsing learning. Moreover, the playback device requirement is low; the entire public computer can play it and no need of dedicated workstations. Moreover, the development cycle is short, the cost is low, the shooting production is faster than 3D production and the timeliness is strong. Table 190.1 is the comparison of object panorama's characteristics with others methods.

190.5 Discussion and Conclusion

190.5.1 Points for Attention in Development

Object panoramic technology combines the photography and media-rich software. In the product development, the image must be clean and detailed to meet the demands of teaching, thus the macro lens are used to satisfy this effect. Moreover, because of the time interval or manual operation during taking images will cause color difference between images and rotation axis deviation of object in the images, it is repaired and adjusted in the image processing software, thus such products in interactive process will not appear beat phenomenon in observation. If the fluency of the 3D objects requires enhancing, during the image taking process, the rotating angle can be reduced and the image numbers can be increased, moreover, the total image number is no more than 36 to prevent excess image increasing the occupancy data space and slowing network download speeds. Anyhow, the principle of panoramic product is not only to satisfy the image detail observation but also to meet the simulation interaction experience requirements.

190.5.2 Application Advantages

Digital 3D specimen can not only reserve the basic characteristic of original specimen but also can infinitely spread by copying, moreover, there is no specimen transportation and use loss, therefore it is very helpful for the pathological files preservation. Also in the medical teaching, the teacher can use digital specimens displayed by multimedia equipment instead of real specimens to give lessons. After courses, the students do not have to go to either the laboratory or the classroom but just using the PC, smart phone or other mobile devices for pathological study in the dormitory or even on the bus for study. It contributes greatly to the mobile learning and cooperative learning which is now often advocated in China.

It has been proved that the object panoramic technology for digital processing of pathologic gross specimen images has the advantages of good process effect, low cost and wide application prospect, which is worth to be popularized in the other subjects of medical field.

References

1. Wei Z, Zhi-yun X (2004) Making, use and manage ways of gross specimen in pathology. J Pract Med Tech 11(1):16–17
2. Shao-hua Z, Li-juan L, Lun-shu G (2007) Construction of digital picture storehouse of pathologic gross specimens and sections for microscope. China Med Educ Technol 21(2):123–124
3. Hong-liu Q, Xue-song C, Jing-hua Q, Bin W (2008) Digitalized construction and innovation of the pathologic experiment teaching. Exp Technol Manage 21(2):123–124
4. Jian L, Dong-Liang C (2010) Apparel presentation on Internet based on object panorama. Comput Eng Des 31(5):1111–1113
5. Wei-ming H, Li-hong L (2009) Implementation 3D display of goods by flash. J Guangdong Univ Technol (Soc Sci Ed). 9(suppl):317–318
6. Guo-qiang L (2010) Techniques of taking pictures of patho-anatomic specimens. China Med Educ Technol 24(1):107–109
7. Shao-hua Z, Li-juan L, Lun-shu G, Yinli S (2007) Construction of digital picture storehouse of pathologic gross specimens and sections for microscope. China Med Educ Technol 21(2):123–124

Chapter 191
Ontology-Based Medical Data Integration for Regional Healthcare Application

Yu-Xin Wen, Hua-Qiong Wang, Yi-Fan Zhang and Jing-Song Li

Abstract The regional information sharing provides the ability to transfer up-to-date patient health information quickly and easily across hospitals and institutes. However, the fact that most systems are developed proprietarily hinders data integration. Most developers solve this problem by employing specific data model standards, leading to system inflexibility and inextensibility. In this paper, we present an ontology-based integration method to cope with data heterogeneity in the regional health information network. To carry out interoperability at runtime and in a non-intrusive manner, we design three-layer system architecture. The semantic layer is used to perform coordination among heterogeneous systems, which can connect seamlessly without changing original data structure. We adopt the hybrid ontology approach that extracts information from heterogeneous databases to establish local ontologies and uses an upper-level ontology to make these ontologies compatible. This paper demonstrates a means of accessing to heterogeneous databases for better regional information sharing.

Keywords Data integration · Hybrid ontology · OWL · Regional healthcare

191.1 Introduction

The development of regional information exchange is viewed as a crucial step in the development of health information technology [1]. The goal of data integration is for information to follow patients, wherever and whenever they seek care, in a private and secure manner so that doctors can provide coordinated and effective care. Unfortunately, most healthcare institutions employ proprietary systems to

Y.-X. Wen · H.-Q. Wang · Y.-F. Zhang · J.-S. Li (✉)
Healthcare Informatics Engineering Research Center, Key Laboratory for Biomedical Engineering of Ministry of Education, Zhejiang University, Hangzhou 310027, China
e-mail: ljs@zju.edu.cn

store, represent information which hinders data integration and makes it very difficult for clinicians to capture the complete clinical history of a patient at a fast speed [2]. Additionally, as the complexity of the health domain is evolving rapidly, these systems contain a large number of raw data, leading to the phenomenon of data exploding while lacking of semantic. Namely information can be readable only by humans but computer itself cannot effectively process or interpret the data present in it. Moreover, The deficiency of information heterogeneity can be found as follows [3]: different resources often provide heterogeneous data formats: structured as databases, semi-structured as XML documents and non-structured as web pages or other type of documents; the existence of synonyms and homonyms. For example, system A stores '1' and '2' in integer formats to represent 'gender'. Instead, system B uses 'F' and 'M' to represent it; the ambiguity of concepts: the term 'insulin' can represent the concept 'hormone' or 'drug' as well; etc.

Some prominent industry standards, such as openEHR, ISO13606, and HL7 CDA, etc., are in use as the most usual approach to solve aforementioned problems. These standards are developed to keep patient records in structured formats, they follow a dual model-based methodology to represent information [4]. Static mapping rules make systems inflexible and inextensible yet. In addition, Healthcare is a many-to-many business, different systems might use different standards, so the heterogeneity problem will remain unsolved unless these standards be merged into a single one. Semantic Web technologies' arrival resulted in new capabilities to match healthcare demands. In this paper, an ontology-based method to medical data integration is proposed.

191.2 Methods

In this paper, the Semantic Web technologies are used to provide data integration in the regional health information network. Ontologies provide the basis for the Semantic Web as a type of controlled vocabulary that attempts to capture the knowledge of a specific domain. They make the relationships explicitly among data types in databases, meanwhile express how data can be exchanged with other resources to deduce redundancy [5]. For example, if two different databases contain the same concept, whereas the concept is represented by different names, ontologies are used to map these names to the same concept descriptor [6]. In general, there are three different ways to use ontologies for data integration: single ontology approaches, multiple ontologies approaches and hybrid ontology approaches [7]. Considering the complexity and variety of data sources in the healthcare domain, we choose the hybrid ontology approaches: the semantics of each source is described by its own ontology, namely local ontology. In order to make the local ontologies comparable to each other, one global shared vocabulary is required. Upper-level ontology contains basic terms for a shared understanding of health data among the healthcare delivery organizations in the given network [8]. The hybrid ontology approach can support dynamic data source integration:

new sources can be easily added with no need to modify existing mappings. Then SPARQL endpoints are built on the upper-level ontology to unify and link the legacy databases, it enables to query information semantically from decentralized resources beyond database boundaries, and allow the detection of new relationships that were previously not detectable.

191.3 System Architecture

The architecture of the regional health information network is shown in Fig. 191.1. It contains three layers: physical layer, semantic service layer, and application layer.

The physical layer consists of distributed data resources dispersed over different healthcare institutes. These databases model their data independently according to their requirements and applications.

The semantic service layer plays a key role in the web-enabled system. The operational components include: The local ontology extraction, upper-level ontology construction, semantic query and reason service, ontology maintenance. This layer is used to perform the necessary translation and coordination between the heterogeneous databases.

The application layer is designed as Web application so that it is accessible from remote locations and at different platforms. It is used to display and retrieve data. Consequently, the implementation of this application is platform-independent and can easily adjustable to new requirements.

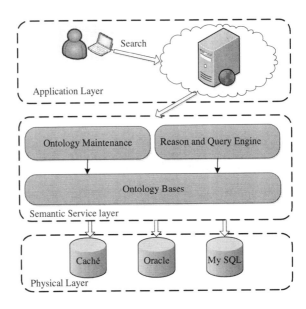

Fig. 191.1 The architecture of regional health information network

191.4 Implementation of the System

Construction of ontologies is the core of this web-based regional health system framework. Currently there are many ways and tools to deal with database to ontology mapping. They can be classified into two main categories: approaches for creating a new ontology from a database and approaches for mapping a database to an already existing ontology [9]. We adopt the first way to construct local ontologies. In our work, we use D2RQ Platform to bridge the gap of legacy databases and the Semantic Web. D2RQ Platform is one of the most prominent tools in the field of relational database to ontology mapping. It allows applications to query non-RDF databases using the SPARQL query language without having to replicate it into an RDF store. This on-the-fly translation allows the content of large databases to be accessed with acceptable response times [10]. There are mainly two steps: first, we need to connect each database by Java Database Connectivity (JDBC) component and generate a corresponding mapping file from each database using the generate-mapping tool. A mapping file is an RDF document written in Turtle syntax which defines mapping rules of the relational data into RDF format.

Figure 191.2 is a fragment of a mapping file which present the map rules of tables 'trnordering' and 'trnpatient' to the corresponding classes in an ontology, 'd2rq: ClassMap' specifies how URIs (or blank nodes) are generated for the instances of the class and 'd2rq: PropertyBridge' specifies how the properties of an instance are created. 'd2rq: join' property means that the table 'trnordeing' has a contact with the table 'trnpatient' through the foreign key 'PatientId'.

The system adopts Eclipse as development platform and the Jena semantic web framework as the knowledge engine. The Jena Framework provides an ontology API for handling OWL ontologies and a rule-based inference engine for reasoning with OWL data sources. Additionally, it includes a query engine compliant with the latest SPARQL version.

Fig. 191.2 A fragment of a mapping file

```
# Table trnordering
map:trnordering a d2rq:ClassMap;
        d2rq:dataStorage map:database;
        d2rq:uriPattern "trnorder-
ing/@@trnordering.OrderNolurlify@@";
        d2rq:class vocab:trnordering;
        d2rq:classDefinitionLabel "trnordering";
.
map:trnordering_PatientId__ref a d2rq:PropertyBridge;
        d2rq:belongsToClassMap map:trnordering;
        d2rq:property vocab:trnordering_PatientId;
        d2rq:refersToClassMap map:trnpatient;
        d2rq:join "trnordering.PatientId => trnpatient.PatientId";
        .....................
# Table trnpatient
map:trnpatient a d2rq:ClassMap;
        .....................
```

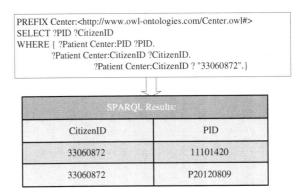

Fig. 191.3 A patient's PID SPARQL query results

Local ontologies above accurately describe the semantic of data in each data resources, but there is still a problem that the relationships between them are not clear, semantic mappings need to be identified between concepts and relations from heterogeneous ontologies to ensure interoperability. Ontology provides rich terminologies such as owl: equivalentClass, owl: equivalentProperty, owl: sameAs, owl: inverseOf to bridge the relationship among different ontologies. We build a unified semantic model, namely upper-level ontology to integrate various local ontologies. It contains basic terms for a shared understanding of health data in the given network. We use OWL DL ontologies to model domain terms. Through analyzing the data structures and local ontologies, we define major OWL classes, including: Patient, Documents, Observations, Order, Variance, Documents Event, Observations Event, OrderEvent. For example, hospital A uses HosA: PerID for representing a patient's identity, whereas hospital B uses HosB: PatientID (where HosA and HosB are namespace URIs for database ontologies), we define Center: PID in the upper-level ontology. Then, HosA: PerID and HosB: PatientID are bridged to the property Center: PID via owl: equivalentProperty.

We show an example of a patient's records retrieval from between hospital A and hospital B. His identity card number (CitizenID) is '33060872'. We construct SPARQL command with upper-level ontology 'Center'. Figure 191.3 shows the patient's PID SPARQL query results:

From Fig. 191.3, the results show that the patient with Patient ID '11101420' in hospital A also has diagnostic history with Patient ID 'P20120809' in hospital B.

191.5 Conclusion and Discussion

To achieve regional information sharing is compromised by the lack of interoperability. The semantic web technology which focuses on the representation of knowledge explicitly brings a more effective approach to achieve data integration. In this paper, we present a three layers' system architecture. The ontology-based approach provides a better mechanism for connecting patient information seamlessly. Compared with current data exchange standards, the framework presented in this paper is more flexible and effective. For this integration, a new information system can be involved at any time simply by producing a corresponding mapping file using the D2RQ Platform and mapping it with the upper-level ontology. It is not necessary to change original data structure. What's more, as ontologies represent domain knowledge in a computable and reusable form, ontologies have become important resources for biomedical research. Ontology-based system architecture also contributes to discovering new knowledge and providing a complete new level of reasoning over medical data that is stored in multiple locations, thus facilitating clinicians and researchers to make decisions effectively.

Acknowledgments This work was supported by the National Natural Science Foundation (Grant No. 61173127) and Zhejiang University Top Disciplinary Partnership Program (Grant No. 188170*193251101).

References

1. Mäenpää T, Suominen T, Asikainen P et al (2009) The outcomes of regional healthcare information systems in health care: a review of the research literature. Int J Med Inform 78(11):757–771
2. Sachdeva S, Bhalla S (2012) Semantic interoperability in standardized electronic health record databases. JDIQ 3(1):1
3. Kienast R, Baumgartner C (2011) Semantic data integration on biomedical data using semantic web technologies
4. Berges I, Bermúdez J, Illarramendi A (2012) Toward semantic interoperability of electronic health records. IEEE Trans Info Technol B 16(3):424–431
5. Rubin DL, Shah NH, Noy NF (2008) Biomedical ontologies: a functional perspective. Brief Bioinfo 9(1):75–90
6. Pérez-Rey D, Maojo V, García-Remesal M et al (2006) ONTOFUSION: Ontology-based integration of genomic and clinical databases. Comput Biol Med 36(7):712–730
7. Wache H, Voegele T, Visser U et al (2001) Ontology-based integration of information-a survey of existing approaches. In: IJCAI-01 workshop: ontologies and information sharing, pp 108–117
8. Raghupathi W, Umar A (2008) Upper-level ontologies for health information systems. Method Inform Med 47(5):435–442
9. Ghawi R, Cullot N (2007) Database-to-ontology mapping generation for semantic interoperability. In: VDBL'07 conference, VLDB Endowment ACM, 1–8
10. Bizer C, Cyganiak R (2006) D2r server-publishing relational databases on the semantic web. In: 5th international semantic web conference, 26

Chapter 192
The Application of Positive Psychology in Effective Teaching

Yu Lin, Yu Jing, He Zhifang and Li Wuiguo

Abstract Positive psychology seek not how things go wrong, but how things go right. Therefore, it gives a new perspective for the teaching of mental health, especially in higher education. The study was to discuss the effect of positive psychology in the mental health education by elective course teaching in Jiangxi University of Traditional Chinese Medicine. 33 undergraduates were given a 12-week elective course teaching, then they were impersonally evaluated by SCL-90 and CMI before and after the teaching. The total points of mental health the after was evidently lower than the before ($p < 0.001$), which shows there is a obvious raise in the total level of mental health; the points of somatization, compulsion, interpersonal sensitivity, depression, anxiety, and paranoid was lower than before ($p < 0.05$), which proves there is a raise in six facets. The positive psychology course is good for the raising of the level of mental health, and students can evaluate themselves and face the life positively.

Keywords Positive psychology · Application · Undergraduates · Effective teaching

Positive psychology studies the virtues and value of human beings, focuses on psychology conditions of every man and attaches importance to the positive aspects of humanity. It overcomes the one-sidedness of traditional psychology which emphasizes psychological disease, and truly retakes the responsibility of psychology. Positive psychology was founded only 10 years ago, yet we have seen the brilliant prospects of it.

Y. Lin (✉) · Y. Jing · H. Zhifang · L. Wuiguo
Jiangxi University of Traditional Chinese Medicine , Jiangxi University, XingWuan Road 28, Nanchang, China
e-mail: lily4868@sina.com

College students were offered "Positive Psychology" as an elective course, and the experiment investigates its effect on the mental health of them. The data which were collected and analyzed are as follows.

192.1 Research Method

192.1.1 Original Data

The subjects of the study are 40 college students who volunteered and have been tested. There are 19 males and 21 females, aged from 19 to 23, and the average age of them is 20.21 ± 0.99. And there are 24 freshmen, 14 sophomores and 3 juniors.

192.1.2 Research Tool

The experiment uses Symptom Check List-90 (SCL-90) and Cornell Medical Index (CMI).

There are 90 items and 10 factors in SCL-90. It uses five levels of score (0–4), which represent negative, light, moderate, serious and extreme respectively. Addition of the scores of the 90 items is the total score, which could reflect the general mental health level of the subject. The score of the factors = the total score of the items which are involved with the factor/the number of the items which are involved with the factor. The seriousness and importance of various symptoms can be observed through it. The higher the score, the lower the level of mental health is. See Appendix 1 for more information.

CMI are divided into 18 parts (from A to R), which contain 195 questions. Only the total score and the score of Part M to R are counted and statistically analyzed. There are only two answers attached to each questions: "yes" is 1 point while "no" is zero. Addition of score of all questions is the total score of CMI, while addition of every items from M to R is the M-R score. The max point of screening in America is 30 points for total score and 10 points for M-R score. The reference value of screening in China is: male: total score ≥ 35 points, M-R score ≥ 15 points; female: total score ≥ 40 points, M-R score ≥ 20 points.

192.1.3 Contents of the Course

The contents of Positive Psychology (12 weeks) include introduction; happiness and enjoyment; love; confidence; potential; optimism and humor; innovational thinking; hope; Forgiveness and gratitude; positive self-suggestion; positively confronting frustration. The contents are separated into three parts: facing the past—gratefully and pleasantly; facing the present—happily, contentedly; benevolently and confidently; facing the future—ambitiously, optimistically and bravely. The teaching procedures are designed in order to improve the students' psychological quality and help them to directly face their lives with smiles. The lecturers focused on cultivating students' interest to the course instead of teaching pure theories. Besides they made efforts to enhance the operability of the experiment. The details of teaching procedure are listed in the Table 192.1.

192.1.4 The Methods of the Research

The main method for this experiment is to compare the mental states of the students before and after taking the course. Through the comparison, we are looking forward to get some materials about the college students' various definition on what is happiness and their reflections to conventional and unconventional emergencies. In doing so, we can validate the theory of some educators that the people living a happy life are more likely to have the positive psychology. 1. They are more optimistic and tenacious. 2. They have proper expectation to their future. 3. They tend to use positive way to live life. 3. They think that they can control their money. 4. They have an expectation the livings in the future. 5. They have confidence to their ability and technique, and can turn the negative to the positive and look at themselves objectively.

192.2 The Process of the Research

192.2.1 Pre-testing

At the beginning of the course, students are evaluated by SCL-90 and CMI. The questionnaires are collected in the class and analyzed promptly.

192.2.2 The Design of the Course

The object of the teaching: To meet the needs of the teaching mental health in a new environment to college students, this course is mainly to improve the students' understanding on Positive Psychology and their mental health, helping them to face the life positively. This can be achieved through classroom teaching, case analysis and discussion, communication on personal experiences, interaction between the teacher and students, practices after the class and etc. And then by

Table 192.1

Unit	Content	Teaching goal
Introduction of positive psychology	1. Test of psychological scale 2. Background of psychology 3. Development of psychology 4. Contents of psychology 5. The necessity of Positive psychology; being positive is human nature 6. Psychology advocates positive explanation to problems	1. Getting a rudimentary knowledge of the students' psychological condition 2. Making the students have a briefly understanding about the background, development and contents of psychology 3. Understanding that being positive is human nature and it is essential for the development of human beings 4. Having a general understanding of the main thoughts of positive psychology
Happiness and enjoyment	Definition of happiness in psychology Pictures of happiness The happiness levels of 4 kinds of people in our lives 1. How to be happier? 2. Definition of being pleasant 3. How to be more pleasant?	1. Making the students have a clear understanding about happiness and enjoyment 2. Knowing thoroughly the happiness levels of different people 3. Learning how to be happy and pleasant 4. Inspiring the students to think and positively find happiness and enjoyment in lives
Love	Definition of love Question of angle: what is love? love in life psychology test love, family and friendship	1. Making the students know the definition of love 2. Helping the students find different kinds of love in their lives 3. Training the subjects to express their love 4. Making the subjects understand love, family and friendship more deeply
Confidence	Confidence and self-abasement Testing your confidence Ways of establishing confidence Testing where is your confidence	1. Helping the students know what is confidence and self-abasement 2. Learning how to test your own confidence 3. Helping the subjects to establish confidence 4. Finding your own confidence
Potential	1. Introduction to potential 2. Different kinds of potential 3. Development of potential 4. Ways of potential development 5. Potential consultation	1. Knowing what is potential and various kinds of potential 2. Knowing how to find one's potential 3. Making the subjects learn the ways of developing potentials 4. Doing potential consultation to the subjects

(continued)

Table 192.1 (continued)

Unit	Content	Teaching goal
Optimism and humor	1. Definition of being optimistic 2. What caused optimism and pessimism 3. Why the society prefer optimism? 4. Definition and kinds of humor 5. Function and Skill of Humor	1. Knowing what is optimism, and understanding what caused optimism and pessimism 2. Making the students know the reasons why being optimistic is popular 3. Helping the students know how to face life optimistically 4. Knowing the definition and contents of humor 5. Knowing how to use humor
Innovational thinking	1. What is innovation 2. How to cultivate innovational thinking 3. How to use innovation 4. Applying innovational thinking	1. Knowing the basic definition of innovation 2. Learning innovation by thinking in a different perspective 3. Knowing how to use your own creativity 4. Making the students use their own innovational thinking correctly
Hope	1. What is hope 2. A hopeful life 3. Discussion how to find hope in a certain situation	1. Knowing what is hope 2. Hopeful life is colorful 3. Helping the students to find and embrace hope in life
Forgiveness and gratitude	1. How to express gratitude 2. The meaning of gratitude 3. Speaking out your gratitude 4. Definition of Forgiveness 5. Learning how to forgive	Being grateful Being grateful makes our life meaningful Understanding the concept of forgiveness Learning how to forgive people and things around you Knowing what needs our forgiveness in life
Positive self-suggestion	1. Definition of self-suggestion 2. Function of self-suggestion 3. Disadvantage of inpositive self-suggestion 4. Facing life positively	1. Making the students know the contents and function of self-suggestion 2. Knowing the advantages of inpositive self-suggestion 3. Knowing the ways of positive self-suggestion, and learning to face the life positively
Positively confronting frustration	1. What is frustration 2. Various of frustrations in lives 3. How to face frustration properly 4. How to face frustration positively	1. Making the students know that frustration is a part of life 2. Learning the right way of facing frustration 3. Facing frustration positively makes our lives complete and successful
Conclusion	1 Review the contents of the course 2. Making the students sharing their understandings 3. Test the students	1. Having a deeper and more complete understanding about positive psychology 2. Creating a more positive atmosphere for students through communication 3. Comparing psychological conditions of the students before and after the course

testing the mental states of the students before and after the course, analyzing and concluding on the data, we can create a firm foundation for the future teaching on Positive Psychology.

The methods of teaching:

1. The teacher explains the topic and guides the discussion.
2. Group discussion on cases. With the help of the teacher, the students are required to find the problem, solve the problem and exchange the experiences by themselves.
3. The students are required to share their feelings and understandings on Positive Psychology in daily life.
4. The students are evaluated by questionnaires and tests.

The measures: This course is mainly to develop the students' ability to face and solve the problems in reality. So we take some measures to improve the teaching.

1. To guaranty the attendance to ensure the consistency of the class.
2. Pay more attention to the understanding and application. Whether the students have grasped the knowledge is not decided by whether they finish the course or not, but by their real talking to their understanding and application in resolving the problems.
3. Greater efficiency inside the class. Let the students study efficiently and happily.
4. Discuss and solve the problems in groups and broaden the horizon of the students through communication (Table 192.2).

Table 192.2

Contents (chapters)	Periods			
	Teaching 授	Discussion 论	Tests	Others
Brief introduction to the positive psychology	2		1	
Well-being and happiness	2	1		
Love	2	1		
Confidence	2	1		
Potency	2	1		
Optimism and humour	2	1		
Creative Thinking	2	1		
Hope	2	1		
Tolerance and thanksgiving	2	1		
Positive self-suggestion	2	1		
Positive reaction to setbacks	2	1		
Conclusion	1	1	1	
Total	23	11	2	36

[a] Periods arrangement of the course

192.2.3 Post-testing

At the end of the last class, students are required to take the SCL-90 and CMI again. The questionnaires are collected inside the class. At the same time, the students are required to write a report after the course.

192.3 Data Analysis and Result

192.3.1 Analysis Tool

The statistic software SPSS 17.0 is adopted to analyze the experience data and the group t test is used to analyze the measurement data.

192.3.2 The Result of Data Collection

There are totally 40 people in this group, except four students who were absent in class more than two times and three invalid questionnaires, 33 people are effective research object, including 15 boys, 18 girls, 19 freshman, sophomore 12, junior 2.

192.3.3 The SCL-90 Scale is Adopted to Test Data before and after Experiments

From the Table 192.3 we can see that the mental health status of posttest score was significantly lower than before ($P < 0.001$), indicating that at the end of the course, the psychological health level of 33 college students were improved

Table 192.3 The analyses of test results by SCL-90 scale before and after experiments

Factor	n	Pre-test	Post-test	Value t	Value p
Somatization	33	1.27 ± 0.26	1.19 ± 0.19	2.44	<0.05
Force	33	1.86 ± 0.44	1.73 ± 0.48	2.43	<0.05
Personal sensitivity	33	1.70 ± 0.52	1.55 ± 0.47	3.03	<0.01
Depression	33	1.60 ± 0.40	1.43 ± 0.42	4.50	<0.001
Anxiety	33	1.46 ± 0.39	1.37 ± 0.30	2.07	<0.05
Hostile	33	1.34 ± 0.30	1.33 ± 0.35	0.15	>0.05
Horror	33	1.31 ± 0.29	1.24 ± 0.34	1.43	>0.05
Paranoid	33	1.52 ± 0.44	1.39 ± 0.41	2.26	<0.05
Psychotic disorder	33	1.49 ± 0.45	1.39 ± 0.41	2.02	>0.05
Total score	33	135.64 ± 26.22	126.42 ± 27.00	4.21	<0.001

obviously, and the posttest scores in somatization, force, interpersonal sensitivity, depression, anxiety and paranoia were lower than before ($P < 0.05$), which means that at the end of the course, 33 students have been improved in the above six aspects; Posttest score and pre-test score had no significant differences in the three factors of hostility, phobia and psychotic disorder (after P values were more than 0.05).

192.3.4 The CMI Scale is Adopted to Test Data before and after Experiments

From the Table 192.4, the total score and M-R score of the pre-test and posttest were both decreased ($P < 0.05$).

192.4 Experiences

In recent years, an increasing amount of attention has been paid on the problems of students' psychological health. The mental health status of university students in China is not optimistic, and the number of incidents of psychological problems is increasing year by year. Investigation on 126000 college students by the relevant departments shows that 20 % of the students have different degrees of psychological problems. All kinds of psychological problems of college students has become a focus of the society, school and family attention. At present, the psychological health education in Colleges and universities is basically the course about psychological health education, supplemented by the diagnosis and treatment of psychological guidance and counseling and mental health education model, which are often in the passive situation, therefore, in terms of the students' psychological health problem strengthening mental health education in college students should not be delayed.

Through this experiment, positive psychology course could change negative cognitions among college students. The innovation is that for the first time through the operation and intriguing teaching, the psychological quality of students could be effectively improved, which has been manifested in: 1. students showed positive illusions; 2. students can absorb the positive significance from the negative events; 3. students could use humor and faith to cope with difficulties; 4. students will not choose a dead end; 5. students will conduct social comparisons and trade-

Table 192.4 The analyses of test results by CMI scale before and after experiments ($\bar{x} \pm s$)

Factor	n	Pre-test	Post-test	Value t	Value p
Total score	33	24.85 ± 13.39	20.33 ± 12.75	2.97	<0.01
M-R score	33	8.09 ± 5.63	6.33 ± 5.41	2.33	<0.05

offs with suitable ways. By the above factors, compared with the traditional model of mental health education, positive psychological education not only can early find and solve the problems of students' psychological health, but also further improve the psychological quality of the students on the basis of the original, so this is undoubtedly of great significance to the effect of teaching.

References

1. Qu L (2010) Chinese culture and positive psychology. School Mental Health Educ 8:21–22
2. Shao Y (2008) On understanding the definition of positive psychology subject. J East China Norm Univ (SOCIAL SCIENCE EDITION) 3:54–59
3. Seligman ME, Rashid T, Parks AC (2006) Positive psychotherapy. Am Psychol 61(8):772–788
4. Yan B, Zheng X, Qiu L (2008) The contribution of self-determination theory to positive psychology research. J Dialectics Nat 25(3):94–99
5. Miao Y, Yu J (2003) Positive psychology: idea and action. J Nanjing Norm Univ 2:81–87
6. Ren J, Ye H (2010) Positive: the core value of the contemporary psychology. J Shaanxi Norm Univ (PHILOSOPHY AND SOCIAL SCIENCES EDITION) 33(4):106–111
7. Zhou Q, Shi G (2006) Introduction of positive psychology. Chin Mental Health J 2:129–132

Chapter 193
The Exploration of Paramilitary Students Management in Vocational Colleges

Wang Haohui

Abstract Good student management work is the guarantee and foundation for Vocational College to train talents needed by our society. The paper focuses on our practice work to explore paramilitary management and the necessity in Vocational College, practical exploration and considerations. We are willing to do something useful for the construction of harmonious campus and strengthening and improving management work in Vocational College.

Keywords Vocational education · Student management · Paramilitary management

Vocational education takes the responsibility for the output of practical talents, so student management not only affects the teaching quality in Vocational College, but also the whole social personnel output quality. There are some general characteristics of students' poor cultural foundation and self binding power. On the other hand, there is more flexible exploring space and significance compared with student management mode in general Colleges and University. We put our many years management experience into with management practice in the Metallurgy and Resources School of Bayin Guoleng Vocational and Technical College to explore the paramilitary management mode in Vocational College.

193.1 The Paramilitary Management

Paramilitary management is one of management patterns in enterprise management. It refers to the usage of military special organization form, acting norms, strict management system and testing means in the enterprise production activities

---

W. Haohui (✉)
Bayin Guoleng Vocational and Technical College, Korla 841000 XinJiang, China
e-mail: 8157309@qq.com

and daily management in order to train staff self-conscious behaviour, good habits, strong characters, team awareness, and work responsible sense. All of these will help to make employees have normative action, standard operation method in the process of safe production and running management so that it makes enterprise achieve a high degree of consistency, improve work efficiency and get the best results.

Paramilitary management in Vocational College refers to one of ways to manage students by setting up strict rules and regulations according to the characteristics of Vocational College and students practice, which uses the military, and enterprise management mode and standard. At present it includes three types Schools implementing paramilitary management: The first is military and police Colleges; with; The second is the emerging "private schools"; The third is the general College without military and police characteristics.

193.2 The Necessity of Paramilitary Management in Vocational College

We can get the general situation of Vocational College students by investigation and analysis. Some of them failed in the College entrance examination; the majority of poor foundation adds even the poor family economical conditions in general. Many students have little self-discipline and uneven comprehensive quality. Even someone surfs on Internet overnight instead of having a good sleep in dormitory, which makes them feel tired in daytime, cut class or fight with other, and many parents and teachers have nothing to do with it. The poor students' management not only seriously impedes to achieve the school education goals, but also affects the entire school management. In adverse greater crisis lie in Vocational College students: younger age, the not yet established value, poor self-discipline ability, dropping self-learning ability, seriously affecting the other students. All of these make more students neglect their studies and face the fact of leaving the school. Faced with this situation, it is evading responsibility with simple persuasion, therefore, we must strength further in the administrative and further explore in the management pattern.

Implementation of paramilitary management is not only necessary for the innovation of management, but also improving the students' comprehensive competitiveness and meeting enterprises employing standard. We need to carry out the paramilitary management to make students build up a good learning attitude, form a good atmosphere of learning, develop learning and life habits. The improving standards of requiring employees in modern enterprise force staff to have obedient consciousness and strong executive power like military and have strict discipline and teamwork spirit. Vocational College needs to keep steps with enterprises employing standard, which also needs to carry out the paramilitary management.

193.3 The Practice and Exploration of Implementing Paramilitary Management

In order to make students paly the main role in the paramilitary management process in the main role of students, achieve the change from the "heteronomy" to "self-discipline", and eventually form a students' independent management team, we establish the following special paramilitary management system scheme in our School.

193.3.1 To Establish Student Vertical Management Mode

Vertical management mode is to imitate the military management mode of authority–cadre–soldiers vertical to form the mode of making Students 'Organization manage student backbone and the backbone manage students'. It can effectively save the management time, improve management efficiency, and prevent direct contradictions between the manager and by-manager in parallel management. We will focus on the establishment of student organizations and student backbone team.

193.3.1.1 To Establish Vertical Student Management Mechanism

The student section—class committee—monitor (vice monitor)—small group leader–student.

193.3.1.2 The Appointment and Removal of Class Committees and Responsibilities

The class committee is made up with five members including monitor, vice monitor, three deputy lead. Monitor and vice monitor are elected by secret ballot difference list (self, students, teacher, or former class committees recommendation), and determined by the class committee vote. Monitor and vice monitor will be elected monthly and the small group leader every two weeks. Monitor and vice monitor cannot take part-time small group leader.

There are at least 30 students in principle each class. Less than 30 students' class will elect their leaders to establish more than 30 student classes, and then elect monitor and vice monitor. The monitor is mainly responsible for daily life, discipline management, helping the vice monitor and small group leader do a good job of class management, and assisting the teacher in charge of class to do some temporary task. Vice monitor is in charge of class learning, culture and physicals, the house health management, and class completed daily management tasks asked by monitor. Small group leader will help monitor and vice monitor to complete daily management tasks.

193.3.1.3 The Appointment and Removal and Responsibilities of the Members in Student Union

The main work of Student Union is to oversight each class's work and makes an evaluation to them. The members of the Student Union are recommended by themselves, class committee and teacher in charge of class and then they can be reported to Student Union after the discussion of class committee. The minister of Student Union will select the section members. The members' election of the Student Union will be done every month. The minister of Student Union is elected from each section meeting recommendation and discussion. President of the Student Union, vice president is elected by the Student Union minister meeting recommendation.

193.3.2 The Formulation and Modification of Student Management System

193.3.2.1 The Formulation of Student Management System

Student management system is drafted by the student section, discussed by the class committee, modified by Student Union, and finally formulated by student section.

193.3.2.2 The Modification of Student Management System

The members of Student Union will collect the opinions of students on monthly regular meetings and discuss or modify the student management system if necessary when 80 % student members agree and student section approves.

193.3.3 Regular Meeting System

Students section will hold a regular meeting weekly for minister of Student Union and the monitor each class. The proceedings is roughly as follows: count the number of students; the ministers of Student.

Union summarize and explain each week's work and make an arrangement for next week's work, and know students ideological situation by meeting. After the regular meeting the ministers will hold the meeting for the members of Student Union, and the monitors hold a meeting for a class committee, and the group leaders hold a group meeting.

193.3.4 Life System Each Day

1. System: count noses in morning exercise, day class and night, and individual study.
2. Report: the group leaders report students' number to monitor on gathering.
3. Summary: monitor must summarize and evaluate in gathering, class activities in front of all class.
4. Class: monitor exactly reports the students' number to classroom teachers about the absent or present numbers. The classroom teachers will tell the student section if some students are absent. Monitor will comment on the students' disciplinary situation in each lesson (90 min) with 3 min left in the class.
5. Count at night: monitor (vice monitor) organizes the count job and inspect work and comment on the day work.
6. Sanitation check: the vice monitor with three small group leaders will check the dormitory sanitation before class every morning, and night lights time.

193.3.5 The Scores of Student Employment

The scores of student employment include the daily score and final term score. Daily score results from daily behavior and management ability. Daily score plus exam score is the final term score.

The small group leader will give the members scores (including discipline, the house divided, grooming) as their daily scores before weekly class committee meeting. Monitor and vice monitor will consult to each group scores. The Student Union will count each class week score according to week class actual scores and taking the monitor and vice monitor's management abilities as class week score and the small leader's management abilities as group week score. The Student Union ministers, deputy minister will consult to the members' dairy scores and chairman and vice chairman will consul to the ministers and deputy ministers' scores for week work. The student section will give the scores to Student Union as the management abilities scores of the chairman and deputy chairman. The office will count each student dairy score each week.

193.4 The Management Effect of Implementing Paramilitary Management

The implementing of paramilitary management played an important role in improving students' abilities in organization and discipline, teamwork and bearing hardships compared with the ordinary management. We take our College as an example in implementing paramilitary management since 2008. The measurement not only makes students enhance their physique and willpower, but makes them learn military discipline, interior management, and other various forces of fine tradition. Many students become stronger in military training thanks to the spirit of hardship in facing difficulties, and they are proud of looking like soldiers. In 2008 the number of freshmen is 602, and the normal graduate is 576, so the turnover rate is 4.3 %; In 2009 the number of freshmen is 565, and the normal graduate is 544, so the turnover rate is 3.7 %. The turnover rate is controlled within 5 %. After graduate 98 % students are willing to go to work in the oil, steel, mining etc. hard working positions, and get high praise from enterprise. Ever some students got the position in human resources department, operation department as monitors or directors. The militarization management was praised and accepted by students' parents. One of student parents said: "My child looks like grow-up after 2 months in experiencing militarization management. He doesn't want to worry about any more. I send him to your school not only for children employment in the future, but for the training of strict and self management" One of students said: "the strict and orderly life makes us develop the habit of when to do, where to do, and how to do".

193.5 The Attentions of Implementing Paramilitary Management

The ultimate goal of paramilitary student management is to realize students' self-management and self-discipline, which is the nuclear issue in the process of paramilitary management, and we should pay more attention to following points:

1. The student main function will be further taken in paramilitary management. The students' enthusiasm of participation should be raised, team spirit should be cultivated, the management should be improved and trained in the process of paramilitary management, and finally an independent management tea should be established.
2. Campus culture construction should be emphasized according to the students' characteristics of Higher Vocational College. The numbers of our College students are continuing to increase, which will bring new vitality to the culture construction. We need to explore and summarize in practice between 'management' and 'freedom' of tension and relaxation.

3. Teaching quality will be improved connecting with teaching work. Teaching work and teaching quality is the foothold of our College's development. The paramilitary management should focus on the teaching center and serve to improve the teaching quality and putting them together. There are still a lot of works to do for us.

In short, the paramilitary management for Vocational College students is still in the exploratory stage, and it needs further adjustment and improvement in practice. We are wishing to make a useful exploration to the construction of harmonious campus and to strengthen and optimize Vocational Colleges' student management work.

References

1. Bai Y (2005) Based on the three facings: to improve Vocational education. J Shihezi Univ (philosophy and social science edition) (1)
2. Jiang D (2007) Vocational education research new points. Education Science Press, Beijing
3. Wang X (2005) The Course of professional technical personnel quality and ability training tut. China Media University Press, Beijing

Chapter 194
Research on a New DNA-GA Algorithm Based on P System

Shuguo Zhao and Xiyu Liu

Abstract In recent years, DNA-GA algorithms, which attracts many scholars' attention, combine the DNA encoding method with Genetic algorithm. It effectively overcomes GA's limitation such as premature convergence, poor local search capability and binary Hamming cliffs problems. In this work, a new DNA-GA algorithm based on P system (PDNA-GA) is proposed to improve the performance of DNA-GA algorithms by combining the parallelism of P system in Membrane Computing. The performance of PDNA-GA in typical benchmark functions is studied. The experimental results demonstrate that the proposed algorithm can effectively yield the global optimum with high efficiency.

Keywords Membrane computing · P system · DNA-GA · Fitness · Genetic operators

194.1 Introduction

Natural computation is put forward and immediately shows a strong vitality when the traditional computing encounters a bottleneck. The natural computation model can vary with its biological level, such as evolutionary computing, neural network, DNA computing and Membrane computing [1].

S. Zhao · X. Liu (✉)
School of Management Science and Engineering, Shandong Normal University, Jinan, China
e-mail: sdxyliu@163.com

S. Zhao
e-mail: sugarlover@126.com

DNA-GA algorithm is a kind of genetic algorithm replacing binary coding with DNA coding. Ding and Ren (2002) firstly proposed a DNA-GA algorithm [2]. After 2005, scholars began to propose improved DNA-GA algorithms [3–7].

P system is the biological model of Membrane Computing introduced by Paun [8]. Roughly speaking, a P system consists of a membrane structure, in the compartments of which one places multisets of objects which evolve according to given rules in a synchronous nondeterministic maximally parallel manner [9].

In this work, we proposed a new DNA-GA Algorithm Based on Monolayer P System named PDNA-GA algorithm to improve the performance of DNA-GA algorithms by combining the parallelism of P system in Membrane Computing. Algorithms are completed in two stages. Stage 1: genetic operation happens within the membrane; Stage 2: genetic operation happens outside the membrane.

194.2 The New DNA-GA Algorithm Based on P System (PDNA-GA)

194.2.1 DNA Coding

A DNA sequence contains Adenine (A), Guanine (G), Cytosine (C) and Thymine (T). It is an effective way to use A, T, G and C to generate representations of individuals. In this work, for better processing we adopt $E' = \{0, 1, 2, 3\}^l$ to denote $E = \{C, T, A, G\}^l$, where l is the length of DNA sequences. According to Watson–Crick complementary principle, the new bonding occurs like this: 1 bonds with 2 and 0 bands with 3. So the solution can be expressed as a quaternary integer string.

Generally, optimization problem can be described as follows:

$$\begin{cases} \min f(x1, x2\ldots, xn) \\ x_{\min i} \leq x_i \leq x_{\max i}, i = 1, 2, \ldots, n \end{cases} \quad (194.1)$$

In the real-world optimization problems, variable x_i represents the integer string of length l. $[x_{\min i}, x_{\max i}]$ is the bound of x_i. $x_{\min i}$ is the decode integer 0 and $x_{\max i}$ is the decode integer $4^l - 1$. The precision variable x_i is $(x_{\max i} - x_{\min i})/4^l$ and the length of each individual is $L = n \times l$.

194.2.2 Fitness Function

In this paper, a fitness function based on exponential transformation is adopted to expand differences in exponential form. The fitness function is described as follows:

$$F(x) = \exp(-C) - \exp[-(f(x) + C)] \quad (194.2)$$

where $f(x)$ is the minimized objective function optimization problems. C is a positive number large enough to ensure $(f(x) + C)$ nonnegative.

After encoding n individuals of the initial population into quaternary sequence, we sort the fitness values by the fitness function value. Choose the individuals with the smallest (optimal) and the largest (worst) fitness value (2 individuals in total) as elite individuals and put the remaining $(N-2)$ individuals into the P system.

194.2.3 P Processing

After the previous step, 2 elite individuals are kept outside. The remaining $(N-2)$ individuals are put into m basical membranes equally. And that forms a P system. We define m as follows:

$$m = \left\lfloor \sqrt{(N-1)} \right\rfloor \quad (194.3)$$

where N is the total number of individuals of initial population, m is the square root of $(N-1)$ (round down).

When adding the membrane structure we define the rules: individuals in m membranes conduct genetic operations. After several times of iteration, each membrane will generate an elite individual. When the termination criteria is met, the membrane structure will dissolve. m elite individuals will be released from m membranes. They will step to next round operation together with the initial 2 elite individuals. Because it involves several elite individuals, P system can effectively solve the problem of getting into the local optimum.

194.2.4 Genetic Operators

194.2.4.1 Crossover Operators

In this paper, we use two kinds of crossover operators: replacement operator and transposition operator [7].

(a) Replacement operator: Firstly, two parent individuals are randomly selected and assumed to be $R^1 = R_1^1 R_2^1 R_3^1 ... R_L^1$ and $R^2 = R_1^2 R_2^2 R_3^2 ... R_L^2$; And then randomly select a subsequence $R_S^1 = R_i^1 ... R_{i+m_1}^1$ from R^1, where R_i^1 is an randomly selected position in R^1 and m_1 is a positive integer and $1 < m_1 + i \leq L$. Similarly, the selected subsequence from R^2 is $R_S^2 = R_j^2 ... R_{j+m_1}^2$ ($1 < m_1 + j \leq L$). Exchange the sequence R_S^1 and R_S^2, and the two new individual become $R'^1 = R_1^1 ... R_j^2 ... R_{j+m_1}^2 ... R_L^1$ and $R'^2 = R_1^2 ... R_i^1 ... R_{i+m_1}^1 ... R_L^2$.

(b) Transposition operator: Firstly, a parent individual $R = R_1R_2R_3R_L$ is randomly selected. And then randomly select an position R_i in R and a positive m_2, so the selected sequence is $R_S = R_i...R_{i+m_2}$ $(1 < m_2 + i < L)$. Randomly select a position R_j $(1 \le j \le L$ and $j \notin [i, m_2 + i])$ in R again. Next, cut off the R_S of R, and insert R_S next to the position R_j. Finally, the new individual become $R' = R_1...R_jR_i...R_{i+m_2}R_{j+1}...R_{i-1}R_{i+m_2+1}...R_L$ $(j < i)$ or $R' = R_1... R_{i-1}R_{i+m_2+1}...R_jR_i...R_{i+m_2}R_{j+1}...R_L(j > i + m_2)$.

In this paper, we adopt the same probability of crossover operator inside and outside the membrane. The probability of replacement operation *pc1* is *0.1*, and the probability of transposition operation *pc2* is *0.1*.

194.2.4.2 Mutation Operator

Mutation operator can effectively prevent the search process from falling into local optimum. In this paper we adopt the ordinary operator but with adaptive probability in membranes [7]. It is described as follows:

We divide the nucleotide bases into two parts: left and right parts. Correspondingly, the adaptive probabilities *pml* (left) and *pmr* (right) are described as follows:

$$\begin{cases} pml = a_1 + \dfrac{b1}{1 + \exp(aa(g - g_0))} \\ pmr = a_1 + \dfrac{b1}{1 + \exp(-aa(g - g_0))} \end{cases} \quad (194.4)$$

where a_1 denotes the initial mutation probability of *pml*, b_1 denotes the range of transmutability. The parameter g is evolution generation, and g_0 denotes the generation where mutation probability will come up with great change, and aa is the speed of change. Outside the membrane, we adopts the traditional mutation probability and define the mutation probability outside as *pm3*.

194.2.4.3 Selection Operator

Selection operator determines the direction of evolution. In this paper, we adopt elitism strategy and choose the fitness function as selection operator. Outside the membrane, we adopt the elitism strategy as well.

194.2.5 Procedure of the PDNA-GA

The procedure of PDNA-GA can be summarized as follows:

(1) Initialize a population with N individuals.
(2) DNA coding and calculate the fitness value of each individual and sort.
(3) Choose the *two* individuals with the best and worst value as elite individual. The remaining $(N-2)$ individuals are put into the P system. Set maximum evolution generation inside the membrane as $T1$.
(4) Conduct genetic operations in each membrane.
(5) Repeat step (4) until the termination criteria inside the membrane is met. m elites are released outside and step to next round operation together with the initial 2 elite individuals. And maximum evolution generation outside the membranes is set as $T2$.
(6) Conduct genetic operations on elite individuals.
(7) Repeat step (6) until the termination criteria outside the membranes is met and finally optimal solution is generated. The PDNA-GA algorithm ends.

194.3 Experimental Simulation

In order to investigate the performance of the PDNA-GA algorithm, we select *three* benchmark functions [7] to have a test (Table 194.1). The three test functions can reflect the optimization performance of the PDNA-GA. The superior performance of PDNA-GA is shown by comparing with RNA-GA and SGA.

In the experiments, the parameters of PDNA-GA are set as follows. The population size is *300* ($N = 300$). The parameters of the mutation operator is set as $g_0 = Gmax/2$, $a_1 = 0.02$, $b_1 = 0.2$, $aa = 20/Gmax$, $pm3 = 0.05$. The number of membranes is *17* ($m = 17$). The maximum evolution general inside $T1$ and outside $T2$ is *500*. For each test problem, we run *50* times for the three algorithms of PDNA-GA, RNA-GA and SGA. The results are shown in Tables 194.2 and 194.3.

Table 194.1 The test functions

The test functions	Optimum solution	Optimal value
$\min f_1(x) = 100(x_2 - x_1^2)^2 + (1-x_1)^2; x_1, x_2 \in [-5.12, 5.12]$	(1,1)	0
$\min f_2 = 1 + \sum_{i=1}^{2} \frac{(x_i-100)^2}{4000} - \prod_{i=1}^{2} \cos(\frac{x_i-100}{\sqrt{i}}); x_1, x_2 \in [-600, 600]$	(100,100)	0
$\min f_3(x) = 0.5 + \frac{(\sin\sqrt{x_1^2+x_2^2})^2 - 0.5}{(1+a(x_1^2+x_2^2))^2}; a = 0.001; x1, x2 \in [-10, 10]$	(0,0)	0

Table 194.2 Precision of optimization

The benchmark functions	PDNA-GA			RNA-GA			SGA		
	F_{max}	F_{min}	F_{ave}	F_{max}	F_{min}	F_{ave}	F_{max}	F_{min}	F_{ave}
f1	1.723E−10	2.423E−23	8.569E−11	2.343E−8	7.247E−10	1.784E−9	3.496E−5	4.452E−9	1.173E−5
f2	3.253E−10	1.334E−18	7.231E−10	0.0004	2.325E−8	0.0001	0.0017	4.569E−10	0.0009
f3	1.172E−10	0	5.275E−10	0.0009	2.397E−4	0.0003	0.0092	2.879E−6	0.0063

Table 194.3 Evolution generations

The benchmark functions	PDNA-GA			RNA-GA			SGA		
	G_{max}	G_{min}	G_{ave}	G_{max}	G_{min}	G_{ave}	G_{max}	G_{min}	G_{ave}
f1	168	17	37.3	500	32	241	500	78	389
f2	48	7	12.4	500	6	373	500	89	402
f3	32	14	19.8	500	21	233	500	23	211

Obviously, conclusions can be obtained from the results of the experiment, PDNA-GA is more reliable than RNA-GA and SGA. Convergence speed and accuracy are important indicators of the algorithm. Experimental results show that PDNA-GA is an effective improvement to DNA-GA algorithm.

194.4 Conclusions

In this paper, a new DNA-GA algorithm based on P system (PDNA-GA) is proposed by combining DNA-GA with P system for the first time. After repeated verifications, the PDNA-GA algorithm performs pretty well when the population size is large enough. The future work is to improve the algorithm efficiency when the population size is small.

Acknowledgments This work is supported by National Science Fund of China (No. 61170038), Science Fund of Shandong province (No. ZR2011FM001) and Social Science Fund of Shandong province (No. 11CGLJ22).

References

1. Huang L (2007) Research on membrane computing optimization methods. Zhejiang University, China
2. Ding YS, Ren LH, Shao SH (2002) DNA computing and soft computing. Science press, China
3. Tao JL, Wang N (2007) DNA computing based RNA genetic algorithm with applications in parameter estimation of chemical engineering processes. Comput Chem Eng 31(12):1602–1618
4. Chen X, Wang N (2010) Optimization of short-time gasoline blending scheduling problem with a DNA based hybrid genetic algorithm. Chem Eng Process 49(10):1076–1083
5. Zhang L, Wang N (2013) A modified DNA genetic algorithm for parameter estimation of the 2-Chlorophenoloxidation in supercritical water. Appl Math Model 37(3):1137–1146
6. Wang K, Wang N (2011) A protein inspired RNA genetic algorithm for parameter estimation in hydrocracking of heavy oil. Chem Eng J 167(1):228–239
7. Dai K, Wang N (2012) A hybrid DNA based genetic algorithm for parameter estimation of dynamic systems. Chem Eng Res Des 90(12):2235–2246
8. Paun G (2000) Computing with membranes. J Comput Syst Sci 61(1):108–143

9. Escuela G, Gutierrez-Naranjo MA (2010) An application of genetic algorithms to membrane computing. In: Proceedings of eighth brainstorming week on membrane computing, pp 101–108
10. Liu XX, Zhang GL (2010) A research on population size impaction on the performance of genetic algorithm. North China Electric Power University, China

Chapter 195
Study on the Assistance of Microblogging in English Literature Teaching

Haixia Fang

Abstract With the development of network technology, Microblogging has become the latest network platform which is widely used in many fields. It is also very useful for college teachers to apply it in teaching English literature. With a solid experience in teaching the course of English literature, the author is trying to provide arguments for using Microblogging as an educational tool, underlining its advantages to counter the predicaments of current English literature teaching. Educated in a Microblogging environment, students can have more opportunities to communicate with teachers, get more helpful information, and extend their learning areas, thus improving their ability of self study and literary appreciation. The article also presents some practical and effective modes that can be adopted in English literature teaching in a Microblogging environment.

Keywords Microblogging · English literature teaching · Predicaments · Teaching modes

195.1 Introduction

In recent years, the mode of large classes is adopted by most Chinese colleges and universities in teaching English because of the paradox between small educational resources and big education scales. Under this condition, the teaching mode is characterized by teachers' one-way infusion and single input language, thus lacking personalization and two-way interaction between teachers and students. Furthermore, this one-way teaching mode can not stimulate students' interest in learning and cultivate students' practical ability of using the English language

---

H. Fang (✉)
School of Foreign Languages, Anhui University of Science and Technology,
Anhui 232001, Huainan, China
e-mail: fang-hx@163.com

effectively. Therefore, a web-facilitated education environment is desperately needed to make up for deficiencies in the traditional teaching methods since it can offer rich input language, reconstruct the interaction between teachers and students and most importantly, stimulate students to acquire the English language and produce the English language actively.

Microblogging is a Web 2.0 technology, and a new form of blogging with two features: the popularity of original content and the many-to-many mode of transmission. It also enables a real-time interaction between users, using different devices, technologies and applications. As a social networking tool, Microblogging lets the users publish online brief text updates within 140 characters and supports multimedia contents such as images, audios, videos, hyperlinks and so on. Conveniently, users can access it through many terminals like computers, cell phones and instant messaging tools. With the development of Microblogging, more and more people are concerned about the value of Microblogging in educational activities. In this paper, according to my own teaching experience, I will explore the feasibility and practicality of this technology used in English literature teaching.

195.2 Advantages of Microblogging Over Other Message Tools

Microblogging has many advantages suitable for its application in English literature teaching. From the perspective of properties, Microblogging is a media platform, subverting the traditional mode of lineal transmission. The distinction between communicators and audiences is obscure. Those who have the willingness to share can communicate, interact and share with others comfortably through Microblogging. Secondly, the content transmitted through Microblogging is microcontent, but it integrates characters with images, audios, videos and superlinks, leading to the strong power of information dissemination. Finally, from the perspective of the transmission direction, the small scale is identified and the wider sphere is scattered like a net. Based on the above features, it is possible that Microblogging is suitable for being applied as a teaching media.

The brevity of Microblogging makes message transmission more efficiently. A blog limited within 140 characters, which requires bloggers to pay more attention to its organization, word choice and thesis statement. This requirement makes the message more concise, concentrated and easier for students to grasp. In this age of instant information, the quick speed of media communication leads to overloaded information and fragmented message. On the contrary, the short and pithy content of Microblogging is an indispensable link of improving study efficiency. So Microblogging plays an important role in speeding up the transmission of teaching messages.

On the other hand, thanks to the multimodal of Microblogging, the transmitted teaching content will be accepted by students more easily. Microblogging supports the contents of different formats such as images, audios, videos and superlinks which can efficiently stimulate students' senses and body participation. This kind of teaching method is in accordance with the learning style of new generation—multitasking generation and help them integrated into study activities comprehensively. The traditional English literature teaching needs this new technology and the new teaching method derived from it greatly to make class activities more colorfully and abundantly.

Moreover, in terms of interaction and sense of distance, Microblogging is better than Blackboard Academic Suite, instant message tools, blog and SNS which are being applied by many teachers in teaching English literature. Compared with Blackboard Academic Suite, Microblogging not only has the functions of synchronized and asynchronous communication but also is quicker in message reception and information feedback. Its functions of calling for attention, comment and forwarding realize the collaborative activities between students and teachers. Microblogging combines every participant in study activities together and makes teaching and learning socialized and collaborative. Compared with blog, though blog can offer more amount of messages for public discussion, the feedback is always delayed and some users are hesitant to say because of the system of comment registration. Fortunately, the transmission mode of Microblogging is face versus back, that is, users can choose unilateral attention, the communication between strangers will be enhanced and discussion and feedback will last. Therefore, debates and collective dialogue will be produced. Compared with the instant message tools such as QQ, Microblogging has the advantage of knowledge management. Its function of storage contributes to knowledge accumulation and the function of micro group can offer people of the same interest to form a small circle and discuss together. Compared with SNS, the relationships between bloggers in Microblogging environment are looser. Microblogging does not lie in the establishment of relationships but broadcast which is more suitable for teaching requirements.

Last but not least, the value of Microblogging applied in teaching can be reflected its filling students' feeling. The birth of Microblogging is to offer a platform for those who communicate unofficially and let people establish social activities in informal situations with equal dialogue and interaction realized. The educational function of Microblogging makes student–teacher relationship free from serious classroom. Students can communicate and interact with teachers through network and then acquire more comprehensive knowledge about each other to promote the development of teaching activities.

195.3 Assistance of Microblogging in English Literature Teaching

195.3.1 Predicaments Faced by Current English Literature Teaching

English literature is a compulsory course for English majors. On the curriculum setting, it is featured by less teaching periods and short teaching cycle. It is usually set in the second half of sophomore year, accounting for about 48 teaching periods. For sophomore students, they lack enough time to read more works because of short teaching cycle and digestive ability is not strong. Students are not ready in terms of psychology, language skills and knowledge reserves. It is a heavy burden for them to read those time-consuming novels because of their vocabulary and reading skills. Lacking basic skills of analyzing texts, students can not appreciate literary works from the perspectives of language, structure and theme which are the essential elements for how to study English literature. On the other hand, in order to fulfill teaching tasks, teachers are anxious for success and neglect to guide students to appreciate the beauties concealed in literary works. In terms of forms of teaching, teachers apply modern teaching technique—the courseware of PPT and present relevant audios and videos to enrich teaching contents and inculcate students with knowledge from multi-angles. But this kind of method often leads to overdo, making students visual and auditory fatigue and lose interest in multimedia teaching. Relying too much on the presentation of PPT, students are in the situation of being passively given and waiting for teachers' answer, thus lacking active questioning and answering, leading to the decline of imagination and the ability of thinking. Besides, the communication between teachers and students cannot be realized because there is no platform for them to talk about literary learning. The only thing teachers can do is to assign tasks but not to supervise students' independent study. Likely, the communication among students is very little. In this environment, they are isolated from each other and teaching cannot benefit teachers and students.

In response to these predicaments that English literature teaching encounters, many universities speed up the pace of educational reforms. With the popularity of networks, web-based instruction is not only a tendency but also a must. The course of English literature complies with this tendency. Based on the construction of elaborate course and integrated with advanced teaching resources at home and abroad, many educational websites for English literature teaching have been established by foreign schools of many famous universities. Excellent teaching resources are assembled in these fine courses including top-ranking teachers, modern information technology and a paradigm of teaching management. The teaching procedures, purposes, methods, courseware, videos and exercises are presented through networks. Moreover, background information, literary criticism and classical works are provided on the network exchange platform, relevant films, lectures and other superlinks as well. In this way, the problem of the shortage of teaching hours is solved. Students can study independently. At the same time, the elaborate courses are open online, realizing resource sharing and using by other universities. However, besides these advantages, we can not neglect that network-based courses pay more attention to knowledge supplies, lack guidance for those who study independently, have nothing to do with students' participation and have no efficient system of network monitoring. Therefore, the networking reform of English literature teaching needs to take one step further and students' participation and supervisory mechanism should be taken into account in reforming English literature teaching. At present, Microblogging seems to be the best way out because it can extend teaching time, expand teaching space, supply real communication environment and more importantly focus on students' participation.

195.3.2 The Application of Microblogging in English Literature Teaching

Microblogging caters to students' individual needs for novelty, odd and wit because of its timeliness, interactivity, convenience, knowledgeablity and interestingness. Students can obtain what they need quickly and directly through Microblogging. Teachers can offer latest information about literary masters and critics through Microblogging to guide students' reading.

Thanks to the timeliness of Microblogging, it is accessible for teacher to extend class to a wider space and assign reading tasks online. According to students' remarks, teachers can check the assignments of students and control the learning process easily. Also, if students have any questions, no matter where they are, in class or after class, teachers can answer them in time. For example, when talking about English literature of English renaissance period, teachers are inevitable to discuss about the politics and economy of Elizabethan society. However, it is difficult for anyone to read, lecture and understand the historical background information of that period because it is so messy and complicated. So teachers can ask students to watch films such as Elizabeth: The Golden Age and Shakespeare in Love before class through Microblogging. In this way, students have a perceptual and rational cognition when teachers explain the background of English renaissance in class and deeply understand the meaning of Elizabeth's famous saying 'I see, but I say nothing'. Through Microblogging, class time will be used more effectively and teaching efficiency will be improved. Moreover, keeping pace with times, Microblogging can provides students with latest teaching resources and new thinking modes. Teacher combines literature with relevant films and comment links to put forward discussion questions. Then, students can watch good films and read famous remarks to improve self-teaching abilities. For example, it is written in a Microblogging that Nobel Prize winner for literature attracts many people while literature itself should draw more attention. Technological advancement changes the way of our reading and writing and literary world as well. Let us present all the technologies that are indispensable elements contributing to literary evolution. This Microblogging start from the latest information about Nobel Prize to discuss technology's influence on reading and writing methods. Therefore, students can not only learn the information about the winner but also fall into thinking whether technological improvements mean the death of traditional literature.

Microblogging can enrich English literature teaching by means of different teaching modes. To solve the predicaments of current English literature teaching, we should explore some pragmatic methods about how to function Microblogging as an educational tool. First, there are some pedagogical applications of Microblogging in English literature teaching to solve the problem of insufficient class time: use for dissemination of teachers' materials, locating original sources of ideas and quotes, getting feedbacks on ideas, fostering professional connections for class chatter, building trust etc. Second, the mode of communication is very important. Students can use it to send out questions and observations to the group while engaged in classroom activities. So the teaching time can be stretched. Moreover, Microblogging promotes writing as a fun activity, fosters editing skills and develops literacy skills. Through it, our students have a chance to express their critical comments on literary works and their cognitive trails will be recorded. And teachers can assess students' responses and know more about students' needs and their cognitive development. Thirdly, an effective mechanism of supervision can be formed through Microblogging. Teachers can keep track of students' study activities and especially give them some points when they are confused in independent study. As a humanity subject, English literature needs teachers to use more individual methods so as to improve students' humanistic qualities and let them absorb more nourishment from classical literary works. That is what English literature teaching aims at.

195.4 Conclusions

As a new social tool, Microblogging is still in its infancy, not mature but full of vigor. Within merely two years, Microblogging has shown its power and potentiality in transmitting messages. With its help, teaching as a special way of transmission can go even further but nearer to students. English literature is a course needing multi-resources to help students understand historical background of each specific era and thus improve students' apprehension of literary works. On these characteristics and the predicaments that current English literature teaching encounters, Microblogging proved to be an effective tool for professional development and for collaboration with students. As a social networking platform, Microblogging can afford us valuable interactions in educational contexts. So teachers should tap the potentials of Microblogging used in teaching fields and improve its service to teachers and students.

References

1. Chai Y, Qin G, Cui L (2006) Study on the assistance of blog in ELT. J CAFLE 111:46–48
2. Karpati A (2009) Web 2 technologies for net native language learners. J ReCALL 21(2):139–156
3. Zhang T (2011) Case study: a probe into the English language teaching strategies in a microblogging environment. J Mod Education Tech 21:96–100
4. Zhao D, Rosson M (2009) How and why people Twitter: the role that Microblogging plays in informal communication at work. In: Proceedings of the ACM 2009 international conference on supporting group work, New York

Chapter 196
Problem-Based Learning of Food Hygiene in Higher University of Traditional Chinese Medicine

Daozong Xia

Abstract Problem-based learning (PBL) has become more widely used in the education of many professionals. This study investigated the effect of PBL on student teaching evaluations in a senior-level food hygiene course, and the pretest/post-test experimental method with an equivalent control group was used. The subjects included the students who were enrolled at the College of Pharmaceutical Sciences in Zhejiang Chinese Medical University. Students attended to Food Hygiene course in the 6th semester. The class taught in the traditional manner was the control group. PBL group attended the PBL course whereas the control group attended the traditional instructor course. A retrospective review of student performance in the food hygiene course was carried out. A cross-sectional survey involving teachers and current food pollution students was also carried out to evaluate learning of food hygiene using the PBL approach. We concluded that integrating PBL into this undergraduate class has a significant effect on the content knowledge acquisition score and thinking skills.

Keywords Problem-based learning · Food hygiene curriculum · Higher university of traditional Chinese medicine · Quality education

196.1 Introduction

Educational research has shown that successful problem solvers possess an organized and flexible knowledge base and master the skills to apply this knowledge for problem solving [1]. Problem–based learning (PBL) was first introduced at McMaster University in Canada in the mid 1960s, and it represents a

D. Xia (✉)
Zhejiang Chinese Medical University, Binwen Road 548, 310053 Hangzhou, China
e-mail: xdz_zjtcm@hotmail.com

major development and change in higher educational practice and continues to be used in diverse ways across different subjects and disciplines worldwide. In most medical schools, the PBL sessions are guided by facilitators so that the students can obtain the learning outcomes [2]. It is emphasized that the role of the lecturer in the PBL process is sometimes referred to as that of a facilitator of learning whose function is to scaffold student learning, by stimulating elaboration, integration of knowledge and interaction between students by asking questions and asking for clarification and application of knowledge [3].

In response to the lack of research on PBL-based food courses, we took a traditional, lecture-based introductory food hygiene course and restructured it into a PBL format. It is believed that the results of this study which aims to compare the impacts of PBL and traditional methods on student teachers' satisfaction in the introductory food hygiene course will contribute to the existing published materials concerned with the teaching of food hygiene.

196.2 Methods

196.2.1 Setting

This study was conducted at the College of Pharmaceutical Sciences, Zhejiang Chinese Medical University, Hangzhou, China.

196.2.2 Design and Procedure

The subjects of this study were 28 third-year student teachers (female = 16, male = 12). Food hygiene is a major course in Food Hygiene and Determination direction of Food Science and Technology profession. In this study, the pre-test/post-test quasi-experimental method with an equivalent control group was used. There were 34 participants that included teachers. Moreover, there was one control group (traditional instruction, CON group) and one experimental group (PBL group), consisting of 14 students and 14 students respectively. The mean ages of the students in the PBL group and the CON group were both 21 years. The students' satisfaction with the introductory food hygiene course was measured using the Student Satisfaction Scale.

The textbook called "21st century teaching material" both in the PBL group and in the CON group. The PBL scenario included a tutor and student copy. The tutor copy is a written copy of all of the steps a student needs to take during the scenario. In the student copy, the previously mentioned parts were left empty for the students to complete. The study was conducted during the 6th semester in the food hygiene course. Initially, workshops for teachers were conducted and objectives for food pollution courses in the food hygiene curriculum were refined. The duration of the study was 6 weeks (18 lessons of lecture time) from March to April. In both of the groups, the students' satisfaction in the food hygiene course was measured before and after the study. The dependent variables were post-test student satisfaction scores on each of the three sub-scales. To examine the implementation of PBL, some key topics in Food Pollution (Physical pollution; Chemical pollution) were chosen for the study. During a 90 min lesson in the PBL group, a sample scenario whose topic was different from the ones targeted in the research was gone through by the teacher and the students. Then, the students were informed about how PBL methods are used. In the CON group, the same topics were covered at the same time using the traditional instruction method [4].

Focus group discussions were conducted to explore in more depth the opinions expressed on the questionnaires by the participants. The questions for the focus groups sought opinions about the incorporation of food pollution courses in the food hygiene curriculum and use of PBL as a teaching approach. The scenario in the module which consisted of six PBL sessions was selected from the textbook. The physical pollution topics previously mentioned were covered in the scenarios and were prepared by the first researcher. In the first five PBL sessions, students were asked to solve three or four new problems (qualitative and/or quantitative problems each connected to each other) working together. In the last session, the scenario consisted of one part and it required the solution of the first problem and revision of all the information learnt. In the CON group, the topics were problems solved during the PBL sessions were solved in the traditional problem solving format in the CON group.

196.2.3 Data Analysis

The data from the Student Satisfaction Scale were analyzed using the SPSS statistical analysis program. Data was both quantitative and qualitative. Means (M) and standard deviations (SD) were calculated. Multi-variate analysis was also used and $p < 0.05$ was adopted for this study.

196.3 Results

Students have consistently excelled in food hygiene course using the PBL approach of learning. Table 196.1 shows the descriptive statistics of student teachers' pre-test and post-test scores on the three sub-scales of the Student Satisfaction Scale. The analysis revealed no statistically significant difference in "satisfaction in learning food hygiene" ($p > 0.05$), "quality of instruction" ($p > 0.05$) and "teaching methods/activities" ($p > 0.05$). Therefore, we found that the two groups were similar to each other with respect to the collective dependent

Table 196.1 Descriptive statistics for student teachers' satisfaction with the food hygiene course

Variable	Pre-test				Post-test			
	PBL group ($n = 14$)		CON group ($n = 14$)		PBL group ($n = 14$)		CON group ($n = 14$)	
	M	SD	M	SD	M	SD	M	SD
Satisfaction in learning food hygiene	40.52	4.16	41.92	4.37	49.62	6.23	42.02	4.83
Quality of instruction	12.35	1.15	11.62	1.03	16.52	2.05	12.14	1.57
Teaching methods/activities	21.62	1.99	21.75	2.13	28.95	2.35	22.08	1.95
Total	74.49	7.30	75.29	7.53	95.09	10.63	76.24	8.35

variable for satisfaction. To compare the groups on each post-measure, again, the tests were conducted between the post-test scores of the PBL group and the post-test scores of the CON group. The analysis indicated that there was obvious significant difference between the groups in the sub-scales satisfaction in learning food hygiene ($p < 0.05$), quality of instruction ($p < 0.05$), and the sub-scale teaching methods/activities ($p < 0.05$). The pre-test and post-test scores relating to quality of instruction ($p < 0.05$) and teaching methods/activities ($p < 0.05$) sub-scales of the students who were in the PBL group showed a significant difference in favour of the post-test.

196.4 Discussion

The present study showed that both students and teachers generally rated the learning of food hygiene by food science and technology students highly. The support for the incorporation of food pollution teaching in the food hygiene curriculum could be explained by various reasons. In addition, the observed group performed significantly better in the test of the first PBL topic compared to the control group. This result could probably due to the fact that the observed group paid more attention during the PBL session [2]. This short-term, problem-based educational intervention was successful in increasing the collective research activities of students.

It is well known, PBL was generally evaluated by teachers as a positive approach which enabled the student to develop skills which were relevant to practice. However, teachers' approaches changed with the stage of the program with greater direction required at first [3]. From this study, some students were probably apprehensive about PBL, but eventually turned out to like it since they had been prepared fully during their orientation and their tutors are available to assist them. Some of the participants in this study felt that students were not always able to challenge each other and evaluate what they had found [5].

PBL as a method and philosophy is a widely adopted and effective approach to fostering autonomy, critical thinking and self-directed learning in undergraduates.

In fact, the ability to understand and use information is emphasized rather than merely possessing it. In this respect, it is crucial for teacher candidates to have these higher order thinking and problem solving skills along with the ability to cooperate and work effectively within a team.

However, there were some aspects that were of concern. The main concern from both students and teachers was the limitation in learning resources for students. There is therefore need to prioritize the issue of learning resources during planning as a way of sustaining PBL. The issue of reliable, valid and cost-effective student ultrasound assessment methods in PBL raised by teachers is another challenge that needs to be addressed. There is need therefore to rethink our assessment methods of food pollution courses to match them with the way students learn. We urge teachers to support the PBL way of learning and not get frustrated because they no longer feel like the authority of knowledge that they previously perceived.

196.5 Conclusion

Food hygiene study using PBL has been successfully implemented. Both teachers and students have expressed satisfaction with the student-centered, problem based learning approach to training. However, this is still an ongoing process and will require the total commitment of both students and teachers.

References

1. Dochy F, Segers M, Van den Bossche P et al (2003) Effects of problem-based learning: a meta analysis. Learn Instr 13:533–568
2. Chuan TY, Rosly NB, Zolkipli MZB et al (2011) Problem-based learning: with or without facilitator? Procedia-Socia Behav Sci 18:394–399
3. Rowan CJ, McCourt C, Bick D et al (2007) Problem based learning in midwifery—the teachers perspective. Nurs Edu Today 27:131–138
4. Selcuk GS, Caliskan S (2010) A small-scale study comparing the impacts of problem-based learning and traditional methods on student satisfaction in the introductory physics course. Procedia-Socia Behav Sci 2:809–813
5. Lin YC, Huang YS, Lai CS et al (2009) Problem-based learning curriculum in medical education at Kaohsiung Medical University. Kaohsiung J Med Sci 25:264–269

Chapter 197
Education Security of Bridgehead Strategic in Southwest China: Concept, Problems and Solutions

Jing Tian and Ling Wang

Abstract Southwest "Bridgehead" construction is a major national strategic in China, which marks a major advance of opening strategy. Education is an important soft power resource. The educational security problem is highlights in the "bridgehead" strategy. This article analysis the problem of education security in the new situation, discusses the development path based on independence, and proposes some relevant recommendations.

Keywords Education security · Southwest bridgehead strategic · China

197.1 Introductions

In 2011, the State Council of China issued "on the support of the Yunnan province to speed up construction the southwest important bridgehead", the document marked that the Yunnan bridgehead construction become to national strategy. The southwest bridgehead was proposed by China's former General Secretary Jin-tao Hu who visited to Yunnan in 2009. No doubt, this can bring more trade opportunities and international capital for Chinese, but it wills also produced profound

J. Tian (✉)
School of Education Science and Management, Yunnan Normal University, Kunming 650500, China
e-mail: jingtian2003003@163.com

L. Wang
Key Laboratory of Nationalities Education Information of Education Ministry, Yunnan Normal University, Kunming 650500, China
e-mail: wanglingyn@126.com

L. Wang
The Development Research Center of Minority Education, Northwest Normal University, Lanzhou 730070, China

influence on China's politics, economy, culture and education and other fields, and has brought new development opportunities and challenges. Yunnan province because of its special geographical conditions, economic characteristics, historical and cultural, ethnic distribution of objective reality has a special education security forms and problems. The implementation of the southwest "bridgehead" strategy highlights the important value to the education safety.

197.2 The Concept of Education Security in the Background of Southwest Bridgehead Construction

Non traditional security can also be called non-military security, the safety factor is very extensive, mainly including: economic, ecological, resource, information, education, terrorism, the spread of the disease, trans-national crimes, illegal immigration, money laundering, etc. Education security is one of them. Research on education security began in early twentieth century in China. Xiao-bo Jin thought that education security is to safeguard the national education sovereignty, protect system of education without external interference, and erosion, and has the right to take measures to protect their interests in education [1]. Fang-ping Cheng have pointed to that the concept of education security contains all kinds of education factors and problem which directly or indirectly affects and restricts safety issues of the national or regional [2]. Scholars have interpreted education security from the international perspective to consider competition, permeability, threat, challenge and whether the loss of sovereignty and development opportunities, also analysis of education security problems which could be lead in the domestic background. Accordingly, the education security is defined as: all kinds of education issues or education crisis involving national security, which are brought by external or internal conflict, challenge, competition, and erosion in the development. Research on education security problems mainly focus on how to maintain the sovereignty, the development right of the national education, enhance the value system of the mainstream education, promoting social stability, ethnic unity, harmonious development etc.

197.3 The Main Problems of Education Security in Bridgehead Construction

Yunnan province is located in the border which is lags behind majority province in China, and neighbouring countries' environment is very unstable, those nationals' development level, social system, religion and culture are different, which would bring uncertain factors about security problems, will directly affect the exchange and development of education, mainly in the following aspects:

Education modernization process is relatively slow, which Mainly displays in: education development is not balanced between urban and rural areas, regional; educational development lagged in the ethnic minority, remote and poor areas; the balanced development of compulsory education have higher pressure; unfair education is more prominent; there is a large gap compared the education investment with the actual demand; internal structure of education and resource allocation unreasonable; the level of scientific research, education quality should be improved; school management is relatively weak etc.

There are 4,060 km land border line in Yunnan province, bordering on Vietnam, Laos, and Burma. Sixteen ethnic groups live across the border. In the promotion of the economic globalization, regional economic integration, along the border area gradually rise of the flow phenomenon of trans-national education of cross-border ethnic children [3]. It shows the importance of cross-border education. In the middle of 1990s, there was appear a phenomenon of students outflow reading in the border areas, this phenomenon could explain the lag problem of cross-border ethnic education development. In 2005, the range of "three free" (free textbooks, free fees, free stationery) expand to all the towns pupils along the border [4]. School running conditions of the cross-border ethnic education have been greatly improved in the border area. The students began to return, many of Burma, Vietnam, and Laos's students flow in Chinese studying. The studying flow situation of cross-border ethnic children related to national social stability in border ethnic areas. However, although the students in border area begin enjoy free compulsory education, but in the edge, border and cross-border ethnic groups living environment change is not big, poverty still plaguing their development.

The implementation of "bridgehead" strategy will further promote China's education opening to the outside world, and strengthen the "going out", "Introduction in" of education. In the "Introduction in", more and more countries will rely on competition strength of education and economic enter into China's education market. The influx of foreign educational resources promotes the diversity of Chinese education development, conducive to learning foreign education experience; to accelerate the process of the development of education, but it would also weaken education resource control. Education is the most effective means to the cultural transmission and preservation. Education and culture are closely related, education security problem also is bound to affect the safety culture, for China. On the one hand is facing the reality shock, how Chinese culture create new, changing excellent ingredients of Chinese national culture tradition into the cultural value resources of world, then make a unique contribution to the world culture; on the other hand, also need to consider some foreign media about the "Chinese cultural expansion" argument, which make the security "dilemma" problem for Chinese culture development.

China as a developing country, educational exchanges have developed from asymmetric to symmetric direction gradually, interdependence has equal gradually. Implementation of the "bridgehead" strategy will enable further internationalization, diversification of Chinese education. Problems related to education security are more extensive, directly and clearly. In the situation of world non-traditional security is becoming more and more complex. China must be up to the level of national security strategy in the international exchange of education, hold overall situation to maintain and promote the overall safety of the country by adapt to development of educational exchanges of the new situation need.

197.4 Countermeasures to Alleviate the Problem of Education Security

In the education security field, the equalization of education needs to gradually achieve in the domestic; to overseas, common safety should be pursuit, and achieve mutual understanding in education ethos, education philosophy with different countries. For the lag problem of Education, educational fund must be increased, supported education of the vulnerable areas and vulnerable groups by the corresponding laws to support and guarantee in employment system, personnel system, management. Continue to improve the literacy and basic education popularization, to support ethnic minority languages teaching, to make the race culture, local value into the classroom. Intensify efforts to adjust the structure of education, encourage the development of private education, and improve the development of occupation education, which closely combined with the characteristics of the local economy, cultural and social development and growth, help the students learn to use. To improve the high school enrolment rate, university enrolment rate, and gradually narrow the gap with the developed areas. Encourage to construct the learning community, to promote the civilization process of local society.

The development of the cross-border education should pay attention to the following points: firstly, to carry out investigations and studies, to speed up the layout and construction of rural primary and secondary schools along the border region. Secondly, the cross-border education should not only attach importance to national identity, but also should pay attention to the sovereignty, national consciousness, national and patriotic education. Thirdly, there are a series of problems need high-level attention which are the shortage of educational resources, the loss of teachers, and lack of bilingual teachers etc., those problems need be taken effective measures to solve. Fourthly, we also need to fully understand the policies of the cross-border ethnic education around the countries, so as to form the communication and interaction of the cross-border education healthy, harmonious border.

Educational sovereignty problem in the course of education internationalization, China whether to create a favourable international environment for self, or to have a louder voice in the international community, must accelerate the pace of integration into the international system, which is one of the important measures to adjust traditional education absolute sovereignty idea, establish new, modern education of sovereignty. Adhere to the development view of educational sovereignty, according to the changes of historical conditions to give timely adjustment and improvement. As a modern idea of education sovereignty, it should insist on sovereignty amortized and hierarchical concept that has the absolute and exclusive legislative power. To meet a "common interest" between countries, education investment rights, running right, information sharing peripheral right and property belong to the elastic, which could give delivered under the principle of the independent, consultation and voluntary. Transfer of education sovereignty should comply with the following principles: Based on voluntary; to respect other countries' education sovereignty.

197.5 Summary

In short, with Chinese development, expand opening to the outside world, education security in the depth and breadth are gradually expanding. Chinese education should emphasize participate actively in the international community. In practice, new educational safe mode should be adopting based on confidence-building measures, emphasizes to strengthen the construction of regional education security mechanism, safeguard national education security could through multilateral cooperation. China should also actively further cooperation with neighbouring countries in education; strengthen the shaping ability, focusing on the institutional framework of comprehensive cooperation of regional education.

Acknowledgments The research reported here is financially supported by the Major project of Key Research Institute of Humanities and Social Sciences Education of Education Ministry of China, Grant NO. 11JJD880023. Part work is supported by the Humanity and Social Science Funds of Education Ministry of China, Grant NO. 10YJC880112.

References

1. Jin X (2004) A preliminary probe into education sovereignty. Int Bus Res 6:3–7
2. Cheng F (2001) Education security problems in the development of west China. Educ Res 9:35–38
3. He Y, Gao H (2010) The education issues of Yunnan cross-border ethnic groups in the perspective of cultural safety. J Yunnan Norm Univ (Philosophy and Social Sciences Edition) 42(4):35–41
4. Li R (2009). The harmony and stability of the relation s between the borderland ethnic groups in Yunnan in the past sixty years. J Yunnan Univ Nat (Social Sciences) 126(15):16–20

Chapter 198
Applications of Network-Based Education in Lifelong Medical Education

Liyuan Sun, Mingcheng Li and Yundong Zhao

Abstract Lifelong medical education extends medical education beyond the limitations of school education, expands the entire living and working spaces for medical workers, and meets the learners' needs for self-development and self-improvement. Online education abandons the traditional education system, gives full play to the network-based educational function and rich medical education resource advantages, provides medical workers with a kind of online teaching and learning environment, and carries out non-face-to-face learner-centered educational activities. Online education has many advantages to meet the desires of various groups of people for knowledge.

Keywords Network-based education · Lifelong medical education · Drawbacks

With the rapid development of science and technology, knowledge and information update faster and faster, and lifelong education is gradually accepted by medical workers. The traditional medical education system that centers on schools, teachers and textbooks can no longer meet the needs of the age and health undertakings. Online education has changed the traditional classroom teaching methods, met desires of various medical workers for knowledge, and provided more people with conditions to receive lifelong education. With the constant progress of network technologies and medical websites, online education has gradually become the best way to achieve lifelong medical education [1].

L. Sun · M. Li · Y. Zhao (✉)
School of Medical Test, Beihua University, Jilin, China
e-mail: jlsunliyuan@163.com

198.1 Lifelong Medical Education

The traditional medical education refers to educational activities based on the needs of social demands to cultivate medical and health talents in a purposeful, planned and organized manner. Generally, it refers to the education at the level of medical colleges and universities. The modern medical education system broadly includes academic medical education, continuing medical education, health care vocational skills training, general medical education, standardized training of resident doctors, and remote medical education [2]. However, faced with busy clinical work after their graduation from schools, medical staff members are very much limited in their learning and professional expertise update. In order to ensure sustainable development of the medical and health services, academic education, continuing medical education and lifelong education must be organically integrated to establish a sound lifelong medical education system, which uses the full range of health and education resources and technical advantages of distance education to carry out various forms of continuing medical education activities and strengthen the management of continuing medical education [3].

198.1.1 Academic Education to Promote Lifelong Education

The national planning outline for mid-term and long-term education reform and development has pointed out the direction for the reform and development of higher education, including medical education. It highlights the people education concept of "moral education first, emphasis on ability and comprehensive development". It requires that medical education highlight quality improvement even more. The most fundamental in improving the quality of medical education is to improve the quality of medical personnel training. It should strive to cultivate personnel with noble medical ethics, superb medical skills, rich humanistic qualifications, a strong sense of social responsibility, and strong innovative spirits. Teachers in their teaching processes should teach the trainees "how to fish" to strengthen their self-learning ability, improve their independent thinking and ability to work independently, and adapt to the development of lifelong education.

198.1.2 Progress of Science and Technology to Drive Lifelong Education

The high-speed update of medical knowledge results in more importance and urgency for continued medical education, and lifelong learning has become the only way to grasp the new diagnostic markers and medical technology. An endless stream of new treatment technologies leads modern medicine toward the multi-disciplinary, multi-technology and multiple-way directions; toward the high-throughput, multi-channel, multi-factor and multi-point directions of comprehensive analysis of complex system development, toward the living-body, dynamic, full-function and whole-process development directions. Medicine in the twenty-first century has become the most extensive realm of the most critical core technological applications, so medical workers must try to keep up the forefront through lifelong learning, vigorously strengthen the acquisition of new medical technologies and their applications to continue raising their professional levels and render better services for people's health.

198.1.3 Institutional Guarantee to Ensure Lifelong Education

The concept of lifelong education requires integration of fundamental medical education, after-graduation education and continuing medical education. While raising the quality of education in schools, we must strengthen the institutionalization and standardization of professional training of resident physicians at the same time, so that the after-graduation education can become a formal medical education system compulsory to all the medical school graduates. The opinions of the CPC central committee and the state council on deepening medical and health system reform has determined the basic objectives and policy measures for deepening the reform of medical and health systems in our country, explicitly proposing strengthening the building of medical and health personnel teams, intensifying team building for high-level scientific research, medical, health management, etc. Actively engaging in continuing medical education, striving to form a modernized medical education system with clear work division among medical college education, after-graduating education and continuing education that communicate with and link to one another, so that medical and health workers can continually develop their intelligence and improve their level of professional skills to promote the development of health services.

198.1.4 Practitioner Licensing to Demand Lifelong Education

In order to strengthen the ranks of the practitioners, improve the physicians' work ethic and professional quality, and protect the health of the people, in June 1998, China promulgated the Law of the People's Republic of China on medical practitioners, providing that no practitioner shall be engaged in medical practice without obtaining the practitioner qualifications. Likewise, traditional Chinese medicine practitioners, public health practitioners, pharmacists, dentists, test technicians, nurses and other medical-related professionals shall also need to pass the practitioner qualification exams before starting work. The mounting pressure on practitioner licensing pushes medical workers to lifelong learning. According to statistics, in 2009 and 2010, the total passing rate of the national practitioner exams was only 20.73 and 25.79 % respectively, and a medical education website reported 75.62 and 79.58 % respectively after it carried out a survey to the students participating in the website tutoring. There is no denying that these two sets of telltale data have revealed some problems.

198.2 Applications of Network-Based Education in Lifelong Medical Education

198.2.1 Online Education

Online education gives full play to various educational functions and advantages of rich online medical education resources, provides medical workers with a network-based teaching and learning environment, delivers digitized contents, and offers non-face-to-face education with learners centered. Online education is mainly dependent on the computer network communication technology and computer multimedia technology, as well as on the use of these technologies to establish a two-way interactive platform of e-learning. It is an educational process that can transmit in real time or make available or online texts, voices, videos, graphics, electronic courseware, etc. across time and space. It provides a rich learning resource for people and creates a good interactive, intelligent and even simulation learning environment—virtual schools, virtual classrooms, virtual laboratories, virtual libraries, etc. It is the best way for medical workers to access to self-education and lifelong education [3].

198.2.2 Application Advantages of Network-Based Education in Lifelong Medical Education

Openness to beneficiary groups: network-based education does not need to teach and learn face-to-face, and openness is its basic feature. Abundant medical professional websites, expert web sites, professional websites of academic organizations, etc. are independent of time and space limitations. They extend, high-quality medical education to every corner of society so that medical workers are given more opportunities to access education [4].

Autonomy of learning behaviors: The teaching model of online education has changed from the original "teaching-centered" to "learning-centered". Choices of learning timeframes, locations, courses, beginning chapters, etc. have become more flexible and free. The learning contents are based on interests and self-development needs. Learners can select various subjects and contents, and adjust their learning schedule according to their own knowledge structures.

Sharing of educational resources: a variety of medical education resources spans through space distance limitations with the help of the networks to achieve equality in education. Medical schools can give full play to their disciplinary advantages and educational resource advantages, spread their best teachers and best teaching results in all directions through the platforms of their quality course and excellent courses, while medical workers, by online telephone, broadband Internet, mobile phone internet, etc., share the rich medical teaching resources of different institutions. Online education platforms will realize resource sharing and complementary advantages immensely, so that quality education becomes accessible to each and every one of the medical workers [5].

Individualized teaching schedule: online education provides individualized teaching with a realistic way to achieve effectiveness. It makes use of the database management technology and two-way interactive features. Targeting the personalized information for each network learner, learning process, knowledge acquisition, etc., the system is able to systematically trace and record them entirely. Meanwhile, the system of teaching and learning services, according to the system records of personal data, can make individualized learning recommendations to different learners.

198.3 Conclusions

With the rapid development of lifelong education of medical workers, we should pay attention to the unbalanced development nationwide, which has resulted in large differences between and among regions, urban and rural areas, disciplines, workplaces, etc. The education forms and contents cannot fully meet the needs of the medical workers. There are still some relatively weak aspects such as education management, supervision, funding and inputs, etc. It is an important approach to create a favorable environment for lifelong education of medical workers, establish lifelong education support platform, develop the education standards consistent with the national situations, improve lifelong education legislation, increase funding and inputs in lifelong education, and constantly improve the management capability.

References

1. Chu W, Lin C (2011) Research on adults' lifelong learning model against the backgrounds of a learning-oriented society. Adult Edu 10:19–22
2. Liu Y, Zhu X (2012) Research and practice of establishing lifelong medical education system by local medical colleges and schools. Edu Vocat 3:166–167

3. Taotao C, Xiaojuan Z (2011) Exploration of network-based adult education innovation model. China Adult Edu 19:117–118
4. Yanyi Z (2010) A survey of students' independent self-learning orientation in open education. Edu Occup 35:60–62
5. Dongchun X (2010) New perspectives in the building of online learning platforms in universities. Edu Rev 02:21–23

Chapter 199
The Application of Informatics Technology in Foreign Medical Undergraduates Teaching

Limei Liu, Taiguang Piao and Wei Li

Abstract As an important part of higher education, international undergraduates' education has become the focus of the education, recently. Parasitology is a basic subject for foreign medical undergraduates. To achieve better effects and apply them advanced development, we give the teaching of parasitology with multimedia and internet communication ways. The results showed that about 94.8 % students accepted this teaching mode. It includes all kinds of teaching methods involve in case analysis, reports and interactive discussion. In this way, the teaching contents were optimized for individuals and were shared with them. They could learn actively. The application of informatics technology shows an important significance in autonomous and lifelong learning.

Keywords Informatics technology · Foreign medical undergraduates · Autonomous learning

199.1 Introduction

In recent years, following the deepening of cultural exchanges and cooperation, the education for International students has now been an important part of the undergraduate medical education, occupied a unique position in the medical education and showed a special significance. In August 2006, approved by the national Ministry of Education, the International education and exchange College of Beihua University attained the privilege for receiving international students sponsored by Chinese Government Scholarship. Our department has taken the responsibility of the parasitological teaching. Now, more than 320 undergraduate medicine students (six batches) had been taught parasitology in English in their

L. Liu · T. Piao · W. Li (✉)
School of Medical Test, Beihua University, Jilin, China
e-mail: bhweili@yahoo.com.cn

undergraduate studying. In order to achieve the intended purpose, a great deal of exploration about arrangement and optimization of teaching content, reformation of teaching methods especially the application of informatics technologies were carried out. Now it was illustrated as follows.

199.2 Optimization of the Contents for Individuals with Multimedia

Parasitology is the basic subject for undergraduates; it involves biology, physiopathology, pathology, immunology and so on. According to the hometown of the foreign undergraduates, we optimized the individualized teaching contents. The tropical parasitic diseases were supplemented, for many students come from Pakistan, Somalia and some countries in Africa. It enhanced the enthusiasm of the students to learn parasitology, because they are very concerned about the parasitic disease endemic in their countries. Considering the customs of Islam, the contents about pork tapeworm were neglect, but when we talked to the students about our arrangements, they did not degree with it. They want to learn more. So we adjust the content into two parts, one was given the details of the tropical parasitic diseases and the other was given a brief introduction of the rare cases. However, to understand the knowledge associated the parasite maybe difficult for them, especially in English. So we give the lecture with digital microscope mutual system in the multimedia-based teaching laboratory.

199.2.1 The Construction of the Digital Microscope Mutual System

The digital microscope mutual system consisted with about 50 sets of digital microscopes, computers and the connections of the net. The morphology of the parasite was shown on the screens of both the teacher's computer and that of the students' through the microscope synchronously. The system even can be connected with internet by route if necessary. The data bank contained PPT document, video, text book, case analysis, electronic courseware and international professional network.

199.2.2 Manipulation and Design of the Class

The director was given to the different batch of students at the class as Table 199.1; the objective is to grasp the parasitological knowledge through reconstructing their knowledge net by autonomous learning, cooperation, analyses

Table 199.1 Construction of the teaching mode

Procedure	For teachers	For students
Induction	Give the requirements, cases and emphases according text book	Understand the arrangement; choose the data by themselves and study
Self-learning and discussion	Supervise the studying of students; Induce the discussion	Studying and submit their question to the teacher; Discuss question with others
Display in class	Organize students to give their shows; Induce students to discuss on it	Give their reports; Listen to the reports and discussion
Summary	Give summary	Construct their own knowledge system Review
Teaching evaluation	Test Give the questionnaire survey	Complete the test Complete the questionnaire survey

and discussion. The results were showed in Table 199.2. About 94.8 % students accepted this teaching mode. And more than 40 % students thought it is helpful for autonomy learning.

199.2.3 Communicate with the International Undergraduates in Network as a Supplement

About 84.5 % students favor of the internet communication methods. The internet informatics allows them to become familiar with their studying content and help them to form the autonomic learning habits [1]. The general modes of internet communication include e-mail, QQ, RenRen, MSN and so on, and E-mail is the most popular Internet service (62.3 %). The teacher could give the review or case report by e-mail, and students might submit their homework. Sometimes some international students contact teacher with QQ, which make them familiar with Chinese living quickly. Companied with the internet communication inside and outside the class, students would be easier in Chinese studying.

199.3 Discussion

The application of the informatics techniques is of great benefits to students and teachers. The operation of the system is simple and convenient. Compared with the traditional teaching methods, it can mobilize the enthusiasm of student greatly and improved the teaching quality and efficiency [2].

Table 199.2 Questionnaire and results of teaching with multimedia

Questions	Results
How about the multimedia?	A. Very good (29.3 %); B. good (65.5 %); C. uncertain (5.2 %); D. bad (0)
What is your attitude to multimedia?	A. strongly supportive (21.4 %); B. supportive (67.8 %); C. uncertain (10.8 %); D. not supportive (0)
Are you interested with the data?	A. Yes (100 %); B. uncertain (0); B No (0)
How much content you can understand?	A. All (30.4 %); B. most (66.4 %); C. part (3.2 %); D. a little (0)
How about the multimedia to autonomy learning?	A. More valid (40.4 %); B. valid (59.6 %); C. not valid (0)
How about the multimedia to the uses of internet data?	A. Highly improved (45.5 %); B. improved (55.6 %); C. uncertain (0)
How about the multimedia to enthusiasm and go-aheadism?	A. More helpful (64.3 %); B. helpful (35.7 %); C. no help (0)
How about the multimedia to the competence of informatics technique?	A. More helpful (31.1 %); B. helpful (68.9 %); C. no help (0)
Compare with the traditional method, how much you can remember?	A. All (3.8 %); B. most (86.4 %); C. part (10.8 %); D. a little (0)
Do you want to continue using multimedia?	A. Yes (100 %); B. No(0)
Which ways of communication do you like best?	A. Direct (15.5 %); B. by QQ (8.5 %); C. by MSN (7 %); D. by email (62.3 %); E. other (6.7 %)
How about the multimedia used in other subjects?	A. Strongly agrees (12.4 %); B. agrees (72 %); C. according to the subject (15.6 %)

199.3.1 Sharing Resources, Improve the Teaching Efficiency

In the class, teacher could share the data with students, including pictures, flash, videos, case reports and so on. The specific images found by the students could be shared with other students or projected apparatus and discussed. Teacher can give homework and review through the system, and supervise the study of the students in the class and reply the students on time. If a student made some mistake, teacher could send a message such as a black flash or words without interrupting others, and reminded him to concentrate on the class. So the multimedia provides more knowledge in the limited time and improved the efficiency of the teaching [3].

199.3.2 Mobilize Students' Enthusiasm to Understand the Class Actively

The lecture was given in English, but sometimes students might had problems in understanding the content because of the medical terms. For example, plasmodium is the emphases and main point. If the teacher give the lecture only by words and pictures, it might be difficult to grasp main points of the development and pathogenesis for so many medical terms, but if it was showed by flash or videos in multimedia, accompanied by explanation, it would be impressed on their memory and easier to be remembered. In the case analysis, students were very actively; the data were attractive and made them thinking which mobilized their enthusiasm of studying. They would actively debate each other and require to be approved by teachers.

199.3.3 Facilitate Autonomous Learning and Long-Life Learning

The aim of higher education is not only to give students knowledge but helps them autonomous learning, which is the base of long-life learning [4]. After graduated from school, they would deal with the problems independently. They should know how to get the knowledge they needed as clinical doctors. So long-life learning is necessary for a doctor. The application of internet informatics technology would benefit for the formation of autonomous learning. It inspirited the students in many ways and facilitates the autonomous learning gradually.

199.4 Conclusion

The internet informatics technology benefits parasitology teaching of international students greatly. However, some problems would be involved, includes the viruses infection and stable system, and as a supervisor, teachers have the responsibility of preventing the students away from the net-games. So how to induce the students is also a big problem. On the other side, the technology of microscope would be ignored in their studying [5]. So we should pay more attention to combine the multimedia with the traditional methods properly.

References

1. Cao L, Zhang T (2012) Social networking sites and educational adaptation in higher education: A case study of Chinese international students in New Zealand. Sci World J, vol 5. doi:10.1100/2012/289356
2. Zhang J, Xu W, Huang F (2010) Experience of the digital interactive system in human parasitology experimental teaching. J Trop Med 10(8)
3. Terndrup TE, Ali S, Hulse S, Shaffer M, Lloyd T (2013) Multimedia education increases elder knowledge of emergency department care. West J Emerg Med 14 (2):132–136
4. Alexander S, Kernohan G, McCullagh P (2004) Self directed and lifelong learning. Stud Health Technol Inform 109:152–166
5. Zhang J, Xu W, Huang F (2010) Experience of the digital interactive system in human parasitology experimental teaching. J Trop Med 10(8):1024–1025

Chapter 200
Discussion on the Reform of Teaching Software Development Training Curriculum Based on Application Store

Yan-jun Zhu, Wen-liang Cao and Jian-xin Li

Abstract With the rapid development of online software application store scale, software application store is not only a development practice platform for students to show themselves, but also a resource platform for teachers to provide much teaching material with real project. Based on the characteristics of software development training courses and software application store. Discussed software development training course on how to introduce the Internet open platform as a real teaching practice platform, according to the software training course teaching objectives, design the whole process of teaching reform.

Keywords Teaching reform · Software application store · Open platform · Practice teaching

200.1 Introduction

In order to improve the students' practice ability and let students can take full use of theoretical knowledge and skills to solve practical problems, the training course is arranged for the corresponding software development course. Training course is a course that requires students to complete a comprehensive experiment under the guidance of teachers in the limited time, combining the teaching theory course and students' practical ability training of organic, it is a benign cycle of the theory and practice, in the cycle, where the knowledge and practice transform each other and students can deepen the related understanding of knowledge. The software development training courses require students to complete the implementation of a system by combining with the corresponding course knowledge that they have

Y. Zhu (✉) · W. Cao · J. Li
Department of Computer Engineering, Dongguan Polytechnic, Dongguan 523808, China
e-mail: zyjun23@gmail.com

learned, just like database, interface design knowledge etc. How to attract the students' interest in learning and provide a better platform for students to display themselves, this paper discusses the reform of teaching software development training curriculum on how to introduce the Internet open platform as a real teaching practice platform into the process of teaching.

200.2 Open Platform and Application Software Store

The Open Platform provides open APIs and packages the website service and content into recognizable data interface, it is also invoked by the third party developers to implement various applications. The Open Platform provides various interfaces to access web resources and complete complex data exchange, the web site convert their site into development platform which is equivalent with operating system. Third party developers can develop various applications to share the site's resources and users based on these existing open API. All programmers and software companies can sell their product, which is developed based on Open API, and obtain corresponding rewarded according to the sites' revenue sharing model.

With iPhone as the representative of the first generation, the intelligent mobile phone has an explosive growth since 2007. In July, 2008, Apple's app store is officially put into operation, in less than 5 years, Appstore has more than 550,000 application. In October, 2008, Google App Store Android Market (now renamed Google Play) has the similar functional architecture, now it has more than 450,000 applications available for download. Following the space of Apple, many IT companies have issued their open platform and corresponding application store. The application store will become the main application sharing platform in the future.

Application of application store involves game, books, entertainment, education, life, tools, travel, music, sports, news, business, reference, efficiency, health, graphics, financial, social, medical, navigation etc. These applications are small and practical application software, which are close to our life. Therefore, these applications can be used as the teaching case, and everyone can obtain these application software with a small fee or free.

200.3 The Concepts and Ideas of Teaching Reform

Software training course requires student to design and develop a software system based on a real subject of social existence, combining various knowledge that they have learned, such as programming language, database, interface design etc. It aims to cultivate students' innovation and the ability of using computer to analyze and solve practical problem. Therefore, the aim of software training course should involve the following items.

Firstly, the course can create innovative atmosphere of learning and train their ability of solving problem. Students are able to actively explore on how to complete individual task in a team.

Secondly, the course should culture students' ability of communication and cooperation. Cooperation is the beginning of communication, in the process of software development, each group and each student can experience that communication and cooperation is a very important thing.

Thirdly, we should respect for the students' personality, pay attention on the individual differences, meet the students' needs. In the whole process of knowledge system, students have their own learning interest, in order to achieve better teaching effect; we must break the traditional teaching mode that take individual task as the center of teaching, the individual task is not choice, closed and follow the pattern, then we should select the teaching mode that take group task as the center of teaching, the group task is selective and opening. It differs from man to man. As a result, the transforming teaching mode can stimulate the enthusiasm of the students, and train students to master and apply knowledge. It make each student can obtain the full development, then we obtain the entire students' development.

200.4 The Design of Teaching Process

Software training courses should take the complete project training as the main content, and take the software development process as the main teaching design, and design the corresponding role for each stage of software development process. In voluntary choice and free combination principle, students choose the corresponding role and set up a team according to their own situation, the team is consisted of project manager, design engineer, develop engineer and test engineer. As a coach,teachers is responsible for guiding the students, setting project scenario, auditing students to complete the project in cooperative ability and professional R&D skills.

200.4.1 The Interaction Patterns Between Teachers and Students

Training course is the process of practice teaching, it takes the individual learning to extend to a team with cooperative learning ability, it is also an exchange platform and interaction process between teachers and students, and its philosophy is communication, understanding, experience and inspiration. Therefore, in the process of teaching, the teacher is just a coach, students are the main role. Firstly, students learn the basic knowledge that is required to complete corresponding task.

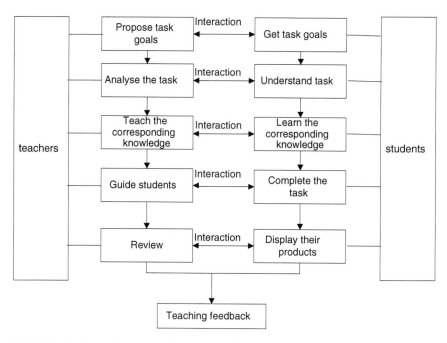

Fig. 200.1 The interaction patterns between teachers and students

Then, with the form of analysis and discussion, students participate in the teaching process to achieve the mastery of the knowledge, the process is consisted of setting up task goals, understanding task, completing task and displaying their product, the interaction patterns between teachers and students as shown in Fig. 200.1.

200.4.2 The Design of Teaching Process

The teaching process usually follow up the teaching process of project teaching, which is divided into six processes: open platform selection, students group, project selection, project development, demonstration and assessment work, review and evaluation.

Firstly, open platform selection, the number of open platform is numerous, the application scope and required skills of each platform are different. For mobile application development, the third developer must master the skill of mobile development, the different development language require for different mobile operating system. For example, For example, application development on the AppStore requires "C" language, while JAVA is required on the Android Market. Therefore, teachers should select an open platform for students according to their interest, specialty and knowledge, for example, for the electronic commerce order class students, we can choose an open platform of electronic business. Then teacher should guide students to search some application software existed in corresponding application store, and guide students on how to use the APIs of open platform.

Secondly, students group, students understand the application scope of open application platform and a variety of existing applications in corresponding application store, then students can have free group based on their interest and experience, each student has a role which had been designed in the group, and they must participate in coding.

Thirdly, project selection, for each class teaching, each group is responsible for the project which must be unique, the project can be an existing application in application store, also can be a new project which the student want to create. But teachers must check and identify if the project can be completed independently within the limited time.

Fourthly, project development, the whole process of development can be divided into five stages: project plan, requirement analysis, software design, code implementation and software testing, students complete the project tasks by free discussion and learning in every stage, while teachers are responsible to solve some difficulties and guide the students on how to use some of the Internet search tools.

Fifthly, demonstration and assessment work, there are corresponding output at every stage of the project development. At each stage, teachers choose several groups which contain good and bad group to comment, and point out the problems in each group, and then students modify the task based on the feedback problem.

Sixth, review and evaluation,for some products with creative or improved existing applications in group, teachers can guide students to publish the corresponding products to open platform, which provide a self-display platform for students, and it makes students enhance their confidence of achievement. At the end of the course, each student does a personal summary about their work in the team, work together with other member of the group to improve work instructions and related documents. The final examination score can divided into five parts: personal summary (30 %), personal performance (20 %), project manager evaluate the personal performance in the team (20 %), the team work and products (30 %), published works to open platforms as bonus. In order to guide students to make better products, for publishing works to open platforms, teachers can give more bonuses.

200.5 Conclusion

In order to improve the students' creativity and learning interest, and to provide students with a more wider self-expression platform and increase their sense of achievement. According to the characteristics of software training course, this paper discusses the reform of teaching software development training curriculum on how to import the Internet open platform as a real teaching practice platform into the process of teaching, and designs the whole process of teaching reform according to the teaching goal of the software training class.

Acknowledgements The work described in this paper was supported by Funds from DongGuan Polytechnic (No. 2012c13).

References

1. Zhang L, Jia Z (2012) Construction of mobile-learning software sharing platform based oil application store. Comput Sci. 39(10):126–128
2. Lu J, Li H,Yang D (2010) Research on software training curriculum reform. Res Explor Lab 29(3):147–148
3. Zhang Y, Zhou Y, Han Y (2008) Cultivating student's innovative spirit and practical ability based on laboratory opening platform. Exp Technol Manag 25(2):23–25

Chapter 201
Research on Construction of Bilingual-Teaching Model Course for Bioinformatics

Dong Hu, Jiansheng Wu, Han Wei, Meng Cui and Qiuming Zhang

Abstract Bioinformatics is an important professional basic course in Biomedical Engineering, which tells about the important theoretical basis of using information technology in modern medicine and biology. In order to build a bilingual model curriculum and bring up the comprehensive talents who can make active learning and have creativity and teamwork spirits, we should actively explore the teaching system that suits the bioinformatics bilingual curriculum and train a high-quality teaching team. In addition, we also need to accumulate teaching resources for students' independent learning, create an independent learning environment, expand the opportunities for communicating the results of course reform.

Keywords Bilingual teaching · Model curriculum · Curriculum system · Bioinformatics CLC number: Q811

201.1 Preface

Twenty-first century is the era of life science, the information age. The bio-informatics has developed rapidly since it was born internationally in 1987. Broadly speaking, bio-informatics is a discipline that uses theories, techniques, methods of mathematical and information science to study the phenomenon of life, organize and analyze the biological data that presents exponential growth [1]. It reveals the biological significance behind the data by acquiring, processing,

D. Hu (✉) · J. Wu · H. Wei · M. Cui · Q. Zhang
School of Geographic and Biological Information, Nanjing University of Posts and Telecommunications, Nanjing, 210046 Jiangsu, China
e-mail: hud@njupt.edu.cn

J. Wu
e-mail: jansen@njupt.edu.cn

storing, retrieving and analyzing them from biological experiments. Bio-informatics is more of the essential tools for all the future biological and pharmaceutical research than just a scientific discipline [2, 3]. Bio-informatics is an important basic course in the biomedical engineering field, which is a course about theoretical basis of using information technology in modern medicine, biology researches. It has realized the organic combination of biotechnology, information technology and some other disciplines. It has also developed the high-throughput, high efficiency and high speed method of extracting biological information, innovation of disease detection, a new method of studying the effect of drugs and targets, the computer processing, and analysis and visualization method of genomic data, proteomics data and structural genomics data. In addition, it has analyzed the relationship between the structure and function of biological macromolecule and improve the level of processing, analyzing and utilizing the biological information, laying the foundation for original innovation of China's life sciences and Biotechnology.

Bilingual teaching means utilizing two languages in class, namely, in teaching links such as teaching courses, use of textbooks, class discussion, homework assignment using both Chinese and foreign language for part or all of the teaching activities [4]. In higher education, bilingual teaching especially means a teaching method using outstanding foreign representative original material and teaching courses by foreign language [5]. With the deepening of reform and opening up in China, All trades and professions' pace of convergence with the international has sped up step by step, national demand of the high-quality and compound talents who are proficient in professional knowledge and foreign language has been increasingly urgent, and culturing the talents who understand both foreign languages and professional knowledge has been a pressing matter of the moment in the higher education in China. The Ministry of education pointed out explicitly in the (2001) document 4 that we should actively promote the bilingual teaching in colleges and universities; undergraduate education should create conditions; and use English or some other foreign languages to teach public courses and specialized courses. Particular emphasis is laid on that some specialties like new materials in the field of high technology, biotechnology and information technology should be one step ahead and we should try to make courses teaching by foreign language account for more than 10 % of the courses that are open. Furthermore, what is especially emphasized is that biotechnology needs a step forward more, of which the fundamental purpose is to put our country's higher education in the context of economic globalization to let it reform and develop, in this way, we can establish an international education platform for the students and make students have the opportunity to directly accept professional education in an international advanced level. Not only in the aspect of knowledge, information, but also in such aspects as education idea, education mode should we affected by the world's most advanced and excellent things and cultivate the students to become the modern talents.

201.2 Analysis of the Current Situation at Home and Abroad

As we all know, at present we are still in lack of the bio-informatics professionals. Genetics professor David Potter in Stanford University pointed out that 'We need the talents who are proficient at computer and biology, just as we need the talents who are proficient at both chemical and biology. In addition, the bilingual teachers of bio-informatics not only need to have strong bio-informatics professional skills, but strong language skills and teaching skills as well. Therefore, domestic universities which have already developed bio-informatics bilingual teaching are now very rare. In order to meet the needs of the cultivating high-quality biological and medical talents with bioinformatics knowledge, we need to change that quickly.

At the moment, after several amendments, many internationally recognized outstanding bio-informatics foreign language textbooks have included latest bio-informatics ideas and researches. Through the bilingual teaching, these foreign language original documents can be passed completely and thoroughly to students with the least time. More significantly, foreign bio-informatics textbooks are mostly written by senior scholars in the field, complied with the characteristics of the discipline of forward-looking and rapid development, showing the unique perspective and the new research methods and conclusions and developing ideas. Meanwhile, they are extremely operable on strict theoretical basis, combining the fact. We can learn from the foreign advanced modern teaching ideas, teaching methods and means from the using of the original teaching materials, getting to know about a new system to cultivate talents of international standards. Therefore, the implementation of bilingual teaching can make bio-informatics realize the leap into the reform on the teaching content and stand directly to the forefront of profession. In the mean time, most information on biological data is shared free globally, mainly including the database of nucleic acid and protein produced by three database system of the United States, Europe and Japan. With the system of whole English interface, only do operators master the correct biological information English terminology, can they easily use the system to study and research in bioinformatics. Therefore, the implementation of bilingual teaching is an effective guarantee to let students obtain biological information knowledge in the shortest possible time. In addition, the students who mastered bio-informatics knowledge and can communicate in English proficiently can be employed easily after graduation and have more opportunities to go abroad for further study.

201.3 Bilingual Teaching Demonstration Course Construction of Biological Information

To promote bilingual teaching and research teaching as an opportunity and cultivate the compound talents of active learning, innovation, teamwork and cooperation, we should create biological information teaching system of bilingual teaching demonstration course actively and provide the independent learning platform for students, bilingual teaching resources for the school teachers and the results of communication curriculum reform as a window of the society.

201.3.1 The Specific Contents of Construction

201.3.1.1 Strengthening the Construction of Teachers' Team

Teachers are the main part of teaching, so the bilingual teachers' quality determines the implementation of bilingual teaching and plays a key role in the realization of the goal of bilingual teaching. Bilingual teachers are not only well versed in the subject content, but also have a high level of foreign languages, skilled at managing foreign language in teaching specialized courses. In order to improve the quality of bilingual teachers, we can carry on the work in the following three aspects:

1. How to actively instruct the bilingual teachers to do some reflective teaching, and achieve self-improvement in reflection.
2. How to strengthen the training of bilingual teachers and establish corresponding incentive mechanism.
3. How to cultivate young teachers with strong scientific research ability to be compound teachers for teaching and scientific research, and take a good 'teaching link'.

201.3.1.2 Arrange the Teaching Content Reasonably

Teaching content refers to the academic quality and organizational structure of the course itself, which is the core element that determines the quality of Bilingual education model curriculum and one of the core content of evaluation index system for the entire. Currently, scientific knowledge about human beings has been increasing about 1-fold every 3 or 5 years. The development and updating speed of the knowledge of bio-informatics is faster than some other disciplines, and its application in various professional fields has been changing with each passing day, which requires teaching to adapt and keep up with development in a timely manner and improve the teaching of bio-informatics in the course of developing. Only in a fresh start or at the forefront of knowledge can we do some pioneering and innovation. Teachers should focus on updating the knowledge structure, and 'learning by teaching as well as teaching by learning'. It mainly includes the following points:

1. Selection of bilingual teaching materials. This is crucial. Writing syllabus according to our own training goals. Finding teaching materials that is acceptable for students' language learning difficulty and have a reasonable structure.
2. Bilingual item pool construction.
3. Course content should include basic knowledge modules (basic theory, basic knowledge and basic skills), practice modules and extension part (trends or developments of the subject) and cannot be confined to the content of textbooks. We should enable students to learn about current hot spots or focus in the study of this discipline through network resources.

201.3.1.3 Research-Based Teaching Exploration of Bio-informatics and Bilingual Teaching's Organic Integration

Europe and the United States's bio-informatics education has penetrated into various subjects of life science. It can follow the discipline's development direction and update knowledge at any time. It lays particular emphasis on cultivating students' ability of doing scientific research so that students have a strong ability to adapt the society. However, there is a big gap between China's current bio-informatics education and the developed countries'. Many domestic colleges and universities have carried out bio-informatics teaching, however, a mature curriculum system has not been formed by now. Students' ability of creativity and researching is in lack of training. Research-oriented undergraduate teaching in colleges and universities is to cultivate innovative talents with international standards and achieve the internationalization of education [6]. It is a new idea, new mode of undergraduate teaching implemented that serves to stimulate students to learn creatively and independently and explore actively. Using research-oriented undergraduate teaching method with exploration, discussion, and students' active participation into teaching science relies on bilingual teaching, because a basic fact is that Europe and some other countries are at the center of development in the field of natural sciences such as biology and the main knowledge carrier of research teaching and learning is English. Bio-informatics is a discipline that develops particularly rapidly and be internationally accepted. Most of its teaching content is from the English literature or English textbooks. Therefore, in the course of the implementation of research-oriented undergraduate teaching, teachers often require students' actively participating in, reasonable scientifically using English literature and databases and using network to trace the frontier and the latest progress of the discipline to carry out research-and-discussion teaching. Obviously, if there is no bilingual education, students and teachers do not have training in listening, speaking, writing and reading English, it will be difficult to carry out research-oriented undergraduate teaching.

201.3.1.4 Construction of Course Websites

Constructing a good course website will provide the students with autonomous learning platform, and provide teachers in and out of schools with teaching resources for bilingual teaching. What's more, it also provides the society with the window of communication course reform results.

201.3.2 Specific Enforcement Steps

We aim at building a bio-informatics bilingual model curriculum teaching system, lying emphasis on cultivating students' capability of active learning and creativity and improving their ability of practice. We want those students who will step into society can adapt the requirement of it and those who are going to purse advanced studies posses stronger scientific research capability. The specific steps are shown in Chart 201.1.

201.3.3 The Demonstrated Significance of Course

The construction of exquisite and demonstrated course is an important part of the teaching quality and teaching reform project of colleges and universities. From a strategic perspective and the perspective of the overall system it is easy to discover that the construction of demonstration course is a long-term and arduous task, which must be based on reality, focused on improving the quality and the level of teaching, putting the construction of course into the whole teaching activities and curriculum system, realize that creating exquisite course is a breakthrough, increase the intensity of the course construction, promote the quality of course construction from the whole, and develop the demonstration effect of bio-informatics bilingual teaching and push both teaching quality and teaching level to a higher altitude.

201.3.4 Compared with the Traditional Teaching

In the university teaching, experiment teaching is often attached to the theory teaching, the traditional experiment teaching focuses on the validation of theoretical knowledge. In order to consolidate and strengthen the knowledge, students perform the verification experiments and summarize the experimental results, with the steps and methods of regulation experimental guide books. Traditional experimental teaching has the following characteristics: (1) Let all the students adopt the same experimental contents, experimental projects, experimental apparatus, experimental times, experimental time; (2) The teaching contents are mostly

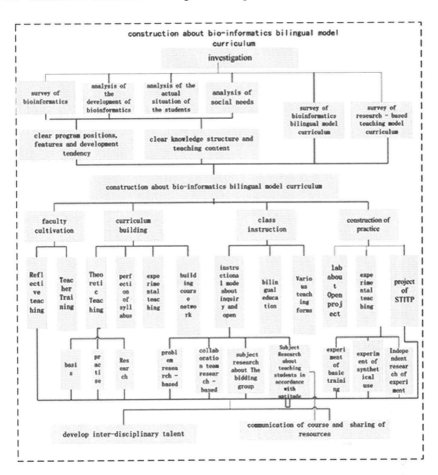

Chart 201.1 Construction about bio-informatics bilingual model curriculum

the verification experiments, much depending on the theory teaching and for theoretical verification methods; (3) The passive learning. The traditional experimental teaching which is much for fixed mode. According to the experimental instructions, the teacher explains the experimental contents, steps and operating demonstrations. And students finish the experiments following the prescribed way. In the whole process of mechanical experiments, students are in the passive learning, where the independent thinking fails. The biggest disadvantage of the traditional experimental teaching is often just like an "assembly" experiment. And the development of students' individual characters is bound to the single and passive aspects of the experiment. It fails to foster the students' independence and innovation. Even if successes, it just fosters an assembler, which cannot exercise and train the ability of students to solve problems. So there can be no innovation to speak of [9]. Innovation laboratory, which focuses on the construction of the opening and innovative experiments, will changes the passive experiments mode that is similar to obtain the medicines according to the prescription completely with the teaching method—"approach, point, dial". In the innovation laboratory, students can propose the problems to be solved and the goals to be achieved, and design an experiment on their own. Other than that, it succeeds in taking initiative and creativity and displaying their individuality with the independent thought and brave practice, which can result in making up the shortage of the current experiment teaching [10].

201.4 Conclusions and Prospect

In "The Notice of Initiating Project About Bilingual Model Curriculum in 2007", the government required that the aim of construction about bilingual model curriculum is to form a bilingual education model that can not only connect with the International advanced teaching theories and methods but also fit into the China's situation with the meaning of demonstration and reference playing an important role in cultivating International competition awareness and ability. As a comprehensive university, Nanjing University of Posts and Telecommunications offers a wide range of courses characterized by information subject and composed mainly of science study. As a cross discipline, bio-informatics not only continues the subject development in the school's information environment, but also magnifies the school's feature. So, it is significant to strengthen the construction and development in bio-informatics bilingual teaching model curriculum under the backdrop of school's information features and driven the need of biology and medical engineering senior specialized compound. "Bio-informatics Guiding Dissertation" is the basic course of biology and medical engineering while less biological course is available in our school. The scientific research in biology is gradually developing through everyone's effort. However, the related courses still lay behind a little. Thus, we want to take advantage of this biding, focusing on the development of specialized basic course to lay the foundation for future related course and promote advancement of major education and subject development. Therefore, we aim for establishing a high level, unique and colorful bilingual model teaching system and gradually forming a bilingual education model connected with the International advanced teaching theories and methods and suitable to the Chinese condition. We aim for making a new, remarkable achievement of all-around improvement of our country's higher education and teaching quality with the help of school's talents majored in information and scientific subject and bio-informatics.

Acknowledgments Foundation item: Nanjing University of Posts and Telecommunications teaching reform research project (No. JG01611JX02 No. JG03212JX67) and Nanjing University of Posts and Telecommunications 2011 lab construction and equipment management research (No. 2011XSG12).

References

1. Tan X, Su Y, Li B (2008) Discussion on bio-informatics teaching. J Shanxi Med Univ (Preclinical Med Educ Ed) (01)
2. Li D (2001) Bioinformatics in the post genome era science. Foreign medical. Physiology. J Pathol Clin Med (04)
3. Lai M (2004) Applications of biological information in medical science research. J Zhejiang Univ (Med Sci Ed) (02)
4. Yang Y, Tian M, Xu L, Chen S (2007) Thinking of the bilingual teaching. Chin J Peking Univ (Philos Soc Sci Ed) (S2)
5. Chen D, Yang M, Yan W (2007) Some understanding of promoting bilingual teaching in colleges. J Peking Univ (Philos Soc Sci Ed) (S2)
6. Yang S (2011) The study of undergraduate teaching and the cultivation of innovative talents. J Guangdong Univ Foreign Stud (02)
7. Wu Z (2001) On the teaching of research study. J Chongqing Educ Coll (05)
8. Zhang Y (2011) Teaching research and training innovative talents. Univ (Acad Ed) (02)
9. Deng W (2011) The integration of multimedia technology and traditional experiment teaching. Teach Instrum Exp (04)
10. Chen S Research methods to improve the classroom teaching efficiency. Teach Instrum Exp 201(04)

Chapter 202
Research on Endpoint Information Extraction for Chemical Molecular Structure Images

Zhao-man Zhong and Yan Guan

Abstract The methods of automatic extracting information of static chemical molecular structure images are introduced in this paper. Endpoint information extraction is the key research contents, and it mainly includes the following two parts: the endpoint character recognition based on BP neural network; the post-processing operation, such as the character combination of endpoint, the endpoint information correction based on dictionary. This is the base for automatically extracting chemical molecular structure images.

Keywords Chemical molecular structure images · Endpoint · BP neural network · Character combination

202.1 Introduction

There are many naming methods of chemical substances, such as systematic name, trade name, common name, the customary name and the CA (Chemical Abstracts), and isomer phenomenon exists among the same molecular formula. In the chemical literature retrieval, it will probably lead to residual error by the name of chemical substances due to incomplete name, and it will also bring difficulty because of no uniqueness in naming. It may cause false detection by the molecular formula because of isomeric. Using the structure of the compound for retrieval is an accurate retrieval approach, and it can avoid ambiguity. At present, the chemical molecular structure information mainly comes from dynamic structure file [1–5], which generated by special tools. The communication between the molecules are based on the chemical molecular structure images, whose format are

Z. Zhong (✉) · Y. Guan
Huaihai Institute of Technology, Lianyungang 222005, China
e-mail: zhongzhaoman@163.com

BMP, TIFF, PNG and GIF in molecular chemistry, patent specification, science magazine and Internet field. Using computer to process the chemical molecular structure images has become urgent need. On the basis of previous research results [5–7], the method of extracting endpoint information for chemical molecular structure images is researched, which will lay the foundation for all structure retrieval and substructure retrieval.

202.2 The Flow of the Chemical Molecular Structure Extraction

Element symbols are atoms and molecules group, and the lines or curves are bonds. All the hydrogen and carbon-hydrogen bonding are needn't to be drawn, the intersections of adjacent line represent carbon atom, heteroatom (non-carbon, hydrogen atom), and group should not be omitted. The extraction of chemical molecular structure is to identify the atom and the chemical bond. The flow of extracting chemical molecular structure is shown in Fig. 202.1.

Because the color information is nonsense for the two-dimensional chemical molecular structure image, binarization is done before information extraction. The

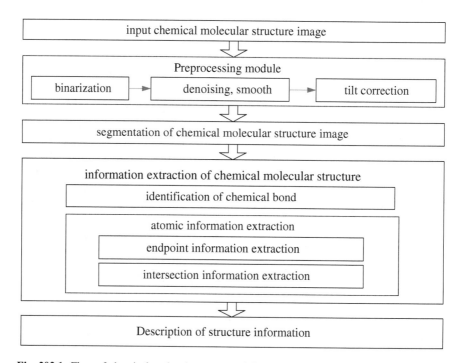

Fig. 202.1 Flow of chemical molecular structure information extraction

chemical molecular structure is composed of toms and bonds. The separation of bonds and atoms is done. We use the segmentation algorithm of chemical molecular structure based on area size and bending degree in literature [6] to segment chemical bonds, heteroatoms and perssad.

Hydrocarbon atoms appear at the intersections of the long chain or loop chain. There are three types: CH_2, CH and C. We can get the form of intersection, according to the type of intersection [5]. The atoms and groups are close to the endpoints, which are said by character, and the endpoint information extraction is key research contents in this paper.

202.3 Automatic Extraction of Endpoint Information for Chemical Molecular Structure Images

202.3.1 Character Recognition Based on BP Neural Network

The English character represents 118 elements in the chemical element periodic table and sixty kinds of groups in organic chemistry. Non-hydrocarbon atoms or groups are near the endpoints of chemical molecular structure image. The endpoint information of 8635 collected two-dimensional molecular structure images are added up, and there are 21 atoms or groups which appear at endpoint. Identification of atom or group is character identification. BP neural network of intelligent pattern recognition is the most active and widely [8–11]. The method based on the BP neural network is used for recognition of the endpoint character in this paper.

The flow of character recognition based on neural network, and the preprocessing includes normalization and feature extraction for character images obtained after the segmentation based on the area size and bending. All the characters are normalized to 24×16. Character features extraction is based on grid characteristics and passage characteristics in this paper.

Grid characteristics: 24×16 binary image is divided into eight squares $S_1, S_2, \ldots, S_8$, each area size is 6×8 pixels, the number $p_i, i = 0, 1, \ldots, 7$ of black pixels in each squares is add up, p_i are 8 dimensional grid features.

Passage characteristics: passage characteristics are calculated from the horizontal and vertical direction. First calculating horizontal direction and the steps are as follows:

(1) The 24 lines image is divided into six regions $S_1, S_2, \ldots, S_6$, and each region includes four rows;
(2) Calculating change times of each row from the white pixel to black pixel $A_i, i = 0, 1, \ldots, 23$;
(3) A_i is used to count the total change times of rows in each region, getting six features $q_0, q_1, \ldots, q_5$, $q_i = \sum_{i=4n}^{4n+3} A_i, i = 0, 1, \ldots, 5$;

The six features are used to calculate $q_{i+6} = q_i / \sum_{i=0}^{5} q_i \times 10 + 0.5$, $i = 0, 1, \ldots, 5$ as the 7–12 features. Similarly getting passage characteristics from the vertical direction and so 20 passage characteristics are generated.

The character feature vector is composed of twenty dimensional passage characteristics and eight dimensional grid features. The training sample characters are from the collected chemical molecular structure images. The upper case and the lower case of some letters is consistent, such as 'c', 'o' and 's', and the atoms represent by them are the same. There are 35 characters in the Table 1, and 25 characters are left after removing repeated characters. The 26 characters are recognized by BP neural network. In the MATLAB environment, training the BP neural network takes 40 s, and the number of iterations is 300 times, 100 chemical molecular structure images are recognized which are random selected from the collected chemical molecular structure images, and the recognition accuracy rate is 79 %.

202.3.2 Post-processing for Information Extraction of Endpoint

The atoms or groups are composed of multiple characters, and the method of character recognition based on the BP neural network is used to identify single character. Subsequent work is to combine the characters of endpoint. Chemical molecular structure image is drawn with professional soft wares, the size of character in the same image is uniform, and the distance between the characters near same endpoints is small. But the distance between the characters near different endpoints is big. So the character combination is based on the distance in this paper, and the setting of distance threshold φ is very critical. In the process of chemical bonds recognition, the coordinate $P_i = (x_i, y_i)$, $(i = 1, 2, \ldots, m)$ of each endpoint is recorded, m is the number of endpoints. Barycentric coordinates of each character is written as: $Z_j = (x'_j, y'_j)$, $(j = 1, 2, \ldots, n)$, n is the number of characters. The specific algorithm is as follows:

(1) Starting from the first endpoint to look for the closest character near the each endpoint, written as: A_k;
(2) Starting from A_k to look for the character of range φ, and if there is, they will be combined, and the operation continue from the combination characters.

Because the types of atoms and molecules are limited, in order to avoid individual character recognition error and reduce the endpoint information accuracy, an atom and group dictionary is made. Each recognition endpoint is compared with the dictionary, calculating distance, and the minimum distance of item will be selected as the final recognition result. If the matching distance is greater than a certain threshold, the recognition result is the final result. The information correction of endpoint t is also the correction of recognition character based on the BP

Table 202.1 The identification results of endpoints

Situation	P	R	F-measure
Without the dictionary	0.78	0.80	0.79
With the dictionary	0.91	0.92	0.915

neural network. We use R (recall rate), P (precision) and $F - measure$ indexes to assess the information extraction algorithm performance of endpoints in the chemical molecular structure. The experimental results are shown in Table 202.1, there are two cases without a dictionary matching and dictionary matching, from the experimental results, the endpoint information extraction accuracy is greatly improved by the method of dictionary matching.

202.4 Conclusion

The information of endpoints is mainly composed of character, the method of character recognition is based on BP neural network, and the characters of endpoint are combined in this paper. In order to improve the accuracy of endpoint information extraction, we make an atoms and groups dictionary, which can correct the endpoint information extraction. Experiment shows that the method of endpoint information extraction in this paper has higher high accuracy.

References

1. Yao JH (1998) Computer handling of chemical structures (II). Internal storage data structures and file formats of chemical structure representation in computers. Comput Appl Chem 15(2):65–68
2. Li X, Song TT, He XF (2007) VF2 algorithm based 2D molecular substructure search. Comput Appl Chem 24(11):1551–1554
3. Karthikeyan M, Bender A (2005) Encoding and decoding graphical chemical structures as two-dimensional barcodes. Chem Inf Model 45(3):572–580
4. Kong DX (2007) Introduction to file formats for storage of chemical structure and their conversion. Comput Appl Chem 24(9):1260–1264
5. Guan Y, Li CH, Zhong ZM et al (2012) Automatic extracting intersection information of static chemical molecular structure images. Comput Chem 29:499–502
6. Guan Y, Li CH, Zhong ZM et al (2012) Segmentation algorithm of chemical molecular structure images. Shandong Univ Technol 42:65–68
7. Sun LL, Li CH, Guan Y (2012) The automatic extraction of the chemical bonds information in the chemical structure images. Shandong Univ Technol 42:18–23
8. Huan CY (2010) Risk evaluation model on enterprises' complex information system: a study based on the BP neural network. J Softw 5(1):99–106
9. Zhu QH, Zhang G (2007) Evaluation model on organizational networking based on artificial neural networks. Appl Res Comput 24(6):239–241

10. Ang JH, Tan KC (2008) Training neural networks for classification using growth probability based evolution. Neurocomputing 71(16/18):3493
11. Zhang CY, Dai WZ (2008). The study and application of improved BP Neural Networks. Zhejiang Sci-Tech University, Hangzhou, pp 442-445

Chapter 203
Using Video Recording System to Improve Student Performance in High-Fidelity Simulation

Wangqin Shen

Abstract *Objectives* To evaluate the effect of video recording system in nursing simulation practice. *Methods* Nursing students in the experimental group (n = 69) participated in the video recording feedback. And the control group (n = 70) participated in the normal teaching methods. Differences of learning competency, communication skills and satisfaction between two groups were measured. *Results* Students in the experimental group got significantly higher scores in catheterization, communication skills, and satisfaction. *Conclusion* This study indicates that the video recording feedback is potentially a useful tool to enhance nursing students' learning in a simulated environment.

Keywords Video recording system · Feedback · Simulation · Nursing students

203.1 Instruction

One of the responsibilities of a nursing school is to provide a safe, controlled environment for students to learn and practice the clinical skills necessary to become clinically competent nurses. However, opportunities for nursing student to practice nursing skills in clinical setting are often limited [1]. Therefore, Simulation-based education has been offered to bridge the gap. Simulation refers to the artificial representation of a complex real-world process with sufficient fidelity to achieve a particular goal, such as in training or performance testing. The aim is to facilitate learning through immersion, reflection, feedback, and practice minus the risks inherent in a similar real-life experience [2]. Simulation-based education

---

W. Shen (✉)
School of Nursing, Nantong University, Nantong, Jiangsu, People's Republic of China
e-mail: fancy@ntu.edu.cn

enables nursing education to acquire and practice an array of tasks and skills in a safe and "mistake-forgiving" environment.

The traditional teaching methods of nursing education mainly include lectures, tutorials, and discussions, which do not facilitate active learning [3]. Recently, video feedback has been widely used as an innovative teaching method for nursing simulation training. This method of self-assessment can provide an opportunity for students to evaluate their own behaviours, such as learning competence, and communication skills.

Feedback is an essential component of simulation learning. Students need to be able to identify what they did well, what they did less satisfactorily, and what else they might have done [4, 5]. Video feedback enabled nursing students to identify good and poor practice with more confidence, and to reflect more carefully on their own and other's practice [6]. Self-evaluation using video enhances knowledge retention, and promotes critical thinking, learning motivation, communication skills [5, 7]. Empirical support for these advantages in teaching clinical skills in courses of fundamental nursing is lacking despite a large amount of literature devoted to reflective learning methods in nurse education [8]. In this study, the effect of video-based feedback of catheterization was assessed for undergraduate nursing students.

203.2 Method

203.2.1 Participants and Setting

Research participants in this study were a cluster sample of 139 sophomore nursing students who were enrolled in the fundamental nursing course of two nursing schools located in Jiangsu province. The participants were randomly divided into experimental group (n = 69) and control group (n = 70). The average age was 19.6 years old. There were 4 male nursing students in experimental group and control group separately. All the students were full-time. The study was conducted in a learning training center equipped with high-fidelity simulators and video recording system equipment.

203.2.2 Measures

Students' competence in catheterization was assessed by a performance checklist developed specially for catheterization. The evaluation criteria were composed of two major components: nursing process of inserting catheter and communication skills. The possible total scores of the nursing process of inserting catheter ranged from 0 to 80; the possible total scores of communication skills ranged from 0 to 20.

The higher scores indicate higher competence. The checklist was validated by professors who were blind to the experiments.

The learning satisfaction of students was measured by the self-rating satisfaction scale of catheterization skill. The possible total scores ranged from 0 to 100 and higher scores indicate a higher level of student satisfaction.

203.2.3 Procedure

All students who participated in the study were verbally informed of the research purpose. Students were told that their participation was voluntary, and non-participation would not affect their academic results or future study. Students in the control group were given the video recording and a chance of self-evaluation after completion of the study.

Catheterization was designed, implemented, and evaluated in scenario. All students in the experimental and control group participated in the same session with their usual course teaching and learning methods. The role of teacher was that of facilitator and observer during the practice and evaluation, respectively. Immediately after the session, experimental participants left the simulation room and watched the video recording. Nursing students were asked to evaluate their learning performance and communication behavior and comment on the usefulness and efficiency of the feedback method. Teachers facilitated a group reflection on how they had enacted the scenario and also gave feedback. All students were required to complete the self-rating satisfaction about the catheterization learning to the researcher at the end of this study.

203.2.4 Data Analysis

Statistical analysis was undertaken using SPSS, version 15.0. Descriptive statistics was used to describe the demographic variables. The independent-samples t test was used to test the difference between the experimental and control groups for the scores on measurement of catheterization, communication skills, and student satisfaction.

203.3 Results

Results showed that students in the experimental group had significantly higher scores for the catheterization, communication skills, and self-reported satisfaction (Table 203.1).

Table 203.1 Learning performance, communication skills, satisfaction differences between experimental and control groups

Variables	Experimental group (n = 69) M ± SD	Control group (n = 70) M ± SD	t	p
Catheterization	67.17 ± 5.43	64.37 ± 5.56	3.004	0.003
Communication	16.80 ± 1.36	16.06 ± 1.43	3.125	0.002
Satisfaction	94.23 ± 4.16	88.72 ± 5.26	4.241	0.000

203.4 Discussion

This article described the feasibility and evaluation of a video recording feedback method design to reflect the catheterization performance, communication skills and learning satisfaction. The results showed that it was an effective way.

Assessment and the provision of feedback are considered essential to students learning [9]. According to the results of this study, the video recording feedback appears to enhance their learning performance. It enhanced the feedback experience for both students and staff. The students, given rich feedback in a short period of time during the session like catheterization, will not acquire all the teaching points in their mind. In the end they will focus on one or two teaching points. And being able to rewatch the whole experience back, they can focus on stuff that they failed to remember. Students can acquire and absorb more detailed information about the simulated scenario than that during the session. On the other hand, the video also enables teachers to receive new information about the timing of actions in the scenario. These results are consistent with the study by [1]. The video recording was also instructive. The session itself was fast paced and it was not easy to totally master. With the video feedback they can find lots of minor details that they had not appreciated before. Therefore, to watch it with the memory of what they were thinking plus the objectively of the video was beneficial.

Good communication is an important skill needed in the health care profession to ensure effective communication between patients and the other healthcare professionals. If the students want to become qualified nurses, it is important for them to acquire special skills in relation to verbal and nonverbal communication with patients. This study proved that communication skills in the simulated scenario, for nursing students in video recording feedback group, had been improved effectively. Several studies found that the form of feedback on providers' actual performance can result in an overall improvement of communication skills of medical students and physicians [10, 11].

When students feel good about themselves as learners, they are willing to take risks and focus on learning. Students are more willing to participate in a class if they believe it will be enjoyable [5]. This is why many teaching programs insist on evaluating the students' satisfaction. The results of this study also found that the students self-report satisfaction scores were significantly higher in the video recording feedback group than those in the control group.

In conclusion, the video feedback is a beneficial instructional method to help undergraduate students improve skill competency, communication skills and enhancing their learning satisfaction. However, the video recording feedback was only used in catheterization. As a result, more other nursing clinical skills should be evaluated in follow-up study.

References

1. Yoo MS, Yoo IY, Lee H (2010) Nursing students' self-evaluation using a video recording of Foley catheterization: effects on students' competence, communication skills, and learning motivation. J Nurs Educ 49(7):402–405
2. Ogden PE, Cobbs LS, Howell MR et al (2007) Clinical simulation: importance to the internal medicine educational mission. Am J Med 120:820–824
3. Carcich GM, Rafti KR (2007) Experienced registered nurses' satisfaction with using self-learning modules versus traditional lecture/discussion to achieve competency goals during hospital orientation. J Nurs Staff Dev 23:214–220
4. Ker J, Bradley P (2007) Simulation in medical education. Association for the Study of Medical Education, Edinburgh
5. Yoo MS, Son YJ, Kim YS et al (2009) Video-based self-assessment: implementation and evaluation in a undergraduate nursing course. Nurse Educ Today 29(6):585–589
6. Bowden T, Rowlands A, Buckwell M et al (2012) Web-based video and feedback in the teaching of cardiopulmonary resuscitation. Nurse Educ Today 32(4):443–447
7. Mazor KM, Haley HL, Sullivan K (2007) The video-based test of communication skills: description, development, and preliminary findings. Teach Learn Med 19(2):62–167
8. Honey M, Waterworth S, Baker H et al (2006) Reflection in the disability education of undergraduate nurses: an effective learning tool? J Nurs Educ 45(11):449–453
9. Crook A, Mauchline A, Maw S et al (2012) The use of video technology for providing feedback to students: can it enhance the feedback experience for staff and students? Comput Educ 58:386–396
10. Yedidia MJ, Gillespie CC, Kachur E et al (2003) Effect of communication training on medical student performance. J Am Med Assoc 290:1157–1165
11. Noordman J, Verhaak P, Dulmen S (2011) Web-enabled video-feedback: a method to reflect on the communication skills of experienced physicians. Patient Educ Couns 82(3):335–340

Chapter 204
Exploration of Vocational Talents Culture Model of "Promote Learning with Competition, Combine Competition with Teaching"

Wen-liang Cao and Xuan-zi Hu

Abstract Profession skills Competition's purpose is to guide the vocational education of "learning by doing, teaching by doing" training model reform, highlight the students' innovation ability and enhance their professional competence and quality of employment. This paper explores the Vocational Talents Culture Model of "Promote Learning with Competition, Combine Competition with Teaching" as the carrier of skills competition, so can develop students' innovation ability.

Keywords Personnel training profession skills competition · Computer applications · Promote learning with competition practical ability · Talents culture

204.1 Introduction

In the year of 2008, the head of vocation education and adult education Huang Yao pointed out "through hold a vocational colleges megagame to make the "combination of learning with working, college-enterprise cooperation, substituted post exercitation "with Chinese characteristics 's experience and method of work which explored step by step from the process of education progress more institutionalization and normalization, this is demand of vocational education adapt to new terrain of the progress of economic social, this is a important institution of design and innovation to our country's educational work at the same time. In 2010, the State Council issued ≪ The national medium—and long-term plan for education reform and development ≫ (2010–2020), reiterated that improve the social

W. Cao (✉) · X. Hu
Department of Computer Engineering, Dongguan Polytechnic, 523808 Dongguan, China
e-mail: cwl2222@tom.com

status and treatment of skilled talents, will increase to award high skill talents who has outstanding contribution, and vocational skills competition were pointed out particularly in chapters of vigorously develop vocational education.

204.2 The Definition of Vocational Skills Competition

Vocational skills contest is based on the national occupational skill standards, carried out in combination with actual production and management work in order to highlight operate skills and solving practical problem skills, organized with emphasis on the competition of mass activities. Vocational skills competition should adhere to the social benefit and the principle of openness, fairness and justice, have close integration with vocational skills training, professional skill appraisal, performance appraisal, technical innovation, and production work. Vocational skills competition generally divided into national, provincial and municipal levels.

204.3 The Characteristics of the Vocational Skills Competition

Skilledness: The training goal of higher vocational education is to cultivate people who can adapt to the demand of production, construction, management and service, highlight the practicability and pertinence of higher vocational education and skills competition must comply with the training goal of higher vocational education. Skilled reflected in competition event and competition content, education departments combination with actual production and management work, according to the national occupational skill standards to carry out the competition event which highlight those event which value operation skills and solving actual problems important, and specialized skill, technique, practical ability become the competition's contend.

Competitiveness: Vocational skills competition itself is a selection activities, can stimulate the motivation of participants, inspiring morale, so produce internal driving force, toward the desired goals. Competition is a basic property of all kinds of game, under the guidance of capture victory, contestants strive to maximize exert potential, study indicate that in the sports competition, people can mobilize 70 % of their body function, and in the fierce competition, can mobilize to more than 90 %. The vocational skills competition is a activity which has the meaning of education, not only skill levels, comprehensive quality competition between players, but also the competition of the level of vocational colleges and teaching achievements. Good competition performance can motivate the competitors, colleges and universities, strengthen the impact on the successful experience, the bad competition results of the student and the school played the supervision role.

Advancement: Advanced nature is refers to the competition focus on new technologies, new techniques, new methods of application. Vocational skills competition only to be advanced can to judging the school and its teachers and students teaching and skills is in line with the current social development needs, through the guidance of vocational skills competition to make the vocational colleges abandon the old contend which don't adapt to the social new technology, new technology, new methods of the development and adopts the new era characteristics and advanced technical content.

204.4 The Purpose and Significance of Promote Learning with Competition and Combine Competition with Teaching

To promote learning with competition can promote students' learning how to conduct oneself, learning how to get along with others and learning skills. To combine competition with teaching can establish "three moves" teaching system they are make students and teachers more interaction, to promote training linkage, driven by enterprise's behavior.

Through taking part in some items of the skills contest even the finals, not only can improve students' professional practice skills, but also can cultivate the students' team cooperation ability, even can provided a chance to students show themselves. The students of vocational college think highly of taking part in skills contest, they desire to be awarded, put the skills competition as a supreme honor, the usual passive students become active learning students. Skills contest emphasize practicality, in order to cooperate with various disciplines, teachers must introduce enterprise's practical solutions, pay attention to practicability and advancement in the usual teaching or in the guidance of the prepare contest. In 2012, for example, the contest of "the computer network application" is to require students to according to the demand of enterprises and the actual engineering application environment to realization the operation of network devices, wireless devices, security equipment, voice communication, and according to the demand of actual engineering business carried out the equipments 'connective and debugging. Will be conducive to the teachers for teaching reform, improve teaching quality, really realize skills contest's concept "let competition to promote teaching and to promote development, to promote learning".

204.5 Competitive Projects of Computer Specialty

In the past, competitors of the national skills contest entry are aim at the secondary vocational students. Since the national vocational skills contest held in Tianjin in 2008, higher vocational academy, the group of the important innovation ability is

Table 204.1 Competitive projects of computer specialty in 2012-2015

Name of competitions	2012	2013	2014	2015
The computer network application (CNW)	√	√	√	√
Robotics applications	√	√		√
Information security technology		√		
Information security management and assessment	√			√
The Internet of things technology application	√	√		√

involved. Competitive form is that all competitive projects in the provinces are carry out qualification trials in advance and then the top 1–2 will be recommended to participate in the national finals. In recent years, competitive projects of computer specialty has more and more, According to the notice of 3 year plan (2013–2015) of the national vocational skills which is issued by ministry of education, higher vocational computer professional students can attend for competitive projects as shown in Table 204.1, Later, which will also gradually add "LTE network and maintenance", "mobile technology application", "mobile Internet applications (APPS) development" and other contests.

204.6 Implementation of Promote Learning with Competition and Combine Competition with Teaching

Skills competition entries in the province basically limited to be two team with 3–6 people, the top 1 or 2 recommended are eligible to attend the national finals, which can't exercise all students. In the process of implementation of promote Learning with competition and combine competition with teaching, we take competition through the teaching process of professional courses and introduce skill results of league matches to graduation test of professional curriculum. On this basis, school select excellent students to prepare to the qualification trials in the province and even nationwide finals. Such a selection system, it can exercise students as well as gather strength for subsequent competition and then get good grades. Place competition of computer network application in the 2012 provincial trials as an example, author accounts for the implementation process in detail.

204.6.1 Introduce Skills League Matches Relying on Professional Courses

In recent years, my department gradually set up concept of talent cultivation the "promote teaching with competition", taking skills competition as one of the important methods to improve the teaching quality, taking skills spec into the professional talent training scheme and the competition content refined integrate into specialized courses teaching content. A same course related the skill competition of different professional direction should keep pace with having class, which will conducive to teachers' synchronous implementation of skills league matches. For example, the course of Networking technologies and network management has eight classes to open simultaneously, On the basis of previous games sample questions of computer network application, We refine six training tasks into the course of experiments such as "planning, configuration, and troubleshooting of computer network", "network equipment and network formation", step by step accomplish in the process of teaching and then grades are given by the teacher. Therefore, through participating in the exercise of skills contest, elites have been selected to participate in qualification trials in the province in the light of scores of skills league matches.

204.6.2 Prepare for Qualification Trials in the Province

Qualification trials in the province are basically held once a year, although the content and the schedule of every megagame will be change, competitions has played a positive role in tracking the latest application of enterprises, enhance students' practical application ability and innovative thinking, team cooperation and so on. Under the support of educational administration department of college, we start with application for competitions, Influenced by relevant premises, equipment etc., every year, a team composed of three students which are probably prepare for one and half months is applied for competition. Firstly, collect information over the year relating to the latest files and test question of the competition. Secondly, tutors are familiar with related document spirit, to interpret historical test questions of contest and grasp all the knowledge points. Thirdly, tutors carry through breakthrough teaching to key and difficult points in order to quickly grasp skilled by students. Fourthly, provide open laboratory for participating students to strengthen guidance and practice operation. Lastly, summarize after the competition in order to accumulation of teaching experience and the gain and loss for subsequent teaching links, eventually improve the students' practical skills and innovation ability.

204.7 Conclusion

With the development of information technology, the demand for computer talents has increased dramatically and requirements for talents quality has also more and more high in IT enterprise. As an important part of higher education, Higher vocational education has trained a large number of skilled talents for IT industry, But there are a serious disconnected issue between a plenty of talents and enterprise needs. So, teaching mode reform for major of computer application has been imminent. After vocational talents culture model of promote Learning with competition and combine competition with teaching puts into effect in our department, students has successively won A number of different awards in national vocational skills competition including a second prize, a third prize and a finalist in the national finals. On this account, we should speed up the pace of teaching reform and innovation personnel training mode.

Acknowledgments This work was supported by Research Project of 2012 Dongguan Polytechnic education reform project (No. CGPY2012008) and Guangdong Province Education Science 12th five Plan Project (No. 2012JK009).

References

1. Cai Q (2010) Practice exploration of the teaching model of "combination of contest with teaching, integrating teaching into contest and fostering reform by contest. Vocat Tech Educ 9
2. Wang X (2012) "Promoting teaching by competitions, promoting learning by competitions" teaching mode reform on office software course. China Educ Technol Equip 12
3. Jia P (2012) "Promote learning with competition,promote competition with learning, combine competition with teaching" research on the teaching model reform of electronic communication course. Comput Telecommun 6
4. Xue M (2011) A study on the production-learning-research operation based on skills competitions. Changzhou Inst Light Ind Technol 1

Chapter 205
Research of Training Professionals in Computer Application Major from the Perspective of the Connection Between Middle and Higher Vocational Education

Xuan-zi Hu and Wen-liang Cao

Abstract The connection between middle and higher vocational education is quite important for the middle vocational graduates to widen their access to further study and to strengthen the attraction of vocational education. The thesis explains in detail the connection mode between middle and higher vocational education in western developed countries and regions, and the current connecting situation between middle and higher vocational domestic education; it analyzes the problems existing in connecting middle and higher education in computer-application major, researches the strategies, explores and builds diversified forms of connecting mold between middle and higher vocational education by utilizing foreign experience in connecting middle and higher vocational education, which is of great significance for our country to improve the system of vocational education and adapt to the lifelong development tendency of vocational education.

Keywords Connection between middle and higher · Computer-application major · Personnel training

205.1 Introduction

In August, 2011, the Education Department issued Guiding Opinions on Boosting the Coordinate Development of Middle and Higher Vocational Education [No. 9 (2011)]. The connection between middle and higher vocational education improves and develops the vocational education Chinese system into a lifelong education system, but also actively respond to the development of society and economy by vocational education system. To build a connecting system between middle and higher vocational education becomes one of our vocational education goals. The connection between middle and higher vocational education in

X. Hu (✉) · W. Cao
Department of Computer Engineering, Dongguan Polytechnic, Dongguan 523808, China
e-mail: huxuanzi@126.com

computer application major is good to training a large group of innovative talents and "application-type" talents of high quality, strong ability and broad vision to adapt to rapid development of IT industry in China.

205.2 The Connecting Mode of Middle and Higher Vocational Education at Abroad

Germany vocational education features as "dual system" through connecting a spiraling educational system and a connecting mode between middle and higher stair-stepped vocational courses. All the higher vocational education is based on the relatively lower vocation education, emphasizing on the students' vocational practice. The graduates from middle vocational school can choose to work or take a higher vocational education. The country provides every middle vocational student with equal opportunity for competition and many ways to further study. As the echelon of vocational education is very obvious, the higher vocational education (including trainings in enterprises and vocational education centers) are based on lower vocational education. The country carries out the dual system, emphasizing the students' vocational practice. People having taken vocational education can find a job by making use of the knowledge and skills learned or take a higher vocational education after taking a dual system vocational practice in order to seek for a better career opportunity. As there are many ways and the time is flexible, all of these totally depend on the personal will and condition. The country and the society provide every middle vocational student with an equal condition for competition and many ways for further study.

The current connecting mode between middle and higher vocational education in England has been set up for 30 years. The National Education Commission established the system that the professional qualification of vocational education is equal to that of general education by local law. The England divided the middle vocational curriculum and higher vocational curriculum into teaching units in order to avoid any repetition. And they classified them into 5 levels according to the depth of teaching, among which the teaching units of middle vocational education covers 3 levels namely level I, II and III, and the teaching units of higher vocational education covers 3 levels, namely level III, IV and V. Teaching units of level I connects the curriculum in middle school, and the units of adjacent levels can connect each other. The diploma can be issued to students according to the minimum total units they have learnt. As the logical order is very clear and the connection is very close without repetition between teaching units, the adaption to teaching connection is good.

205.3 The Connecting Mode Between Middle and Higher Vocational Education at Home

In recent years, the reform of vocational education in China is to lay "flyovers" for middle and higher vocational education so that the graduates from middle vocational school can take a further study besides starting a career. To make the "flyovers" more convenient, different structures of middle and higher education system and the connecting mode are being explored, which can be classified into the following three groups:

Coherent Schooling Mode. A structure of education system and connecting mode results from an overall arrangement and design of middle and higher vocational education, which can be 4-year system, 5-year system and 6-year system. "4-year system" means 1-year middle vocational education and 3-year higher vocational education. "5-year system" can be divided into two modes, namely, "3 + 2" and "2 + 3", which means taking (2 or 3 years) higher vocational education on the base of (3 or 2 years) middle vocational education and issue them correspondent middle vocational diploma and higher vocational diploma. "6-year system" means 3-year middle vocational education and another 3-year higher vocational education.

"3 + 2" Complete Model. Higher vocational colleges in this mode recruit junior middle school graduates directly. In the first 2 years, these students will take education according to the teaching plan of secondary school, then those whose scholastic attainment and comprehensive performance in these 2 years are good will be partially selected to college and take 3-year vocational education to complete their higher vocational education. Those having passed the examinations can be awarded junior college diploma; those who don't enter college have to study 1 or 2 year more according to the teaching plan of secondary school, and they will be awarded secondary school diploma.

Normal Mode. There is not any cooperation or business relationship between middle vocational schools and higher vocational schools. They educate their students according to their own length of education system respectively. The students graduated from middle vocational school can enter higher vocational school to receive vocational education through entrance examination. Students graduated from middle vocational school can freely choose and apply to higher vocational school and the higher vocational school can recruit students in middle vocational school and those in ordinary high school as well.

205.4 Problems in Connecting the Middle and Higher Vocational Education of Computer Application Major

Curriculum is the most important carrier in training professionals, however, no specific national or local requirements on how to build a system of professional courses connecting middle and higher vocational education has been put forward. The main problems are: first, the content of curriculum is repetitive. There is no specific unified curriculum criterion whether in the country or in the local places. There is a lack of unified teaching books connecting middle and higher vocational education, especially proprietary textbooks. The middle vocational school and the higher vocational school set up their own curricular system and teaching content respectively, thus some content are repeated in proprietary curriculum during the period of middle and higher vocational education. Second, the public basis courses get disjointed. When the students graduated from middle vocational school enter the higher one, they have difficulties in learning cultural courses, especially in mathematics, computer, English etc., which is obviously related to the tendency of "focus on skill while belittle cultural course, focus on operation while belittle theory" in many middle vocational school. It in fact reflects the difference of guiding ideology in curriculum structure design at middle and higher vocational school.

205.5 The Strategy Study in Connecting the Middle and Higher Vocational Education in Computer Application Major

Target of Training Professionals: To achieve the successful connection between middle and higher vocational education, the first step is to locate the training target. Higher vocational education in fact enlarge the knowledge structure of middle vocational education, improve their vocational ability and professional skills. As the computer application major is highly comprehensive and practical, middle vocational education, in order to improve the students' ability, should train the students of basic scientific literacy and necessary cultural knowledge, professional knowledge and experienced professional skills based on comprehensive quality. But the computer application major in higher vocational education should focus on enlarging the students' knowledge, training them the innovation consciousness, improving their communication capability and the comprehensive quality including morality, culture, psychological quality, physical quality etc., the ability to take further study and the ability to adapt to the job changes.

Curriculum System and Curriculum Provision: The curriculum between middle and higher vocational education should be of continuity and development. Higher vocational school should study the curriculum provision of middle vocational school and study the curriculum support system to achieve the professional training target so that the connection between middle and higher vocational education can be achieved more successfully. In detail, the curriculum of middle and higher vocational education should be looked as if it is a whole unit, and all the parts of this system should be subject to the overall training target that the curriculum provision aims at. We should carefully define the role of each course in the teaching plan, reasonably arrange the implementation of teaching plan and remove any repetition or old content of this course.

Teaching Management: Higher vocational education should take the quality difference of different resources into consideration so that they can more efficiently solve the problems in connecting middle and higher vocational education. It is advised that we should change the traditional credit system of scholastic year into complete credit system. According to the knowledge structure of sources, the score requirements of professional course, cultural course and technical skill class set by the school should show some difference. The students from ordinary high school have weak bask professional knowledge and strong cultural base, while the students from middle vocational school have a relatively weaker cultural base and a relatively strong professional knowledge. Therefore, the score in professional courses of students from ordinary high school are lower than that of students from middle vocational school, while the score in cultural courses of ordinary high school students are higher than that of middle vocational school students. So we'd better strengthen students' (from the ordinary high school) learning in professional course and improve their cultural knowledge, meanwhile we'd better strengthen the students' (from middle vocational school) cultural knowledge and improve their professional knowledge. Only in this way can students of different sources achieve the final target.

Student Management: As for students in higher vocational school from middle vocational schools, a large percent of who are of poor activity in learning, poor learning ability and low comprehensive quality because the middle vocational schools they stayed before are not strict with them and neglect the management of the students. As most of the leaders and teachers in middle vocational school think that the students in middle vocational school can find a job as long as they learn one technical skill. It's not necessary that the student should be strict with them, or pay much attention to teaching quality. Some middle vocational school may think themselves as the transmission of "3 + 2" system, thus the students' quality is of little relations to them. The key to solve this problem is to change the middle vocational schools' thought and they should realize that the bad habits formed there may influence their study in higher vocational school directly and the students' job choosing, which in turn will influence the recruit of middle vocational students. The middle vocational school should carry out the quality oriented education, insist the job-oriented and ability-based, focus on the total development of students, strengthen the teaching of culture base and improve the humanistic spirit as well.

205.6 Conclusion

To build a complete teaching system of middle and higher vocational education should obey the principle of "Based on middle vocational education and dominated by higher vocational education". The basic task of middle vocational education is to train and send qualified junior or intermediate professional laborers for economic construction and social development. Some middle vocational students will take a job and step into the front line of production, business and service; others will go to higher vocational school for further study. Therefore, middle vocational school should try to improve the teaching quality and take these as their training tasks: to train practical junior and intermediate technicians for the society and to send qualified sources for higher vocational education.

Acknowledgments This work was supported by Research Project of the General Topic in 2012 Research Association of Guangdong Higher Vocational Education Project (No. GDGZ12Y091) and Guangdong Province Education Science 12th five Plan Project (No. 2012JK009).

References

1. Zhang X (2000) Overview of dual system in vocational education. Hainan Press, Hainan
2. Yang H (2011) The connecting problem in middle and higher vocational education and the strategies from the perspective of system theory. China Electr Educ 7
3. Liu Y, Zhou F (2011) The connection between middle and vocational curriculum: appeal out of practice. China Vocat Tech Educ 24
4. Li X, Zhang Y (2009) Thinking about the connection between middle and higher vocational teaching. Sci Educ Cult 5

Chapter 206
Meta Analysis of Teachers' Job Burnout in China

Jian-ping Liu, Zhi-fang He and Lin Yu

Abstract Objective: Job burnout is an exhausted status due to long-hours or high intensity working, which results from the pressure of work environment. Nowadays, job burnout of teacher has been becoming one of the core issues in the areas of occupational stress. To investigate teachers' burnout and mental health, we carried out a meta-analysis of published studies on teachers' burnout (using MBI-ES scale) in mainland China. Methods: Based on the inclusion and exclusion criteria, there were 23 studies in our analysis. The retrieval time was range from the January 31, 1979 to March 10, 2013, and the RevMan 5.1 was used for the Meta analysis. Results: Firstly, emotional exhaustion of male teachers were significantly better than that of female teachers. Secondly, the shorter years the teachers work, the better health they got in emotional exhaustion. Conclusion: The teachers' burnout is prevalent. In particular, the female teachers and senior teachers are in more bad situations, which is consistent with the theory of emotional gender stereo-types and collective self-esteem in social psychology and the theory of career plateau in educational psychology.

Keywords Teachers · Job burnout · Meta analysis

J. Liu (✉)
School of Psychology, Jiangxi Normal University, Nanchang 330022, China
e-mail: Liujianping@jxnu.edu.cn

Z. He · L. Yu
School of Humanities, Jiangxi University of Traditional Chinese Medicine, Nanchang 330004, China

206.1 Introduction

The concept of job burnout was proposed by Maslach in 1974. Job burnout is an exhausted status due to long hours work, overload work and high intensity work [1]. It results from the pressure in the long-term and heavy work environment. The field of education began to focus on the study of burnout in the 1980s. In the mid-1990s, teachers' burnout has become one of the core issues in the areas of occupational stress at home and abroad [2]. Domestic scholars researched different aspects of the main factors affecting teacher burnout in the content of teacher burnout. And in the form from the research point of view, the researches were divided into theoretical speculation and empirical researches, which did not involve secondary researches and systematic reviews. In this study, a comprehensive analysis in the decade of teacher burnout research is studied by systematic reviews, meta-analysis, which provides a scientific basis for the study of teacher burnout and mental health problems.

206.2 Data Sources and Methods

206.2.1 Literature Research

The study retrieved the articles from full-text database of journals, VIP Chinese and Wan fang database technology academic journal by computer. Search keywords were "teacher burnout and MBI-ES Scale", and search time were from January 31, 1979 to March 10, 2013. 81 documents were retrieved initially.

206.2.2 Inclusion Criteria

- Using the Maslach Burnout questionnaire (MBI-ES). The questionnaire was 22 questions, and it was divided into three dimensions: emotional exhaustion (nine questions), de-personalized (five questions) and low personal accomplishment (8 questions) [3].
- Object is Chinese teachers.
- Empirical research. The study finally included 23 studies.

206.2.3 Data Extraction

Two researchers screened and extracted data by inclusion criteria independently. Differences which they encounter would be resolved by discussion.

206.2.4 Statistical Analysis

Meta-analysis was used in the study by RevMan5.1 Software. And the combined statistics was represented by Standardized Mean Difference (SMD).

206.3 Results

206.3.1 Included Literatures

Based on the literature inclusion criteria, 23 articles were finally included. The specific data are shown in Table 206.1.

206.3.2 Meta analysis Results

206.3.2.1 The Compared Results of Different Gender

The comparative results have significant heterogeneity, Therefore, the study using a random effects model to calculate the combined statistics SMD. As can be seen from the Table 206.2, the results show that the status of job burnout for male teachers is significantly better than that for female teachers in the dimensions of emotional exhaustion, and there is no significant difference in the dimensions of depersonalized and low sense of accomplishment for both gender groups.

206.3.2.2 The Results of Different Titles

From the Table 206.3, the results showed that the junior titles teachers significantly better than intermediate grade teachers in the dimensions of emotional exhaustion and both of them had no significant difference in the dimensions of depersonalized and low sense of accomplishment. In addition, from the Table 206.4, the results showed that the intermediate titles teachers significantly better than the senior titles teachers in the dimensions of depersonalized and both of them had no significant difference in the dimensions of emotional exhaustion and low sense of accomplishment.

Table 206.1 Twenty-three included literature list

No	Study id	School type	Study areas	No	Study id	School type	Study areas
1	Zhao Yufang (2003)	High school	Sichuan/Chongqing	2	Liu Changjiang (2004)	High school	Shandong
3	Hu Yongping (2004)	High school	Jiangxi	4	Liu Weiliang (2004)	Primary/secondary school	Beijing
5	Lu Xiaoyan (2007)	University	Hunan	6	Zhang Guoqing (2007)	Primary/secondary school	Henan
7	Nin Wanmei (2007)	High school	Guangdong	8	Sun Shujing (2008)	High school	Shandong
9	Huang Peiseng (2008)	University	Sichuan	10	Du Zhenyao (2009)	University	Shandong
11	Shun Lihong (2009)	Primary school	Hubei	12	Zhang Ji (2009)	University	Guizhou
13	Lei Jing (2009)	University	Chongqing	14	Wu Yanping (2009)	Primary/Secondary school	Hebe
15	He Xing (2010)	University	Henan	16	Zhang Xiaowen (2011)	University	Jiangxi
17	Chang Guangchui (2011)	High school	Anhui	18	Li Xiang (2011)	University	Guizhou
19	Zhou wei (2011)	University	Hunan	20	Yu Ping (2012)	University	Jilin
21	Wu Yanan (2012)	Primary/Secondary school	Hebe	22	Wang Li (2012)	University	Shanxi
23	Wu Sumei (2012)	Primary/Secondary school	Guangxi				

Table 206.2 The results of different gender

Dimension	Number of male	Number of female	Test of differences effect sizes			Test for heterogeneity		
			SMD	95 % CI	Z values	Chi^2 values	P values	I^2 %
Emotional exhaustion	3878	4203	−0.21	−0.43,0.00	1.99*	330.13	0.00	93
De-personalized	3878	4203	0.19	−0.27,0.65	0.83	1431.84	0.00	98
Low sense of accomplishment	3878	4203	0.19	−0.27,0.65	0.83	1431.84	0.00	98

206.4 Discussions

Our findings suggest that gender differences only exists in the dimensions of emotional exhaustion of college teachers, that is to say, male teacher's emotional control and management are better than that of the female teachers. This conclusion is consistent with the theory of emotional gender stereo-types, which is an emerging field of gender stereotypes. The areas included that people held a particular belief when the male and female experienced and performed specific emotional [4]. That women were more emotional than men was one of the most enduring gender stereotypes, if didn't distinguishing between specific emotions [5]. Some other studies also showed that people thought female in the Eastern culture were more sentimental and emotional [6]. Moreover they were also more concerned about family and everyday life than men. Whereas, Men had good control and management, and they focused more on career and social responsibility than women. Results of other study that did not conform to our criteria of time frame, dependent measures, or different subject investigated also point to the same outcome of us. For example, a meta study of primary and secondary school teachers found that the degree of burnout of male teachers were bad than female teachers, but the difference was not significant. Thus far, the gender was not the main factors which affected the teacher burnout [7].

From the point of view of the different titles of the teachers, the junior titles teachers significantly better than intermediate grade teachers in the dimensions of emotional exhaustion and the intermediate titles teachers significantly better than the senior titles teachers in the dimensions of depersonalized. Compared to junior titles teachers, intermediate titles teachers were exposed to bigger pressure from the teaching, scientific research and competition. Meanwhile, they had the pursuit of a higher goal. Therefore, they had the higher emotional exhaustion. Compared to the mediate titles teachers, the senior titles teachers had a greater age difference, a deeper generation gap and there are certain objective obstacles to communication and exchange with university's students. Furthermore, the senior titles teachers had entered the career plateau, which referred the stop of the individual's career's development and formation of a kind of take for granted-set mentality. Another published study employing different inclusion criteria and a somewhat divergent

Table 206.3 The compared results of junior and intermediate titles teachers

Dimension	Number of junior titles	Number of intermediate titles	Test of differences effect sizes			Test for heterogeneity		
			SMD	95 % CI	Z values	Chi^2 values	P values	I^2 %
Emotional exhaustion	1386	1756	−0.27	−0.40,−0.13	3.93**	21.74	0.01	53
De-personalized	1386	1756	0.36	−0.13,0.86	1.43	304.43	0.00	97
Low sense of accomplishment	1386	1756	0.01	−0.15,0.17	0.11	31.64	0.00	72

Table 206.4 The compared results of senior and intermediate titles teachers

Dimension	Number of intermediate titles	Number of junior titles	Test of differences effect sizes				Test for heterogeneity		
			SMD	95 % CI	Z values		Chi2 values	P values	I2 %
Emotional exhaustion	1756	903	0.07	−0.09,0.22	0.86		23.77	0.01	58
De-personalized	1756	903	−0.73	−1.26,−0.19	2.65**		302.26	0.00	97
Low sense of accomplishment	1756	903	0.11	−0.21,0.42	0.65		109.25	0.00	91

strategy also provides additional support that the teacher's titles is an important factor influencing teachers' burnout [8]. From the theory of social psychology, the higher titles teachers maybe get higher collective self-esteem and more likely to feel burnout [9].

There are 6986 subjects in this research, which are widely distributed in China. Therefore, the research results are representative. However, due to the classification of teaching experience, working age, education, income, and other factors in original studies vary greatly, meta-analysis can not be carried out. For this reason, our meta-analysis does not involve these factors.

This study attempts to review and reflect the teachers' burnout carried out by Chinese scholars in this field during the past 30 years. The teachers' burnout phenomenon is prevalent in the group of teachers, especially female teachers, intermediate and senior titles teachers. This conclusion is consistent with the theory of emotional gender stereo-types and collective self-esteem in social psychology and the theory of career plateau in educational psychology. Future researches which should be included more literatures can conclude the more comprehensive and convincing results.

Acknowledgement This work was financially supported by College of Humanities and Social Science Fund project in 2012 of Jiangxi province (XL1207) and the Twelfth Five Years Educational Planning Fund of Jiangxi province (12YB139).

References

1. Zhang L, Wang D et al (2007) Foreign teachers' burnout factors Influencing new progress. Psychol Sci 30(2):492–494
2. Chen Y (2011) Retrospect and prospect of teachers' burnout in domestic. J Teach Manag 6:10–11
3. Enzmann D, Schaufeli WB, Janssen P et al (1998) Dimensionality and validity of the burnout measure. J Occup Org Psychol 71(4):331–352
4. Durik AM, Hyde JS, Marks AC et al (2006) Ethnicity and gender stereotypes of emotion. Sex Roles 54:429–445
5. Williams JE, Best DL (1990) Measuring sex stereotypes: a multi-nation study. Sage, Newbury Park
6. Zhang Y, Zuo B et al (2011) The attributed explain of emotional gender stereotypes. J Chinese Clin Psychol 19(5):578–581
7. Liu X, Chao H (2003) Realistic analysis of primary and secondary school teachers Job burnout. Prim Second Sch Teach Train 21(10):68–70
8. Zhao Y, Bi Z (2003) Burnout and influencing factors of the primary and secondary school teachers. Psychol Dev Educ 26(1):44–47
9. Bulter SK, Constaintine GM (2005) Collective self-esteem and burnout in professional school counselors. Prof Sch Couns 2005(5):55–62

Chapter 207
Similar Theory in Material Mechanics Problem

Luo Mao and Song Shaoyun

Abstract Similar on guidance the experimental and organize experimental data, analysis the similar modulus material mechanics, given the large circular sheet surrounding stepping up the load evenly distributed around the degree of the problem.

Keywords Similar theory · Similar modulus · Mechanics of materials · Application

207.1 Similar Modulus and the Law of Similarity Theory

Similar conditions can be expressed with equal relationship between the various physical quantities and between two similar systems, they are called for similar modulus, that is similar to the conditions of the first system and the second system is similar modulus equal. The number of similar modulus is actually dimensional analysis. Dimensional analysis in number and may not be suitable for the physical equations, it is often not the only, major weakness of dimensional analysis. In a similar theory, these numbers are selected by physical equations, therefore, similar modulus for physics equations π number.

Similar on the first law: when the similarity of the two phenomena not only these two phenomena similar have a certain similarity constant, and there are similar modulus equal, similar to its modulus is generally called Newton modulus.

L. Mao (✉) · S. Shaoyun
Information Technology Engineering Institute, Yuxi Normal University, Yuxi, Yunnan, China
e-mail: luomao@yxnu.net

S. Shaoyun
e-mail: mathsong@126.com

Similar phenomenon is represented by the equation of physical quantities, these algebraic equations must be $x_1^{\alpha_1} x_2^{\alpha_2} \ldots x_n^{\alpha_n}$ in the form of a homogeneous equation. This physical phenomenon similar conditions is represented by (1) conditions. These similar conditions with similar modulus can be written as:

$$\frac{N_{i1}(x_1, x_2, \ldots, x_n)}{N_{ir}(x_1, x_2, \ldots, x_n)} = k_{i1}, \frac{N_{i2}(x_1, x_2, \ldots, x_n)}{N_{ir}(x_1, x_2, \ldots, x_n)} = k_{i2} \ldots, \frac{N_{i(r-1)}(x_1, x_2, \ldots, x_n)}{N_{ir}(x_1, x_2, \cdots, x_n)} = k_{i(r-1)},$$

$$(i = 1, 2, \ldots, m) \quad (207.1)$$

Total $m(r-1)$ modulus, these algebraic equations, can be used with similar modulus is expressed as:

$$1 + \sum_{k=1}^{r-1} k_{ik} = 0, \quad (i = 1, 2, \ldots, m) \quad (207.2)$$

In other words, the dimensionless equations items is similar modulus. So as long as the differential operator equation similar phenomenon can direct them written in dimensionless form, that they can become similar modulus modulus equation. Since the similar phenomenon similar modulus is the corresponding equal, so that their modulus equation is also the same.

But contains many physical equations differential form, have differential form can not simply Kasei (207.2) as the form. Have proven in the literature [1]: is the physical phenomena expressed by using the same text equations, the necessary conditions for similar phenomena is also similar modulus are equal, and also have the same modulus equation.

The second law of similarity theory: similar phenomenon similar modulus must be equal, the modulus modulus equation must be equal.

207.2 Application Examples

Large round sheet tightening around evenly distributed load deflection.

A set of thin circular plate a radius a, the flexural rigidity D around the degree of w, diameter of the thin film force N_r, the Young's modulus of E, sagittal diameter r, a thickness of h, a load of q (Fig. 207.1 shown).

Around the degree plate due to deformation by elongation and tensile force occurs, these tension also bear part of the load, its balance equation [1]:

$$D \frac{d}{dr} \frac{1}{r} \frac{d}{dr} r \frac{dw}{dr} - N_r \frac{dw}{dr} = \frac{1}{2} qr$$

207 Similar Theory in Material Mechanics

Fig. 207.1 The basic parameters of the thin circular plate

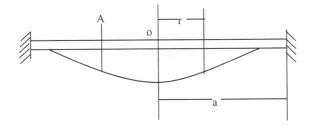

There $N_r \frac{dw}{dr}$ is part of the tension loads, because the tension is due to tensile deformation after bending and deflection, this relationship is to coordinate equation, it can be written as:

$$r \frac{d}{dr} \frac{1}{r} \frac{d}{dr}(r^2 N_r) + \frac{Eh}{2}\left(\frac{dw}{dr}\right)^2 = 0$$

The clamping varying boundary conditions:

If $r = a$ then $w = 0$, $\frac{dw}{dr} = 0$; $r\frac{dN_r}{dr} + (1-v)N_r = 0$

If $r = 0$ then $\frac{dw}{dr} = 0$, $\frac{dN_r}{dr} = 0$

There v is poisson's ratio, the introduction of a dimensionless quantity, assume N_0, w_0 are rally and around the degree of the center: $\frac{r}{a} = \rho$, $\frac{N_r}{N_0} = S$, $\frac{w}{w_0} = y$. Then merge the above equation to get:

$$\frac{w_0}{h} = \frac{d}{d\rho}\frac{1}{\rho}\frac{d}{d\rho}\rho\frac{dy}{d\rho} - \frac{N_0 a^2}{D}\frac{w_0}{h} S\frac{dy}{d\rho} = \frac{1}{2}\frac{qa^4}{Dh}\rho$$

$$\frac{N_0 a^2}{D}\rho\frac{d}{d\rho}\frac{1}{\rho}\frac{d}{d\rho}(\rho^2 S) + 6(1-v^2)\frac{w_0^2}{h^2}\left(\frac{dy}{d\rho}\right)^2 = 0$$

Clamping varying boundary conditions are:

If $\rho = 1$ then $y = \frac{dy}{d\rho} = 0$; $\rho\frac{dS}{d\rho} + (1-v)S = 0$

If $\rho = 0$ then $\frac{dy}{d\rho} = 0$, $\frac{dS}{d\rho} = 0$

It has been applied the expression of the bending stiffness of the $D = \frac{Eh^3}{12(1-v^2)}$.

By above a few formulas, there are three similar modulus $\frac{w_0}{h}$, $\frac{N_0 a^2}{D}$, $\frac{qa^4}{Dh}$.

No single value condition similar modulus, because this is the differential automatic similar problems.

Assume $\frac{w_0}{h}y = \frac{w}{h} = W^*$, $\frac{N_0 a}{D}S = \frac{N_r a^2}{D} = N^*$. Then the above equation can be simplified to $\frac{d}{d\rho}\frac{1}{\rho}\frac{d}{d\rho}\rho\frac{dW^*}{d\rho} - N^*\frac{dW^*}{d\rho} = \frac{1}{2}\frac{qa^4}{Dh}\rho$

$$\rho\frac{d}{d\rho}\frac{1}{\rho}\frac{d}{d\rho}(\rho^2 N^*) + 6(1-v^2)\left(\frac{dW^*}{d\rho}\right)^2 = 0$$

Fig. 207.2 Uniform thin circular plate under load the center the Rao degrees of experimental data

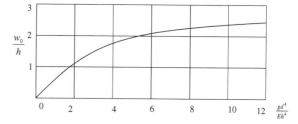

The boundary conditions are:

If $\rho = 1$ then $W^* = \frac{dW^*}{d\rho} = 0, \rho \frac{dN^*}{d\rho} + (1-\nu)N^* = 0$

If $\rho = 0$ then $\frac{dW^*}{d\rho} = 0, \frac{dN^*}{d\rho} = 0$

In these two equations, W^*, N^* are equivalent to X^*, which are the single variable modulus. (23) In under the condition of (24), the integral obtained solution can be written as: $W^* = f(\frac{qa^4}{Dh}, \rho), N^* = g(\frac{qa^4}{Dh}, \rho)$. Among $\frac{qa^4}{Dh}$ is the only similar. Analog digital W^*, N^*, ρ are variable modulus, the above formula is the modulus equation. If $\rho = 0$ then the Centre in thin pull is $W^*(\rho)_{\rho=0} = w^*(0) = \frac{w_0}{h}$, So get $\frac{w_0}{h} = f(\frac{qa^4}{Dh}, 0) = f_1(\frac{qa^4}{Dh})$. If the experimental value of A and B is plotted. Obtained experimental points should be in a curve, the experimental results fully confirmed that, in the customary $\frac{qa^4}{Dh}$ this modulus is represented by $\frac{qd^4}{h^4 E}$, $d = 2a$ Is the diameter of the circular plate, two modulus only by a constant factor $3/4(1-\nu^2)$. MoPherson, AE 744 kinds in the United States National Aeronautics and Consulting Association (NACA) report (1942) published data (11 different sizes of circular plates under different loads experimental record). $\frac{qa^4}{Eh^4}$ and $\frac{w_0}{h}$ as analog-to-digital finishing results, as shown in the figure below. (Fig. 207.2 shown).

207.3 Conclusion

The analysis of the mechanics of materials with similar theory calculations can get more reliable data. Stepping up from a uniform distribution of load surrounding large circular sheet analysis and calculation of the deflection can be seen similar to the importance of the theory in the mechanics of materials.

References

1. Qian W (1993) Applied mathematics. Anhui Science and Technology Press, China
2. Liu Y (2012).Local rigid body of thinking in material mechanics. Jilin Province, College of education

3. Huang J (1999) Optimization design method in mechanics of materials. Natural Science, Jimei University, China
4. Xiong Z (2010) Similar mechanical properties of metallic materials and application. Paper presented at The steel engineering research ⑧ — China steel association, structural stability and fatigue branch 12th (ASSF-2010) academic exchanges conference. China, 28 Aug 2010
5. Li Y (2012). Maple material mechanics - to draw complex load beam shear force diagram and bending moment diagram mechanics and engineering application. Meeting 10 Aug 2012

Chapter 208
Some Reflections on the Course Teaching of Physical Oceanography

Hao Liu and Song Hu

Abstract The course of Physical Oceanography is the important curriculum generally designed in the ocean universities or colleges to cultivate the practical professionals embarking on a career in the marine sciences. This course mainly introduces the physical processes and the dynamic mechanisms happening in the ocean. Based on the course content and feature, also in conjunction with our teaching experience, we suggest that the class teaching should regard both theory and practice as equally important, and both the teacher and students jointly construct the subject of this course. What is more, only the learning interests are initiated by means of various teaching skills or methods would the students be able to think and consult independently. It is very important for students to better understand and master the knowledge of this course.

Keywords Course of physical oceanography · Content of teaching · Teaching method

208.1 Introduction

The twenty-first century is thought to be the oceanic century. As the limited land resources seem not fit to the rapid development of the society and economy, the ocean is becoming the natural substitute. Furthermore, the maritime countries have to face such tough problems as how to utilize the ocean resources effectively to serve the social and economic development without disturbing the marine environment.

H. Liu (✉) · S. Hu
College of Marine Sciences, Shanghai Ocean University, 999 Hu-Cheng-Huan-Lu
201306 Shanghai, China
e-mail: haoliu@shou.edu.cn

According to the report given by United Nations Educational Scientific and Cultural Organization (UNESCO), the coastline length of china ranks the fourth place among all countries, which is about 1.8×10^4 km long, the sea area of the continental shelf and the nautical mile exclusive economic zone rank the fifth and the tenth place, respectively in the word. Therefore, it can be seen that China is a big ocean country absolutely. On the other hand, China was never a maritime power, and more often than not China was regarded as a continental country. In fact, the large scale of research, exploitation and utilization of the ocean just began two decades ago in China, which is owing to the rapid promotion of the economic strength. Another major reason that limited the development of the oceanic entertainment is the lack of enough professionals. Based on the incomplete statistics, there are only two universities in China, namely Qiangdao Ocean University and Xiamen University, which had established the synthetic courses concerning the marine sciences. This situation is very different from that in USA, since the department of oceanography or the college of marine sciences is almost established in each comprehensive university. During the last decade, our government began to promote the research and development of the ocean to the national strategy. Accordingly, some native colleges and departments which had some relationships with the marine sciences updated their name to the ocean university, and then began to construct the subject of marine sciences. In order to live up to the name, the disciplines and courses concerning marine sciences like physical oceanography, chemical oceanography, biological oceanography, and so on, have to be established and developed. Meanwhile, new undergraduates and postgraduates are also enrolled in these new subjects, which aim to cultivate enough professionals embarking on a career in the field of marine sciences.

The subject of Physical Oceanography is the fundamental discipline of the marine sciences. Except the several traditional ocean universities or colleges, it is inevitable that these newly established ocean universities are lack of the inside information of this subject, and then there are lots of improvements and modifications for the course design and construction. Therefore, in this paper we shall introduce the content and feature of this course teaching firstly, and then discuss the problems that the teacher and students may face in this course. Our final purpose is to improve the teaching quality earnestly and construct this course as an excellent course of the Committee of Shanghai Education.

208.2 Course Content and Feature

In the course of Physical Oceanography, the thermodynamic and thermohaline characteristics of the seawater is introduced first, and then the heat budget and water balance in the global as well as in the regional seas are described, at last various movements of the ocean are illustrated, which includes the movement type, the equation of motion and the dynamic mechanism governing the sea movement. The course content generally constitutes the physical base of the marine sciences, and the purpose of this course is set to help students to understand the key hydrodynamic processes happening on the surface as well as in the interior of the seas. The higher target is to require students to comprehend the dynamic mechanisms that control the sea movement and to present the reasonable explanation for the phenomenon of the physical process in the ocean.

In terms of the comprehensive course hierarchy, the courses of Calculus and Introduction to Marine Science should be arranged in front of this course. The course of Calculus presents a mathematic tool for students to understand and fathom the equations of motion. According to the teaching program, the courses of Introduction to Marine Science and Physical Oceanography seem not very different. However, the genuine contents of teaching are distinct. The former course mainly focus on describing the physical phenomenon in the ocean, hence it can also be regarded as Descriptive Physical Oceanography, in which the mathematic skills are not requested for students. The course of Physical oceanography aims to introduce how the physical process happened in the ocean, and the formula derivations are the important method to illustrate such problems. Therefore, this course may be called as Dynamical Oceanography, and it is oriented for the undergraduates of higher grade or postgraduates, whereas the former course is characterized by the general education course and oriented for the undergraduates of lower grade.

The teaching content of Physical Oceanography covers a wide range, and each knowledge point may be expanded to an independent course. Take the ocean circulation as an example, it comprises geostrophic currents, inertial currents, wind-driven currents, compensation currents (upwelling and downwelling), thermohaline currents, and so on. The joint interactions of several currents generate the western boundary current like the kuroshio and the gulf streams. In addition, the interactions between the oceanic and atmospheric currents may even create the El Nino, the La Nina, or other extreme weathers. In the strict sense, the above knowledge belongs to the scope of Physical Oceanography. However, it seems impossible to introduce each knowledge point to students using the limited class hours. Therefore, lecturers have to make their choice on the teaching content based on the students' subject and the actual class hours.

208.3 Teaching Matters Needing Attention

As related previously, the course of Physical Oceanography needs the strong speciality, which means that students should have accumulated enough knowledge about calculus and descriptive physical oceanography before this course. Even so, lecturers should make the necessary review of the conception, characteristics, principle and method on the physical phenomenon happening in the ocean. In this course, much attention should be paid on the explanation and analysis of the dynamic mechanisms so that students are able to draw inferences about other cases from one instance by grasping the key and difficult point. Lecturers should link theory with practice when teaching. Aiming to the common phenomenon of the physical oceanography, lecturers should describe the dynamic process using the mathematic language, lead students to derive formula, and inspire students to understand thoroughly and think independently. In addition, lecturers may enlarge the information about the content of teaching by means of multimedia to initiate the students' interest.

This course is a typical foreign subject. Its knowledge hierarchy and professional architecture are relatively perfect in the western developed countries, and the accumulated materials and methods are more abundant and sound than ours. Therefore, lecturers should pay much attention on the introduction and utilization of the professional English so as to help students to enrich their professional knowledge by reading English texts and references.

In terms of teaching method and style, lecturers should utilize the multimedia sufficiently, and present the observed or simulated temperature, salinity and vector fields by means of MODIS picture or other visual methods so as to inspire the students' interest. It is suggested that diverse teaching styles should be adopted. The theoretical knowledge could be introduced through the traditional teaching, and the case study could be conducted through the interactive teaching. For example, in the chapter of ocean circulations, teachers can ask a variety of questions, like what circulation it is, what is the major driving force to a kind of circulation, what is basic feature about this circulation, and so on. Some simple questions can be answered by students quickly, and as for the question no one can answer in the classroom, teachers encourage students to think and resource the answer in the spare time and organize discussion in the next classroom. Also only like this, the learning ability can be cultivated and the learning method can be trained.

It is necessary to cultivate the students' subjective initiative, which is conducive for students to absorb the knowledge in the classroom and use the knowledge in their future career. Concerning the important equations, teachers should make the formula derivation on the blackboard to help students to understand. Additionally, in order to keep the course teaching continuously, it is suggested that teachers should make a simple revision about the knowledge point of the last classroom in the beginning and make a concise conclusion on the teaching content before dismissing this class.

Besides completing the normal classroom teaching, lecturers should set moderate homework in the end of each paper. In fact, arranging students to think, resource and prepare the questions in the spare time and then to discuss these questions in classroom can help students to cultivate the ability of learning. Furthermore, the learning ability is not only essential for students to understand and master the knowledge in the classroom, but also helpful for students to expand their own scope of knowledge and to trace the recent advance of this subject. Generally speaking, the common quantity of homework should not be less than 10 class hours.

As for the assessment method, examination is still the necessary tool to evaluate students' learning, since this course is defined as an important professional course.

However, this course emphasizes the knowledge understanding, so the ability of mechanical memorizing is not requested in examination, which means that the form of examination should be improved.

At last, it needs to be pointed out that the lack of a suitable textbook is the serious problem that has puzzled the course construction. The currently existed book with the same name as the course was either published long time ago, or more professional in terms of the content. Therefore, lecturers should choose those sound and recognized concept, terminology and theory as the main content when they design the teaching program, determine the teaching content and write or edit the teaching notes. On the other hand, lecturers also need to update the knowledge based on the recent scientific fruit so as to expand the students' horizon on this subject.

208.4 Conclusions

In this paper, we have introduced the content and feature of the course of Physical Oceanography. Furthermore, we present the possible problems encountered when teaching, and give some constructive countermeasures in order to perfect the teaching hierarchy and improve the teaching quality of this course.

Acknowledgments This study is financially supported by the 085 course construction of Shanghai Education Administration (B5102110401).

References

1. Jiang DC (2005) Engineering and environmental oceanography. China Ocean Press, Beijing
2. Ye AL, Li FQ (1992) Physical oceanography. Press of Qiangdao Ocean University, Qingdao
3. Feng SZ, Li FQ, Li SJ (1999) Introduction to marine sciences. Higher Education Press, Beijing
4. Li FQ, Su YS (2000) Analysis on water mass of oceans. Press of Qiangdao Ocean University, Qingdao
5. Stewart RH (2005) Introduction to Physical Oceanography. A&M University, Texas
6. Pickard GL, William JE (1990) Descriptive physical oceanography, an introduction. Butterworth-Heinemann, Oxford
7. Pond S, Pickard GL (1983) Introductory dynamical oceanography. Butterworth-Heinemann, Oxford

Chapter 209
A Neural Tree Network Ensemble Mode for Disease Classification

Feng Qi, Xiyu Liu and Yinghong Ma

Abstract A neural tree network ensemble model is proposed for classification which is an important research field in data mining and machine learning. Firstly, establishes each single neural tree network by using an improved hybrid breeder genetic programming, and then more neural tree networks are combined to form the final classification model by the idea of ensemble learning. Simulation results on two disease classification problems show that this model is effective for the classification, and has better performance in classification precision, feature selection and structure simplification, especially for classification with multi-class attributes.

Keywords Neural tree network · Breeder genetic programming · Ensemble learning · Disease classification

209.1 Introduction

Classification problem is an important research field in data mining and machine learning [1]. Currently, Bayesian method [2], decision tree method [3] neural network method [4] and support vector machine [5], etc. are widely used for classification problem. Among them, the neural network method, especially multilayer feed-forward neural network (MFNN) is always used and studied in classification and can be trained by standard BP algorithm, the additional momentum and self-adaptive learning efficiency based BP algorithm (BPX) or Levenberg–Marquardt method (LM), etc. [6]. But these algorithms have several disadvantages, such as low learning efficiency, slow convergence speed, easy to

F. Qi (✉) · X. Liu · Y. Ma
School of Management Science and Engineering, Shandong Normal University, Jinan 250014, China
e-mail: qfsdnu@126.com

fall into local optimum for complex problem, hard to decide number of nodes in hidden layers and fixed structure in training process.

And then, it is necessary to find a new classification model with quicker training speed, not easier to fall into local optimum, simpler network structure and higher classification accuracy. Neural tree network model (NTNM) [7–10] is a kind of neural network similar to MFNN with tree coding. The structure of NTNM can be evolved by tree-based evolutionary algorithm [7–10], while parameters of NTNM can be optimized by classic search algorithms [7–10]. By combining the above structure and parameters algorithms, the defects in structure and algorithm design in MFNN can be effectively solved. So a neural tree network ensemble model (NTNEM) is proposed for solving classification. This model uses an improved hybrid breeder genetic programming (IHBGP) for its structure and parameters optimization and it combines single NTNM to form the final classification model by the idea of ensemble learning. Experimental results show that this model is effective and especially for the complex classification with multi-class attributes.

209.2 Neural Tree Network Model and

In NTNM, there exists only two types nodes: function node and terminal node. The function node set F and terminal node set T are described as follows: $S = F \cup T = \{+_2, +_3, \ldots, +_N\} \cup \{x_1, x_2, \ldots, x_n\}$, where $+_i$ denote the function nodes with i arguments. x_i are the terminal nodes correspond to the input of issues.

When building NTNM, if a function node $(+_i)$ is selected, i real values are randomly generated as connection weights between $+_i$ and its children. In addition, two real numbers a_i and b_i are randomly created as flexible activation function parameters which is defined as $f(a_i, b_i, x) = e^{-((x-a_i)/b_i)^2}$.

The performance of NTNM mainly depends on accuracy and parsimony. For accuracy, Mean square error (MSE) is applied as the fitness function of IHBGP and defined as $Fit(i) = \frac{1}{N}\sum_{j=1}^{N}(y_1^j - y_2^j)^2$, where, N is the number of samples, y_1^j and y_2^j are the actual and NTNM output of jth sample. $Fit(i)$ denotes the fitness value of individual i.

209.3 The Improved Hybrid Breeder Genetic Programming

In order to find an optimal or near-optimal NTNM and avoid the noisy fitness evaluation problem, a hybrid evolutionary algorithm based on breeder genetic programming [11] is proposed.

The main procedure is described as follows, initial population $A(0)$ with S individuals is generated randomly from F and T. For gth generation, fitness value

$Fitness_i(g)$ is calculated by the training set. If the termination condition is satisfied, the algorithm stops. Otherwise, S pairs of individuals in gth population are chosen into the mating pool $B(g)$ by roulette wheel algorithm. For each individuals in $B(g)$ undergoes a hybrid encoded next-ascent hill climbing algorithm which is described later. The $(g + 1)$th generation with size S is generated by using crossover operation (the same as classic genetic programming) on randomly chosen individuals from $B(g)$. As the BGP algorithm, elitist strategy is also applied by replacing the worst individual $A_{worst}(g + 1)$ in $A(g + 1)$ by the $A_{best}(g + 1)$ of $A(g)$. A new population is generated repeatedly until an acceptable solution is found or the maximum number of generations reaches G_{max}.

Further, two newly mutation operators are introduced: (1) Real-parameter mutation operator. Real-parameter contains connect weight ω, activation function parameters a and b. Here exponential mutation operator [12] is applied: $v'_i = v_i \pm R_i 2^{-K\eta}, \eta \in [0, 1]$, where, R_i denotes the maximum mutation steps, η is a uniform random over [0, 1], constant K determines the shape of the exponential function. (2) Terminal node mutation operator. The selected terminal node $x_i \in T$ is replaced by another terminal node $x_j \in T$.

Based on the next-ascent hill climbing algorithm [13], a hybrid encoded next-ascent hill climbing algorithm is proposed for optimizing parameters and terminal nodes. First, all the terminal nodes and weights are formed a hybrid vector L. For each element $l_i \in L$ belongs to parameters or terminal nodes corresponding to parameter and terminal node mutation, respectively. For each time, after mutation on $l_i \in L$, the fitness of the individual will be evaluated by using L', if the fitness of L' is less than that of L, then L should be replaced by L' for the new hybrid vector, otherwise L' will be discarded.

209.4 Neural Tree Network Ensemble Model

By considering the characteristics of classification and NTNM, a neural tree network ensemble model based on simple binary code for classification is proposed and the framework and workflow of the model is shown in Fig. 209.1.

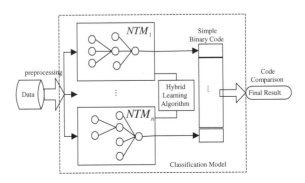

Fig. 209.1 The framework and workflow of the proposed model

The simple encoding rules are defined as follows, the ith bit of the binary string S_i of class i is set to 1 and the others are 0. After fixing the encoding forms, the data set DS_i for each $NTNM_i (i = 1, 2, \ldots, n)$ can be obtained in the following way: the class label of the sample belongs to class i is set to 1 and the other samples are set to 0. Finally, each NTNM is obtained by the above proposed algorithm on corresponding data set and then the ensemble model is constructed.

209.5 Simulations and Analysis

The performance of the proposed NTNEM is testified on two data sets: lung cancer and breast cancer obtained from UCI database. In experiment, each simulation is repeated 10 times. All the results are average classification accuracy (ACA), average training error (ATE), average number of network connections (ANNC) and training time is the total training time (TTT) of 10 times.

Detail settings are list as follows: (1) Training set and testing set are created randomly with proportion 1:1; (2) Classification accuracy $E = CN/|TS|$, where CN denotes the number of samples correctly classed in testing set; (3) IHBGP algorithm: $S = 50$, $G_{\max} = 400$, $Depth_{\max} = 4$, $k = 10$;

Table 209.1 Simulation results for lung data (*left*) and cancer data (*right*)

Models	ACA (%)	ATE	TTT (s)	ANNC	ACA (%)	ATE	TTT (s)	ANNC
BP	75.86	5.85×10^{-2}	198.62	236	95.65	2.79×10^{-2}	148.63	192
BPX	83.30	7.17×10^{-4}	59.033	236	97.19	9.87×10^{-3}	16.878	192
LM	89.13	4.81×10^{-4}	38.825	236	95.89	6.23×10^{-3}	13.063	192
NTNEM	93.21	3.19×10^{-4}	70.261	86	97.56	8.71×10^{-3}	50.850	69

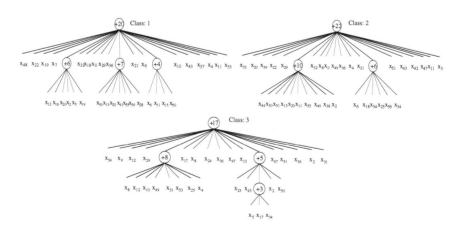

Fig. 209.2 Classification model created by NTNEM for lung data

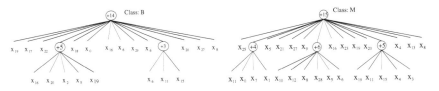

Fig. 209.3 Classification model created by NTNEM for cancer data

Simulation results are list in Table 209.1. It is clear that NTNEM has the highest classification accuracy and the least number of connect edges. Figures 209.2 and 209.3 are the final NTNEMs for Lung and Cancer data sets, where $F = \{+8, +9, \cdots, +25\}$, $T = \{x_0, x_1, \cdots x_{55}\}$ and $F = \{+5, +6, \cdots, +15\}$, $T = \{x_0, x_1, \cdots x_{29}\}$ are used, respectively. NTNEM maintains the classification accuracy under choosing some more important attributes, which greatly reduces the complexity of the structure and is a very promising classification model.

209.6 Conclusion

A neural tree network ensemble model based on simple binary code for classification is proposed and each single neural tree network is evolved an improved hybrid breeder genetic programming. Simulation results show that this model is effective for the classification, and has better performance in classification precision, feature selection and structure simplification, especially for the complex classification with multi-class attributes.

References

1. Han JW, Kamber M (2007) Data mining: concepts and techniques, 2nd edn. Machine Press, China
2. Friedman N, Geiger D, Goldszmidt M (1997) Bayesian network classifiers. Mach Learn 29(2–3):131–163
3. Breiman L, Friedman J, Olshen RA, Stone CJ (1984) Classification and regression trees. Wadsworth, Belmont
4. Zhang GP (2000) Neural networks for classification: a survey, systems, man, and cybernetics. IEEE Trans Syst C Appl Rev 30(4):451–462
5. Cortes C, Vapnik V (1995) Support-vector networks. Mach Learn 20(3):273–297
6. Sanchez VD (2003) Advanced support vector machines and kernel methods. Neurocomputing 55(1–2):5–20
7. Chen YH, Yang B, Dong J (2004) Nonlinear systems modeling via optimal design of neural trees. Int J Neural Syst 14:125–138
8. Chen YH, Yang B, Dong J (2004) Evolving flexible neural networks using ant programming and PSO algorithm. In: International symposiums neural networks (ISNN'04), Dalian, China, LNCS3173, pp 211–216

9. Chen YH, Yang B, Dong J, Abrahama A (2005) Time series forecasting using flexible neural tree model. Inf Sci 174(3–4):219–235
10. Chen YH, Abraham A, Yang B (2006) Feature selection and classification using flexible neural tree. Neurocomputing 70:305–313
11. Zhang BT, Muhlenbein H (1993) Genetic programming of minimal neural nets using Occam's razor. In: Forrest S (ed) Proceeding of fifth international conference on genetic algorithms, Forum, vol 1. Morgan Kaufmann, pp 342–349
12. Zhang BT, Ohm P, Muhlenbein H (1997) Evolutionary induction of sparse neural trees. Evol Comput 15:213–236
13. Muhlenbein H (1992) How genetic algorithms really work. Mutation and hill-climbing. In: Parallel problem solving from nature PPSN II, vol 1. North-Holland, pp 15–25

Chapter 210
Application of PBL Model in the Teaching of Foreign Graduate Student

Songzhu Xia, Xiaoyong Cao, Guisheng Yin, Haibo Liu and Jianguo Sun

Abstract The PBL model which focuses on the problem solving, as it can stimulate the initiative of student, is the more popular teaching method in the international. This paper establishes the specific embodiment of PBL model for the foreign graduate student from the perspective of teaching.

Keywords PBL · Foreign graduate student · Teaching

With the continuous improvement of teaching quality and an increase in foreign exchange, more and more foreign students studying in China, International student education has become an important part of higher education in china. Foreign student education has become an important indicator to measure a school of education level.

Foreign student education can enrich the school teaching system and increase the school's foreign exchange, it also enhance the school's international reputation. In the education for international students, we should pay attention to cultivating high level foreign graduate student with independent scientific research ability.

210.1 PBL Teaching Model

PBL is abbreviation of problem-based learning, which was pioneered at McMaster University School of Medicine by the American Academy of Neurology Professor

---

This work is sponsored by the Basic research and operational funding projects of central college under grant number HEUCF100602.

S. Xia · X. Cao (✉) · G. Yin · H. Liu · J. Sun
College of Computer Science and Technology, Harbin Engineering University,
Harbin 150001, China
e-mail: xiasongzhu@hrbeu.edu.cn

Barrows in 1969. PBL teaching has changed the textbook-centered learning methods in the past, but to develop the ability to use knowledge, PBL emphasizes the use of textbooks and the outside of the information resources to solve the problem. Student is the main body of this kind of teaching method, teachers no longer act as the role of the sources of information and knowledge, but as a student learning guide, to promote students' self study. Due to the particularity of graduate education, the teacher must according to the characteristics of students, the teaching method is take the student as the main body. PBL according to the teaching content and students learning to design a series of questions, which is consistent with the purpose of the study in graduate education, give full play to the initiative of the students [3].

PBL is very different with the traditional teaching method based on subjects. In traditional teaching emphasizes teacher-centered, PBL stressed to solve the problem of combining as the center, a variety of approaches to learning, emphasizing teamwork, emphasizing the support and guidance. Students active learning mode to acquire knowledge through a variety of ways to solve practical problems to stimulate students' interest and enthusiasm, to obtain a large number of opportunities to apply knowledge, focus on training students to master the ability to apply knowledge to enable students to benefit from life. 1980s, PBL teaching mode is more popular in North American universities after the 1990s, the European part of the school also launched of PBL, PBL is a teaching method that has become more popular. The implementation of the PBL can be divided into three levels: single course level of PBL, interdisciplinary aspects of PBL, college level of PBL. PBL teaching method is a more effective than the traditional model of curriculum design, it can effectively promote students' autonomous learning and cooperative learning, and improve the students' self satisfaction, and professional identity.

210.2 Study in Graduate and PBL Teaching Mode

Foreign graduate students of our school are from the Third World and the neighboring countries in Asia. These countries are less-development in economic and science and technology, their basic knowledge is slightly weak and uneven. Because of the social, cultural, educational and other differences, foreign graduate students compared with domestic students, they are free and lively, dare to express their views, it can form a good interaction with the teachers in class, their English with a thick accent.

PBL has the following several factors: (1) By students personally involved in the problem put forward, so as to arouse the students' interest in exploring innovation and brave to ask questions, the consciousness of thinking and habits. Foreign graduate students in the classroom are thinking active, and daring to ask questions. Student is the center of learning, they have to shoulder the responsibility of the study, PBL teaching practice lay particular stress on group cooperative learning and autonomous learning. This is conducive to the implementation of the different countries and different learning backgrounds graduate teaching, to improve their ability to social development and collaboration skills. (2) The teacher plays the coaching and support role in the critical moment. Teachers are no longer the only the Knowledge Base, but a facilitator of knowledge construction, subject experts, information consultant [1]. Teachers train students' thinking ability, logical level and the strong style of study, at the same time, they improve their enterprising spirit and improve their own knowledge structure, get new technologies and methods for teaching, so as to improve the teaching level [3, 5].

Traditional teaching based independent series of courses, Students can get credits through the assessment of these courses. The basic teaching: classroom teaching, reading, experiments, jobs and separate examinations of several parts. Single course of PBL only involves classroom teachers, it Need to consider the following questions: Group work—how many people in each group, free combination or teacher assigned; Topic—student in the definition of the framework free topic or the teacher assigned; Content selection—which is completed in the classroom, which is completed on the link of PBL; Counseling and support—how guidance and support to the student in PBL; Assessment methods—the traditional examination mode is suitable for PBL mode or not, if isn't, what kind of assessment method should be use (Fig. 210.1).

Interdisciplinary aspects of PBL need to consider the following questions: Goal—Goal usually should be set for more abstract, its purpose is to guide students to choose learning method according to the learning objectives; Group work—how many people in each group, free combination or teacher assigned; Organization—interdisciplinary courses to solve the open topic provides a better condition for students, but it need to have a clear theme; Content selection—what is taught in the classroom, it must be compressed to lecture time, otherwise the students won't have enough time to complete the project; Counseling and support—how guidance and support to the student in PBL; Assessment methods—the traditional examination mode is suitable for PBL mode or not, if isn't, what kind of assessment method should be use [2] (Fig. 210.2).

Our college implements PBL mode in a single course level and cross-program level.

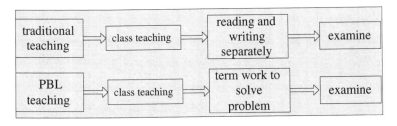

Fig. 210.1 Traditional teaching and PBL teaching

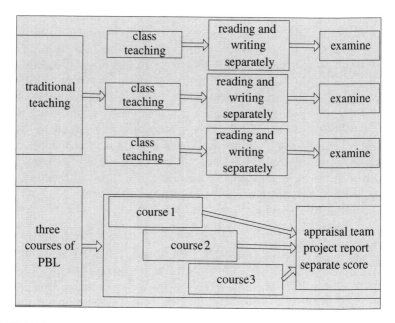

Fig. 210.2 Three courses of PBL

210.3 Implementation of the Program

210.3.1 Course PBL Mode

According to the characteristics of foreign graduate students, course PBL mode should use the mode of free combination, form a group composed of 3–5 students study groups, each group choose a team leader, the team leader responsible for the group discussion and division. The teacher put the question to students a week early, let them have enough time to solve this problem. According to their own division of labor, they start to understand the background of the problem, to gather information, and to find a solution to the problem. The group discussion is an important link in the PBL teaching, students can exercise expression ability, communication skills and teamwork skills. IN group discussion, each group member express what he do to solve the problem, then is fully discussed in the group, everyone express his view, and finally get a perfect solution. Each student collected a lot of information in this process, in the group discussion, they took their own newly acquired knowledge sharing to everyone, students will have a great harvest in every discussion. After students have mastered the method to solve problem, and then to explore the knowledge of the problems contained. PBL teaching method to make students change from passive learning to active learning, stimulate their interest in learning, their knowledge is more comprehensive and solid. Teacher in this process plays a supporting and coaching role, do not have to explain each knowledge point, at the appropriate time to guide the direction of student discussion, or when they are dispute over the their problem, teacher help them to solve the problem. After a group discussion, let each group sent a representative to report their solutions, the other members of the group added to speak. Such exchange of views and the collision among groups will inspire more thinking spark and active classroom atmosphere, and enrich students' way of thinking. Finally, teachers made a conclusion on this issue. PBL model assessment is based on a comprehensive assessment of the times and quality of students to speak in every discussion, and data review and written report. The mentor assess the results of a personal, at the same time, the other team members also assess him. According to the nature of the course to arrangements a written examination or to writing an essay at the end of the course, scientifically judge the actual effect of the course, and form a benign circulation.

210.3.2 Project PBL Mode

Computer as a very practical subject, students just around the book knowledge is not enough, they must do a lot of practice. In the process of solving a problem will encounter many problems, the experimenter will master the methods and the knowledge of the difficulties contained with solving these problems. More importantly, in this process, the experimenter's thinking is diverging, by a problem in another thought, in this development thinking guidance, the problem will become more rich and specific, the experimenter can make the original single rich knowledge points up, let the dead knowledge become a method to solve the problem. Foreign graduate student as a scientific research ability and innovation spirit of high-quality talent, should put more effort on research and projects, to scientific research as the guide, based on project, use knowledge to solve practical problems. To learn new knowledge in the process of doing the project is consistent with the PBL teaching mode. We use PBL teaching mode in research projects, and to further reform the culture of foreign graduate student.

When foreign graduate students' basic knowledge and research capacity is enough, 2–3 students form a group, then they select a team leader, the mentor assigned a small project (may be a part of the project has been completed.) to each team. Each team start from the understanding of the project background and knowledge, make a clear division of labor, find information, and then work separately. Then discuss in groups, they should make a clear system requirements, and give the system outline design and detailed design, and then according to their own division of labor to complete the system. When students have problems, he can refer to the use of knowledge, and make full use of network resources. If he is unable to solve the problem, he raised it in the group discussion, with the wisdom of all team members to overcome the difficulties. Student with problems to study, and learning based on the problems, such learning is more purposeful and more efficient. In this process, the teacher still play the role of supporting and guiding the overall guidance of each team's project to help them solve the problems encountered. Such teaching methods to let the students use their knowledge to solve practical problems, and in the process of project to do enrich their knowledge, also exercise their team cooperation ability, stimulate their innovation spirit, improve their scientific research ability, to lay the foundation for later study and work.

After the foreign graduate students' ability to get plenty of exercise and improve, tutor will make them to do scientific research project. One mentor and 2–3 foreign graduate students form a team to complete a research project or part of a project, the mentor head worked as team manager. Foreign graduates' solve the problem in a real environment, which can check their deficiencies, and to add new knowledge and innovation in the work to improve the research capability. In the teacher work together with foreign graduate students, which can improve the affection between teachers and students, and also make the teacher know more about each student's characteristic, the mentor is more targeted to guide the foreign graduate students.

210.4 Summary

Learning based problem and project is an important means of cultivating foreign graduate student. PBL teaching mode can enhance the penetration and comprehensive interdisciplinary and expand students 'knowledge. It can improve comprehensive ability of students. Teachers and students can benefit from the PBL teaching mode. Study adopts the model of PBL, students not only get the disciplines related to the specific skills, but also won comprehensive skills applied to jobs.

References

1. Belland B, French B, Ertmer PA (2009) Validity and problem- basedlearning research: a review of the instruments used to assess intended learning outcomes. Interdisc J Probl Based Learn 3(1):59–89
2. Du Y, Kolmos A, Holgaard JE (2009) PBL: university curriculum reform and innovation. Res High Educ Eng 2009 (3): 29–34
3. Guo F, Lin J, Liu P (2009) Exploration and practice of the PBL teaching mode in the teaching of foreign students. Med Educ Res 7:773–775
4. Ioan D (2001) How-to- do guide t o problem—based learning. University of Manchester, UK, p 5
5. Liang R (2001) Study on problem-based learning mode. China Educ Technol 173(6):15–17

Chapter 211
The Influence in Bone Mineral Density of Diabetes with Deafness in Different Syndrome Types by Prescriptions of Hypoglycemic Preventing Deafness

Ruiyu Li, Kaoshan Guo, Meng Li, Jianqiao Li, Junli Yan, Liping Wu, Weihua Han, Qing Gu, Shuangping Wei and Yanfu Sun

Abstract *Objective* To study the influence in bone mineral density of diabetes with deafness in different syndrome types by Prescriptions of hypoglycemic preventing deafness. *Methods* We treated 42 patients (84 ears) of diabetes with deafness in different syndrome type by prescriptions of hypoglycemic prevent deafness. Then determinate bone gla protein (BGP), calcitonin (HCT), parathyroid hormone (PTH) and bone metabolic index of these patients before treatment and after treatment. We also maesured the bone mineral density of lumbar spine, femoral, arm, heel of these patient in treatment group. There were 40 normal people in control group. *Results* We compared the bone metabolism of patients with different syndromes in group treatment before the treatment with the normal people. Results show that BGP, HCT of patients with Yin scorching has no obvious statistical significance ($P > 0.05$). PTH of patients had gawped higher ($P < 0.05$). BGP, HCT of patients before treatment had more obvious changes than normal person ($P < 0.05$). All indices of patients with different syndrome types after treatment except the HCT has more significantly decreased ($P < 0.05$).

R. Li (✉)
Institute of Integrated Traditional and Western Medicine, Second Affiliated Hospital Xingtai Medical College, No. 618 Gangtiebei Road, Xingtai, Hebei Province, China
e-mail: Liruiyu651021@163.com

K. Guo · W. Han · Q. Gu · Y. Sun
Second Affiliated Hospital of Xingtai Medical College, Xingtai, Hebei Province, China

M. Li
Health Team of Hotan Prefecture Detachment of Chinese Armed Police Force in Xinjiang, Xinjiang, China

J. Li
Chinese Medicine Hospital of Luquan City, Luquan, Hebei Pronvince, China

J. Yan · L. Wu
Xingtai People's Hospital, Xingtai, Hebei Province, China

S. Wei
Xingtai Medical College, No. 618 Gangtiebei Road, Xingtai, Hebei Province, China

We compared the bone mineral density of patients with different syndromes in treatment group before treatment with the normal people. The results shown that the bone mineral density of lumbar spine, femoral, heel, BUA, SOS and so on of patients in Yin scorching had no significant statistical significance ($P > 0.05$). Patient in qi and Yin deficiency, deficiency of Yin and Yang have obvious changes ($P < 0.05$). The bone mineral density of patient in Yin scorching, qi and Yin deficiency, Yin and Yang deficiency type had more improved in the after e treatment than before ($P < 0.05$). The bone mineral density of forearm was improved after treatment, but had no significant statistical significance ($P > 0.05$). *Conclusion* Prescriptions of hypoglycemic preventing deafness can improve the bone metabolism and bone mineral density of diabetes patients with deafness in different syndrome types. It can provide basis for diabetes-kidney-bone-ear integration hypothesis.

Keywords Prescriptions of hypoglycemic preventing deafness · Diabetes · Deafness · Bone metabolic · Bone density

211.1 Introduction

The relationship between diabetes and osteoporosis have been studied [1–3], but the relationship between sensorineural deafness of diabetes with syndrome type in traditional medicine and osteoporosis is rarely reported. According to the theory of "kidney governing bone", "kidney opening at the arc" and our work that had been done [4–7], we conclude the scientific hypothesis of "diabetes-kidney-bone-ear". In order to further research on the subject, we will further discusses the relationship between deafness of diabetes in different syndrome types and bone metabolism and osteoporosis in this article. It is reported as follows.

211.2 Data and Methods

211.2.1 General Data

There were 42 patients (54 ears) who have non insulin dependent diabetes mellitus (NIDDM) with deafness. 17 patients are male and 25 patients are female. Their average age are 51.6 years old (36–73 years old). Their average course of the disease were 4.8 years (1–11 years). Standard of diagnosis is According to the international standards organization (ISO) that were published in 1954. There was 9 mild deaf ears, 14 moderate deaf ears, 17 more moderate deaf ears, 8 severe deaf ears and 6 more severe deaf ears.There were 34 patients who had one ear of deafness and ten patients with deafness. There were 12 patients who had Sudden deafness and 42 patients who had gradual deafness. According to traditional medicine there were 15 patients with Yin scorching and 11 patients with Yin deficiency and 16 patients with Yin and Yang deficiency. There were 40 healthy persons in control group. Among them 26 people were male and 14 people were female. Their average age are 59.4 years old (34–59 years old). These people have not disease of kidney, diabetes, disease of cardiovascular.

211.2.2 Main Symptoms

The patients who have non insulin dependent diabetes with deafness felled thirsty, hungry, more urine, excessive weakness and debility of lumbar accompanied with all kinds of deafness.

211.2.3 Diagnostic Standard

The patients were diagnosed to non insulin dependent diabetes according to diagnostic standard putting forward by the world health organization (WHO). Dialectical classification of traditional medicine reference to the new medicine (TCM) guiding principle about treatment of diabetes (collateral) in clinical research [8]. Diagnosis standard of osteoporosis used diagnosis standard recommended by WHO in 1994.

211.2.4 Exclusion Standard

(1) The patients excepted for brain injury, toxicosis diseases, deafness from noise and so on. (2) The patients have used hormone and immune inhibitor in recent a month, or have use medicine that affect bone metabolism in recent 3 months. (3) The patients were pregnancy or breast-feeding women, or had metal illness. (4) The patients had disease of spinal and joint with seronegative and rheumatoid disease that can cause osteoporosis. (5) The patients had severe malnutrition or heart disease, brain disease, kidney disease, hematopoietic system disease. (6) The patients had alcohol dependence, sulfa drug allergies.

211.2.5 Measure Method

Indicators of the bone metabolism: bone gla protein (BGP) and calcitonin (HCT) were measured by radioimmunity method that provided by the research office of isotopes in the institution of atomic energy in China. Parathyroid hormone (PTH) were measured by enzyme-linked immunoassay method that were produced by the Diagnostic Systems, Laboratories, Inc. We measured the bone density of lumbar spine, left femoral neck, left Ward's triangle, left femoral trochanter, left forearm (distal radius 33 %) in two groups before the treatment and after the treatment using DEXA method and instrument of DPX-L bone mineral density instrument that was produced by U.S. LUNAR company of America. Error of the lumbar spine is less than 1/1,000, Error of the femoral neck is less than 3/1,000.We used QUS methods that is detected the bone mineral density of calcaneus by ultrasonic. These instruments that was belong to ultrasonic bone strength tester of Achilles QUS system were produced by the United States GE company's. Its error is less than 2 %. The main parameters is ultrasonic transmission speed (SOS) and degree of broadband ultrasound attenuation (BUA). Safety and adverse reaction is monitored by checking blood, urine, liver and kidney function, electrocardiogram and so on. At the same time we will observe records and adverse reactions of drug.

211.2.6 Treating Method

The patient of diabetes with deafness in treatment group eat capsules that can lower glucose and prevent deafness (including puerariae, salvia miltiorrhiza, rhizoma ligustici wallichii, cooked rehmannia root, Chinese yam rhizome, poria cocos, cortex moutan, rhizoma alismatis, dogwood, magnet). These capsules are combined of the above thing and have 0.5 g. The patient eat five softgels capsules every time and have three times a day.

According to dialectical diagnosis of Chinese medicine we choose from 1 to 3 sort capsules. Patients belong to Yin scorching type eat 1 sort capsules (mading from plaster, rhizoma anemarrhenae, rhizoma coptidis, scrophulariae). Patients belong to Qi and Yin deficiency type eat 1 and 2 sort capsules (mading from astragalus membranaceus, straight ladybell, radix ophiopogonis, trichosanthis). Patients belong to Yin and Yang deficiency type eat 1, 2 and 3 sort capsules (mading from epimedium, monkshood, cassia, medlar). From 1 to 3 sort capsules are combined of the above thing. Each capsule has 0.5 g. The patient eat 3–5 softgels capsules every time and have three times a day.

The patient in treatment group were measured by above methods before treatment. After treating them with above drug for 150 days, then compared them between before treatment and after treatment.

211.2.7 Statistical Methods

We analyzed the above results using SPSS 11.0 statistical software. The measurement data was showed with mean ± standard deviation ($\bar{x} + S$). We use t test comparing mean of between groups.

211.3 Results

We compared the patients with different syndromes in treatment group before treatment with normal people. The result was that BGP, HCT of the patients with Yin scorching had no obvious statistical significance ($P > 0.05$). PTH of the patients with Yin scorching was higher ($P < 0.05$). BGP, HCT of the patients with Yin scorching before treatment had obvious differents with normal people ($P < 0.05$). Excepting the HCT of patients had no obvious change after treatment ($P > 0.05$), other index had significantly decreased than before treatment ($P < 0.05$) as shown in the Table 211.1.

We compared between patients with different syndromes in treatment group before treatment with normal people. The result was that bone mineral density of lumbar spine, femoral, heel, BUA, SOS and so on of patients with Yin scorching had no significant statistical significance ($P > 0.05$). Patients with qi and Yin deficiency, deficiency of Yin and Yang have obvious changes ($P < 0.05$). Bone mineral density (BMD) of patient with Yin scorching, qi and Yin deficiency, Yin and Yang deficiency type had higher than before treatment ($P < 0.05$). BMD of forearm had improved after treatment, but hadn't significant statistical ($P > 0.05$). It shown in the Table 211.2.

211.4 Discussion

Lee in Columbia University found that bone gla protein was Focused on because it may participate in pathological formation process of type two diabetes [9]. Patient with diabetes has different degree of kidney deficiency. Tonifying kidney can not only improve the symptoms above kidney empty of diabetic patients, also can increase osteoblast proliferation that can promote bone gla protein secretion. Bone gla protein can improve insulin secretion, insulin sensitivity and prevent fat accumulation [9]. Bone gla protein levels of patients with type two diabetes was negatively correlated with blood sugar of patients with type two diabetes [10]. Osteoblast (OB) coming from leaf stem cells can produce collagen, bone matrix proteins that is not collagen (e.g., bone gla protein, etc.) and cytokines (such as BMP, etc.). Osteoblast (OB) can also transport calcium and dressing to the calcification sites through the mitochondrial in order to promote calcification. It is

Table 211.1 The results measured about bone metabolism of normal people and diabetic patients with deafness belong to each card type before and after the treatment ($\bar{x} + s$)

Index	Normal people (n = 40)	Yin scorching (n = 15)		Both qi and Yin deficiency (n = 11)		Deficiency of Yin and Yang (n = 16)	
		Before treatment	After treatment	Before treatment	After treatment	Before treatment	After treatment
BGP (ng/L)	0.40 ± 0.23	0.41 ± 0.25Δ	0.61 ± 0.41	0.34 ± 0.16※Δ	80.55 ± 0.27	0.29 ± 0.24※Δ	0.51 ± 0.40
HCT (pg/L)	2.59 ± 2.25	2.55 ± 2.26	2.31 ± 2.18	2.41 ± 2.19	2.34 ± 2.20	2.46 ± 2.37	2.54 ± 2.22
PTH (ng/L)	46.37 ± 35.64	67.36 ± 35.62※Δ	43.76 ± 28.32	68.32 ± 35.58※Δ	43.72 ± 28.10	69.40 ± 36.71※Δ	44.55 ± 29.58

※ Compared with normal group $P < 0.05$; Δ Comparison of before and after treatment $P < 0.05$

Table 211.2 The results measured about BMD of normal people and diabetic patients with deafness belong to each card type before and after the treatment ($\bar{x} + s$)

Index	Normal people (n = 40)	Yin scorching (n = 15)		Both qi and Yin deficiency (n = 11)		Deficiency of Yin and Yang (n = 16)	
		Before treatment	After treatment	Before treatment	After treatment	Before treatment	After treatment
A	1.299 ± 0.170	$0.971 \pm 0.222\triangle$	0.296 ± 0.180	$0.963 \pm 0.282\ast\triangle$	1.276 ± 0.184	$0.944 \pm 0.274\ast\triangle$	1.287 ± 0.172
B	1.123 ± 0.216	$0.980 \pm 0.129\triangle$	1.122 ± 0.211	$0.840 \pm 0.250\ast\triangle$	0.982 ± 0.158	$0.833 \pm 0.200\ast\triangle$	1.012 ± 0.214
C	1.132 ± 0.211	$0.935 \pm 0.243\triangle$	1.035 ± 0.201	$0.754 \pm 0.250\ast\triangle$	0.927 ± 0.245	$0.747 \pm 0.265\ast\triangle$	0.947 ± 0.234
D	1.115 ± 0.135	$0.902 \pm 0.1.37\triangle$	1.105 ± 0.127	$0.703 \pm 0.185\ast\triangle$	0.892 ± 0.145	$0.692 \pm 0.177\ast\triangle$	0.901 ± 0.135
E	1.128 ± 0.115	0.955 ± 0.179	1.119 ± 0.148	0.872 ± 0.253	0.924 ± 0.180	0.884 ± 0.230	0.951 ± 0.204
F	129 ± 19	$90 \pm 21\triangle$	110 ± 19	$89 \pm 21\ast\triangle$	107 ± 18	$88 \pm 20\ast\triangle$	110 ± 19
G	130 ± 20	$122 \pm 22\triangle$	130 ± 20	$96 \pm 24\ast\triangle$	129 ± 20	$95 \pm 25\ast\triangle$	95 ± 19
H	1765 ± 37	$1586 \pm 35\triangle$	1655 ± 34	$1367 \pm 38\ast\triangle$	1585 ± 36	$1360 \pm 39\ast\triangle$	1587 ± 38

A The lumbar spine (L1–L4); B The femoral neck; C Ward's triangle; D Femoral trochanter; E The forearm; F Heel bone strength index; G BUA (dB/MHz); H SOS (m/s)
※ Compared with normal group $P < 0.05$; $\triangle$ Comparison of before and after treatment $P < 0.05$

the main cell that involved in bone metabolism [11]. Tonifying kidney in traditional Chinese medicine (TCM) contribute to combining bone cells. It mainly express to promote osteoblast proliferation. As same time it can promote the bone cells to mineralize of bone matrix and can correct the kidney essence and kidney deficiency that existed disorder and hypofunction of two gene regulation in nerve-endocrine-immune and nervous-endocrine-bone metabolism [12]. According to "kidney advocate bone" and "kidney begin to understand the ear" theory and our previous work, we put forward "diabetes-kidney-bone-ear" integration hypothesis. In this paper we discusses effect of prescriptions about hypoglycemic preventing deafness on patients with diabetes different syndrome of bone metabolism and bone mineral density according to this scientific hypothesis types.

Prescriptions of hypoglycemic preventing deafness is come of radix puerariae, salvia miltiorrhiza, rhizoma ligustici wallichii, cooked rehmannia, Chinese yam rhizome, tuckahoe, alisma, magnet, etc. Both rhizoma ligustici wallichii that pass twelve meridians and salvia miltiorrhiza has the promoting blood circulation to remove blood stasis. Puerarin has growing hair and clear yang, as the same time it has made medicine running. Cooked rehmannia is soft and sweet. It can supply blood and make kidney well and vital essence sufficient. Chinese yam rhizome can make spleen strong and benefit stomach to digest. Poria cocos can make spleen and body wet. Dan skin can make liver excreting waste. Dogwood can make liver and kidney better. Quality of magnet is heavy. It can make kidney Yin strong. It is mainly made of four iron oxide. Patient of kidney empty, deafness and blurred vision use dogwood in "Ben cao yan yi". Prescriptions of hypoglycemic preventing deafness can nourish kidney Yin, activate blood, enhance SOD, lower blood sugar, blood lipids and fibrinogen, enhance and improve NIDDM with deafness hearing, and so on. Prescriptions of hypoglycemic preventing deafness have not only main party but also side path. It reflects the principle of treatment based on syndrome differentiation of Chinese medicine and individual differences.

We studied bone metabolism and bone mineral density of patients who had different syndrome types of the diabetes with deafness in this article. We compared the bone metabolism measurement results of patients who have different syndrome types in the treatment group before the treatment with the bone metabolism measurement results of the normal people. Results show BGP, HCT of patients with Yin scorching has no obvious statistical significance ($P > 0.05$). PTH of patients had increased higher ($P < 0.05$) BGP, HCT of patients before treatment were different with normal people ($P < 0.05$). All index except the HCT of patients has no obvious change in treatment groups ($P > 0.05$) and it had decreased lower than before. We compared the bone mineral density of patients who have different syndrome types in the treatment group before the treatment with normal people. The bone mineral density in lumbar spine, femoral, heel, BUA, SOS and so on of patients with Yin scorching had no significant statistical significance ($P > 0.05$). Patients with qi and Yin deficiency, deficiency of Yin and Yang have obvious changes ($P < 0.05$). The bone mineral density of patients with Yin scorching, qi and Yin deficiency, Yin and Yang deficiency type was obviously higher though treatment ($P < 0.05$). The bone mineral density in the forearm of is higher than before, but had no significant statistical significance (P > 0.05). These express that prescriptions of hypoglycemic preventing deafness can improve bone metabolism, bone mineral density of patients with diabetes with deafness of different syndrome types. As the same time it can provide objective basis for diabetes-kidney-bone-ear integration hypothesis.

References

1. Wang Y, Li BX, Liu Y et al (2011) Bone reconstruction study about rats of NIDDM diabetes with osteoporosis. Basic Med Clin 31(7):777–782
2. Wang J, Shu YQ (2012) The new study of steoporosis pathogenesis of NIDDM. Tradit Chin Cedicine Clin J 24(2):183–184
3. Li HH, Jiang T (2011) The bone mineral density and its related factors of elder NIDDM with nephropathy. J Geriatr Med Chin 32(13):2711–2713
4. Li RY, Wu LP, Song N et al (2000) The TCM treatment of diabetic an loss: an audiological and rheological observation. J Tradit Chin Med 20(3):176–179
5. Li RY, Li M, Wang R et al (2008) Jiang Tang Fang Long Jiao Nang in treating non-insulin dependent diabetes mellitus with an LOSS. J Otol 3(1):45–50
6. Li RY, Li B, Guo YJ (2009) The influence of prescriptions of hypoglycemic preventing deafness to blood insulin c-peptide and glucagon of diabetes with deafness in different syndrome types. Tradit Med Chin Liaoning 4(4):510–511
7. Li RY, Guo YL, Liu JW et al (2011) The influence of prescription of tonifying kidney to diabetes with deafness [J]. J Mod Tradit Chin West Med 20(6):654–656
8. Ministry of health of the People's Republic of China (1993) Guiding principle of traditional medicine and new drug in clinical research, vol 1, Beijing, pp 215–217
9. Lee NK, Sowa H, Hinoi E et al (2007) The endocrine regalation of energy metabolism by the skeleton. Cell 130(3):456–469
10. Tao L, Xue X, Li DK (2003) Related factors analysis of NIDDM and osteocalcin level in serum. J Mod Med China 13(1):21–22
11. Liu JP, Cheng Y (2010) The research of traditional medicine promoting osteoblast working and ALP activity. J Tradit Med Coll ShanXi 33(1):7–8
12. Shen ZY, Chen Y, Huang JH et al (2006) Two gene network regulating map of kidney empty drawn by the drug. J Tradit W Med Chin 26(6):521–525

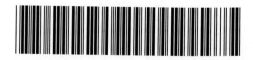

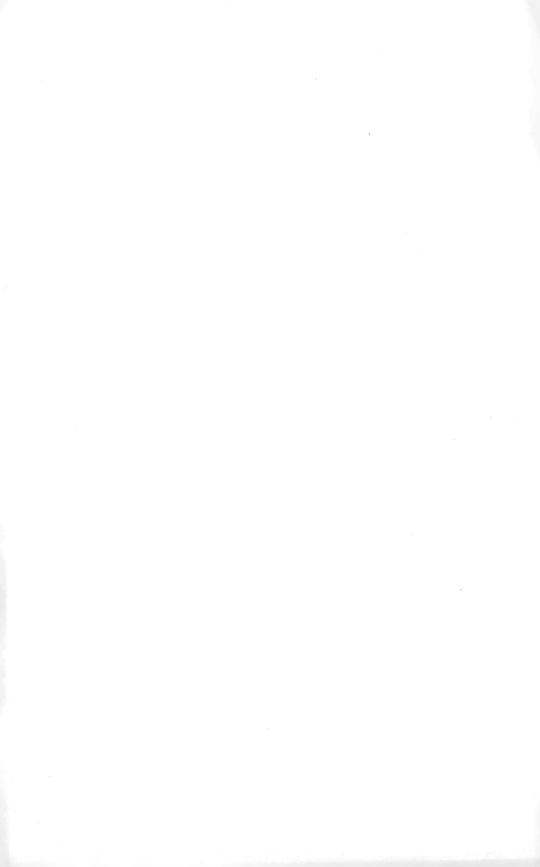